Neuropsychopharmacology

Fundamentals
of Neuropsychopharmacology

Robert S. Feldman
UNIVERSITY OF MASSACHUSETTS, AMHERST

Linda F. Quenzer
UNIVERSITY OF CONNECTICUT HEALTH CENTER, FARMINGTON

Sinauer Associates, Inc. • Publishers
Sunderland, Massachusetts

FUNDAMENTALS OF NEUROPSYCHOPHARMACOLOGY

Library of Congress Cataloging in Publication Data

Feldman, Robert Simion, 1918–
    Fundamentals of neuropsychopharmacology.

    Bibliography: p.
    Includes index.
    1. Neuropsychopharmacology.   I. Quenzer, Linda F.
II. Title.   [DNLM: 1. Nervous system—Drug effects.
2. Behavior—Drug effects.   QV 76.5 F312f]
RM315.F43   1983   615'.78   83-14937
ISBN 0-87893-178-3

Printed in U.S.A.

5

We dedicate this book, first, to our students, whose needs and interests led us to create courses to explain the interaction of chemical substances with mood and behavior.

We also dedicate this book to the scientists, many of whom are named in the bibliography, who have created and developed the science of neuropsychopharmacology.

Contents

Preface

For thousands of years, probably including prehistoric times, humans have used drugs. Often the drug selected to cure an illness had only the most superficial relationship to the symptoms or the nature of the illness. Extracts or teas brewed from willow bark were consumed to relieve the pain of rheumatism, simply because of the abundance of willow trees in swampy areas where the symptoms of aching joints were common. The snake root was used to treat snake bite because the root looked like a poisonous snake. In fact, willow bark is a source of salicylic acid—the active ingredient in aspirin—and snake root contains reserpine, an effective drug for reducing cardiovascular hypertension. The growth of scientific and medical knowledge about drugs and their effects has resulted in the decline of beliefs in their magical powers, and today rational thought prevails in the prescription and use of drugs in modern society.

The central theme of this book is the mechanisms of action of drugs that amplify or modify neural function and how these processes cause change in mood and behavior. These drugs are known as psychotropic agents. They are studied by examining their chemical properties, their biochemical action, their effects on nerve cells, and the resulting changes in behavior. Several disciplines are involved in this approach, which can be called neuropsychopharmacology.

Because students come to this field from quite different backgrounds, the authors have felt a need for a single volume on the fundamentals of neuropsychopharmacology, a book which would present the material at a level that college upperclassmen and beginning graduate students with some background in the physical, biological, and behavioral sciences can readily comprehend. To fill

that need we have attempted to provide fundamental knowledge about pharmacology, behavior, neurophysiology, and neurochemistry, and to show how this knowledge is applied in the study of brain function and in the treatment of behavioral disorders. Additional, advanced information is provided so that interested students can proceed confidently to advanced courses, the research literature, advanced reviews, and ultimately to careers in research and clinical applications.

Although this book is primarily for students in behavioral pharmacology, we also intend that it appeal to the interests of students in the neurosciences, pharmacology, and the medical disciplines. We believe that selected chapters will be of interest to physicians, psychiatric nurses, and clinical psychologists who frequently encounter users of psychotropic drugs (licit and illicit) and who would find it useful to know how such drugs exert their effects.

In the writing, we have tried to maintain a neutral course with respect to the use or avoidance of the drug substances we discuss. We have tried to make it clear that most drugs are prescribed on the basis of a cost-benefit ratio: cost, referring to the financial, physiological, and psychological burdens associated with the drug; and benefit, referring to the improvement in health and well-being. In most cases this ratio is determined by physicians for individuals. Obviously, we would not be in this position with respect to our readers. The one exception to this rule is our strong stance against the use of tobacco. We are in agreement with those who do not find any redeeming features from a health standpoint to support the use of this substance.

This book is organized into four main parts. The first

part covers the principles of pharmacology, i.e., how drugs act upon biological systems (Chapter 1). Chapter 2 describes the techniques of behavior analysis which lead to the accurate assessment of the behavioral effects of drugs.

The next part deals with neuron morphology and neurophysiology, including the structure and function of the nervous system with emphasis on cellular activity (Chapter 3). Chapter 4 presents the unique features of nerve cell function (neurophysiology), and Chapter 5 is a detailed description of the ways nerve cells interact among themselves (synaptic morphology and function).

Detailed information about neurotransmitters (substances, synthesized and secreted by nerve cells, that are involved in neuron–neuron and neuron–effector organ interactions) are presented in the third part. Chapters 6 through 10 discuss acetylcholine, catecholamines, serotonin, amino acid transmitters, and peptide transmitters, respectively, as well as discussing a number of drugs that exert specific effects upon the transmitters.

The final part describes drug effects on neurotransmitter systems for three psychotropic drug classes that have significant behavioral effects of therapeutic value. Chapter 11 discusses anxiolytic drugs (drugs that attenuate anxiety). Chapter 12 deals with drugs used to relieve the symptoms of mental illnesses such as the depressive and schizophrenic states; and Chapter 13 presents a discussion of drugs that attenuate pain, especially those drugs derived from opium. The biochemistry of endogenous opiatelike substances is also discussed in detail.

A reading list follows each chapter to lead the interested student mostly to reviews of research literature. We have also provided an extensive glossary for ready access to definitions. It includes, for example, definitions of neuro- and general anatomical structures, the morphology and microstructures of nerve and other types of cells, and neurophysiological processes and research procedures. It also includes medical terms for normal and pathological physiology and for normal and pathological psychology. Chemical names are supplied for some drug classes, and chemical terms, chemical analytic procedures, and pharmacological and psychological testing methods are described. Typically we have resorted to abbreviations

and acronyms that refer to many chemical entities in this book; the abbreviations and their derivatives are listed in a separate section.

We have attempted to provide an overview of neuropsychopharmacology to students and health sciences practitioners with diverse backgrounds. In a field that is so multifaceted, it would be impossible to include in one volume in-depth explorations of all relevant topics. Thus, some educated guesses have been made about what was essential to include in the book. We hope our readers appreciate our dilemma and will favor us with suggestions about what choices might have been better ones.

Acknowledgments

First, we wish to express our thanks to those students who over a decade ago asked us to offer a course in drugs and behavior because they wanted to understand drug abuse and to help those who had fallen prey to that unfortunate circumstance. Their request and their acceptance of our efforts in that regard led to the development of the course that was the nucleus of this book. There were also graduate students who acquainted us with many areas of drug research when they independently did in-depth studies for psychopharmacology seminars. We owe much to our colleagues, whom we frequently consulted. We are especially grateful to Dr. Jerrold Meyer for sharing with us his erudition in neurochemistry, to Dr. Neil Carlson whose ability to write clearly about neurophysiology served as a model for us, and to Dr. Russell C. Leaf of Rutgers University whose careful reading and comments about the entire manuscript were a major contribution toward clarification and updating of many sections of the text.

Among contemporary students, John F. McElroy has been a constant source of ideas about content and clarity of presentation. He has patiently explained the whys and wherefores of chemical nomenclature and its symbolic representation, and he has generously given us access to the products of his literature searches and his research manuscripts that we wanted to include in our book. We are indeed indebted to Jodi L. Simpson whose editing not only significantly improved the writing style of the text, but whose technical knowledge proved extremely valuable. We deeply appreciate the efforts of Carlton Brose, who patiently kept us on track, reined in our excesses, and argued for high standards in the development of the book. We are very grateful for his efforts in our behalf.

Finally, we want to acknowledge the efforts of Pat McGuinness who escaped the boredom of an appointments telephone by offering to arrange and type our reference list. We extend unbounded praise to Christina Decoteau whose superlative typing was more than matched by her sunny disposition, even after many rush jobs, as she typed hundreds of pages that she felt had no end. And we extend sincere thanks to Carol Wigg who tried to make certain that everything was in place, and everything we wrote made sense, before the manuscript went off to the printers. She did a fine job. Yet, it almost goes without saying, despite all the support we had in this venture, ours is the final responsibility for the contents therein.

RSF
LFQ

Neuropsychopharmacology

CHAPTER ONE

Principles of Pharmacology

Pharmacology is concerned with both drug effects and drug action. *Drug effects* are alterations in the normal function of an existing biological process. Drugs can increase heart rate, slow down reaction time, and reduce pain. They almost always have several simultaneous effects. Amphetamine, for example, will increase motor activity, increase heart rate, and decrease appetite.

Drug action refers to how and where a drug ultimately produces its effect. An example will demonstrate that the site of action is not necessarily near the site of drug effect. Atropine and morphine each alter the size of the pupil of the eye. Atropine has a site of action near the pupil of the eye, and external application of the drug to the eye increases the size of the pupil—a condition frequently desired during routine eye examinations. In contrast, the application of morphine to the eye produces no effect on pupil size. However, morphine administered internally decreases the size of the pupils (frequently referred to as "pinpoint" pupils). In the case of morphine, we know that it acts on areas of the brain that modify the pupillary response to light. Thus, although both drugs have an effect on pupil size, their site of action and their neurochemical mode of action are quite different.

Determinants of Drug Action

The ultimate goal of neuropsychopharmacology is to understand the neurochemical action of drugs that yield a specific behavioral effect. This chapter describes the variables that help to determine the characteristics of drug action in general: where the drug acts, how quickly it acts, and for how long it acts.

In the interval between administration of a drug and a measurable change in nervous system activity and behavior, many physiological processes occur. Figure 1 shows the routes followed by drug molecules after administration. Each drug must be absorbed into the bloodstream and be transported to its site of action, or TARGET SITE. These processes are similar for any pharmacological agent, whether it acts on the brain, heart, or other organs. Thus, we must consider the dynamic processes that influence drug action and determine its characteristics. Among these processes are:

1. Routes of administration. How and where a drug is administered will determine how quickly the drug is absorbed and how completely it gets into the bloodstream.
2. Absorption. Because a drug rarely acts where it initially contacts the body, it must pass through a variety of cell membranes and be distributed to fluid compartments prior to its binding at a target site or a nonactive storage depot.
3. Binding. Once transport has occurred, the drug binds to a specific cellular receptor that modifies the biological activity of the cell, for instance, by increasing or decreasing enzyme activity or by altering membrane properties. The action of many psychoactive drugs on specific metabolic processes in nerve cells will be the topic of much of this textbook.
4. Inactivation. Drug inactivation, which occurs through metabolism or excretion, must be included with the study of drug action. Inactivation determines the intensity and duration of drug effects.

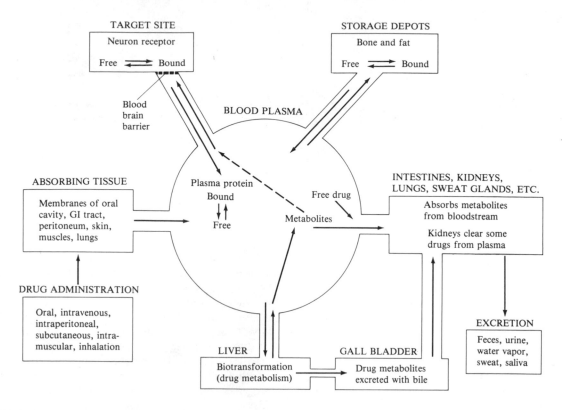

FIGURE 1. TRANSPORT AND FATE OF NEURO-TROPIC DRUGS. After injection into the bloodstream or absorption through membranes of the GI tract, skin, muscles, etc. the drug molecules are distributed in blood plasma throughout the whole body. Some drugs bind to plasma proteins, such as albumin, maintaining an equilibrium between bound and free drug. Free drug that can pass the blood brain barrier forms complexes with neuronal receptor sites to initiate drug action. An equilibrium is established between the receptor-bound and free drug in the plasma. An equilibrium is also maintained between plasma levels of the drug and that stored in bone and fat. The drug that is circulated in the liver may be metabolized and the metabolites collected into the gallbladder, emptied into the intestines with bile, and excreted with feces. Liver metabolites may also return to the bloodstream to be absorbed by the kidneys, lungs, etc. and excreted, or they may be active agents that will stimulate neuronal receptors. The kidneys, as well as the lungs and glands, may clear some drugs directly from the blood plasma.

5. Adaptation. Finally, because many drugs are administered over long periods of time, we will discuss adaptive changes in the organism (tolerance) that alter drug action with repeated administration.

Most of the phenomena discussed in this chapter are not limited to psychoactive drugs but describe the essentials of drug action in general. Examples will be used that emphasize behavior-modifying agents, but much more detail regarding these drugs follows in later chapters.

Route of Administration

The route of administration of a drug determines how much drug reaches its site of action and how quickly the drug effect occurs. Intravenous (i.v.) injection is the most rapid method of drug administration as the agent, in active form, is placed directly into the blood to be carried to the site of action. By delivering the drug into the blood, the time of passage through cell membranes, for example the gastric wall and blood vessel membranes, is eliminated. In addition, the amount placed in the blood is readily known, unlike the highly variable amount resulting from absorption from the gastrointestinal (GI) tract after oral administration. Intravenous administration is used when a substance to be injected is irritating to tissue or when a rapid effect is required. The speed of drug effect is a potential hazard with this method because an overdose or allergic reaction will be rapid in onset, leaving little time for correction.

An alternate injection procedure is intramuscular (i.m.) injection, which has the advantage of slower and more even absorption over a period of time. However, absorption is usually quicker after i.m. injection than after oral administration because the drug does not have to pass through the GI tract to the site of absorption. Absorption can be slowed by simultaneous administration of a vasoconstrictor, because rate of absorption is dependent upon rate of blood flow to the muscle. In addition, the drug may be injected as a suspension; this method provides slow and even absorption and sustained action. As a rule, i.m. injection is not good with irritating substances.

The most common methods of administration to animals are subcutaneous and intraperitoneal injections. Subcutaneous (s.c.) administration requires that the drug be injected just below the skin. In laboratory animals such as rats or rabbits, the drug is injected in the scruff of the neck. Absorption is fairly slow and even with this method. Injection of a drug in a nonaqueous solution (such as peanut oil) or implantation of a drug pellet further slows the rate of absorption. Implantation of drug-containing pellets is most often used to administer hormones. The pellets release their contents subcutaneously at a rate dependent on the surface area of the pellet, its rate of erosion, and the solubility of the drug in body fluids. The implanting of a drug pellet has also been used successfully to produce a state of drug dependence in research animals without the need for frequent injections and the prolonged treatment that is cumbersome in the research environment.

Intraperitoneal (i.p.) injection deposits the drug into the body cavity (peritoneum) from which it must be absorbed into blood. This route of administration avoids passage through the GI tract and absorption is fairly rapid. The blood level of drug achieved, however, is variable, depending upon the injection site. Although it is the most frequent method of treating research animals, much of the experimental variability can be attributed to uneven drug absorption. I.p. injection is rarely used in humans because of the danger of peritoneal infection.

Because the route of administration significantly alters rate of absorption, blood levels of the same drug administered by several different routes vary significantly. Figure 2 shows the very rapid rise in blood level of a drug administered intravenously and the rate of decline, which reflects drug metabolism or elimination. A much lower blood drug level is achieved after subcutaneous administration of the same drug, but there is a longer duration of its presence in the blood. Because absorption is slow, metabolism of part of the active drug can occur before absorption is completed. Thus, no peak occurs, and a lower blood drug level is maintained over a longer period of time.

A special injection method must be used for some drugs that act on nerve cells because a cellular barrier (the blood brain barrier) prevents or slows the passage of the drugs from the bloodstream into neural tissue. This special method is used clinically when spinal anesthesia is administered directly in the cerebrospinal fluid (CSF) surrounding the spinal cord of the mother during childbirth. For the laboratory animal, a stereotaxic apparatus and microsyringe or cannula are employed and enable precise injection into discrete areas of the brain. In this way experimenters can study the electrophysiological, biochemical, or behavioral effects of drugs on particular cell groups.

Oral administration is the most popular administration method for clinical treatment because it is safe, self-administered, and economical. To be effective, a drug must be soluble in stomach fluid, pass to the intestine, and move through the intestinal lining into the

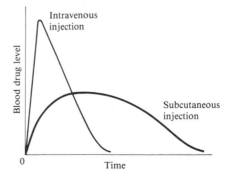

FIGURE 2. BLOOD DRUG LEVEL following single intravenous and subcutaneous injections.

blood. However, there are many factors that affect absorption from the GI tract, so blood levels of drugs administered orally are often irregular and not easily predicted. For example, the solubility of the drug in the stomach will alter absorption, as will the presence of food in the stomach (which slows gastric emptying). Drugs that can be destroyed in gastric acid or by digestive processes obviously cannot be administered effectively by the oral method, for example insulin. Several of these absorption difficulties can be avoided for some drugs by sublingual administration. This method of administration provides more rapid and more even absorption than from the GI tract because it avoids destruction of drug by liver enzymes and gastric factors. An example of a very fast-acting drug is nitroglycerin, which when placed under the tongue rapidly relaxes the smooth muscle of the cardiovascular system. The muscle relaxation increases the blood supply to the heart muscles and subsequently reduces the pain of angina pectoris. Clearly, neither irritating nor bad-tasting drugs can be administered this way.

The principal goal of any drug regimen is to constantly maintain the desired blood levels of a drug. As blood drug level at any given moment is a result of absorption and degradation (or elimination), one would expect an inconstant level over time. For instance, after oral administration, the blood level of a drug that is readily absorbed increases rapidly. Figure 3 shows that drug administration at time A produced a high drug level in the blood , shown at peak 1. Almost immediately, however, the drug begins to disappear from the blood because of metabolism, excretion, or redistribution to inactive sites (e.g., fat). By time B, the blood drug level has fallen to one-half the peak 1 value. That rate is expressed in terms of DRUG HALF-LIFE,* that is, the time it takes for the blood drug level to fall to half its peak level. For many drugs, the next dose should be administered before the blood drug level has fallen significantly. For those drugs whose half-life is short, administration must be frequent.

This illustration, at its extreme, suggests that intravenous infusion is the only method capable of producing stable blood drug levels. However, the subcutaneous pellet implantation is a reasonable substitute and has become technically more sophisticated in recent years (Blackshear, 1979). In addition to the development of implantation materials (e.g., silicone rubber

*Also called "half-time."

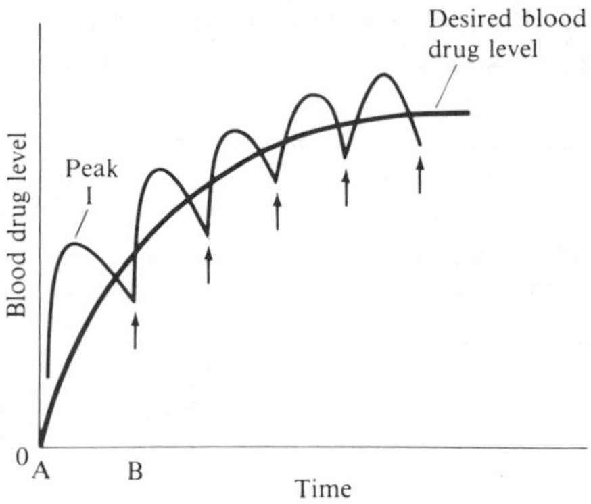

FIGURE 3. CHANGES OF BLOOD DRUG LEVEL during continuous infusion and repeated administration. The smooth line depicts the drug accumulation in blood during continuous intravenous infusion. The scalloped line demonstrates the pattern of accumulation during repeated administration (at arrows) of the same drug. The shape of the scallop is dependent upon both the rate of absorption and the rate of elimination.

capsules) that release drug at a constant rate for up to 13 months, other researchers have developed implantable infusion pumps that can deliver drug to a specific target area. Particularly exciting was the development of a pump implanted under the skin of the scalp and connected with the brain reservoir (ventricle), which contains CSF. On the side nearest the skin, the tank has a self-sealing membrane that can be repeatedly punctured with a hypodermic needle for refilling with drug or for sampling of the CSF. This system has been used to treat meningitis with high concentrations of antibiotics that normally would not reach the CSF through the blood brain barrier. As more is learned about the neurochemical basis for neurological and psychiatric disorders, a drug delivery system that can administer drug to specific and localized sites within the brain has tremendous potential.

Drug Absorption and Distribution

Once the drug has been administered, it is absorbed from the site of administration into the bloodstream to be circulated throughout the body and ultimately to the brain, which is the target site of utmost importance for psychoactive drugs. The rate of absorption is dependent on several factors. Clearly the route of administration alters absorption because it determines the area of the absorbing surface, the number of cell layers between site of administration and blood, the amount of drug destroyed by liver metabolism or extreme acidity (e.g., in the stomach), and the extent of binding to food or inert complexes. Absorption is also dependent on solubility and ionization of the drug, drug concentration, and variables of the organism such as age, sex, and body size.

Effects of Age, Sex, and Body Size

Because drug effects are directly related to the amount of drug reaching the target site, the volume of body fluids is a significant determinant of drug action. Thus, the larger the individual, the more diluted will be the drug in the larger fluid compartment, and less drug will reach the receptor sites. The sex of the individual also plays a part in determining blood drug level because adipose tissue, as compared to water, represents a larger proportion of the total body weight in the female. Thus, the fluid compartment, which contains the drug, is generally smaller in women than in men, producing a higher drug concentration at the target site in women. It should be obvious also that the smaller fluid volume of a child means that a standard dose of drug will be more concentrated at the target site and therefore, will produce a larger pharmacological effect. However, in the very young, as well as in the elderly, the rate of drug metabolism (inactivation) is perhaps a more significant factor in determining the blood drug level. Because liver metabolism is generally much slower in those age groups, blood levels of certain drugs tend to be much higher for a longer period of time.

An important example of these general rules is provided by the action of ethyl alcohol (ethanol), a drug whose effects in the central nervous system (CNS) on thinking and behavior are directly related to the level of drug in the blood. It should not be surprising that the effects of equal amounts of alcohol will be much different for a 100-pound female as compared to her 200-pound husband. After 1.0 ounce of pure alcohol (in the form of 2 ounces of spirits or 2 cans of beer), the female in our example may have a blood level of alcohol of approximately 0.09 mg ethanol/100 ml blood. In contrast, under the same experimental conditions, her husband, at 200 pounds, may have a blood level of 0.037 mg/100 ml. Clearly, these two individuals can expect quite different effects on behavior (such as instability of gait, slurred speech, and delayed reaction time) following the same dose of drug.

Drug Transport Across Membranes

Perhaps the single most important factor in achieving therapeutic blood drug levels is the rate of passage of the drug through the various cell layers (and their respective membranes) between the site of administration and the blood. Membranes maintain the integrity of cells by selectively regulating the migration of materials into and out of the cells.

Passive Diffusion. This process is characterized by the movement of a dissolved substance through a biological barrier (a membrane) in a direction from higher to lower concentration so that an equilibrium is ultimately reached. The concentration gradient directs the movement, and no energy is required. An example of this is the passage of ethanol across the membrane from intestine to blood. As the ethanol moves from the intestine, it passes to the bloodstream, where its concentration is lower. From there it is circulated in the blood away from the intestine. Thus, the level of alcohol on the blood side of the barrier remains low, and passive diffusion continues at a constant rate. For many drugs, diffusion is that simple and depends only on the concentration gradient and the blood flow to the absorbing area. However, the selective permeability of the membrane prevents many molecules from passively penetrating, regardless of the concentration gradients that exist. Therefore, passive permeability also depends upon the drug's molecular shape and weight, its lipid solubility and its degree of ionization (charge).

Lipid Solubility. Membranes have a high lipid content (Chapter 3). Lipids are molecules that have the characteristics of fats. Thus, it is reasonable that drugs that are lipid soluble will more readily permeate a lipid membrane, just as oil of turpentine will readily mix with oil-base paint. (Conversely, substances that are soluble in water, such as sugar, will not dissolve in oil.)

The lipid solubility of a given substance can be estimated in the following way. A radiolabeled drug can be mixed with water. The mixture is then added to the same volume of oil, such as olive oil, and again thoroughly mixed. After settling, the oil and water form two distinct layers. The oil floating on top can then be drawn off and the radioactivity of the oil and water can be measured separately. The amount of radioactivity in each solvent is directly related to the amount of drug dissolved in that solvent. The ratio of the drug concentration in oil divided by its concentration in water is the oil/water PARTITION COEFFICIENT. It is the relative affinity of the drug for either oil or water that determines whether it can leave the water in the blood or stomach juices and enter the lipid layers of membranes. The partition coefficient also determines how readily a drug will pass the lipid barriers to enter the brain. For example, the abused narcotic drug heroin is a simple modification of the parent compound morphine. Heroin, or diacetylmorphine, is more soluble in lipid than is morphine, and thus penetrates into brain tissue more readily and has a quicker onset of action.

The Ionization Factor. To facilitate an understanding of the role of ionization in transmembrane diffusion, let us first briefly review some basic concepts in chemistry. We are all aware that some substances dissolve quickly and completely in water, whereas other substances do so slightly or not at all. Thus, water solubility, like lipid solubility, is a relative matter. Water solubility and ionization are associated phenomena because the molecules of soluble substances are formed by ionic bonding of atoms. For example, common table salt (sodium chloride) is formed by combining an atom of sodium, which can readily give up one of its electrons (a negative charge), and an atom of chlorine, which can readily accept the negative charge. These bonds are relatively strong in the crystalline state but are weak in water solutions because the dissociated atoms of water (H^+ and OH^-) pull these molecules apart to form ions. The more soluble a substance, the more easily it can be pulled apart by the dissociated atoms of water. Thus, the sodium atom, having lost one of its electrons, has a net positive charge of 1 (Na^+; a cation), whereas the chlorine atom has, by addition of an electron, a net negative charge of 1 (Cl^-; an anion). Thus, ions are defined as atoms or groups of atoms (molecules) that have gained an electric charge (+ or −) after dissociating from a stable configuration. The extent of ionization of a substance is a property of the molecule and depends upon the electron attraction and repulsion of various atoms in the molecule.

Ionization also depends on the acidity or the alkalinity of the solvent, which is expressed as pH. pH is defined as the negative logarithm of the concentration of hydrogen ions (H^+) in solution. For example, distilled water has a concentration of hydrogen ions of 10^{-7} M (0.0000001 moles/liter). This pH level of 7 is called neutral because the concentration of H^+ equals the concentration of OH^- ions. Acids have a lower pH, signifying a larger concentration of H^+; for example, vinegar has a pH of 2.2 ($10^{-2.2}$ M). Solutions having a higher proportion of OH^- to H^+ ions are called alkaline or basic and have pH numbers higher than 7. Thus, a saturated solution of magnesium hydroxide $[Mg(OH)_2]$, has a pH of 10.5, indicating a smaller concentration of H^+ ions in solution. (Magnesium hydroxide is commonly used as an antacid, i.e., to neutralize stomach hyperacidity.)

Because transmembrane diffusion of a drug molecule depends upon ionization, which in turn is dependent upon the pH of the solvent, it is important to note that the different body compartments differ in their respective pH levels. For example, gastric juice is very acid (pH 1.0), whereas the contents of the small intestine may vary from a pH of 5.0 to 6.6. Blood is slightly basic (or alkaline) with a pH of 7.4; and kidney urine is acidic, its pH varying from 4.5 to 7.0. As will be seen, the differences in pH that exist between these compartments play an important role in drug transfer from one compartment to another, for example, from the stomach to the bloodstream or from the bloodstream into the kidney urine.

Lipid Solubility–Ionization Interactions. Those drugs that are lipid soluble, and hence relatively insoluble in water, are usually also those having very little charge, that is, they are un-ionized. Consequently, they mix freely with lipid layers that are nonpolar, that is, having no electrostatic charges. On the other hand, drugs that are ionized are bound to water molecules by the electrostatic attraction between the drug and water ions and do not readily move from the aqueous to the lipid components of the membranes. Because many drugs are either weak acids or weak bases, they are capable of ionizing at a particular range of acidity or alkalinity (pH). The extent of ionization of a drug is expressed as the pK_a of the drug. The pK_a is the negative logarithm of the acid dissociation constant and is equal to the pH of the aqueous solution in which that drug would be 50 percent ionized and 50 percent un-ionized. Drugs that are weak acids ionize more readily in an alkaline environment and become less ionized in an acidic environment. The reverse is true of drugs that are weak bases.

If we put the weak acid aspirin* (acetylsalicylic acid), which has a pK_a of 3.5, into the stomach, we would have the equilibrium:

$$\text{COOH} \rightleftharpoons \text{COO}^- + \text{H}^+$$

Un-ionized   Ionized

Acetylsalicylic acid

From chemical principles we know that by increasing H^+ (from HCl in the stomach) we drive the reaction to the left, or increase the nonionized form of the drug. The reduced charge increases the lipid solubility of the drug. Thus, aspirin is readily absorbed from the stomach into the blood, which carries it to the target sites, where it reduces pain. In the intestine, where the pH is around 5 to 6.6 and the H^+ concentration is low, the reaction is driven to the right, toward dissociation. Thus, the ionization of aspirin in the intestine reduces its absorption through that membrane.

Although we might expect a drug to pass back and forth freely across the membrane, the pH of the compartment's fluid and the degree of ionization of the drug determines where the greatest concentration of drug occurs. Returning to our example, aspirin in the acidic gastric fluid is primarily in the un-ionized form and thus passes through the stomach wall into the blood. In blood (pH 7.4), however, aspirin becomes ionized, and so it is said to be "trapped" within the plasma compartment and does not return to the stomach.

In contrast, drugs that are weak bases, for example, morphine, will be more ionized in the stomach where the pH is low and will, therefore, not readily pass the gastric wall. In the intestine, however, where the pH is more basic, weak bases will be less ionized and will be more readily absorbed. Upon reaching the plasma pH (7.4), the drug becomes even less ionized and so may pass back through the membrane to the intestinal fluid. Moreover, the pH difference is not very great between intestine and blood, and so absorption is usually slow or incomplete.

It is important to recall that other factors also have a part in absorption. For instance, any drug that will be absorbed from the intestine must be resistant to the very low pH and the digestive processes in the stomach. Also, despite our earlier argument emphasizing the importance of ionization, the much greater surface area of the small intestine, as compared to the stomach, provides tremendous opportunity for absorption of weak bases or weak acids. In addition, passage of orally ingested material through the intestine is much slower than through the stomach, further increasing total absorption time. Thus, the rate at which the stomach empties into the intestine very often is the significant rate-limiting factor. For this reason, medication is often prescribed to be ingested before meals and with sufficient fluid to move the agent through the stomach and into the intestine.

Once the drug has entered the bloodstream, it is carried throughout the body and can have an action at any number of receptor sites. In general, those parts of the body that are well vascularized will have the highest concentration of drug. For this reason, high concentrations of a lipid-soluble drug will be found in the heart, brain, kidneys, and liver. As the brain receives perhaps 20 percent of the blood that leaves the heart, lipid-soluble drugs are readily distributed to brain tissue. However, as a result of the existence of the blood brain barrier, permeability by passive diffusion of water-soluble or ionized molecules is low.

Blood Brain Barrier. Because of our primary interest in the effects of drugs on neural tissue, it is important to understand the unique characteristics of drug transport to the brain. The concept of the BLOOD BRAIN BARRIER (BBB) arose from the observations of Paul Ehrlich in 1882. He noted that the acidic protein trypan blue (TB), when infused into the bloodstream, infiltrated most tissues but was not significantly taken up by brain tissue. However, when trypan blue was infused into the cerebrospinal fluid, the amount found in the brain was substantial. Ehrlich proposed that a selective barrier existed between the circulatory system and brain tissue and excluded substances that might in-

*The six-sided ring structure seen in the aspirin molecule is a common feature in many organic compounds found in biological systems as well as in drugs. It is a typical cyclic hydrocarbon because it consists of hydrogen and carbon atoms arranged in a ring. The alternating single and double bonds are not static but are constantly interchanging. A carbon atom is present at every angle and a hydrogen atom is attached to the carbon (unless another atom or group of atoms is indicated). There are hundreds of thousands of organic compounds consisting of combinations of these and other rings, some with fewer sides and angles, some with more. Also, many other atoms, either singly or in chains, can be attached to these rings at the angles.

terfere with brain function. Actually, there is no intrinsic barrier to trypan blue. The effect Ehrlich discovered was later found to be due to albumin binding of trypan blue in the blood plasma, with little or no free trypan blue remaining to traverse the capillary membranes between the bloodstream and neural tissue. The binding of trypan blue to a specific component in the blood is, in principle, the same as the binding of lipid-soluble substances to the fatty brain. The importance of binding at inactive sites, such as to albumin, with respect to the effectiveness of a drug is discussed in greater detail in the section on silent receptors. Nevertheless, Ehrlich's basic concept of a selective barrier between the blood and neural tissue was correct.

In looking for the anatomical or structural features that might explain the physiological action of the BBB, it was proposed that the barrier was a function of the extracellular space. The extracellular space in brain tissue was found to be minimal, as examination of brain tissue revealed a dense packing of neural and glial elements with virtually no space between them. However, later studies showed that artifacts of tissue preparation accounted for this apparent finding. At present, there is general agreement that an extracellular compartment does exist in the CNS, although there is some disagreement about its comparative volume. The amount of space is presently estimated to be between 20 and 25 percent of the total brain volume (Davson, 1972). A schematic diagram (Figure 4) of the spatial relationship between capillaries, glial cells, and neurons shows the numerous aqueous INTERCELLULAR CHANNELS. These channels provide to molecules leaving the capillaries the most direct access to neurons. Thus, contrary to the older view that all organic molecules must pass through the glial cells before reaching the neurons (Levine, 1973), more recent evidence shows that small molecules (having a molecular weight of 2000 or less) are able to move freely through the intercellular channels to reach the neuron (Kuffler and Nicholls, 1976). Thus, the physiological and metabolic blood brain barrier for smaller molecules cannot be explained by the presence of glia or the nature of the intercellular space.

The factors that now seem to account for the existence of the BBB became clearer when the morphology of brain capillaries and adjoining structures were examined. Figure 5 illustrates the structures of general (or nonneural) and brain capillaries. Capil-

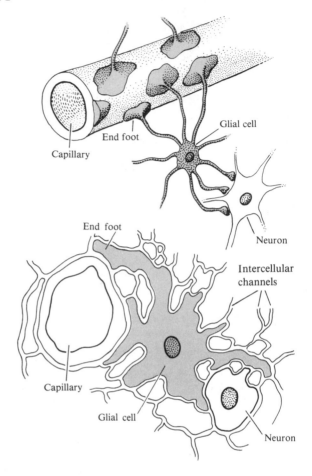

FIGURE 4.   SPATIAL RELATIONSHIPS AMONG CAPILLARIES, GLIA, AND NEURONS. The intercellular channels between the cells allow the small molecules that diffuse through the capillary wall to reach the neuronal surface. (From Kuffler and Nicholls, 1976.)

laries are made up of endothelial cells one layer thick (about 1 μm*) surrounded by an amorphous mucopolysaccharide matrix called the BASEMENT MEMBRANE. The latter forms a layer about 50 nm** thick, which contributes to the permeability of the capillary. The endothelial layer of general capillaries has small gaps (clefts) between adjacent cells or where the cells

*μm = micrometer; 10^{-6} meter, or 10^{-3} millimeter
**nm = nanometer; 10^{-9} meter, or 10^{-6} millimeter

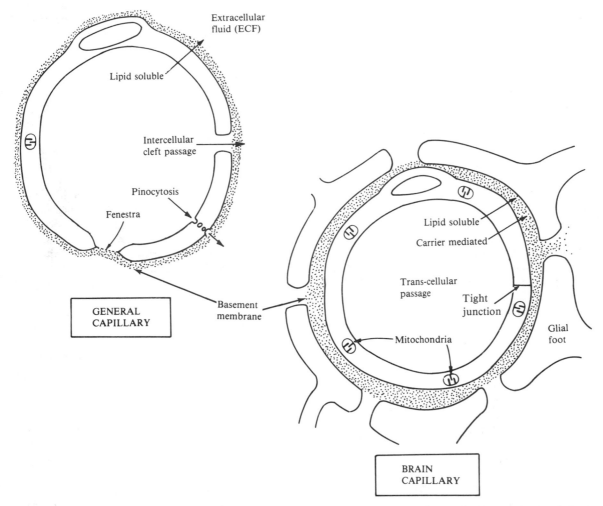

FIGURE 5. GENERAL (NONNEURAL) AND BRAIN (NEURAL) CAPILLARIES. Small molecules can pass by diffusion from the blood of general capillaries through the intercellular clefts to the extracellular fluid. Fenestrae are typically found in capillaries through which fluids pass in high volume, such as in the kidney. Pinocytosis, though somewhat ineffi- cient, is the mechanism for passing large molecules. In brain capillaries, intercellular clefts are replaced with tight junctions that block the passage of water-soluble molecules, even of small size; fenestrae are absent and pinocytotic sites are rare. (From Oldendorf, 1975.)

circle upon themselves. There are also fenestrae (openings) about 9–15 nm wide in capillaries, such as those found in the kidney. Through these openings small molecules can pass. In addition, general capillaries have PINOCYTOTIC VESICLES that envelop and trans- port large molecules through the capillary wall. In contrast, in brain capillaries, the intercellular clefts are absent because the adjoining edges are fused, forming tight junctions. Also, fenestrae are absent and pinocy- totic vesicles are rare. Surrounding brain capillaries are numerous ASTROCYTIC PROCESSES, or GLIAL FEET (see Chapter 3), covering about 85 percent of the basement membrane that fills the gap between the endothelial cells and the glial feet.

It is now apparent how molecules having a molecular weight (MW) as large as 20,000–40,000 can equilibrate in nonneural tissue between blood plasma and the extracellular fluid (ECF) in half-times of 10 to 30 seconds following an intravenous injection. That is, within 10–30 seconds, half of the molecules have left the blood and entered the ECF. Larger molecules, such as albumin (60,000 MW), remain in the blood plasma much longer, with a half-time of several hours. In the brain, however, because of the absence of clefts and fenestrae, water-soluble molecules having molecular weights as low as 2000 cannot enter the brain ECF from capillaries. These molecules escape from blood capillaries by crossing the inner endothelial cell membrane, then the endothelial cell cytoplasm, and finally the outer endothelial membrane to reach the brain ECF.

However, the blood brain barrier is selectively permeable rather than impermeable. The barrier reduces diffusion of water-soluble or ionized molecules but does not impede lipid-soluble or un-ionized molecules. In addition, water-soluble materials that are moved by specific transport processes, (e.g., glucose and other sugars, and amino acids) are not impeded by the barrier. (See facilitated diffusion in Chapter 3.)

Finally, the BBB is not "intact" along the entire capillary–brain ECF interface. There are places where fenestrations in the capillary endothelium permit proteins and small organic molecules to pass into brain ECF and thus presumably to interact with neurons. Examples of these areas (Figure 6) are the AREA POSTREMA, a highly vascularized strip of tissue found in the medulla along the lateral border of the caudal end of the fourth ventricle; the MEDIAN EMINENCE of the hypothalamus; the line of attachment of the CHOROID PLEXUS; and the PINEAL GLAND. The area postrema is adjacent to the CHEMICAL TRIGGER ZONE, otherwise known as the "vomiting center." Because toxic substances in the blood are stimuli for vomiting, the less hindered passage of materials from blood to this area of the brain provides a coupling of stimulus and response. Similarly, the hypothalamus has profound effects on the regulatory processes of the body (such as temperature control, feeding, and drinking) because it has extensive neural connections to other parts of the nervous system and the hormonal system. Thus, the lack of a barrier permits the receptors in the hypothalamus to monitor the level of hormones in the blood and subsequently to regulate hormone synthesis and release.

The choroid plexus synthesizes and secretes the CSF, which fills the cisterns, the lateral, the third and fourth ventricles, and surrounds the brain and spinal cord. CSF is similar to the brain ECF and differs significantly from blood plasma. Waste products from the brain pass into the CSF and then pass into the blood (the so-called "sink" function of the CSF) to be excreted. Thus, in addition to providing mechanical protection to the brain, the "sink" function may provide benefits that also depend on a blood monitoring feature. The pineal gland also has a close relationship to the blood vessels, and its role in mammalian sexual behavior may require that it also have a monitoring function of the blood (Katzman, 1976). The pineal gland is discussed in more detail in Chapter 8.

Placental Barrier. A second unique barrier is one that occurs between the maternal vascular system and her fetus. Drug transfer, as with vital nutrients and waste materials, is dependent on the passage of the substance across several layers of epithelial and endothelial cells separating maternal and fetal circulation. These barriers are not themselves unique and transfer occurs as for any epithelial barrier. However, the importance of recognizing the potential for transfer of drug from mother to child should be emphasized. The thalidomide disaster dramatically demonstrated that agents that were safe for an adult individual could penetrate the placental barrier and harm the fetus (*Medical News*, 1975). Also it is well known that opiates such as heroin readily reach the fetal circulation, and newborn infants from heroin- or methadone-addicted mothers experience many of the signs of opiate withdrawal.

Silent Receptors

A high concentration of drug may be found in various organs that are well supplied with blood. In addition to these reservoirs, drug binding also occurs at inactive binding sites where no measurable biological effect is initiated by the binding. Such sites, sometimes called "silent receptors," include plasma protein, muscle, and fat. The binding of a drug to inactive sites (DEPOT BINDING) may slow the onset of drug ac-

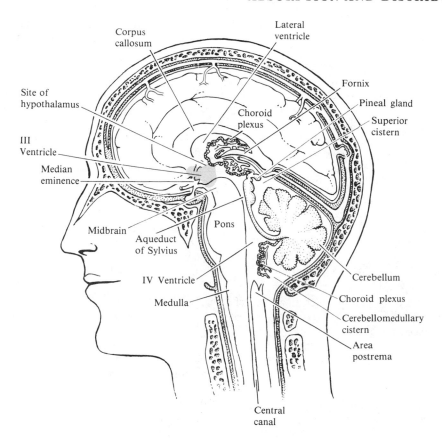

Corpus callosum

Lateral ventricle

Site of hypothalamus

Fornix

Pineal gland

Choroid plexus

Superior cistern

III Ventricle

Median eminence

Midbrain

Pons

Aqueduct of Sylvius

IV Ventricle

Medulla

Cerebellum

Choroid plexus

Cerebellomedullary cistern

Area postrema

Central canal

FIGURE 6. MIDSAGITTAL VIEW OF THE BRAIN. The blood brain barrier is breached at the choroid plexi, the median eminence, the hypothalamus, the pineal gland, and the area postrema. This means that some chemical components of the blood can escape from capillaries and influence cells in those areas. The shaded area represents the location of the hypothalamus, which is lateral to this midsagittal view.

tion, prolong drug action, or prevent it from occurring. Depot binding effectively reduces the concentration of drug at its sites of action as only unbound drug can readily pass across membranes. However, as the unbound drug leaves the circulation, the inactive drug complex begins to dissociate (unbind) and makes more unbound drug available for diffusion. Thus, if binding to silent receptors occurs rapidly, the onset of drug action at its active sites is dependent on its release from inactive sites and is slowed.

Depot binding may also prolong drug action. As unbound drug is eliminated from the body, more drug is dissociated from the inactive sites to enter the circulation. In contrast, it is possible to have an agent that so readily forms inactive complexes that its release into blood is too slow to produce an effective plasma concentration, preventing any drug action from occurring.

It may be found that the initial small doses of a drug may produce very little effect because most of the drug has been sequestered by the storage sites. Once these sites have been filled, however, blood drug levels more closely resemble the dose administered. An example of this occurs with the drug chloroquine, which is used to counteract the malaise associated with malaria. Chloroquine readily binds to the liver. Therefore, the liver sites must be saturated before a blood drug level effective in treating malaria can be attained.

The depots may also be responsible for terminating a drug's action, as in the case of barbiturates, which are CNS-depressant drugs. Thiopental, a barbiturate used for intravenous anesthesia, is highly lipid soluble and readily passes from the blood to various tissues. Its initial very rapid action after i.v. infusion is due to the drug's rapid binding to organs with the greatest vascularity, which includes the brain as well as the heart and liver. Its effect is of very short duration, however, because there is a shift of the drug from the plasma to other tissue compartments with less blood circulation (e.g., muscle, fat). Within 30 minutes of administration, the brain may give up as much as 90 percent of the initial peak concentration to various inactive binding sites. High levels of thiopental can be found in the brain 30 seconds after i.v. infusion, whereas 15–30 minutes are required to find the drug in muscle, and more than an hour is needed for the barbiturate to redistribute to fat (Harvey, 1975). Thus, thiopental induces sleep very quickly but is effective for only a short period of time.

These examples emphasize several of the pharmacological factors contributing to the final drug effect. To understand how a drug produces a biological effect, we have been considering what happens to the drug between administration and binding to an active receptor at the target tissue. Of importance are (1) the route of administration, (2) factors that regulate the passage of drug across cell membranes and through various fluid compartments, and (3) binding of drug to inactive sites ("silent receptors"). In the next section we explore the relationship of the drug to its site of biological action.

Receptor Binding

A RECEPTOR is a physiological entity present in cells and is a site of action of any biologically active agent that alters cellular function. Thus, before producing a change in a cell (which ultimately alters body function or behavior), a drug must physically interact with a specific cellular component. Receptors are generally quite specific, and those drugs that have the best "fit" tend to produce the most response from the cell. In the following section, we will consider the relationship of any drug to its receptor.

Law of Mass Action

Once the drug has reached a specific tissue receptor, in the simplest case, the response is proportional to the fraction of receptors occupied. The binding represents a dynamic state, with drug molecules constantly binding to and breaking away from the receptor. In other words, the binding is reversible. The law of mass action best sums up drug–receptor interaction:

$$D + R \rightleftharpoons DR \longrightarrow \text{pharmacological effect}$$

It says that the drug (D) and free receptors (R) must combine to form an active complex (DR), which leads to a pharmacological response in proportion to the fraction of receptors occupied. The active form (DR) is in equilibrium with the inactive components (D, R). Thus, the drug associates with the receptor and then dissociates, much as we described for the drug binding to silent receptors. The fact that the binding is reversible implies that the binding between the drug and the receptor is IONIC or ELECTROSTATIC. That is, a bond forms between charged groups in the receptor molecule and oppositely charged groups on the drug. Bonds of this type are less strong than some other types of bonds and, therefore, are reversible.

Dose–Response Relationships

From the law of mass action ($D + R \rightleftharpoons DR$) and elementary chemistry, we know that when we increase the concentration of drug (D) we drive the reaction to the right, thus forming greater amounts of drug–receptor complex (DR) and attaining greater pharmacological effect. The DOSE-RESPONSE CURVE, which describes the amount of pharmacological effect for a given drug concentration (DOSE), is shown in Figure 7. With increasing drug concentration (which, in turn, increases the amount of DR complex), there is an increase in pharmacological effect, until the maximum effect is achieved. Based on our equation, the maximum effect is achieved when receptors are fully occupied.

If we were to graph the effects of a family of drugs with similar molecular structure, we would expect a relationship similar to the one shown in Figure 7. That figure shows the dose–response characteristics for hydromorphine, morphine, and codeine—all drugs from the opiate analgesic class that reduces pain. For each drug, increasing the concentration produces greater analgesia (elevation in pain threshold) until the maximum response is achieved. The difference among the three drugs is in potency. By arbitrarily selecting a fixed dose of 10 mg (dotted line), they can be compared. At that concentration the analgesic effect of hydromorphine is maximal. For morphine, the same dose produces a much smaller elevation in the pain threshold; and a 10 mg dose of codeine produces no analgesic effect. Even at ten times the dose (100 mg),

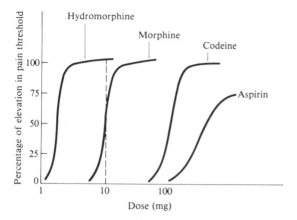

FIGURE 7 DOSE-RESPONSE RELATIONSHIPS FOR FOUR ANALGESIC AGENTS. Each curve represents the increase in pain threshold as a function of the dose. The pain threshold is the magnitude of painful stimulus required to elicit a response. (From Levine, 1973.)

the same. Thus, a larger amount of codeine will be as effective as either of the other drugs administered at a lower dose. The fact that the curves are identical in shape and approach the same maximum suggest that the drugs act at the same receptor. When we look at the dose–response curve for aspirin in Figure 7, we see that it is not parallel to the other three and does not reach the same maximum regardless of how high a dose is administered. Although aspirin also reduces pain, it acts on a different receptor and works by a different mechanism.

The structural specificity of the receptor determines the relative potency of a family of drugs. We can infer from the example that hydromorphine fits the opiate receptor more closely than does morphine. A minor molecular modification of morphine produces codeine, which shows less effectiveness in lowering pain. Such specificity has been utilized by organic chemists, who have synthesized a wide variety of morphine-like pain killers, hoping to produce a drug that is more effective than morphine.

Drugs are absorbed and distributed throughout the body. Therefore, drugs have multiple sites of action (receptors) and multiple pharmacological effects. Furthermore, because the receptors may not have identical characteristics, the order of potency for structurally similar drugs is not the same for each pharmacological effect. Thus, we may see a distinct family of curves, depending on the pharmacological effect we are measuring. Table I shows the multiple effects of several

codeine does not produce its maximal action. Because of this difference, we would say that hydromorphine is more potent than morphine, and each is more potent than codeine. POTENCY is determined by the affinity of the drug for the receptor, as well as the accessibility of the drug to the receptor.

Despite great differences in potency between the three drugs in Figure 7, the maximum effectiveness is

TABLE I   Relative Pharmacological Activity of the Xanthines

| | XANTHINE | | |
	Caffeine	Theophylline	Theobromine
CNS and Respiratory Stimulation	1*	2	3
Cardiac Stimulation	3	1	2
Coronary Dilation	3	1	2
Smooth Muscle Relaxation	3	1	2
Skeletal Muscle Stimulation	1	2	3
Diuresis	3	1	2

*1 = most active.   (From Ritchie, 1975b)

drugs in the xanthine class: caffeine, theophylline, and theobromine. Notice that the order of potency for the three drugs in stimulating the CNS is caffeine > theophylline > theobromine. In contrast, theophylline (which is found in tea) is most potent in cardiovascular stimulation compared to either of the other two, whereas caffeine (found in coffee) stimulates the cardiovascular system least.

One more point should be mentioned that is relevant to the subject of drug dose and potency. Frequently a drug is administered as a salt, meaning that the free base or active drug is ionically bound to an inorganic salt. This is usually done to make the drug more soluble in aqueous solutions, the salt being pharmacologically inert. Thus chlordiazepoxide (Librium) is frequently given as chlordiazepoxide HCl. To determine the proportion of active drug that is administered as a salt solution one must know the molecular weight (M.W.) of the free base, the M.W. of the salt anion, and the proportional number (N) of free base molecules to salt molecules. Furthermore, the salt must be specified as hydrochloride because each salt such as sulfate or bitartrate has a different molecular weight. A formula for the determination of the proportion of active drug in a solution is below (Seiden and Dykstra, 1977):

$$\frac{N(M.W. \text{ free base})}{N(M.W. \text{ free base}) + N(M.W. \text{ salt ion})} =$$

drug proportion (mg/ml)

Side Effects and the Therapeutic Index

Frequently the usefulness of a drug must be balanced with the extent of undesirable effects (SIDE EFFECTS). For instance, amphetamine-like agents may be prescribed for short-term weight reduction because they significantly reduce appetite; but because they also stimulate the CNS, a major side effect is sleeplessness. Under other conditions, for example, in the treatment of narcolepsy (an illness characterized by uncontrolled, sudden lapses into sleep), the alerting properties of amphetamine are the desired therapeutic action while loss of appetite in the treated individuals may be a serious side effect. A discussion of side effects reemphasizes the fact that drugs have neither a single site of action nor a single pharmacological effect. Drugs that have actions on the CNS also almost certainly have potent peripheral effects. Thus, amphetamine acts on the CNS, causing alertness, hyper-

activity, and appetite suppression, but in addition, it may cause cardiac arrhythmias and hypertension and produce dry mouth, diarrhea, and a host of other changes following peripheral stimulation. Recall, however, that all drugs that have peripheral effects do not act on the CNS because the blood brain barrier effectively excludes many chemicals from neural tissue.

In a therapeutic situation, the extent of side effects must be carefully considered as part of the therapeutic index. For example, in Figure 8 you can see the dose-response curves for two distinct pharmacological effects of drug A which is prescribed to induce sleep.

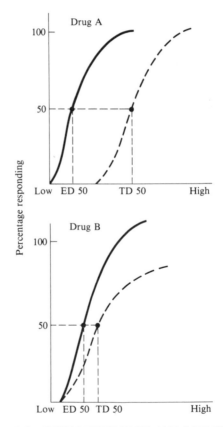

FIGURE 8. DRUGS WITH HIGH AND LOW THERAPEUTIC INDICES. Comparisons between the dose-response curves for an effective dose (sleep induction, solid curve), and a toxic dose (respiratory depression, dotted curve) for the same drug. In A, the difference in average dose for the two effects (ED 50, TD 50) is large enough for the drug to be considered fairly safe. This is not true in B.

The solid curve shows the number of individuals who fall asleep at various doses of the drug. The dotted curve shows the number of people suffering respiratory depression at various doses of the same drug. By comparing the dose at which 50 percent of the people fall asleep (effective dose 50 = ED 50) with the dose at which 50 percent of the population tested show respiratory depression (toxic dose 50 = TD 50), you can see that for most individuals the toxic dose is several times higher than the dose producing the desired effect. Pharmacologists would say the drug has a relatively good therapeutic index, which is the ratio of the dose TD 50 to that of the ED 50 (therapeutic index = TD 50/ED 50), that is, it is fairly safe. In contrast, drug B has a poor therapeutic index because the toxic dose (TD 50) is not very different from the therapeutically useful dose (ED 50). Thus, the danger of serious side effects (respiratory depression) is much higher for drug B and the margin of safety is small. In the case of therapeutics, potential benefit must clearly outweigh potential hazard. For this reason, given a choice of drugs, the one with the safer therapeutic index would be used. However, in the case of a drug without an alternate, one must ask whether the disorder is sufficiently severe to warrant the risks of medication.

Receptor Antagonists

Thus far, the picture of drug–receptor interaction has been quite simple. However, few drugs follow the simple rule without modification. Some drugs bind to an activatable receptor but produce no pharmacological action. These drugs are called ANTAGONISTS because, although they have no effect *per se*, they can effectively block the action of an AGONIST, a drug that binds to the receptor and does have pharmacological effects. Among the antagonists discussed in later chapters is naloxone, which blocks the effects of morphine, heroin, and other opiates. Antagonists as well as agonists have receptor specificity. Thus, naloxone will block the effects of morphine or heroin but will not directly affect the action of aspirin.

One further complication requires that we distinguish between COMPETITIVE and NON-COMPETITIVE ANTAGONISTS. Figure 9A demonstrates the effect of a competitive antagonist (naloxone). The solid line shows a typical dose–response curve for the analgesic effect (as measured with the hot plate test) of morphine given i.p. in rats. When the rats were pretreated (i.p.) with 10 mg naloxone per kg body weight, the

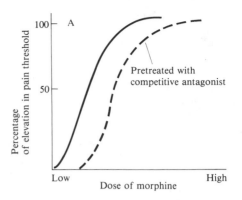

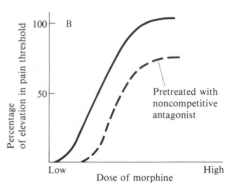

FIGURE 9. COMPETITIVE AND NONCOMPETITIVE DRUG ANTAGONISM. The effect of a competitive antagonist (naloxone) on the analgesic effect of morphine. (A) Pretreatment with naloxone decreases the potency of morphine, as shown by the shift of the dose-response curve to the right. The maximum effect of the drug can be achieved by increasing the dose of morphine. (B) The noncompetitive antagonist not only decreases the potency of the drug, but the antagonism cannot be entirely overcome by increasing drug dosage.

dose–response curve shifted to the right (dashed line), demonstrating that for any given dose of morphine, the naloxone-pretreated rats showed less analgesia. Thus, the addition of naloxone makes morphine less potent. The figure also shows that the inhibitory action of naloxone can be overcome by increasing the amount of morphine administered, that is, the same maximum effect (analgesia) can be achieved, but more drug is required. Because the competitive antagonist binds to the same receptors as the active drug, it is reasonable that increased concentration of active drug can compete more effectively for the fixed number of receptors.

A noncompetitive antagonist cannot be overcome by increasing the amount of agonist (Figure 9B). Thus, not only is the curve shifted to the right, but the maximum effect achieved is also reduced. A noncompetitive antagonist may bind to the same receptor as the active drug, or it may bind to the cell in such a way as to prevent the agonist–receptor coupling. Much of this discussion will sound familiar to those persons acquainted with the principles of enzyme kinetics.

There are drugs that act as mixed agonist–antagonists. These agents possess some of the pharmacological effects of an agonist, but when administered with that agonist, reduce the agonist's potency. One such drug is nalorphine, which has some analgesic action and produces certain autonomic effects resembling those produced by morphine. However, it is not constipating and tends to produce dysphoria rather than euphoria. In addition, it can antagonize morphine-induced analgesia, euphoria, drowsiness, vomiting, miosis (pinpoint pupils), and many other pharmacological effects. Further discussion of mixed agonist–antagonists and their relationship to drug receptors can be found in the chapter on opiates.

Biotransformation and Excretion

A final biological process affecting the amount of drug–receptor interaction at any one time is the rate of biotransformation and/or excretion. Drugs are eliminated from the body either unchanged or as metabolites. The most important organ of elimination is the kidney, although small amounts of some drugs are eliminated from the lungs, in the sweat, saliva, and feces, or in milk. Although the excretion in milk is usually an insignificant route of elimination for the mother, it may be of consequence to a nursing infant, who may take in a significant amount of drug. The young child, much like the unborn fetus, may have underdeveloped metabolizing enzymes in the liver and thus will be unable to effectively handle a dose of drug intended for its mother.

Renal Excretion

The kidneys are a pair of organs each about the size of a fist and are responsible for filtering out products of metabolism and maintaining appropriate blood levels of various ions and other substances. The kidney excretes the end products of body metabolism (e.g.,

urea), as well as excess sodium, potassium, and chloride. However, the organ conserves water, sugar, and necessary amounts of sodium, potassium, and chloride.

The anatomy of the kidney facilitates maximum interaction between the internal and external environment. The functional unit of the kidney is the NEPHRON (Figure 10), which contains a long, unbranched tubule that begins in a capsule-like structure (Bowman's capsule) that encircles a network of capillaries called the GLOMERULUS. There are approximately one to three million nephrons per kidney, with a total of about 35 miles of tubules. With approximately 1300 milliliters of blood passing through each kidney per minute, the pressure of the blood in the glomeruli causes the fluid constituents of the blood to leave the capillaries and flow into Bowman's capsules (as the glomerular filtrate) at the rate of 125 milliliters per minute. Because the capsules are continuous with the tubules, the filtrate passes into the tubules, from which 124 milliliters are reabsorbed into the blood as the

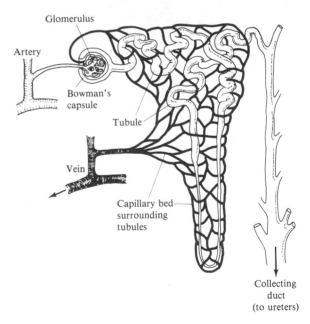

FIGURE 10.   SINGLE NEPHRON WITHIN A KIDNEY. This highly magnified view shows how the large surface area of the tubules and the close relationship of the blood vessels to the tubule enable maximum internal/external fluid exchange. (From Julien, 1981.)

fluid flows through the various segments of the nephrons and collecting ducts, leaving only 1 milliliter to be excreted as urine. Within the reabsorbed fraction is virtually all of the sodium chloride, glucose, amino acids, proteins, and other substances necessary for the body. Left in the tubules are some chemical substances (such as some drugs, end products of metabolism, urea, uric acid, and creatinine) that are of little or no use to the body, as well as substances that are exchanged for sodium (such as potassium, hydrogen, and ammonia). Hormones from the hypothalamus regulate the amount of water and sodium that is reabsorbed, thus determining the concentration of the urine that passes via the collecting ducts and ureters to the urinary bladder for excretion (Bloom and Fawcett, 1968). Most drugs are readily filtered unless they are bound to plasma proteins or are of large molecular size. The reabsorption of water from the tubules produces a drug concentration gradient so that the drug is more highly concentrated in the kidney than in the blood plasma. Because of this gradient and because many drugs are small molecules with little charge, they also are often reabsorbed into the bloodstream. For this reason, kidney clearance of unaltered drugs is rather ineffective.

In order to eliminate drugs from the body more readily, the reabsorption process must be reduced. The ionization of drugs will reduce reabsorption (from kidney to blood) because it makes the drug less lipid soluble. Most drug metabolism alters an essentially nonionic drug molecule into a metabolite with a greater charge. This process of drug metabolism or biotransformation occurs primarily, but not entirely, in the liver.

Tubular reabsorption, like diffusion across other membranes, is pH dependent. When tubular urine is made more alkaline, weak acids are excreted more rapidly because they become more ionized and are reabsorbed less well, that is, they are "trapped" in the tubular urine. If the urine is acidic, excretion will be less. The opposite is true for a weakly basic drug. This principle of altering urinary pH is frequently used in treatment of drug toxicity, when it is highly desirable to remove the offending drug from the body.

Drug Metabolism

The process of drug metabolism or biotransformation can occur in the kidney, blood, or brain. However, the greatest amount of drug metabolism occurs in the liver. (The discussion in this chapter will deal primarily with metabolism within the liver, but in later chapters we will discuss drug metabolism within the brain.) Biotransformation of a drug usually produces an inactive metabolite that is more ionized and therefore is reabsorbed from the kidney into blood less well and excreted more readily. In some instances liver metabolism produces an active metabolite from an inactive drug. An example of this occurs with tremorine, which is converted to oxotremorine. Oxotremorine, when injected into mice, produces shaking and tremors of the whole body. However, if the parent drug is administered along with a metabolism inhibitor, no tremors occur. Thus, metabolism converts the inactive drug (tremorine) into an active metabolite (oxotremorine).

In other cases, a variety of metabolites are formed because several enzymes metabolize the same compound. One such drug is diazepam (Valium).* This commonly used minor tranquilizer is metabolized into a large number of compounds, some of which are active tranquilizers themselves and others of which are inactive drugs. In this case, the formation of active metabolites helps to explain the long duration of the drug's potent antianxiety effects.

The ability of an enzyme to alter a drug is dependent on the formation of an enzyme–drug complex, which may be described as

$$E + D \rightleftharpoons E \cdot D \rightarrow P + E$$

where: E = enzyme, D = drug,
$E \cdot D$ = enzyme–drug complex,
P = products of metabolism.

This formula is very much like the drug–receptor interaction described earlier, and in fact, one might consider that the receptor in our earlier discussion is an enzyme. Many of the principles of enzyme–drug inter-

*Drugs that are sold commercially, either by prescription or over the counter, have a chemical name that indicates chemical composition, a generic name that is a much shortened form of the chemical name but still can be unique for it, and one or many trade names. For example, the popular antianxiety drug known by its trade name Valium (always capitalized) has a chemical name, 7-chloro-1,3-dihydro-1-methyl-5-phenyl-2H-1, 4-benzodiazepin-2-one, and a generic name, diazepam. Sometimes a generic name is so widely recognized that it is also used as a trade name. Thus acetylsalicylic acid is known almost solely by its generic name, aspirin. In fact almost all chemical compounds have a generic name such as salt, lime, milk of magnesia, penicillin, and so on.

action are similar to those for receptor activity. For instance, the enzyme and drug combine in a reversible fashion and the bonds formed are primarily ionic bonds, that is, are electrostatic in nature. Furthermore, the drug–enzyme complex produces a sequence of events that lead to an end product. Also, although enzymes usually show some specificity based on the conformation of "active sites," the specificity is not absolute. Often an enzyme can act on drugs that are structurally similar to a naturally occurring substrate; however, some enzymes show very little specificity at all.

Synthetic Reactions

There are two principal ways in which a drug molecule can be modified: SYNTHETIC REACTIONS and NONSYNTHETIC REACTIONS. The synthetic reactions, also called CONJUGATIONS, involve the chemical coupling of the drug with some molecule provided by the body. An enzyme acts as a catalyst for the coupling reaction. (The catalytic activity of an enzyme is characterized by the fact that the enzyme is required for the reaction to occur, but no part of the enzyme molecule itself is incorporated into the new product. The formula in the preceding section shows that the enzyme–substrate interaction produces several products of metabolism plus unaltered enzyme, which can rebind to new unmodified drug.)

Synthetic reactions most often make the drug more water soluble and less lipid soluble, and usually the end product is pharmacologically inactive. The chemical groups on the drug that provide sites for conjugation are carboxyl (COOH), hydroxyl (OH), amino (NH_2), or sulfhydryl (SH). In order for conjugation to occur, one of these groups must be present. Drugs that have no site for conjugation may undergo a nonsynthetic reaction first before undergoing a synthetic reaction. Drugs that have multiple sites for conjugation will produce a variety of metabolites, depending on the site altered.

The most common synthetic reaction is conjugation with glucuronic acid, $C_6H_{10}O_7$, an acid derived from glucose. For example, aspirin (Figure 11) is first converted to salicylic acid by a nonsynthetic reaction (step 1) and then can undergo conjugation with glucuronic acid (step 2) at two sites. Thus, two metabolites have been formed. Both of the glucuronide-modified molecules produced are highly water soluble and ionized and so are rapidly excreted by the kidneys. It should also be mentioned that salicylic acid can

undergo a variety of other metabolizing reactions at the same sites, for example, conjugation with glycine.

It is important to recognize that salicylic acid is an active metabolite of aspirin. In fact, aspirin was derived from salicylic acid for systemic use because the acid is extremely irritating and can only be used externally. Furthermore, if the nonsynthetic metabolism of aspirin were inhibited, its pain-killing effects would be greatly reduced. If the conjugation with glucuronic acid were inhibited, the analgesic effect of salicylic acid would be prolonged. Clearly, drug metabolism can produce active or inactive metabolites.

In other synthetic reactions, different chemical molecules are attached at the conjugation sites. Among the most common additions are two amino acids (glutamine and glycine) and sulfate. In addition, both acetylation and methylation are conjugation reactions in which an acetyl group ($O = C—CH_3$) and a methyl group ($—CH_3$) are added, respectively.

Nonsynthetic Reactions

Nonsynthetic reactions are those in which the parent drug is modified by oxidation, reduction, or hydrolysis. These reactions differ from conjugation in several respects. The products of these reactions are not necessarily inactive and, in fact, may be made active (sometimes more active than the parent drug). On the whole, drugs that undergo nonsynthetic reactions are not eliminated from the body but undergo a conjugation reaction in a second step. In the example of aspirin metabolism (Figure 11), the first step is a nonsynthetic hydrolysis. The product of that step, salicylic acid, is as active as the parent compound. As in conjugation reactions, nonsynthetic reactions are dependent on the presence of an appropriate chemical group, but the presence of the group does not guarantee that a particular nonsynthetic reaction will occur.

Liver Microsomal Enzymes

A large number of drug metabolizing reactions are catalyzed by liver enzymes located on the SMOOTH ENDOPLASMIC RETICULUM, which is a network of tubules within the liver cell cytoplasm. These enzymes catalyze many of the oxidation and reduction reactions and some of the hydrolysis reactions. They also catalyze one synthetic reaction: conjugation with glucuronic acid. They are often called MICROSOMAL ENZYMES because, when liver cells are homogenized and the cell constituents separate by sucrose gradient cen-

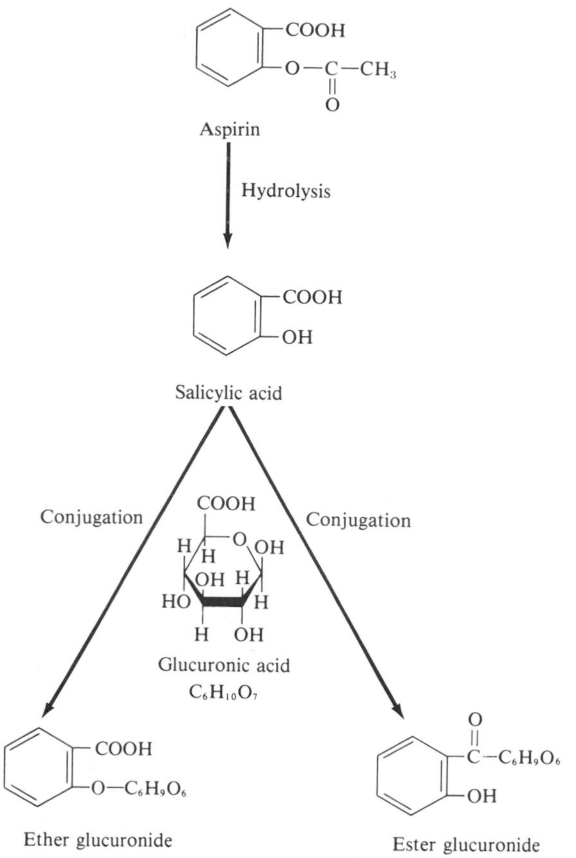

FIGURE 11. METABOLISM OF ASPIRIN. Alternative routes of the two-step metabolism of acetylsalicylic acid (aspirin). Aspirin first undergoes nonsynthetic hydrolysis to form salicylic acid (an active metabolite). The second step is the conjugation with glucuronic acid (synthetic reaction), which produces two highly water-soluble metabolites that are readily excreted from the body.

trifugation, the enzymes are found in the microsomal fraction. The MICROSOMAL FRACTION contains primarily smooth endoplasmic reticulum with some contamination by membrane fragments from other organelles.

The microsomal enzymes lack a great deal of specificity and can metabolize a wide variety of compounds. They do not seem to metabolize naturally occurring substances, possibly because they best catalyze reactions involving compounds that are lipid soluble. Lipid solubility improves the penetration of a drug

into the endoplasmic reticulum and its binding with the enzyme system.

The metabolizing enzymes of the liver are particularly important to psychopharmacologists because a large number of drugs altering mood and behavior cause an increase in liver enzyme activity. For example, repeated use of barbiturates, which are used to elicit sedation and sleep, increases the capacity of the liver enzymes to metabolize the administered drugs into inactive compounds. With chronic use, the pharmacological effect of the barbiturates is apparently diminished. Thus, changes in drug metabolism explain in part why some drugs lose their effectiveness with repeated use—a phenomenon known as tolerance.

Tolerance

TOLERANCE is defined as diminished response to drug administration after repeated exposure to that drug. In other words, tolerance has developed when increasingly larger doses of a given drug must be administered to obtain the same magnitude of pharmacological effect observed with the original dose. It is well known, for example, that the daily administration of morphine must be gradually increased in order to maintain a quantitatively similar degree of analgesia (relief from pain).

We should be aware that not all pharmacological effects of a particular drug demonstrate tolerance equally. This can sometimes be beneficial, such as in the case of the minor tranquilizer chlordiazepoxide (Librium). In animal studies, it has been shown that initially this drug has both sedative and antianxiety properties, but with repeated administration, tolerance develops for the sedative effect but not for the antianxiety effect. Therapeutically, this property is of significance for those who need the reduction in anxiety but who must continue to function without sedation. The reduction in sedation occurs only with chronic use of the drug. As with most drugs, tolerance disappears after a period of abstinence. Thus, for an individual who uses the drug infrequently, the sedative effect will be apparent.

Another example of the differential development of tolerance occurs with the use of the barbiturates. Although the sedative property of barbiturates shows the tolerance reaction, the respiratory centers in the brain stem that are depressed apparently do not show the same extent of tolerance. Consequently, after repeated administration of the barbiturate, the dose that effectively produces sedation and the lethal dose become more similar, and the probability of lethal overdose becomes significantly greater.

We should also keep in mind that for some drugs tolerance can appear at the second administration, whereas for others repeated doses over a period of many days is required. Furthermore, the appearance of tolerance is related to the amount of drug administered, as well as to the temporal sequence. Thus, a drug administered in large doses at short intervals will produce more tolerance than smaller doses of the same drug at longer intervals. Keep in mind that tolerance is reversible. When drug administration is stopped, tolerance disappears gradually, its rate depending on the particular drug involved.

Cross Tolerance

The development of tolerance to one drug administered over a period of time can diminish the pharmacological effectiveness of a second drug. This phenomenon is called CROSS TOLERANCE and is the basis for a number of drug interactions. It is known that the effective anticonvulsant dose of phenobarbital is significantly larger in a patient who has a history of chronic alcohol use than in a patient who has not developed tolerance to alcohol. Because tolerance to alcohol diminishes the effectiveness of the barbiturates, we say that cross tolerance exists between alcohol and phenobarbital. Cross tolerance also exists among several hallucinogenic drugs, for instance, LSD, psilocybin, and mescaline.

Drug Disposition Tolerance

Based on our previous discussion of the importance of the receptor for pharmacological activity, we will assume that the quantitative effect of a drug is determined by its concentration and chemical reaction at a specific receptor site. By the law of mass action:

$$\text{drug} + \text{receptor} \rightleftharpoons \text{drug–receptor} \rightarrow \text{response}$$

Tolerance is defined as a diminished response to drug administration after repeated exposure. We can see from the preceding equation that there are only a few ways in which an individual can become tolerant to a drug. Tolerance can be the consequence of (1) a decrease in the effective concentration of the agonist at the site of action, (2) a reduction in the normal reactivity of the receptor, or (3) a change in the response elic-

ited because of activation of a homeostatic mechanism.

In the first case, tolerance can develop if, with repeated drug administration, there is a reduction in the concentration of the drug at its receptor. DRUG DISPOSITION TOLERANCE (metabolic tolerance) occurs when a drug produces effects that reduce its own absorption, increase its binding to an inert complex, alter its rate of transfer across a biological membrane, or increase its own rate of elimination.

The only well-documented way of reducing the drug concentration at the receptor is by increasing the rate of drug metabolism. Drug disposition tolerance can be shown for drugs like the sedative pentobarbital, which increases its own rate of biotransformation through stimulation of liver microsomal enzymes.

In one experiment it was shown that rabbits respond to pentobarbital treatment by falling asleep. Rabbits pretreated with pentobarbital for 3 days slept a much shorter time after an intravenous test dose than did controls (Remmer, 1962). Because the blood drug levels were the same for each group at the moment of awakening, the reduced sleeping time can be attributed to an increased metabolism without a change in the animals' sensitivity to a given drug concentration. The biological half-life of pentobarbital in the tolerant animals was 26 minutes as compared to 79 minutes for those that were not pretreated. Clearly, the metabolism of pentobarbital was much greater in the pretreated animals. The increased rate of metabolism was not due to more efficient enzyme activity but was due to an increase in smooth endoplasmic reticulum in liver cells, the structure associated with drug-metabolizing enzymes. Thus, treatment with selected drugs over a period of time can increase the amount of liver microsomal enzymes, which then reduces the blood drug level and hence reduces the pharmacological effect. Because evidence suggests that the enzyme induction involves new protein synthesis, high blood drug levels have to be maintained for that length of time needed to enable an increase in the amount of liver microsomal enzymes. This characteristic is demonstrated by the finding that mice and rabbits, which metabolize drugs very rapidly, have to be given the drug several times daily for several days in order to see an increased rate of metabolism. Dogs, which metabolize drugs much more slowly, develop tolerance at a faster rate.

One interesting aspect of drug disposition tolerance is that its appearance is dependent upon the route of administration of the drug. Intravenous administra-

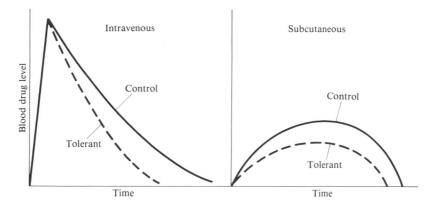

FIGURE 12. EFFECT OF TOLERANCE ON BLOOD DRUG LEVEL. Blood level of a drug administered intravenously or subcutaneously to tolerant and nontolerant individuals. The difference in peak blood drug levels and the duration of drug in the blood is related to the method of administration and the metabolic rate in each individual.

tion of the drug to a tolerant and a nontolerant animal should produce the same maximum effect because absorption is rapid and the dose should reach the same drug concentration in both animals (Figure 12). However, because the rate of metabolism of the drug in the tolerant animals is greater, it is expected that the pharmacological effect should be terminated sooner. This same relationship would not be true if the drug is administered subcutaneously because the slow rate of absorption means that the peak drug concentration is a balance between absorption rate and elimination rate. Thus, tolerant animals that are metabolizing faster would have a lower effective drug concentration at any one time than would nontolerant animals.

As mentioned earlier, liver microsomal enzymes are not very specific for their substrate, that is, they metabolize a variety of drugs. Therefore, cross tolerance between many drugs is possible. However, the occurrence of cross tolerance is not solely related to rate of metabolism. For many drugs, pretreatment with one agent diminishes the response of the nervous system to a second drug.

Pharmacodynamic (Cellular) Tolerance

The most dramatic form of tolerance that develops to the central actions of certain drugs cannot be explained on the basis of altered metabolism or altered concentration of drug reaching the brain. Thus, some change in receptors might be expected: a change in the number of receptors, perhaps, or in their affinity for the drug. No mechanism has been determined as yet to explain the appearance of cellular tolerance, and so we speak of adaptation of the cells to the presence of the drug. This type of tolerance occurs for the barbiturates (e.g., pentobarbital) and is manifested by a decrease in drug-induced sedation with repeated doses. Cellular tolerance also occurs for ethanol. (Notice that any one drug, such as ethanol, may demonstrate several types of tolerance.)

Tolerance to the opiates (e.g., morphine, heroin) is characterized by a shorter duration of action, a reduced intensity of the analgesic and sedative effects, and a significant increase in the average lethal dose. Although some metabolic tolerance may occur, it has been shown that at equal brain drug levels, tolerant animals show much less analgesic and sedative effect than nontolerant animals. A biochemical basis for the reduced effectiveness of these drugs has been suggested. By examining growing cells in a cell culture medium, Sharma et al. (1975a) have been able to determine both the acute effects of morphine as well as the effects after several days of exposure to the drug. They found that by attaching to its receptor, morphine initially reduces the activity of adenylate cyclase, an enzyme that directs cellular processes. After several days of treatment with morphine, however, the adenylate cyclase was no longer easily inhibited by the drug; much more morphine had to be added to the cells to produce inhibition. Apparently, adaptive changes in the receptor (or in the enzyme regulated by the receptor) occurred after prolonged exposure to morphine. (For further discussion, see the chapter dealing with opiate dependence.)

Behavioral Tolerance

Many drugs with CNS effects, particularly those that are abused, cause a tolerance reaction of the cellular adaptation type. Often tolerance is manifested in a task in which learning plays some part. For example, a psychotropic drug might disrupt the performance of a task (such as maze running for food reward) initially, but repeated administrations may have less and less effect. The improved performance could be identified as a type of tolerance, but the apparent tolerance could be due to the learning of a new skill (the ability to run a maze in the drug state), which we would expect to improve with practice. One example of this is the alcoholic who learns to maneuver fairly efficiently while highly intoxicated to avoid detection, whereas a less experienced drunk with the same blood alcohol level may appear behaviorally to be quite intoxicated (see Krasnegor, 1978).

State Dependent Learning

Tasks learned in the presence of a psychotropic drug may subsequently be performed better in the drug state. Conversely, learning acquired in the nondrug state may be more available in the nondrugged state. This phenomenon has been called "state dependent learning" and demonstrates the inability to transfer learning from a drugged to a nondrugged condition. An example of this is the alcoholic who during a binge hides his supply of liquor for later consumption but is unable to find it while he is sober (in the nondrugged state). Once he has returned to the alcoholic state, he can readily locate his cache.

One explanation for state dependency is that the drug effect may become part of the environmental "set," assuming the properties of a stimulus itself. A drugged subject learns to perform a particular task in relationship to all the internal and external cues in the environment, including, it is argued, drug-induced cues. Thus, in the absence of the drug-induced cues, performance deteriorates much the same as if the test apparatus were altered. It has been shown in animal studies that the decrease in performance is very much related to the change in environmental cues. That a particular drug state does provide discriminable cues has been well documented (Overton, 1971). (Further

discussion of the cueing properties of drugs follows in the section on behavioral pharmacology.)

The appearance of state dependent learning quite probably has great importance in clinical pharmacology. It would not be surprising, for example, if a new behavior acquired during psychotherapy by a patient who is receiving psychotropic drug medication, does not transfer to the nondrug state when the drug is discontinued.

Tolerance by Indirect Mechanisms

Looking once again at the law of mass action, we can see that tolerance might also occur at the final step in the drug–receptor interaction sequence—at the response stage— as a consequence of the operation of homeostatic adjustment.

An example of this type of tolerance occurs when the drug does not produce all of its effects by direct action but instead is responsible for releasing an endogenous, physiologically active substance from its storage vesicles. If stores of the endogenous substance become depleted because the interval between doses of drug that release them is too short to allow reaccumulation, then tolerance to that drug will appear. Tolerance of this type develops to morphine-induced dilation. One effect of morphine is the release of stored histamine, which produces a dilation of cutaneous blood vessels and in man is seen as flushing in the face, neck, and upper thorax. If small doses of morphine are administered to an animal over several weeks, very little tolerance to peripheral vasodilation occurs because stores of histamine can be replenished. With larger doses, tolerance develops rapidly because stores of histamine become depleted, that is, histamine synthesis cannot keep up with demand. When tolerance of this type occurs very rapidly, it is called TACHYPHYLAXIS.

A second example of a physiological, homeostatic adjustment to a drug effect is the response to treatment with thyroid hormone. When thyroid hormone (a "drug" that increases cellular metabolism) is administered to a normal individual, it circulates to the pituitary. The pituitary, in turn, signals to the thyroid gland to stop releasing natural thyroid hormone. Thus, although initially the administration of the hormone leads to high blood drug levels (and increased cellular metabolism, with a perception of increased vigor and energy), the body very quickly responds by turning down the normal hormone release, thus restoring the usual level of thyroid hormone in the blood (hence restoring normal rates of cellular metabolism and perhaps eliciting a feeling of fatigue).

Summary

Drugs are chemical substances that cause changes in physiological systems. This chapter attempted to show the mechanisms by which drugs are able to reach and affect organ function with reasonable efficacy and safety. The principles of drug administration, distribution, dose requirements, duration of action, metabolism, excretion, and tolerance, apply to all drug treatment. The same mechanisms must be considered for drug therapy and research applications. For example, lipid solubility determines absorption and onset of action, while rate of metabolism modifies the duration of action.

A unique concern in psychopharmacology is the effect of drugs upon behavior. It must be appreciated that drugs do not create behavior—rather, they affect behavior that is already in existence. The behaviors alone are complex because they are the consequence of highly varied experiences as well as variations in physiology both within and between species. Thus, behavioral pharmacology systematically begins with standard procedures and measurements to establish a norm (baseline behavior) against which to compare behavioral drug effects. These techniques are the subject of Chapter 2.

Recommended Readings

Goodman, L.S. and Gilman, A. (Eds.) (1980). *The Pharmacological Basis of Therapeutics*. Macmillan, New York. One of the outstanding medical reference texts dealing with virtually every class of drugs in terms of their development, mode of action, and clinical application.

Levine, R.R. (1973). *Pharmacology: Drug Actions and Reactions*. Little, Brown, Boston. A concise and beautifully written pharmacology text within the grasp of undergraduates with some biology and chemistry background.

Krasnegor, N.A. (1978). *Behavioral Tolerance: Research and Treatment Implications*. NIDA Research Monograph No. 18. U.S. Government Printing Office, Washington D.C. A collection of papers dealing with the role of learning in reactions to narcotics, ethanol, marihuana, stimulants, and depressants.

CHAPTER TWO

Principles of Behavioral Pharmacology

Behavioral pharmacology has three distinct goals. First, researchers use drugs with a known mechanism of action to study the neurochemical or physiological basis of behavior. With these tools, they may also examine the action of other drugs whose mechanism is unknown. Second, behavior may be used to screen families of drugs, to identify their relative potencies, their spectrum of behavioral effects, their structure–activity relationships, and so forth. In both cases, other tools such as brain lesions or electrical stimulation of the brain may be used along with drug administration. Third, behavioral pharmacologists use drugs on animals to provide models of pathological conditions in humans that cannot be studied directly in a patient population.

There is a close relationship in psychopharmacology between clinical research and laboratory studies with animals. Animal studies clearly have several advantages over clinical studies using patient populations. The most obvious advantage is that of allowing rigorous and objective experimental controls; the living conditions of animal subjects can be regulated far more precisely than those of humans. In addition their past history as well as their genetic background is well known. Furthermore, drugs can be administered to animal subjects in ways not generally appropriate for humans. For example, drugs can be administered to animals over a long period of time to determine toxic effects or the potential for addiction. Finally, animal subjects are most appropriate for the study of the mechanism of drug action, as both electrophysiological and neurochemical bases of drug effects require invasive techniques that are unsuitable with human subjects.

Based on these investigative advantages, it would seem reasonable that the development of new drugs would occur first in the laboratory, followed by preclinical (animal) testing, and, finally, testing with a human subject in a therapeutic setting. Despite the efforts of preclinical researchers, however, many, if not most, of the useful psychotropic agents have been discovered as a result of fortunate clinical observation. For instance, the effective antischizophrenia drug chlorpromazine was originally used as a supplement with conventional anesthetic agents to prevent surgical shock. The observation that the drug had a calming effect on surgical patients prompted its use in psychiatry. Only after its effectiveness in reducing psychiatric symptoms was discovered clinically was a thorough analysis made of its chemical structure, its neurochemical and electrophysiological effects, and its action in various animal behavior tests. Gradually a family of drugs related structurally to chlorpromazine was developed and matched to the patient's needs (for a discussion of the phenothiazines see Chapter 12).

In addition, drug testing on humans uncovered subtle or unusual drug effects that animal tests had been unable to reveal. It is very difficult, for example, to develop animal tests to screen drugs that alter a purely cognitive aspect of human activity. Many of the manifestations of psychiatric disorders and the drug action related to the disorders are described in uniquely human terms, such as facial expression, altered mood, manner of speech. Nevertheless, psychopharmacology has evolved to the point where distinct classes of drugs have been found to alter one or several measurable animal behaviors in a predictable fashion.

Some animal tests evaluating drug effects on physiology closely approximate their human counterparts, particularly when the drug-induced changes can be recorded in physical terms such as blood pressure, muscle tension, or body temperature. However, for many drug effects this is not the case, and the animal response does not resemble the human condition. In these instances, a correlated, quantifiable measure in an animal is substituted for a more cognitive human behavior. Should such a correlation be close, a drug that modifies rat behavior in a predicted way can be useful in altering a particular human behavior, even though the two behaviors seem unrelated. (Thus, if a new drug were to reduce mouse killing by rats, tests on humans might show it to be an antidepressant.) To be optimal, a behavioral test on animals should meet three criteria (Glick, 1976): (1) It should be specific for the class of drug being screened, that is, other types of drugs should not have the same effect. (2) It should be sensitive to all drugs having the desired pharmacological effect. (3) The rank order of potencies of drugs in the screening test should match the order of potency in therapeutic action. Unless these criteria are satisfactorily met, the results of the screening procedure must be evaluated cautiously.

Primary Evaluation

In general, drug evaluation proceeds in two distinct steps: primary evaluation followed by secondary testing. Primary evaluation usually begins with observation and/or simple behavioral measures that utilize untrained animals and a minimum of instrumentation, for example, measures of activity changes. Among the observations made are measures of tremors, ptosis, salivation, defecation, catalepsy, hyper- or hyporeflexia, responsivity to tail pinch, and changes in eating or drinking. The screening method developed varies for different species, depending on the usual behavior of each species. For example, the rotarod is a test to measure motor coordination (Watzman and Barry, 1968) and is frequently used for rodents but rarely used for larger animals such as dogs or monkeys. Animals are placed on a slowly rotating rod and the time it takes to fall-off is measured. The difference between the pre- and postdrug scores gives an indication of ataxia, coordination, vestibular control, and muscular strength.

To further characterize behavior, measures of catalepsy are made. CATALEPSY is the abnormal maintenance of distorted postures, often called "waxy flexibility." Animals demonstrating catalepsy will remain in bizarre postures when positioned by the experimenter. The time to restoration of normal posture may give an indication of the extent of catalepsy. The use of catalepsy as a test to identify drugs that alleviate the symptoms of schizophrenia demonstrates the usefulness of screening tests that are unrelated to human behavior. The relative potency of some drugs in producing catalepsy in rats parallels their relative potency in clinical treatment of certain forms of mental illness. This characteristic action has been the subject of controversy because some individuals have suggested that the production of catalepsy in rats is a measure of a drug's therapeutic effectiveness, whereas others suggest that the production of catalepsy is correlated with the drug's production of undesirable side effects in humans (e.g., tremors and movement disorders). This argument has not been resolved and serves as a demonstration of one of several potential pitfalls in attempting to correlate drug effects in animals and man.

Measures of Motor Activity

If CNS effects are seen during initial testing, primary evaluation is continued with measures of motor activity. In addition to identifying drugs that produce sleep or ANESTHESIA (loss of consciousness from which one is not easily aroused), activity measures also determine loss of coordination and sedation. Spontaneous motor activity is measured using a variety of tests that measure unrestrained movement within a prescribed area. A JIGGLE CAGE, for example, is a box balanced on a single central pivot point; a switch closes and activates a counter whenever movement of the animal brings the cage edge in contact with the sensors located on the periphery. An alternate method employs infrared light beams (invisible to rodents) directed across the cage which, when broken, activate a counter that records one movement. These automated counting procedures enable measurement of animal activity in a setting that is not disruptive to normal behavior, that is, it can be done in the dark and without the presence of the investigator. Also, more than one activity cage can be operated simultaneously so that the activity of more than one animal can be measured at the same time. Some devices can be programmed to discriminate ambulatory behavior from stereotyped head bobbing or scratching. Discrimination between the behaviors is based upon the principle that stereotyped movements cause multiple interruptions of the same beams whereas ambulatory movements interrupt consecutive beams. A less automated technique involves placing the animal subject in a prescribed area that is divided into squares. Here the investigator must be present to record the number of squares traversed in a unit of time. However, one distinct advantage of the nonautomated technique is that observation of animal behavior in an unstructured environment may provide important information about drug effects quite apart from general motor activity.

The importance of nonautomated observation is demonstrated for the CNS stimulant amphetamine. Amphetamine at low doses significantly increases general motor activity in rats, whereas at higher doses their activity score is much lower. This reduced activity, however, is not due to a cessation of all behavior. Rather, the animals behave stereotypically (i.e., showing repetitive sniffing, licking, and gnawing) with only infrequent bursts of locomotor activity. Clearly, the stereotypy is significant drug-induced behavior, but in motor activity tests that are not responsive to small movements of the head and neck, the behavior may go unrecorded. Thus, activity measures used alone may give a misleading picture of drug effects on behavior.

Interactions with Other Drugs

Much drug screening involves interactions with other drugs. In many cases, when administered alone, drugs do not produce a characteristic behavioral effect in animals except at very high doses. For example, in general, antidepressant drugs do not have unique behavioral effects alone but do interact with selected drugs in unique ways. Antidepressant drugs, for instance, potentiate (or accentuate) the increase in body temperature produced by treatment with amphetamine; alone the antidepressants have no effect on body temperature. The probable mechanism for this interaction will become clearer when the drug's effects on the chemical signals of the brain are discussed in Chapter 12.

A more intuitively reasonable test for antidepressants is determination of their interaction with reserpine. Reserpine, a drug initially used to treat hypertension, was found to cause depression in patients. In animals, low to moderate doses produce calming and sedation; higher doses eliminate all motor activity. The behavior depressant action of reserpine is frequently used as a model of human depression. The classical antidepressant drugs antagonize the effects of reserpine on animal activity but do not increase motor activity when given alone.

The most widely used initial test to identify anti-anxiety drugs (Chapter 11) is the prevention of pentylenetetrazol-induced seizures in mice. In an unprotected animal, i.v. infusion of pentylenetetrazol produces an almost immediate onset of CLONIC SEIZURES (alternating contraction of opposing muscles causing limb shaking). Pretreatment with an effective anti-anxiety drug, such as diazepam, is said to protect against the seizure if such activity fails to occur for a given time interval. Relative potency in this animal test generally parallels the clinical pattern of anxiety reduction.

Secondary Evaluation

The remainder of the procedures described in this chapter are considered techniques of secondary evaluation, and each of them is more complex than the simple observational methods described thus far. The methods of measuring aggression are based largely on the methods of ethology—observation of animals in their natural environment. These naturalistic observations of animal aggression have evolved into quantifiable measures of aggression in a controlled environment. However, despite the advantage of objective quantification, the relationship to human aggression is rather remote. In contrast, the tests for analgesia in animals were techniques modified from tests originally developed for humans. Animal and human data obtained by similar test procedures for measuring analgesia are generally in agreement; thus, the analgesia tests provide a more rational basis for prediction of drug effects than do the aggression tests.

Tests of Aggression

Although aggression tests are not highly useful screening devices, animal models of aggressive behavior may be used to elucidate some basic components of human aggression. Human aggressive behaviors, in addition to appearing in many forms, have widely differing etiologies and neural mechanisms. Animal models of aggression have the advantage of being quantifiable and modifiable in a controlled environment. However, animal models have also been divided into several categories based on such parameters as the attack stimulus, characteristics of the attack behaviors, the target of attack, and underlying biochemical correlates. Aggressive behaviors most often studied include predatory aggression (as exemplified by mouse-killing behavior in rats), irritable aggression, and intermale aggression, which are three of the seven forms of aggression originally described by Moyer (1968). In addition, drug-induced or brain lesion-induced aggression is also frequently utilized for pharmacological manipulations.

Predatory Aggression. The examination of drug effects on animal aggression has not been a particularly useful method of screening new pharmacological agents. One exception is the use of muricide (mouse-killing) behavior to identify antidepressant drugs. In this test (Karli et al., 1969), male rats are isolated and deprived of food for 24 hours before a mouse is placed in each rat's home cage. Investigators observe the rats to see if they kill the mice and, if so, how quickly. Depending on the strain of rat, from 10 to 70 percent of the rats will kill the mice by biting through the cervical spinal cord. Food deprivation facilitates killing behavior in some animals, but satiation does not suppress it. It has been shown that antidepressant drugs antagonize muricide behavior at a dose that does not cause ataxia or other motor impairment (Horovitz et al., 1966). In contrast, tranquilizers reduce muricide only at doses that cause sedation and ataxia (Quenzer and Feldman, 1975). However, not all drugs that selectively reduce muricide are effective antidepressants; thus, muricide testing in the rat does not provide a completely valid or highly selective test for antidepressant drugs.

Irritable Aggression. Irritable aggression is elicited by the application of an inescapable noxious stimulus. Shock-elicited aggression is the most frequently used test. In these experiments, two animals are confined in a small test chamber and exposed to electric shock presented through the grid floor. After initial attempts to escape the box, the animals assume a species-specific attack posture accompanied by boxing-like paw movements, vocalizations, and biting responses toward the other animal's snout. When the shock ends, the animals return to normal postures. This type of aggression testing (developed by Ulrich and Azrin, 1962) is popular because the behavior is easy to elicit and can be controlled by varying the shock parameters. In addition, the aggressive responses can be readily quantified by counting the number of responses during a series of discrete shock presentations.

Thus, drugs that either increase or decrease the number of aggressive responses can be studied. One criticism of the method is that the responses made are probably defensive and submissive reactions rather than being attack or threat behavior (Miczek and Barry, 1976).

Isolation-Induced Aggression. Isolation-induced aggression between male mice is a test developed by Yen et al. (1959). It requires isolation of male mice in individual cages for a period varying from 1 day to 8 weeks before the animals are allowed to interact in the test cage. When two strange male mice encounter each other, they frequently demonstrate distinct, stereotyped aggressive and submissive behaviors. In general, the experimental measures made are latency to fight, fight duration, or the number of animals that fight. Occasionally the intensity of fighting is assessed by a rating scale. Although the use of a rating scale increases subjective evaluation, it provides information on the complex structure and sequence of behaviors (e.g., predatory stalk, attack, defense, and kill) that constitute "aggression" and also identifies the differential behavior of individual animals (i.e., dominance and submission). It is clear, however, that such detailed analysis of aggressive responses is more appropriate for the ethologist than for a psychopharmacologist involved in routine drug screening, where readily identifiable, repeatable, and quantifiable measures must be made.

Lesion-Induced Aggression. The pioneering work of Wasman and Flynn (1962) demonstrated that distinct components (e.g., biting, stalking, vocalizations) of aggression could be elicited by electrically stimulating discrete areas of the brain of awake cats with chronically implanted electrodes. Many others (Fried, 1972, 1973) have shown that destroying some areas of the brain (e.g., septal nuclei) leads to rage, hyperemotionality, or hyperirritability, whereas destroying other areas of the brain produces passivity in a previously aggressive animal. Although a large number of investigators have examined lesion-induced aggression and concomitant changes in brain chemistry, the complex nature of the response does not lend itself well to routine drug screening.

It is important to keep in mind that drug effects on aggression are dependent on a number of parameters including (1) form of aggression tested, (2) drug dose, and (3) regimen of drug administration and testing. For instance, amphetamine seems to facilitate intraspecies aggression (e.g., isolation-induced aggression) at low doses, but at higher doses it apparently suppresses it (Welch and Welch, 1969). In addition, the drug has distinct actions depending on whether it is administered to the more dominant or to the more submissive rat in the pair (Miczek, 1974).

Measures of Analgesia

ANALGESIA is the reduction of pain without loss of consciousness. PAIN is a sensation arising from excessive stimulation of a number of sensory modalities and can be elicited by heat, extreme cold, electrical impulses, chemical irritation, and so forth. In general, pain is considered to have two distinct components: the physiological sensation and the emotional response to the physiological sensation. A separation of the two components is demonstrated by the athlete who sustains a serious injury during the heat of competition but is unaware of the pain until the arousal surrounding competition subsides. (For a more detailed discussion of the phenomenon of pain, see Chapter 13.)

Because of the dual nature of pain, the quantification of pain (and hence of analgesia) is difficult using human self-report techniques in the clinical setting, where anxiety and anticipation of more pain influence a patient's response. Analgesia testing with humans in the laboratory setting is also frequently misleading because the response to some types of experimentally induced pain is quite different from that to chronic or pathological pain. In other cases, when the induced pain is a very good model, it is understandably difficult to secure subjects.

An alternate method for measuring analgesic properties is the use of animal models. We cannot know whether the animal "feels pain," but we can measure the animal's avoidance of a noxious stimulus and we can call this avoidance a "pain reaction." The responses that the stimulus elicits might really measure a "sensation" threshold rather than a pain threshold. Of greatest value in analgesic testing would be a method to measure the loss of severe and continuous pain, such as in carcinoma, a goal that is not met with animal testing. Nevertheless, animal testing does allow more controlled measures and eliminates some of the complications of the human emotional response.

Those measures of analgesia in animals that are most popular include the tail-flick test, the hot plate test, the jump–flinch test, the acetic acid writhing test, and the operant titration test.

Tail-Flick Test. This test is designed to measure drug-induced analgesia and was developed by D'Amour and Smith (1941). In this test, a beam of light, the intensity of which is controlled by a rheostat, is focused on an ink-blackened portion of the rat's tail. The latency between onset of stimulus and the removal of the tail from the beam of light is assumed to be correlated with pain intensity. The test was originally developed for use with human subjects with whom the light was focused on a blackened spot on the forehead. Determinations were repeated every 30 seconds at increasing intensities until an intensity was reached at which the subject just perceived pain. A similar threshold technique can be used for animals and eliminates the problems normally associated with subjective reports on pain from human subjects in the laboratory setting. However, an important control procedure when using tail measures is to consider the age of the rats tested, because age-related increases in epidermal cornification raise pain thresholds.

Before the development of the tail-flick test, popular methods of producing experimental pain included piling weights on a cat's tail or heating the skin by means of hot water passing through tubes. The behavioral measure in such tests is vocalization. The earliest of these tests was hampered by lack of precision and large individual differences in the subjects' responses. Another drawback was that the stimulus applied often had to be quite intense in order to reach the nociceptive (pain) threshold, and thus subsequent determinations in the same area were altered.

The tail-flick test is not adequate for determining analgesic properties of compounds under conditions of severe, protracted, pathological pain, but there is a good relationship between analgesic effect as measured with the tail-flick and the efficacy of various analgesic agents. In addition, the test is both simple and rapid and shows a relatively small individual variability.

Hot Plate Test. Another method for measuring analgesic drug action, using thermal stimuli, is the hot plate test introduced by Woolfe and Macdonald (1944). The animal to be tested is placed in a cylinder on a metal plate maintained at a constant temperature, which can be varied between 55° and 70°C. Most often the animal's initial responses are to sit on its hind paws and lick its forepaws. Because that response can easily be confused with the common grooming response, drug evaluation is based on the second, more delayed, response of kicking with the hind paws or attempting to escape the cylinder. The sensitivity of this test is not very good and is approximately equal to that of the tail-flick test. However, this method seems to produce reliable and fairly stable pain thresholds with which to measure analgesic activity.

Acetic Acid Writhing Test. Intraperitoneal injection of a caustic compound, such as 0.6 percent acetic acid (Koster et al., 1959) or phenylquinone (Siegmund et al., 1957) produces repeated characteristic stretching movements that may last several hours. Although it is not clear whether writhing is closely associated with "pain," the potency of various analgesic agents in reducing the writhing response correlates well with the clinical efficacy of the drugs.

Flinch–Jump Procedure. This test, which was developed and modified by Evans (1961) is based on the finding that electric shock delivered to a rat's feet through the grid floor of a testing apparatus will elicit two distinguishable responses. At low shock intensities, the animal will be startled or "flinch" but show no signs of agitation. At higher intensities, the animal will remove two or more paws from the grid at the time of the shock onset (called a "jump"); the jump is often accompanied by vocalization, running, and other signs of a highly emotional reaction. One might consider the possibility that if the flinch response reflects the first perception of pain by the animal and the jump response reflects an emotionally aroused reaction to the pain, then the method might provide information on the two factors believed to contribute to the human response to pain. As a rule the animals are administered a series of shocks (1 second in duration) varying from 0.1 to 3.4 mA in both ascending and descending order. The effect of various analgesic drugs can be readily determined over a range of shock intensities and with great sensitivity. Clearly, it is impossible to determine whether the "flinch" response indicates the first recognition of pain or just the perception of electric shock. Furthermore, although electric shock is

easy to apply, it is quite difficult to control. Even when voltage is known, biological tissues offer impedance that cannot be controlled. Other tests that apply electric shock to the tooth pulp or the tail have been used, but in most cases these tests show considerable variability and therefore do not have the sensitivity of the flinch–jump test.

Schedule-Controlled Behavior (Operant Conditioning)

Within the past few years, great interest has developed in the use of various conditioned behaviors to study drug effects. The technique entails the selection of a small portion of a complex behavior pattern that can be clearly defined and modified by changing elements in the environment and by drug action. An example of such a behavior is lever-pressing by a rat. Although the behavior examined is not a normal component of a rat's behavioral repertoire, it has been shown that the behavior can be readily quantified and avoids an anthropomorphic interpretation of animal behavior.

The underlying principle of operant conditioning is that "reinforcement" controls behavior. An animal performs because it is reinforced for doing so. Reinforcement can be positive (food or water for a hungry or thirsty animal) or negative (electric shock that can be avoided if the animal makes the correct response). Animals learn to respond to obtain rewards and avoid punishment.

The experiments are carried out in a Skinner box (named after B. F. Skinner, the father of the theory of operant conditioning). The box is a soundproof chamber with a grid floor that can be electrified (for shock delivery), a food or water dispenser (for rewards), lights or loudspeaker (for cue presentation), and levers (one or more) that the animal can press (Figure 1). The equipment is almost always automatically controlled so that cues (if used) are presented at specified times; the lever-pressing is converted to an electric signal to enable automatic counting of responses and reinforcement delivery. The responses are frequently recorded graphically, with their distribution over time plotted on a cumulative recorder. The recorder is a paper moving over a drum at a set speed with a pen marking a step across the paper whenever a lever-press is made. Delivery of reinforcement is also recorded on the page (Figure 2). Thus, the animal is conditioned to press the lever to obtain rewards or avoid punishment. Because the ex-

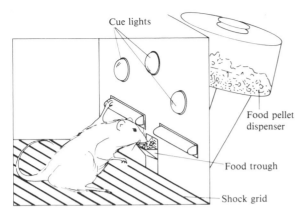

FIGURE 1. RAT IN A SKINNER BOX can be trained to press the bar (response) which activates a food delivery mechanism (reinforcement). Schedules can dictate that 10 responses are necessary for reinforcement (FR-10), or that reinforcements occur after variable time intervals, the average interval being 40 seconds (VI-40). An animal can also learn to bar-press to terminate or postpone shocks that can be delivered by the grid floor.

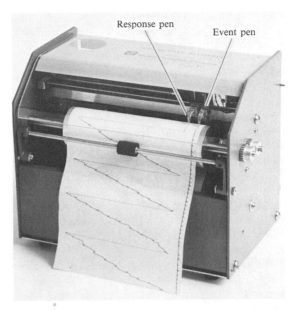

FIGURE 2. CUMULATIVE RECORDER. The paper unrolls under the two pens at a constant speed (5 mm/min). Each occurrence of a bar-press moves the response marking pen a small increment to the left. Reinforcements are indicated by a short diagonal slash on the cumulative record, or by a similar mark made by the event pen on the right. The event pen can also be used to indicate additional events during an experimental session, such as the onset of a discriminable stimulus—a light or a sound. (Courtesy of Gerbrands Corporation, Arlington, Massachusetts.)

periment must occur rapidly with precise timing and with many repetitions, accurate automatic programming and recording of the experiments is important.

The behavior required is not "natural" (that is, the behavior does not appear in the animal's environment) and so must be trained ("shaped"). Because the behavior is trained, it can be similar for diverse species both in its form and its consequences. When hungry, the animal makes many responses in rapid succession, one of which may be pressing a lever. The animal must learn that pressing the lever produces a desirable result (e.g., food). The experimenter helps by presenting the reinforcer immediately after the correct response and before another behavior can occur.

The arrangement of times or circumstances when lever-pressing produces reinforcement is called the SCHEDULE OF REINFORCEMENT. There are many known schedules for studying behavior. Representing behavior as a temporal distribution of responses allows us to examine precisely the action of a drug on the patterning of behavior. Also, drug–behavior interaction can be analyzed by determining how changes in the schedule modify the effect of the drug. Because there are a large

number of possible reinforcement schedules, each eliciting a distinct pattern of behavior, the combinations of drug and operant schedule are very numerous and represent many volumes of research. The present chapter identifies only the most elementary and most commonly used operant behavior techniques and uses examples of drug effects that are explained more thoroughly in later chapters.

Positive Reinforcement Schedules

The two basic types of schedules of reinforcement are based on time and frequency of reinforcement.

Continuous Reinforcement Schedule. Perhaps the simplest schedule is CONTINUOUS REINFORCEMENT

(CRF), which means that each lever-press is reinforced by delivery of a food pellet (or other reinforcer) regardless of how often the animal responds.

Fixed Ratio Schedules. A variation of the CRF schedule is the FIXED RATIO (FR) SCHEDULE, which requires a fixed number of responses before a reinforcer is delivered. Thus, an FR-3 schedule means the animal must press the lever three times to receive one food pellet. Changing the fixed ratio, from 3 to 20 or 45, will tell us how hard the animal is willing to work for the reinforcement. As a rule, animals respond at fairly continuous high rates when working on an FR schedule. A typical cumulative recording of response under an FR schedule is shown in Figure 3, which shows the steady rate of pressing and regular delivery of reinforcement.

The simple FR schedule has been used very effectively in identifying drugs that have abuse potential, that is, that are capable of bringing about psychological dependence. The procedure requires that the reinforcement for lever-pressing is injection of drug rather than food. The injection site must be directly into the bloodstream or into the brain so that the reinforcing effect can be perceived rapidly by the animal. The drug self-administration method is a very accurate indicator of abuse in humans. For instance, morphine and amphetamine are readily self-administered by animals and certainly are abused by humans, whereas drugs in the phenothiazine class are neither self-administered

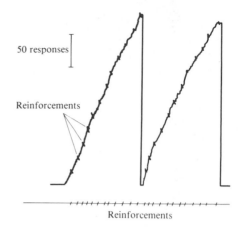

FIGURE 3. CUMULATIVE RECORD OF FIXED RATIO RESPONDING. The FR-20 schedule produces a high, steady rate of responding by a rat for liquid food reinforcements. Reinforcements occur after every 20 responses. Note the brief pause that usually follows a reinforcement. The pen resets to the baseline after 240 responses.

by animals nor abused by humans. More detail on the self-administration method appears in Chapter 13. It is used frequently and is an excellent example of the utility of animal testing to predict human behavior.

Fixed Interval Schedules. On the FIXED INTERVAL (FI) SCHEDULES, reinforcement is available at fixed times after the last reinforcement only if the animal makes a

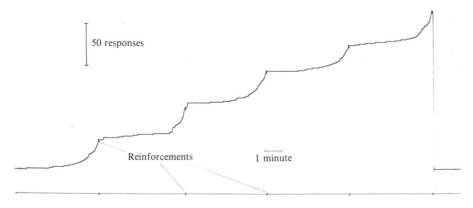

FIGURE 4. CUMULATIVE RECORD OF FIXED INTERVAL RESPONDING. A trained rat learned that reinforcements only occur after the first response following a 5-minute interval (FI-5). Thus there is little responding at the beginning of the interval and a burst of responding toward the end of the interval. This accounts for the "scalloped" appearance of the cumulative record. The pen resets after 5 reinforcements.

response. Thus, on FI-2, reinforcement follows the first response that an animal makes after 2 minutes have elapsed since the last reinforcement; responses made during the 2-minute interval are "wasted," that is, they elicit no reinforcement. After some experience with the schedule, the pattern of responding that an animal makes is called "scalloping." A typical record of scalloping is shown in Figure 4. Immediately after a reinforcement, little or no responding occurs; responding accelerates as the time for the next reinforcement approaches.

The behavior in the case of the FI schedule is based in part on temporal discrimination. Humans tend to create a "clock" by counting during the interval between responses. If their counting is disrupted, then their response patterns resemble those of other animals; the responses are clustered toward the end of the interval but are not as close to optimum responding as when a "clock" is used. In a classic study, Weiss and Laties (1964) provided a "clock" for pigeons working an FI-5 schedule by projecting five different symbols on the response key to correspond to 1-minute intervals. The response characteristics under the "clock" and "no clock" conditions are shown in Figure 5. You can see that in contrast to the skewed, but dispersed responding with "no clock," the pigeons responded most efficiently when the "clock" was presented by key pecking only during the last 1-minute interval.

A second influence on the behavior is the distribution of reinforcement. On the FI schedule, responding that occurs early in the interval is not closely followed by reinforcement, thus the behavior is less likely to occur again. If the response occurs later in the interval, the closer temporal association with reinforcement increases the recurrence of the behavior. Thus, the responses of an experienced subject tend to be clustered at the end of the interval.

From this discussion it should be clear that even the simple behavior that occurs during an FI schedule may be regulated by several factors. When the effects of drugs are tested on response behavior, a number of interesting changes in that behavior can occur. Weiss and Laties (1964) found that amphetamine increased the total number of responses made during a test session. The drug did not increase the response rate but merely caused the pigeon to start responding earlier in the interval. However, the increased responding was much less during test sessions when the "clock" was available. Thus, an external timing cue could offset the

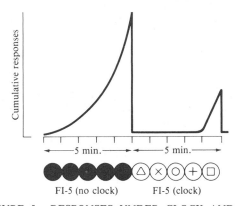

FIGURE 5. RESPONSES UNDER CLOCK AND NO-CLOCK CONDITIONS. The cumulative records above the symbols represent typical performance during the two conditions. During the no-clock condition, the key was illuminated by a red light; during the clock condition, the key was illuminated by symbols which changed at 1-minute intervals. (From Weiss and Laties, 1964.)

disruptive effects of amphetamine. In contrast, chlorpromazine (a drug that is effective in treating schizophrenia and produces sedation) disrupted the FI-induced behavior in the presence or the absence of the "clock." Perhaps, based on this subtle difference in performance, it is possible that an essential difference in these two classes of drugs can be identified. Weiss and Laties and others have concluded that chlorpromazine reduces the ability of stimuli (both internal and external) to influence behavior. Of interest is that this conclusion correlates with the frequent clinical observation that chlorpromazine reduces the impact of environmental stimuli on the schizophrenic's behavior. Amphetamine, on the other hand, may act by strengthening the weakly maintained behavior early in the interval because it enhances the retroactive effect of reinforcement. Thus, even relatively simple behaviors can be modified in distinct ways by various drugs.

Differential Reinforcement of Low Rates. A modification of the FI schedule yields the schedule that produces DIFFERENTIAL REINFORCEMENT OF LOW RATES OF RESPONDING (DRL). In the DRL schedule, reinforcement is programmed to occur after a period of time has elapsed since the previous response. If a response occurs during this interval, not only is no reinforcement delivered, but it also resets the interval timer and a new waiting period must begin. If the waiting time exceeds the specified period, a lever-press produces reinforcement. Thus, the DRL schedule produces very low rates of responding.

As you might guess from our earlier discussion, amphetamine tends to disrupt efficient performance of DRL behavior by shortening the waiting time that the animal demonstrates. However, the effects of amphetamine are not simple. It is well known that increases in the rate of responding occur after low or moderate doses of amphetamine, but at higher doses, behavior tends to be depressed (Dews, 1958). Furthermore, the baseline rate of responding also modifies the effects of amphetamine.

Clark and Steele (1966) showed that when responding is very low amphetamine increases the rate of responding in a dose–dependent manner (curve A, Figure 6). When response rate is moderate (as for an FI-4 minute schedule), low doses of amphetamine increase responding and high doses decrease it (curve B). At doses up to 1 mg/kg,* the response rate increases, whereas from 1 to 4 mg/kg, a gradual decline in responding occurs. When response rate is high (as for an

*Doses of drugs are usually expressed in milligrams (mg) or micrograms (μg) per kilogram (kg) of body weight of the recipient. Thus the term mg/kg.

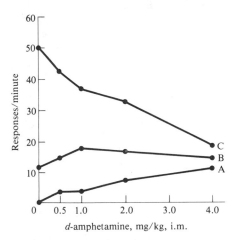

FIGURE 6. RESPONSE RATE–DRUG EFFECT INTERACTIONS. Mean rates of responding on 3 schedules of reinforcement are modified by the effects of d-amphetamine. Curve A illustrates the drug's effect on a low rate of responding with no reinforcement; curve B, responding under FI-4 minutes; curve C, responding at high rates under a FR-25 schedule. (From Clark and Steele, 1966.)

FR-25 schedule), amphetamine tends to decrease the rate as a function of increasing dose (curve C).

Many CNS stimulants have been tested under the same conditions and the results compared to the effects of amphetamine. One striking finding is that nicotine has very many of the same effects on schedule-controlled behavior as amphetamine, although it suppresses responding briefly after administration, unlike the latter drug. This similarity in action of the two drugs may have important implications for the biochemical and behavioral bases of drug abuse for this class of drugs.

Variable Interval Schedules. Another modification of the fixed interval schedule is the VARIABLE INTERVAL (VI) SCHEDULE (Figure 7). Reinforcement following bar-pressing under a VI schedule is dependent upon the amount of time elapsing since the previous reinforcement. Unlike the FI schedule, the interreinforcement delays in the VI schedule vary around a mean value, which is used to describe the schedule. For instance, a VI-2 minute schedule has a mean interreinforcement time of 2 minutes. As you might suspect, the uncertainty of reinforcement inherent in this schedule produces a high and sustained rate of responding. The VI schedule is frequently incorporated into multiple schedules.

Multiple Schedules. MULTIPLE SCHEDULES are created by combining two or more schedules in a regular pattern. Most often the two schedules (e.g., FI and FR) are alternated during a test session. Frequently each schedule is signaled by the appearance of a colored light or other cue. Thus, a typical multiple schedule might begin with a green light to signal a FI-2, which lasts for 20 minutes. At the end of that period, a red light may signal the start of the FR-8, which may last for 10 minutes. Several alternations between schedules may occur and each time the animal adjusts his response rate to optimize reinforcement. The greatest advantage of a multiple schedule is that a drug effect can be tested on behaviors with different baseline rates. From our earlier discussion it should be clear that the ongoing behavior frequently modifies drug effects. One of the more popular multiple schedules employs the Geller procedure.

Negative Reinforcement and Punishment

The simplest schedule of negative reinforcement involves the use of the lever press to terminate the aver-

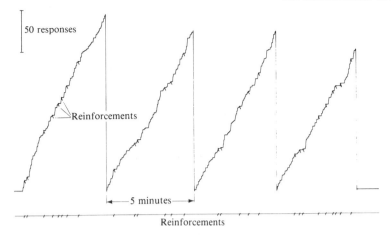

FIGURE 7. CUMULATIVE RECORD OF VARIABLE INTERVAL RESPONDING. Reinforcements occur after a response following variable time intervals that average 45 seconds. Note the different intervals between reinforcements recorded by the event pen (bottom). The response pen resets after every 5 minutes.

sive condition. Once again the schedule can be an FR, so that after a given number of responses the negative reinforcer (usually electric shock) is terminated. The schedule may be an FI or VI, in which termination depends on a response occurring after an interval of time has elapsed.

Negative reinforcement techniques are relatively recent devices for testing the analgesic properties of drugs. The methods may have an advantage over those previously described because they depend upon a learned response of the subject. The learned response may correlate better with the human response to pain, which certainly has a complex learned component based on previous experience. In the titration schedule (Weiss and Laties, 1961), the animal is first trained to perform a particular operant response (most often a lever-press) in order to reduce a noxious stimulus, such as foot shock. The experimenter applies the nociceptive stimulus in increasing intensities until the animal responds at the "aversive threshold." The intensity of the shock at this point indicates how much "pain" will be tolerated by the subject. The method is very sensitive even to mild analgesics such as aspirin. However, without an independent measure of behavioral depression, it is not clear whether the change in threshold is due to the test drugs' analgesic effects or to general behavioral depression.

Signaled Avoidance-Escape. A popular experimental design uses avoidance or postponement of noxious conditions rather than escape or termination. One of the best-known screening tests for psychotropic drugs is based on this type of behavior. In this test, called the signaled avoidance–escape procedure, rats are placed in a box with a grid floor through which an electric shock can be delivered. A vertical climbing pole in the box provides a means of avoiding the shock. A trial consists of sounding a buzzer and subsequently delivering a foot shock, at which time the rat can escape the shock by climbing the pole. After several pairings of buzzer and shock, the rat climbs the pole when the buzzer sounds. If the rat fails to climb the pole when the buzzer sounds, it can climb the pole when the shock is delivered and thus escape.

When drug effects were tested in this design, it was found that drugs that act effectively in reducing symptoms of schizophrenia (such as the phenothiazines) blocked only the conditioned avoidance response. In contrast, other depressants of the CNS that are not effective against schizophrenia (such as the barbiturates) depressed the conditioned avoidance response but also depressed the escape response. Thus, the antischizophrenic drugs showed selective blocking action, whereas the others tested slowed all behavior.

Sidman Avoidance Procedure. A variation on these schedules, the SIDMAN AVOIDANCE PROCEDURE or continuous advoidance procedure, has no signal to mark the onset of shock (Sidman, 1953). A shock is delivered to the animal which lasts for 1–2 seconds at regularly spaced intervals (the shock–shock interval). The presentation of shock can be delayed by a fixed time interval if the animal makes the appropriate response. For example, a shock is presented every 5 seconds unless a lever-press occurs. If the animal makes the response, no shock occurs again until 15 seconds after the response. By optimally spacing the lever-pressing, an animal can avoid receiving any shocks. This behavioral test has not been used as frequently as the signaled avoidance because training is significantly more difficult. The difficulty arises from the fact that when shock is applied the animals will frequently "freeze," behavior that is incompatible with lever-pressing.

Conditioned Emotional Response. The "freezing" response has been utilized by other investigators to provide a behavioral measure of anxiety or fear. In these tests, an animal first develops regular responding based on an appropriate schedule. Once the behavior is stable, a signal is introduced and is followed by electric shock. Because the shock can neither be avoided nor escaped, the signal produces a suppression of responding after several pairings of signal and shock. The CONDITIONED EMOTIONAL RESPONSE (CER) is an effective test to identify anxiety-reducing drugs such as diazepam or chlordiazepoxide. Anxiety-reducing drugs are highly effective in increasing behavior that is suppressed by punishment.

Although this procedure is frequently used, its parameters have not been clearly identified. Among the parameters that alter the degree of suppression are the relative durations of the presence and absence of the preshock signal, the schedule of reinforcement used to maintain behavior, and the previous experimental history of the subject (Kelleher and Morse, 1964).

Geller Procedure. Perhaps the best example of the use of immediate punishment to suppress behavior is the procedure developed by Geller (1962). The subject is trained to press a lever for food on a VI schedule. Once the behavior is established, shock is introduced in such a way that lever-press produces both reward and punishment. By varying the intensity of punishment, the response rate can be closely regulated. A further modification of the method is a multiple schedule that alternates signaled periods when (1) responding is followed by positive reinforcement alone, and (2) bar-

pressing produces both reward and punishment. With this design, the effects of a drug can be studied on both types of behavior. Its usefulness as a screen for anti-anxiety agents is discussed more fully in Chapter 11.

Discriminative Stimuli

A DISCRIMINATIVE STIMULUS is a stimulus that signals reinforcement for a subject performing an operant task. It is usually designated S^D. Thus, a green light may signal reinforcement available following the appropriate response. In the same experiment, a red light may signal reinforcement unavailable regardless of the operant response made. The nonreinforcement condition is called S^Δ. An animal that learns to lever-press in the presence of the green light but not the red light clearly can discriminate between the two. Its behavior is said to be "under stimulus control." The specificity of discrimination can be tested by presenting stimuli that vary in larger and smaller amounts from the training S^D. As you would expect, the more similar the test stimulus to the original training stimulus (S^D), the greater is the likelihood that the animal will respond. This phenomenon, called STIMULUS GENERALIZATION, is shown graphically in Figure 8. In this experiment, monkeys were trained to press a lever when one specific light intensity (S^D) out of eight possible intensities illuminated the experimental chamber (Hearst, 1964). The arrow in the figure marks the training intensity. The amount of bar-pressing was related to the similarity or difference of the test stimuli to S^D. The more similar the intensity, the greater the generalization to S^D and the more the responses occurred.

Discrimination training allows the researcher to evaluate sensory processes in subjects that are unable to communicate verbally. Thus, color vision can be studied if an animal is trained to respond to one color and not to respond to another. Furthermore, the effects of drugs on sensory perception can be tested with the same procedure.

Although discriminative stimuli are usually changes in physical environment (e.g., lights, patterns, or tones), interoceptive stimuli have been found to be significant environmental cues. The ability of subjects to discriminate altered internal states has been utilized to study drug effects. In most experiments, the subject is trained to emit one response (e.g., press the left lever of a pair) to obtain reinforcement in one drugged state and to make a different response (press the right lever)

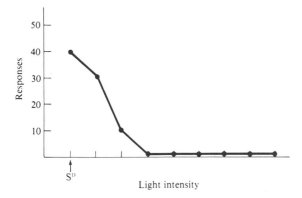

FIGURE 8. STIMULUS GENERALIZATION GRADI-
ENT. The curve shows the number of responses as a function
of the intensity of several cues. S^D indicates the intensity of
light that was the training cue. (After Hearst, 1964.)

for reward in a nondrugged or different drugged state.
The animal's response is dependent on discriminating
among internal cues produced by the drug.

Just as physical stimuli fall along a curve of stimulus
generalization, so too do internal (i.e., drug-induced)
cues. Thus, if an animal is trained to respond to 5 mg
of morphine, maximum responding occurs at 5 mg,
and the response rate falls off in a predictable fashion
as the dose deviates from 5 mg. The drug clearly provides a cue that follows the laws of stimulus generalization. Following training with morphine as the cue(s),
the specificity is such that all other drugs in the morphine class (the narcotics) can substitute for morphine
as an S^D in those animals trained on morphine discrimination. However, other drugs that act on the
CNS (e.g., amphetamine or marijuana) are treated by
the animals as S^Δ. Clearly, morphine and the narcotics
provide a cue that is unique to that class of drugs.

The precise mechanism for the narcotic cue is not
known. However, as a first attempt, drugs that alter
CNS neurochemistry can be tested for their ability to
antagonize or disrupt the narcotic S^D. For instance, the
drug cue is challenged by increasing doses of a
suspected antagonist until the cue has lost its effect. If
the antagonist acts in a competitive manner with the
drug cue, the dose–response curve will be parallel but
shifted to the right. If the antagonist does not act specifically at the drug cue receptor site, then the dose–
response shifts are not parallel. In the case of the morphine cue, a specific antagonist which is known to bind

to the morphine receptor also disrupts the cue effects
of morphine (Lal et al., 1977).

These techniques can also support hypotheses regarding the mechanism of a drug's action. For example, the anxiolytic drug chlordiazepoxide (CDP)
(Librium) is believed to block the release of serotonin,
a neurotransmitter, from axon terminals. If this is true
then serotonin agonists (drugs that *increase* the release
of serotonin) should diminish the effect of CDP. An
experiment using CDP as a discriminative stimulus
tested that hypothesis.

Rats were trained to discriminate CDP (2.5 mg/kg)
from saline in a two-lever Skinner box. Pressing one of
the levers on a drug day on a FR-10 schedule led to
food reward, and the same result occurred on a saline
treated day when the opposite lever was pressed. Pressing the inappropriate lever only resulted in no reward.
This discrimination was easily mastered. Next, the
animals were tested with increasing doses of serotonin-
releasing drugs that were given concomitantly with
CDP. The drugs were p-chloroamphetamine (PCA),
p-fluoroamphetamine (PFA), and fenfluramine (FEN).
These CDP + serotonin agonist tests were always preceded by four alternating days of tests with CDP or
saline to maintain the discrimination. On CDP + se-
rontonin agonist tests, the first lever that was pressed
10 times was reinforced. Each animal's score was the
percentage of CDP-lever choices at the time of the first
reinforcement. Thus, 1 response on the saline lever and
10 responses on the CDP lever gave a ratio of 10/11 or
91 percent, and 1 response on the CDP and 10 responses on the saline lever gave 1/11 or 9.1 percent.
Consequently, high scores indicate a rat was responding as though it were a "CDP" day, low scores indicate a "saline" day.

Figure 9 shows that as the doses of the serotonin
agonists rose, the rats pressed the CDP lever less and
the saline lever more. Thus, these drugs are competitive antagonists of CDP and suggest that serotonin
blockade plays a role in the discriminative properties
of CDP (McElroy and Feldman, unpublished study).

To further evaluate the neurophysiological basis of a
drug discrimination, the drug may be injected into discrete areas of the brain. Another approach to studying
mechanisms of drug action is to mimic a drug cue by
electrically stimulating a specific brain area. Alternatively, it should also be possible to modify the cue by
making specific brain lesions at the drug's site of
action.

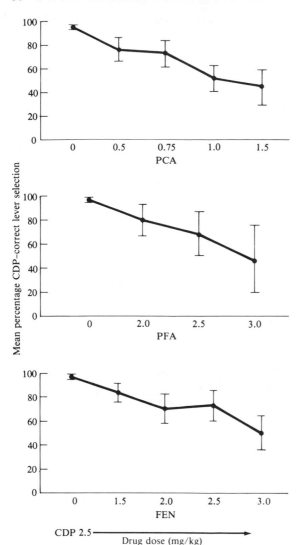

FIGURE 9. THE DISCRIMINATIVE PROPERTIES OF CDP are blocked by drugs that enhance the release of serotonin from nerve terminals. As the dose of the drugs was increased, the animals responded less often to the CDP lever. CDP, chlordiazepoxide; PCA, p-chloroamphetamine; PFA, p-fluoroamphetamine; and FEN, fenfluramine. The bars represent the mean ± S.E.M. for 10 rats.

The use of drug cue discrimination testing has increased over the last few years. It has been found useful in identifying new drugs that have similar therapeutic effects and also for examining the neurochemical basis for drug action. Discrimination testing, along with operant conditioning and the other behavioral methods described in this section, provide the basic tools for the investigator in neuropsychopharmacology.

Summary

Behavioral pharmacology attempts to assess the effects of drugs on behavior. The testing is done in a controlled and systematic way to enhance the reliability and the validity of the measurements. When studying the effects of drugs on animals, baseline behavior (behavior in the no-drug state) is carefully assessed before behavior is assessed in the drug state in the same animals or concomitantly, in drugged animals that are carefully matched to the no-drug controls.

Primary evaluations are made of possible drug-induced ataxia, tremors, general sedation, etc., and drug effects upon behaviors that require no training, such as locomotion, food and water ingestion, reactions to novel environments and noxious stimuli, and sleep. Secondary evaluations are made of the effects of drugs on animals that are trained in various ways to respond to food or liquid rewards, to sensory discrimination, or to pain avoidance. These behaviors, called operant responses, are controlled by reinforcement contingencies known as schedules of reinforcement.

Schedules of reinforcement make it possible to utilize a wide variety of behaviors in which the antecedents of those behaviors are precisely defined. The testing of drugs under these conditions probably provides the most objective assessment of drug effects on behavior. To be sure, a gap exists when animal testing is used to evaluate drugs designed to restore disordered thought and mood to normal limits in humans. Nevertheless, when the mechanisms of drug action are assessed by neurochemical and behavioral methods, insights concerning the basis of a drug's therapeutic benefits in humans are possible.

Usually drugs are researched in humans after animal studies reveal no physiological or behavioral toxicity and establish an effective range of doses. Objectivity is maintained in research on humans by double-blind techniques wherein the evaluators of the drug effects are unaware which subjects received the drug and which received the placebo. Imprecision in establishing the value of human medication occurs because of difficulty in matching control and experimental groups, in establishing diagnostic criteria, and because human subjects vary in the durations of illnesses, previous histories of medication and substance abuse (e.g., alcoholism), lifestyle, nutrition, age, sex, and placebo effects. Nevertheless, the methods of behavioral pharmacology can improve the quality of the pharmaceuticals available for the disabling conditions that are so prevalent among us.

Recommended Readings

Donahoe, J.W. and Wessells, M.G. (1980). *Learning, Language, and Memory*. Harper & Row, New York. A survey of the conceptual and empirical work on operant conditioning including schedules of reinforcement.

Honig, W.K. (Ed.) (1966). *Operant Behavior: Areas of Research and Application*. Appleton-Century-Crofts, New York. A wide assortment of papers dealing with operant conditioning techniques.

Lal, H. (Ed.) (1977). *Discriminative Stimulus Properties of Drugs*. Plenum, New York. A series of papers showing the use of this technique to investigate the mechanism of action of psychotropic drugs.

Reynolds, G.S. (1975). *A Primer of Operant Conditioning* (Revised). Scott, Foresman, Glenview, Illinois. A well-written beginning book, easily comprehended by undergraduate students.

CHAPTER THREE

The Cytology of Nerve Cells

An understanding of the effects of drugs on behavior must include knowledge of drugs; that is, their chemistry, how these chemicals affect nervous tissue, and how the chemically-induced neural effects lead to behavioral changes. A thorough knowledge of the entire picture also requires a firm familiarity with the structural units of the nervous system, the neurons (or nerves), and the way they carry out their functions.

General Organization of the Nervous System

The nervous system has been systematically studied for a long time, but contemporary investigators, using techniques and instruments developed only recently, are providing us with a prodigious amount of new information about it. With the aid of the high resolution of the electron microscope, we are able to observe cellular details that at one time could hardly be imagined. We are able to record electrical activities in the brain involving a change of only 1 or 2 millivolts (mV). Chemical changes can be detected by the sophisticated use of radioactive labeling and the isolation and identification of substances existing in amounts less than a billionth of a gram are now possible. We can now fractionate cells into their components—cytoplasm, nuclei, membranes, organelles, end processes and identify physiological events that are specific to each of them. Electrodes with diameters small enough to penetrate a nerve cell without seeming to injure it make recordings of interior activities while the cell is subjected to a wide variety of stimuli. Thus, with technological assistance, a great deal has recently been learned about the structure and function of this system.

The nervous system can be thought of as an information input, processing, storage, retrieval, and output system. The condition of the internal environment of an organism is constantly monitored by cells of the nervous system and adjustments are directed by other neurons to maximize the efficiency of the nonneural physiological systems that sustain life. For example, sensory cells track the presence or absence of food in the stomach or intestine, and effector neurons control the amount of activity in the gastrointestinal tract. Similarly, the rate of respiration is regulated according to the oxygen needs of the body. The external environment also provides input into the nervous system. The amount of this input depends upon the complexity of the environment, and its overall effect depends upon the state of awareness of the organism. For example, a sleeping person would still make adjustments to a change in temperature—he or she might curl up if too cold and stretch out if too warm—but the sound of his or her favorite tune would have little effect on behavior.

The nervous system is not a homogeneous structure like the liver or spleen. Rather, it is a collection of anatomically distinct subsystems that are highly integrated to receive information about the external and internal environment of the body, and under usual conditions the differing actions of these separate systems ultimately lead to the execution of glandular and muscular responses that contribute to the well-being of the body. Different parts of the nervous system serve different functions. For example, the thalamus serves to process and relay sensory information, whereas the corpus striatum, in conjunction with the cerebellum, modulates and controls muscle action. To be sure, these two neural systems do interact in significant ways, but their cells are clustered in different places, different chemical substances stimulate them, and their connections differ. The different cells of the liver, on the other hand, although serving many functions, are found in similar ratios uniformly throughout its volume. A physician who suspects liver disease may perform a biopsy and excise a few grams of liver tissue for analysis. What is found in these samples would usually apply to the whole structure. This would not be true of the nervous system; a few grams of cortical tissue from one area would not be likely to reveal neuropathology typical of some other part of the central nervous system.

The functional unit of the nervous system is the individual NEURON. Neurons and neuroglia (which support neurons physiologically) make up the bulk of the brain and other parts of the nervous system. NERVE CELLS (another name for neurons) are distinctive in that they rapidly transmit excitation, thus exciting other neurons or cells of effector organs. Nerve cells are stimulated by impulses that arise either from sense organs that have been stimulated by energy changes in the internal or external environment, by other nerve cells that have been so stimulated, or by neurons that have the ability to respond spontaneously. The cells of the endocrine glands (such as the thyroid gland, the pancreas, and certain parts of the ovaries and testes) also stimulate other cells, but they do so by releasing hormones into the bloodstream, which carries the hormones to their respective receptor sites. However, neural communication takes much less time than hormonal communication, and in most instances it is much more specific.

The junctions over which communication from sense organ to neuron and from neuron to neuron occurs are known as SYNAPSES. The junctions between neurons and effector organs (muscles and glands) are known as NEUROEFFECTOR JUNCTIONS. Membranes that circumscribe the nerve cell as a whole, as well as those that surround substructures within the cell, also play important roles in neuronal activity. Indeed, it can be said that both the membrane interface at the junction between cells and the membrane surface within cells are areas of greatest significance in neuronal function.

Neurons are organized into peripheral bundles called NERVES and a central system usually referred to as the BRAIN. The peripheral nerves are distributed to all sense organs, muscles, and glands on the surface of the body and to smooth and cardiac muscles and glandular tissues within the body cavity. The nerves are either AFFERENT (carrying nerve messages from sense organs to the central system) or EFFERENT (from the central system to the muscles and glands). The CENTRAL NERVOUS SYSTEM (CNS), located within the skull and the vertebral column, receives the afferent messages and directs them either to appropriate muscles via efferent nerves for simple reflexes or to higher levels of the CNS for integration at increasing levels of complexity.

The nervous system can be divided into autonomic and somatic divisions. The AUTONOMIC NERVOUS SYSTEM consists of peripheral and central neurons that control the functions of the relatively involuntary visceral organs. For example, this system controls the overall metabolic rate, the pupillary response, salivary and gastrointestinal responses, respiration rate, blood pressure, and heart rate. The autonomic system can be subdivided into sympathetic and parasympathetic divisions. The SYMPATHETIC NERVOUS SYSTEM "dominates" visceral activity during strong effort, excitement, or stress, speeding up respiration and heart rate and inhibiting gastrointestinal activity. The PARASYMPATHETIC NERVOUS SYSTEM is more influential during moderate levels of activity, decreasing blood pressure, increasing gastrointestinal activity, and so forth. These two systems are always involved in a delicately balanced interplay that tends to optimize the functions of the visceral organs (see Figure 1, Chapter 6).

The SOMATIC NERVOUS SYSTEM includes those neural systems that respond to external stimuli (such as the skin senses, audition, and vision) and directs responses of the somatic musculature for overt activity. It should be emphasized that the autonomic and somatic systems are not independent. Rather there is significant interaction between these systems that serves to convert the needs of the body (such as replacement for metabolized and excreted food products) into overt behaviors like seeking, hunting, or overcoming competition. Moreover, acts such as hunting are accompanied by a high level of sympathetic activity to insure that the energy output will increase the probability of success. The conscious awareness of these high levels of autonomic activity is known as feelings and emotion. In humans, these autonomic substrates of emotion may easily be aroused by symbolic stimuli such as invasion of territory and threats to dominance, and even by racial and political differences.

The somatic system may initiate heightened autonomic activity in a hostile environment, aiding attack or flight, or possibly the reverse, expressed as submission, passivity (hiding or "playing possum"), or fainting. On the other hand, changes in the visceral organs because of disease and physiological imbalances or deficiencies may also come into awareness as changes of mood and emotion. For example, PHEOCHROMO-CYTOMA (a tumor of the adrenal gland) causes sudden release of epinephrine, which gives rise to PAROX-YSMAL TACHYCARDIA (a sudden increase in heart rate). This is very stressful because it produces feelings of impending disaster. These symptoms can be alleviated by the drug α-methyl-p-tyrosine, which blocks the synthesis of epinephrine. The pharmacological manipulations of these interacting neuronal systems are of key importance in psychopharmacology.

At all levels of neural function, neurons make contacts (synapses) with other neurons—either with a few or many thousands—and influence them by secreting special substances called NEUROTRANSMITTERS (chemicals involved in transmitting messages between nerve cells and between a nerve cell and an effector organ). In this way, the cells are organized into circuits because a given neurotransmitter may stimulate some cells but not others. A circuit may be as simple as a monosynaptic reflex that involves only one synapse between the afferent and efferent nerve (e.g., the raising of the lower leg in response to a tap on the patellar tendon of the knee), or it may be a polysynaptic circuit of almost unimaginable complexity controlling skillful movements, sensory and perceptual processes, memory, language, intellectual activities, and emotion.

The effects of drugs upon these circuits are our immediate concern in neuropsychopharmacology. For example, consider some of the effects of amphetamine. This drug heightens arousal, reduces boredom, increases attention, and combats fatigue. Physiologically, amphetamines intensify the action of norepinephrine (NE) and dopamine (DA) in the central nervous system. (NE and DA are neurotransmitters that stimulate or inhibit neurons in diverse parts of the central nervous system.) Although we still do not know all the details of the effects of amphetamine on behavior, we know that we should focus our attention upon those brain structures that are sensitive to NE and DA.

Neuron Types

Neurons can be classified in several ways. Golgi, the famous Italian histologist (1844–1926), classified neurons in terms of whether they had long axons with a few branches (Type I) or short axons with many branches originating near the cell body (Type II). Both of these types are found in the gray matter of the brain and spinal cord (Figure 1A and B). Neurons are also classified according to the number of branches that extend from the cell body: there are unipolar, bipolar, and multipolar cells. The unipolar cells have the function of conveying exteroceptive information from the periphery to the spinal cord. The unipolar cell bodies are in the spinal ganglia. These cells have a single extension that divides some distance from the soma into a peripheral and a central branch (Figure 1C). The peripheral branch extends to sense organs in peripheral structures such as muscles, tendons and joints, and the skin. The central branch enters the spinal cord and communicates with other neurons that are involved with reflexes, sensory awareness, and motor control. The peripheral branch differs from the usual form of dendrite in that it is considerably longer and conducts action potentials or nerve impulses in an all-or-none fashion. Typically, dendrites convey a signal of graded intensity that is much weaker than an action potential.

Bipolar neurons receive inputs from the sense organs of vision, hearing, and smell, and from the equilibratory sense mediated by the vestibular apparatus (Figures 1D and E) (i.e., these neurons convey sensory information to the central nervous system.)

Multipolar neurons have many short, branched dendrites, such as those of motoneurons (Figure 2), the Golgi Types I and II (Figure 1A and B), or the Purkinje cells of the cerebellum (Figure 1F). The elaborate branching of the dendritic tree of the Purkinje cells enormously increases its synaptic surface, making it possible for these cells to receive inputs from many other cells and to exert excitatory or inhibitory influences. Because these neurons coordinate body and limb movements, a reduction of inhibitory influences upon these cells causes convulsions and an excess of inhibition causes ataxia (a loss of coordination). Figure 1G shows the soma of a neuron from the hypoglossal nucleus in the medulla, which controls tongue movements.

Morphology of Neurons

Because of the wide variety of neurons in the vertebrate nervous system, it is not possible to describe a typical neuron in a way that encompasses all the morphological features that exist (Bodian, 1962). Therefore, we will describe in detail only one type of neuron—motoneurons of the spinal cord that activate

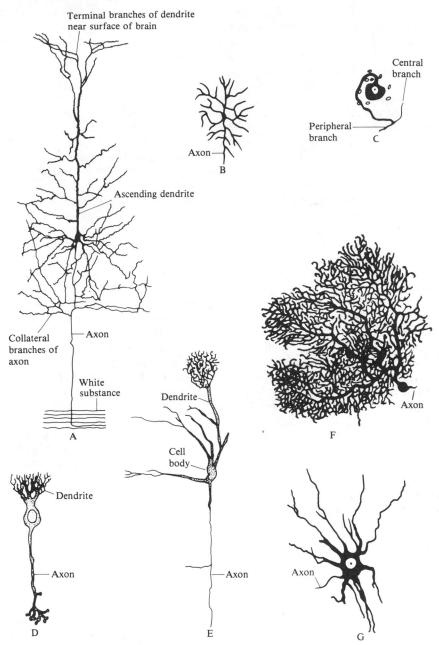

FIGURE 1.   SHAPES OF NEURON TYPES. The neurons shown were drawn to different scales in order to show their structures. (A) A pyramidal cell from the motor cortex of a rabbit (Golgi Type I). (B) An interneuron (Golgi Type II) of the kind found in the gray matter of the brain and spinal cord. (C) A unipolar cell body of a sensory branch of a spinal nerve. (D) A bipolar cell from the retina of a dog. (E) A mitral cell (bipolar) which serves as a relay neuron in the olfactory bulb of a cat. (F) A multipolar Purkinje cell from the cerebellar cortex of a monkey—a cell that may receive inputs and form synapses with 100,000 other neurons. (G) A multipolar cell body from the nucleus of the hypoglossal nerve of a human. (Only small parts of the axons of the Purkinje cell and the hypoglossal nerve cell are shown.)

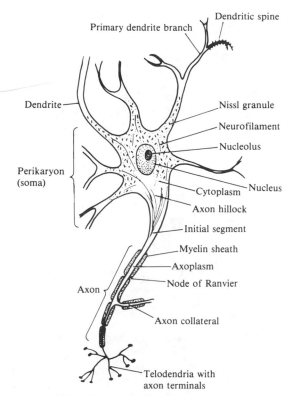

Primary dendrite branch
Dendritic spine
Dendrite
Nissl granule
Neurofilament
Nucleolus
Perikaryon (soma)
Cytoplasm
Nucleus
Axon hillock
Initial segment
Myelin sheath
Axoplasm
Node of Ranvier
Axon
Axon collateral
Telodendria with axon terminals

FIGURE 2. SPINAL CORD MOTONEURON. For illustrative purposes, the axon depicted is shorter and heavier than that of an actual nerve cell. Also, the internodal segments of the myelin sheath are shortened; normally they are about 100 to 200 times longer than the neuraxon diameter.

skeletal muscles. These neurons have most neuronal features and function in many typical ways, and thus illustrate the concept of a neuron quite well. A MOTONEURON (Figure 2) has a cell body (frequently called the SOMA or the PERIKARYON); branched twig-like extensions called DENDRITES, which convey electrical changes toward the soma; and an AXON, which conveys nerve impulses away from the cell body to the axon terminals. At the axon terminals, changes are initiated that induce contractions of the skeletal muscle cells.

Dendrites

Typically the primary, secondary, and tertiary branches of the dendrites of multipolar cells have smooth surfaces, whereas the more distal branches are covered with many fine spines or GEMMULES (Figure

3). The number of spines on a single Purkinje cell of a cat, monkey, or human may number 100,000 or more and thus provide a combined synaptic surface of more than 400,000 square microns.

It is possible that dendritic spines may be of special significance in learning and memory. It has been reported that there were more spines on the dendrites of the pyramidal cells of the cortex of rats that were exposed to an enriched environment than in litter mates that were exposed to an impoverished environment (Rosenzweig et al., 1972). (The pyramidal cells receive nerve impulses from other parts of the brain and direct impulses to the somatic musculature of the head and the body.) There may be a correlation between the absence of normal dendritic spines and the presence of abnormal ones in cortical neurons of some mentally retarded persons (Purpura, 1974). Normal spines are divided into three types: thin, stubby, and mushroom-shaped. In mentally retarded persons, there is a marked absence of the stubby and mushroom-shaped types, depending upon the age and severity of the developmental retardation. Instead there are many long, fine, and sometimes entangled spines with prominent terminal heads. It is possible that these abnormalities in the dendritic spines may have profound effects on the ability of the cells to integrate their neural input.

Internal Structure of the Perikaryon

The cell body of a neuron has many internal features in common with other cells of the body. Within a neuron cell body are a number of cell inclusions such as the nucleus, nucleolus, mitochondria, Golgi apparatus, endoplasmic reticulum, neurofilaments, microtubules, and ribosomes (Figures 4 and 5). The neurofilaments and tubules extend into dendrites and axons, and the terminals of the axons contain vesicles of secretory material (the neurotransmitters) that play a vital role in synaptic action.

Nucleus. The nucleus is a centrally located, spherically shaped structure 3 to 18 μm in diameter. It is surrounded by a double membrane, the outer layer having openings that communicate with the endoplasmic reticulum. The nucleus contains nucleoproteins and DEOXYRIBONUCLEIC ACID (DNA), the chemical substances of the genes. In cells other than neurons, DNA controls the transmission of hereditary characteristics during cellular multiplication, but in the mature nervous system of warm-blooded species there is little nerve cell multiplication under ordinary circum-

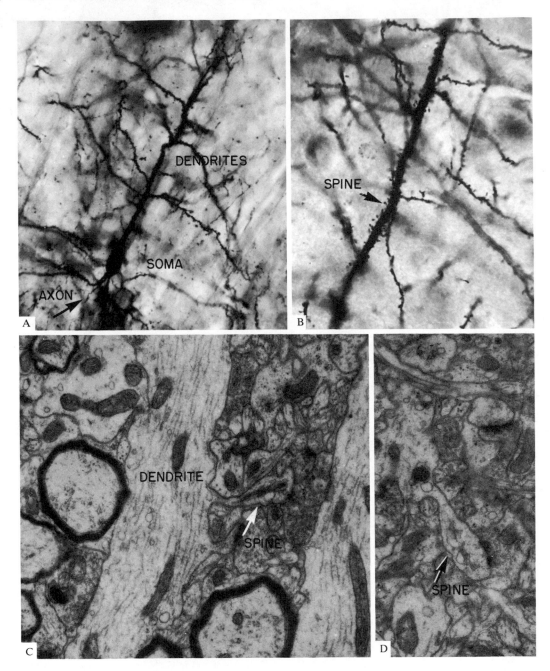

FIGURE 3.   GOLGI TYPE I CELLS. Stained neurons with long axons in the motor cortex of the rat. (A) The entire cell with its soma, axon, and dendrites (Golgi stain x100). (B) Dendritic spines (Golgi stain x250). (C) and (D) Electron micrographs of dendritic spines (x30,000). (From Jacobson, 1972.)

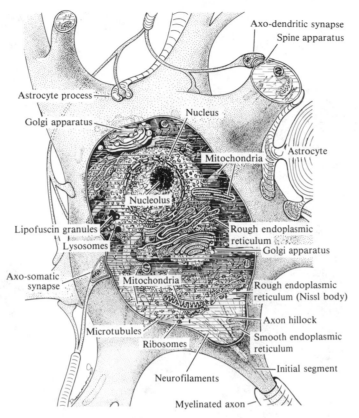

FIGURE 4. INTERNAL STRUCTURE OF A PERI-KARYON. Many terminals from myelinated axons form synapses upon the outer surface of the soma and upon the dendrites. In this figure, their number is tremendously reduced. Only one astrocyte is shown; normally there might be hundreds. The cutaway view reveals the cell inclusions, such as the nucleus and nucleolus, the mitochondria, and the Golgi apparatus. The initial segment is located on the axon at the lower right, just above the first myelin segment. (From McGeer et al., 1978.)

stances. This fact probably accounts for the permanent loss of function that follows extensive loss of neural tissue as a result of trauma or disease. DNA also participates in the formation of RIBONUCLEIC ACID (RNA). RNA is distributed throughout the cell and participates in the synthesis of cellular proteins, some of which are the enzymes that take part in energy production and the synthesis of substances that are involved in synaptic transmission. Some RNA is clustered within the nucleus to form a nucleolus. There is a considerable body of evidence implying that DNA–RNA mechanisms participate in the nerve cell changes that make learning and memory possible. For example, changes have been detected in protein synthesis during learning, and drugs that interfere with protein synthesis in the brain appear to block memory retention (Agranoff et al., 1978; Seiden and Dykstra, 1977).

Mitochondria. Mitochondria are elongated oval structures about 1000–3000 nm (nanometer; 10^{-9} meter) long and are scattered throughout the cell body, dendrites, and axons. They are even found in the smallest branches and end terminals of the nerve cell. They are synthesized in the cell body and are especially numerous where there is intense metabolic activity, such as at synapses. The mitochondria, by a process called oxidative metabolism or oxidative phosphorylation, utilize nutrients and oxygen in the presence of enzymes to produce large amounts of energy-rich ADENOSINE TRIPHOSPHATE (ATP), which diffuses

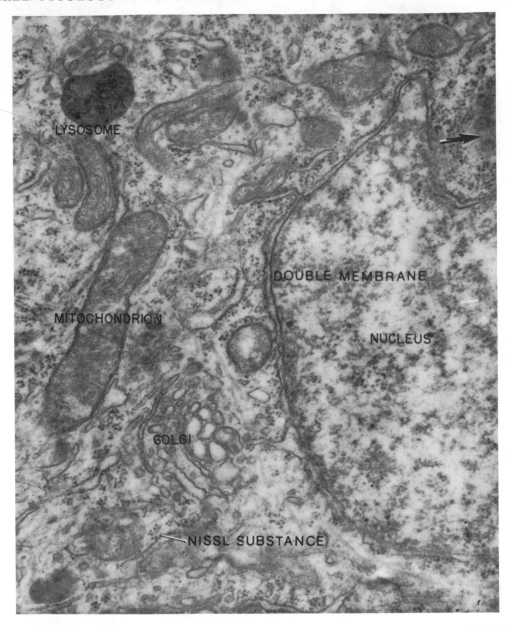

FIGURE 5. ELECTRON MICROGRAPH OF A PERI-KARYON of a small pyramidal cell in the cerbral cortex of a rat. Some of the neuron organelles are identified as well as the double membrane of the nucleus and the Nissl substance. (From Jacobson, 1972.)

throughout the cell and releases its stored energy for celluar functions. It is estimated that a single mito-chondrion may contain as many as 15,000 respiratory enzyme units, each of which contains a dozen or more separate enzymes. For this reason, mitochondria are known as the powerhouses of the cell.

ATP is used in three important cellular functions, namely, membrane transport, synthesis of chemical substances within the cell, and mechanical work. The excitability of neurons and the propagation of nerve impulses depends upon the transport of ions across the neuron membrane. Synaptic action depends upon the synthesis of transmitter substances, which are released at axon terminals to stimulate adjacent cells; and it takes mechanical work to transport substances such as proteins and neurotransmitters or their precursors within the neuron from the cell body to the axon terminals (Ochs, 1972; 1981). Drugs [such as 2,4-dinitrophenol (DNP)] that block the formation of the high energy compound ATP disrupt phosphorylation and block the functions of the mitochondria, causing neuron function to cease.

Mitochondria in cells of the nervous system, as well as those in the liver, kidney and intestines, have attached to their outer membrane an enzyme called monoamine oxidase (MAO), which participates in the metabolism of neurotransmitters and related substances.

Endoplasmic Reticulum. The ENDOPLASMIC RETICULUM is a tubular network filled with an endoplasmic matrix, a fluid substance different from the cytoplasm (the fluid of the cell body). With the aid of the electron microscope, the space inside the endoplasmic reticulum is shown to be continuous with the space between the two layers surrounding the nucleus, as mentioned earlier. Some areas of the endoplasmic reticulum have a large number of small granular particles called RIBOSOMES (consisting mainly of RNA) attached to its outer surface. These parts of the endoplasmic reticulum are called the ERGASTOPLASM or ROUGH ENDOPLASMIC RETICULUM, and are devoted to protein synthesis by linking amino acids together.

Before the advent of the electron microscope, clumps of the endoplasmic reticulum were known as NISSL GRANULES, chromophil substance, or tigroid bodies. These dark-staining granules were well distributed within the perikaryon but were notably absent in the axon hillock (that section of the perikaryon just before the emergence of the axon) (Figure 4). Later this substance was identified as being similar to ribosomes containing RNA which serves to synthesize proteins that need to be restored because of normal attrition or because of disease or injury. During the latter conditions, the granules become finely divided and dispersed, a process called CHROMATOLYSIS. Another part of the endoplasmic reticulum is free of ribosomes and is known as SMOOTH ENDOPLASMIC RETICULUM. It may extend from the perikaryon into the axons and dendrites, and may function as a transport system for substances needed for normal maintenance and function of the extensions of the neuron (Droz, 1975). Smooth endoplasmic reticulum is also the site for the synthesis of lipids (fatty substances that form part of the cell membranes).

Golgi Apparatus. The Golgi apparatus is highly developed in nerve cells. Under high power magnification with the electron microscope, it appears like a stack of a half-dozen or more pancakes, which are actually membrane-bound cisternae (cavities) about 1 μm in diameter. Along the rim of the Golgi apparatus small vesicles 5 to 10 nm in diameter are seen. The vesicles either bud off or fuse to the cistern membranes (Figure 5). Within the cisternae are particles presumably consisting of protein molecules that are in the process of synthesis. These platelike cisternae are contiguous with the endoplasmic reticulum (ER), and each of them is functionally distinct because the density of the intramembrane particles changes from one to the next (Figure 6).

The stack is an asymmetric structure in that the cisternae nearest the cell nucleus and the ER (designated as the *cis* face) receive the precursors of the proteins from the ER and subject them to different chemical treatments. Treatments include glycosylation (incorporation of sugar molecules), proteolysis (hydrolysis of proteins to simpler forms), sulfation (incorporation or treatment by sulfuric agents), phosphorylation (the addition of phosphate groups), and addition of fatty acids. Which of one or more processes occurs depends upon the ultimate destination of the proteins (e.g., the cell membrane, secretion vesicles, lysosomes, and so on). In addition, membrane proteins from the ER that have accompanied the newly synthesized proteins are removed in the *cis* compartment and incorporated into budding vesicles, which flow back to be reincorporated into the ER.

The proteins that have undergone these refinements pass to the last one or two cisternae (designated as the *trans* face or compartment), where they undergo a final sorting for further distribution to the cell. It is not known precisely how the proteins proceed from layer to layer within the stack. It could occur by diffusion or by budding vesicles that go from one cistern to the next. Finally, the whole process appears to be analogous to a distillation tower, which accepts raw materials and in a step-by-step process refines a variety of materials that are collected for distribution else-

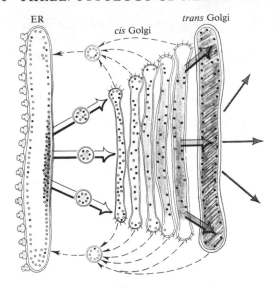

FIGURE 6.   PROTEIN REFINING IN THE GOLGI AP-
PARATUS. The density of shading portrays the progressive
transport of exported proteins from the endoplasmic
reticulum (ER) through the *cis* and *trans* cisternae. The
closed circles represent some of these exported proteins. The
open circles represent ER membrane proteins that most likely
will be removed from the rims of Golgi cisternae by budding
vesicles that then fuse with the ER (dashed arrows). The thick
arrows represent transport steps in which exported proteins
are transported into the *cis* and *trans* Golgi compartments
and then to appropriate places in the cell (thin arrows).
(From Rothman, 1981.)

where (Rothman, 1981). The final distribution of the
protein material may be by way of the smooth endoplasmic reticulum, as mentioned earlier.

Microtubules and Neurofilaments. MICROTUBULES
are very slender filaments consisting of helical or spiral
arrays of neurotubule protein (TUBULIN) of approximately 24 nm in diameter and are found throughout
the cell body, axon, and dendrites. In the cell body,
they tend to cross and interlace, whereas in axon and
dendrites, they tend to run in parallel. They do not
seem to be involved in the propagation of the nerve impulse; that function is the property of the cell membrane. Rather they seem to be implicated in the rapid
transport of substances necessary to keep nerve fibers
viable and in the transport of those substances involved in the synthesis of neurotransmitters.

The NEUROFILAMENTS seem to be constructed of
material similar to that of the microtubules but are
somewhat thinner helical chains about 8 nm in diameter. The functional significance of these structures is
not known. Microfilaments made up of a contractile
actin-like protein have also been identified in axons.
(Actin is a contractile protein associated with muscle
fibers.) They are shorter than the microtubules and run
circumferentially as well as longitudinally (Schwartz,
1980).

Lysosomes. Finally there are cellular inclusions
known as LYSOSOMES within the cytoplasm of the cell
body. They are very small (between 250 and 700 nm in
diameter) and are surrounded by a membrane. They
consist of an aggregate of enzymes capable of digesting
organic compounds. For example, they are involved in
converting proteins into amino acids and glycogen to
glucose (which is the basic nutrient of nerve cells).
Many lysosomes become converted to lipofuscin
granules that accumulate with age and are regarded as
neuronal refuse.

Neuraxons

The NEURAXON, or simply, axon, is the message-
bearing part of the nerve cell and in some ways may be
compared to an electric cable. But there the analogy
ends because the electrical signal transmitted by the
neuraxon travels much more slowly (between 1 and 100
meters per second), whereas electric signals in a copper
wire travel almost at the speed of light. The transmission of a nerve impulse is not by simple conduction but
rather by a built-in amplifying and relay system.

In many large neurons, the axon arises from the
axon hillock (Figures 2 and 4), and from this point the
axon is covered by a membrane known as the AXO-
LEMMA that is similar to the cytoplasmic membrane of
the cell body. The axon hillock is free of Nissl granules
and other cellular inclusions, and the neurofilaments
in the axon hillock seem to be clustered together in
fascicles before proceeding along the axon proper. It is
unlikely that all neurons have an axon hillock, especially those that are comparatively small and have very
fine axons. Typical of many neurons with relatively
thick axons is a short section of the axon known as the
INITIAL SEGMENT (Figure 4). The diameter of this portion of the axon is slightly reduced and is also free of
Nissl granules and other cellular inclusions. Functionally, the initial segment plays a significant role in
the propagation of nerve signals. It is here that excita-

tory and inhibitory influences combine either to promote the discharge of a nerve impulse or to impede it.

Myelin Sheath. Beyond the initial segment, the axolemma in most axons is covered by an insulating fatty material, the MYELIN SHEATH. Along peripheral nerves (e.g., the sensory nerves or motor nerves that run from the spinal cord to muscles), the myelin is formed by

sheath cells, or as they are frequently called, SCHWANN CELLS. These somewhat flattened cells wrap themselves around the axon as shown in Figure 7A. Then the membrane of the cell elongates and burrows under itself so that it completely encircles the axon. This burrowing continues around the axon, thus forming many layers of Schwann cell membrane (Figure 7B). In the process, most of the cytoplasm of the Schwann cell is

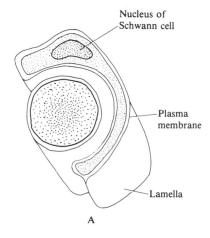

A

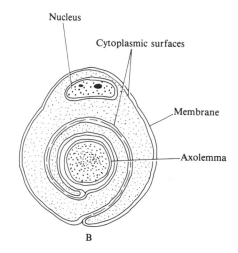

B

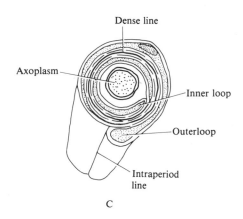

C

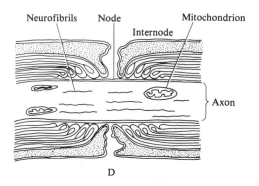

D

FIGURE 7 FORMATION OF MYELIN SHEATHS around axons of peripheral neurons. (A) A Schwann cell encircles the axon by elongating its membrane. (B) One edge of the Schwann cell membrane burrows under the other edge, making a complete rotation around the axon to form layers. (C) Illustration of three rotations of the Schwann cell membrane around the axon membrane, the axolemma. Dense lines are formed where the inner surfaces of the cell membrane are joined and intraperiod lines are formed where the outer surfaces of the lamellae are joined. The cytoplasm remains only in the inner, outer, and lateral loops. (D) A longitudinal cutaway view of a node of Ranvier.

squeezed out so that it is found mostly in the innermost and outermost loops. Where the cytoplasm is displaced, the cytoplasmic (inner) surfaces of the top and bottom membranes come together to form the dense line; where the outer surfaces come together as a result of the wrapping activity of the cell membrane, the intraperiod line is formed. Thus, the myelin sheath appears to be built up from the inside out. Each layer of myelin between the intraperiod lines consists of double thicknesses of Schwann cell membranes about 8.5 nm thick. There may be only a few myelin layers (Figure 7C), or as many as a hundred, forming a concentric insulating cover about 4 μm thick. The thicker the myelin cover, the more effectively it serves the functions of the neuron (Morell, 1978; Morell and Norton, 1980).

However, the myelin sheath for the whole axon is discontinuous; it is made up of segments with an interval of about 4 μm of naked axon membrane between segments. These points of naked axon are called the NODES OF RANVIER (Figure 7D). The length of the myelin segment is proportional to the thickness of the fiber. In fibers that range from 3 to 18 μm in diameter, the myelin segments range from 400 to 1500 μm (0.4 to 1.5 mm) in length. Thus, the myelin segments range from 100 to 400 times longer than the nodes, or in some cases they may be 200 times the diameter of the neuraxon. Mitochondria are congregated at the nodes of Ranvier because relatively higher levels of metabolic activity concerned with the propagation of nerve impulses occur at these points.

In the central nervous system, myelinization is much the same except that it is accomplished by a type of OLIGODENDROGLIA (glial cells) instead of by Schwann cells. A single glial cell sends out many sail-like extensions that envelop nearby axons. The leading edge forms an inner loop that rolls itself up around the axon in a manner similar to the way a window shade would roll itself around a roller if the roller remained stationary while the inner edge of the shade rotated around the roller, pulling the rest of the shade around it (Norton, 1976; Morell and Norton, 1980).

In general, axons have branches (COLLATERALS) that originate either in the initial segment or at nodes of Ranvier and that distribute nerve signals to different destinations. For example, the branches may extend backward to influence the source of its own stimulation. These backward-running branches are called RECURRENT COLLATERALS. An example of this phenomenon is shown in Figure 8. Here a branch from a moto-

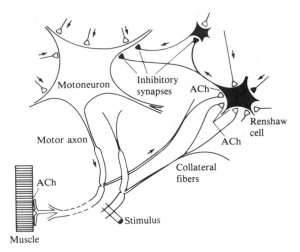

FIGURE 8.   ACTION OF AXON COLLATERALS. Renshaw cells are found near motoneurons in the spinal cord. The motoneurons send long axons to the muscles of the trunk and limbs, as shown schematically. The motoneurons receive excitatory inputs from many sources, as depicted by the open synaptic endings. Collateral fibers that emerge from the nodes of the motoneuron axons go to the Renshaw cells and stimulate them, the transmitter being acetylcholine (ACh). The Renshaw cell axons return to the motoneurons, forming inhibitory synapses (solid terminals), the transmitter being glycine. A stimulus applied to the axon (as shown at the bottom of the figure) would cause a nerve impulse to go to the Renshaw cell. Such stimulation has a strong inhibitory action on the motoneurons. The Renshaw cells receive excitatory and inhibitory inputs from other sources as well. (From Eccles, 1967.)

neuron runs backward to synapse upon a cell, known as RENSHAW CELL, which in turn synapses back upon the motoneuron. Presumably this circuit exerts negative feedback control because the output of these cells inhibits motoneurons and prevents them from firing too rapidly, thus distributing the workload more evenly within the neuron population.

Dimensions of the Axon. Axon length can vary considerably. Some axons are very short, extending for only several cell-body diameters, whereas others may extend over several thousand cell-body diameters. The phrenic nerve, which innervates the muscles of the diaphragm, originates from cell bodies in the brain stem near the base of the skull. In the giraffe, the axons of these cells terminate on the diaphragm 15 feet below the skull. In a 6-foot man, the axons that extend from cell bodies in the spinal cord to the muscles of the big toe may be 5000 cell bodies long. By comparison, if the cell body were as large as a football, the axon would extend the length of 15 football fields (Schwartz, 1980). In mature nerve cells, the volume within their axons may be hundreds to thousands of times that of their perikarya. It is thus apparent that the movement of substances that are synthesized in the perikaryon to the distant parts of the nerve cell is of major physiological importance.

The diameter of the axon is maintained throughout its length, but near the distal end the axon may divide into few or as many as a few thousand fine branches with terminal enlargements. These enlargements form the synaptic connections to other neurons or to cells of effector organs. Axons of the sympathetic and parasympathetic neurons have fine terminal branches with synaptic swellings (VARICOSITIES) along their length and can form thousands of junctions with effector cells. The serially placed synaptic swellings are also seen within the central nervous system and make synaptic contacts with thousands of other neurons.

Axoplasmic Transport

It should be evident that an essential part of nerve function depends upon a number of different products that are synthesized in the perikaryon and subsequently transported to other parts of the cell and the axon terminals. This transport process is known as AXOPLASMIC FLOW. A number of structures participate in this function, including the microtubules, the Golgi apparatus, and the endoplasmic reticulum. Figure 9 shows the relationships among these structures and illustrates some of the mechanisms of axoplasmic flow.

Slow Axoplasmic Transport

The flow of substances from one part of the neuron to the other takes place at different rates, depending upon the material to be transported and the mechanism of transport. Slow axoplasmic transport (between 1 and 2 or 1 and 10 mm/day—estimates differ) mostly involves the movement of newly synthesized protein from the perikaryon to the axon and the nerve endings. This protein, which can be synthesized only in the perikaryon by the ribosomes (Nissl granules) or free polyribosomes, is needed to replace the protein that has been catabolized to peptides and amino acids in the production of energy for action potentials, to provide enzymes for mitochondrial ac-

tivities, and to provide protein for nerve growth in developing organisms and for the general maintenance of nerve fibers. Furthermore, the release of neurotransmitters also involves an accompanying loss of enzyme, and this too has to be replaced. Slow axoplasmic transport apparently takes place within the AXOPLASMIC MATRIX, the area that surrounds the microtubules and other inclusions of the axon. The amount of protein transported by this system is about four times greater than that transported by fast axoplasmic flow. However, very little of it reaches the nerve terminal because most of it is utilized within the axon. Eighty percent of the protein being transported by this process is for buildup and repair of microtubules, neurofilaments, and microfilaments; the remainder comprises enzymes of various kinds. The rate of flow is determined by the axon length—the longer the length, the faster the flow. It is not known what provides the driving force for this process, though some observers have suggested that there are peristaltic waves that affect the axon as a whole (Droz, 1975; Schwartz, 1980).

Fast Axoplasmic Transport

Fast axoplasmic transport occurs at a rate between 50 and 400 mm/day. It requires energy, which is supplied by ATP, and oxygen. Substances such as cyanide or dinitrophenol block this process. Covering a small section of a nerve with a plastic strip covered with petrolatum (Vaseline) produced an anoxia that blocked fast axoplasmic transport, as shown by a damming of radiolabeled protein proximal to the plastic strip and the absence of the labeled material distal to it. When the plastic strip was removed after periods of up to 1.5 hours, fast axoplasmic flow resumed after insignificant delays (Ochs, 1981).

The rate of flow is also temperature dependent, doubling or tripling with each increase of 10 degrees C. The rate of movement is not dependent on the length or diameter of the axon, and the flow is maintained, at least for a time, even if the cell body is disconnected from the axon. The substances transported include membrane proteins for the maintenance of the axolemma and for the formation of synaptic vesicles and enzymes involved in the synthesis or catabolism of neurotransmitters. During fast transport, vesicular movement is more independent than axoplasmic movement during slow transport, i.e., vesicles that may enter as a group soon become dispersed as they move down

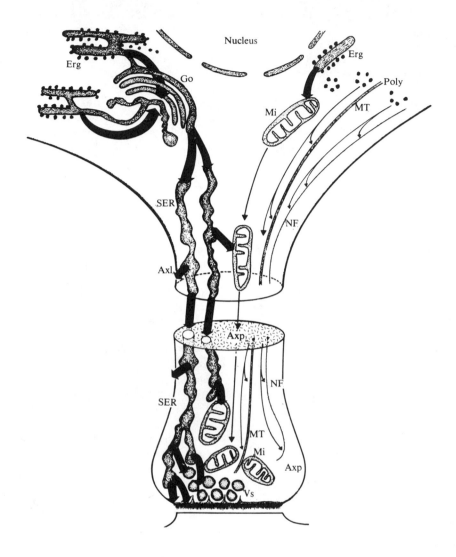

FIGURE 9. AXOPLASMIC TRANSPORT. Fast axoplasmic transport involves the structures and thick arrows on the left. Proteins are synthesized in the ergastoplasm (Erg) and are transferred to the Golgi apparatus (Go) for further synthesis and storage. These and other synthetic products may be enclosed in vesicles and transported to the axon via axonal extensions of the smooth endoplasmic reticulum (SER). Transport in this system is fast and yields membrane components for the axolemma (Axl) and mitochondria (Mi). Other products such as transmitter substances, trophic fac-tors (see text), and mitochondria are carried to the axon terminal. Synaptic vesicles (Vs) may be carried by the transport system or they may "bud off" the SER in the axon terminals. On the right, the thin arrows point to substances that move by slow axoplasmic transport. Polyribosomes (Poly) synthesize and release proteins that are slowly transported in the axoplasm (Axp). The interaction between the SER and the microtubules (MT) and the neurofilaments (NF) is not shown, nor is retrograde axonal flow shown. (Adapted from Droz, 1975.)

the axon. The vesicles also seem to move in jumps, as though they were encountering a force-generating system. Experiments in snail neurons show that the more crowded the vesicles are, the faster they move and vice versa. This keeps the vesicles moving at a constant rate: if one jumps ahead, it slows down; if slowly moving vesicles pile up, they begin to move faster (Schwartz, 1980).

In addition there seem to be trophic substances, so far unidentified, that are transported to the terminals of the axons and are released to modify the functional state of the postsynaptic cell. For example, Miledi and Slater (1970) found that sectioning motor nerves in rats led to a loss of responsivity of the muscle fiber to the nerve ending and that the loss occurred sooner if the nerve was cut close to the muscle rather than farther from it. They estimated that the trophic factor was moving at a rate of 360 mm/day, which is fairly close to the 410 mm/day observed for the movement of radiolabeled proteins in the same nerves. Another trophic factor seems to control protein synthesis in postsynaptic cells. It is well known that cutting motor nerves frequently leads after some time to a supersensitivity of the muscle to a neurotransmitter applied artificially. This is believed to occur because of a compensatory increase in receptor sites for the transmitter. This increase can be blocked by drugs that block protein synthesis (actinomycin D). Therefore, it is believed that a trophic factor from the motoneuron acts to repress receptor protein synthesis at the DNA level.

Retrograde or Reverse Axoplasmic Flow

There is also evidence that the flow of cell products occurs in the opposite direction as well, that is, from the axon terminals to the perikaryon. This activity may be part of an elaborate "feedback" system by which the axons and dendrites send signals to the cell nucleus, regulating the rate of synthesis and transport of proteins, lipids, and neurotransmitters (Ochs, 1975). It may also serve to recycle the products of cell metabolism into new substances needed for the cell. This process seems to be mediated by lysosomes, which are a major component of retrograde axoplasmic flow. These organelles presumably engulf used fragments of membranes and degrade them while transporting them back to the cell body. Retrograde transport is also temperature dependent but occurs at roughly one-half to two-thirds the rate of forward transport. Reverse

axoplasmic flow may also carry the "signal" for chromatolysis (Nissl granule dispersion following axon severing).

By the process of endocytosis, fragments of the terminal membranes are carried into the cytoplasm and presumably engulfed by the lysosomes for transport back to the cell body. (See Figure 19 in Chapter 5.) Small amounts of extracellular fluid (ECF) are also taken up along with any substance that may be dissolved or in suspension in the ECF. The enzyme horseradish peroxidase can be injected into neural tissue, where it is taken up by active end terminals and carried back to the cell bodies. Chemical treatment of tissue containing this enzyme produces a dark precipitate that can be detected easily. Thus, cell bodies that lie far from their axon terminals can be located by this method (Schwartz, 1980; Hammerschlag and Roberts, 1976).

Propelling Mechanism for Fast Axoplasmic Transport

According to Droz (1975), fast axoplasmic flow takes place within the axonal extensions of the smooth endoplasmic reticulum (Figure 9). As the propelling mechanism, Droz proposed an interactive process involving the endoplasmic reticulum and the microtubule–neurofilament system; but the precise nature of this interaction has not been made clear. On the other hand, it is quite certain that the microtubule–neurofilament system plays a significant role in fast transport. There is substantial evidence showing that the drugs colchicine and vinblastine, which disrupt neurotubules by binding to the protein subunit tubulin, interrupt fast axoplasmic transport (Dahlström, 1970). Interestingly, these drugs only slightly affect the conduction of nerve impulses along the axon, but transmission across synapses is strongly impeded.

The Transport Filament Hypothesis

Another proposal that is in some ways compatible with that of Droz is the "transport filament" hypothesis of Ochs (1981). This hypothesis suggests that fast transport is a microtubule–mediated process whereby mitochondria, vesicles, nonvesiculated proteins, and polypeptides are attached to transport filaments that are carried along the microtubules by a series of microtubule attachments called side arms, one set for anterograde transport, another for retrograde transport (Figure 10). Slow transport, rather than requiring a

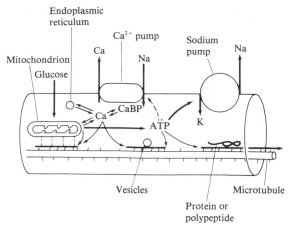

FIGURE 10. TRANSPORT FILAMENT HYPOTHESIS.
Glucose enters the nerve fiber where it is converted within
mitochondria to ATP. ATP fuels the sodium pump which
controls the balance between Na^+ and K^+ within the fiber,
and supplies energy to the side arms (the small appendages to
the microtubule). The side arms move the transport filaments
(shown as black bars). Mitochondria, vesicles, and proteins
and polypeptides are bound to the transport filaments, and
move by fast axoplasmic transport. Ca^{2+} (Ca) is shown participating in transport filament movement. Ca^{2+} is sequestered within mitochondria and the endoplasmic
reticulum, and is bound to Ca^{2+} binding protein calmodulin
(CaBP). The Ca^{2+} pump controls the influx of calcium.
(After Ochs, 1981.)

separate mechanism, is presumed to be the result of a
drop-off and local redistribution of the materials
transported by fast axoplasmic flow.

Calcium (Ca^{2+}) is necessary for this process because
it activates a calcium–dependent enzyme ATPase
which makes energy available from ATP. Axoplasmic
transport is blocked in neurons placed in Ca^{2+}
depleted environments. Intraneuronal Ca^{2+} is sequestered in mitochondria and in the endoplasmic
reticulum, and is regulated by a Na^+–Ca^{2+} exchange
apparatus (a Ca^{2+} pump). Ca^{2+} is transported within
the axoplasm at rates consistent with fast transport
(410 mm/day). Studies have shown that Ca^{2+} is bound
to calcium–binding protein (CaBP) calmodulin. It is
proposed that calmodulin is bound to or part of the
transport filament itself. It could activate the ATPase
on the side arms to utilize the ATP–supplied energy required for movement of the transport filaments. At the
present time the nature of the transport filament is
unclear (Ochs, 1981).

Hormone-Secreting Neurons

From the foregoing, it is evident that nerve cells
function as secretory cells in that they possess
mechanisms for synthesis, transport, and release of
transmitter substances. In addition, there are certain
glandlike neurons in the vertebrate brain that serve as
links in the chain that join the neural to the endocrine
system. These neurosecretory cells are found in the
hypothalamohypophyseal system. The cell bodies are
found in the supraoptic and paraventricular nucleus of
the hypothalamus (Figure 11).

The cells in the supraoptic nucleus synthesize
vasopressin, the antidiuretic hormone (ADH), which is
transported down the axon and secreted from the axon
terminals in the posterior pituitary gland. There it is
accumulated in storage cells and then passes into the
bloodstream to control the absorption of fluid from
the bloodstream by the kidneys. An insufficient synthesis or release of ADH from the posterior pituitary,
results in low reabsorption of water from the kidney
tubules which will cause polyurea and polydipsia (excessive urination and thirst), a condition known as
diabetes insipidus (Moses, 1980). Alcohol (ethanol)
blocks the action of ADH, leading to the same effects
but to a milder degree. Vasopressin also raises blood
pressure by causing contraction of small blood vessels.

The cells in the paraventricular nucleus produce oxytocin. After it is transported and stored in the pituitary
gland, it enters the bloodstream and under appropriate
circumstances causes contractions of the uterus and
ejection of milk from the mammary glands. Because
the hypothalamus receives stimuli via the nervous system from the external as well as the internal environment, it is affected by stress, which can cause alterations in normal kidney function that lead to excessive
urination, or which can interrupt milk flow in nursing
mothers. Conversely, drugs that block the neurotransmitters acting upon the hypothalamus can significantly reduce the physiological effects of stress.

FIGURE 11. HYPOTHALAMOHYPOPHYSEAL SYS- ▶
TEM. Cells in the paraventricular and the supraoptic nuclei
secrete hormones, which are released in the posterior
pituitary gland, are absorbed by the blood vessels within the
gland, and are distributed to sites of action. Other inhibiting
and releasing factors are secreted from the hypothalamic cells
into the median eminence, where they are absorbed and carried by the portal veins to the anterior pituitary gland to control the release of pituitary hormones. (From Frohmann,
1980.)

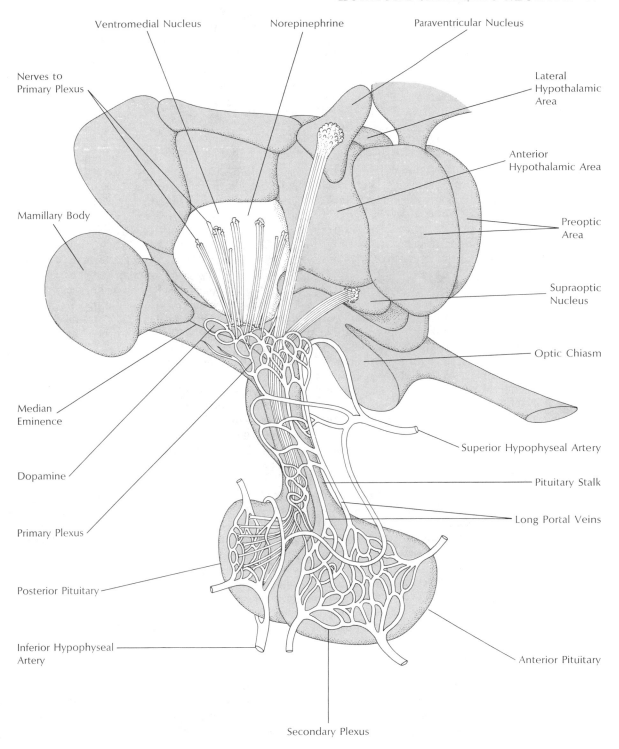

Ventromedial Nucleus

Norepinephrine

Paraventricular Nucleus

Nerves to
Primary Plexus

Lateral
Hypothalamic
Area

Anterior
Hypothalamic Area

Mamillary Body

Preoptic
Area

Supraoptic
Nucleus

Optic Chiasm

Median
Eminence

Superior Hypophyseal Artery

Dopamine

Pituitary Stalk

Long Portal Veins

Primary Plexus

Posterior Pituitary

Inferior Hypophyseal
Artery

Anterior Pituitary

Secondary Plexus

It has also been discovered that neurons in the hypothalamus are capable of releasing a wide variety of substances known as peptide inhibiting and releasing factors or hormones. Peptide hormones, which exist in very small amounts, are secreted into blood vessels and are carried to the anterior lobe of the pituitary gland, where they influence the release of pituitary hormones. The pituitary hormones regulate metabolism, growth, sexual cycles, and so on. There is strong evidence that similar peptide hormones are secreted in many other parts of the brain and have functions quite independent from their hypothalamic counterparts. For example, they have complex interactions with many drugs and neurotransmitters. They are also involved with motor effects, mood, sleep, drinking, appetite, sexual behavior, learning and memory, and blood pressure. These peptides are discussed more fully in Chapter 10.

Nerve Cell Membrane

As with virtually all cells, a membrane surrounds all the parts of the neuron: the perikaryon, the dendrites, and the axon. This membrane is referred to as the CYTO-PLASMIC MEMBRANE to distinguish it from the membranes that surround the organelles such as the nucleus and the mitochondria. The cytoplasmic membrane, approximately 8 to 10 nm thick, plays a crucial role in all cells, but in neurons it has a special ability to transmit information rapidly along the sometimes lengthy extensions of the cell and to other cells.

Membrane Function

The usual function of cytoplasmic membranes is to serve as sturdy envelopes to maintain the identity of the cell and its parts. They also serve as discriminating gates, allowing the passage of some molecules in or out of the cell and excluding others. Membranes also contain structures that function as "pumps," forcing substances against a concentration gradient (that is, from an area of low concentration to one of high concentration). For example, normally there are more sodium ions (Na^+) and fewer potassium ions (K^+) on the outside of a nerve cell than on the inside. It would be expected that Na^+ would tend to flow into the cell and K^+ to flow out, but membrane pumps force Na^+ out and pull K^+ into the cell. These membrane pumps and other related functions are responsible for the fact that there is an electrical charge that exists across the membrane, the RESTING POTENTIAL—a fact of great

importance, as we shall see, in nerve functioning. The cell membrane also controls the passage into the cell of oxygen, nutrients, and precursors (preceding substances; "raw materials") of the neurotransmitters, as well as the passage out of the cell of carbon dioxide and other waste products, which enter the bloodstream and are excreted.

Membrane Structure

Structurally, membranes are composed of two classes of molecules: proteins and lipids. The proteins also serve as enzymes and give the membrane its distinctive character with respect to its gating functions. Lipids (molecules that make up fats and waxes) provide the main structural characteristics of membranes. In nerve cells, small amounts of carbohydrate (sugar) are associated with protein to form GLYCOPROTEINS, and with lipids to form GLYCOLIPIDS. Lipids constitute approximately 40–50 percent of the mass of most membranes, and proteins about the same, with glycoproteins and glycolipids usually constituting less than 10 percent. In the brain as a whole, lipids constitute about 50 percent of the dry weight, compared with 6 to 20 percent in other organs.

Membrane Lipids. Membrane lipid molecules have three parts: a polar head (so designated because it carries an electric charge), a glycerol "backbone," and two tails of long-chain hydrocarbons (similar to those in oil molecules), making up fatty acids, which are nonpolar.

The polar head contains phosphate and other constituents; thus these lipids are known as PHOSPHOLIPIDS. Figure 12 shows the molecular arrangement of the lipid molecule phosphatidylcholine, a lipid commonly found in membranes. Note the negative charge ($-$) on the phosphate group (PO_4).

Lipids known as CEREBROSIDES (Figure 13) are found on neuronal membranes. They contain both a sugar and an amino alcohol called SPHINGOSINE. These lipids are classified both as GLYCOLIPIDS and as SPHINGOLIPIDS. SPHINGOMYELIN is a lipid that is a constituent of the myelin sheaths of nerve cells. Other lipids known as GANGLIOSIDES are found in the cytoplasmic membrane of nerve terminals. They have very large heads made up of complex sugars. Also, they have an affinity for the calcium ion (Ca^{2+}) (which plays an important role in membrane function) and are thus involved in the excitability of neurons.

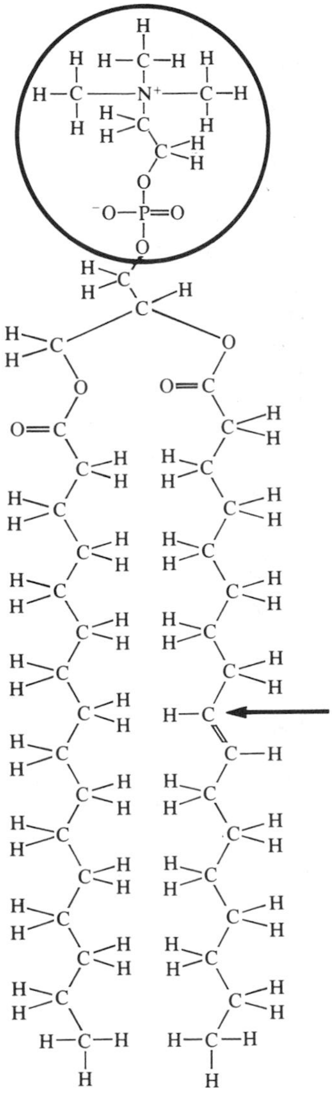

Sphingomyelin

A cerebroside

CH₃
CH₃—N—CH₃ (Choline)
CH₂
CH₂
O
C=P—O⁻ (Phosphoric acid)
O
CH₂
HO—C——C—H
CH   NH
HC   C=O
CH₂   CH₂
CH₂   CH₂
CH₂   CH₂
CH₂   CH₂
CH₂   CH₂
CH₂   CH₂
CH₂   CH
CH₂   CH
CH₂   CH₂
CH₂   CH₂
CH₂   CH₂
CH₃   CH₂
       CH₂
       CH₂
       CH₂
       CH₃

Sphingosine

Fatty acid

(Cerebroside right structure, sugar ring)
H—OH
H—OH   CH₂OH
HO—H   O
H—O
OH   CH₂
H—C———C—H
CH   NH
HC   C=O
CH₂   CH₂
CH₂   CH₂
CH₂   CH₂
CH₂   CH₂
CH₂   CH₂
CH₂   CH₂
CH₂   CH₂
CH₂   CH₂
CH₂   CH₂
CH₂   CH₂
CH₃   CH₂
       CH₂
       CH₂
       CH₂
       CH₂
       CH₂
       CH₂
       CH₂
       CH₃

Sugar

FIGURE 12. MOLECULE OF PHOSPHATIDYL-CHOLINE. Note the negative charge on the phosphate group in the polar head. The fatty acid tail on the left is saturated, meaning that every carbon atom is linked to two or three hydrogen atoms. The tail on the right is unsaturated, with a double bond between carbon atoms at the point indicated by the arrow.

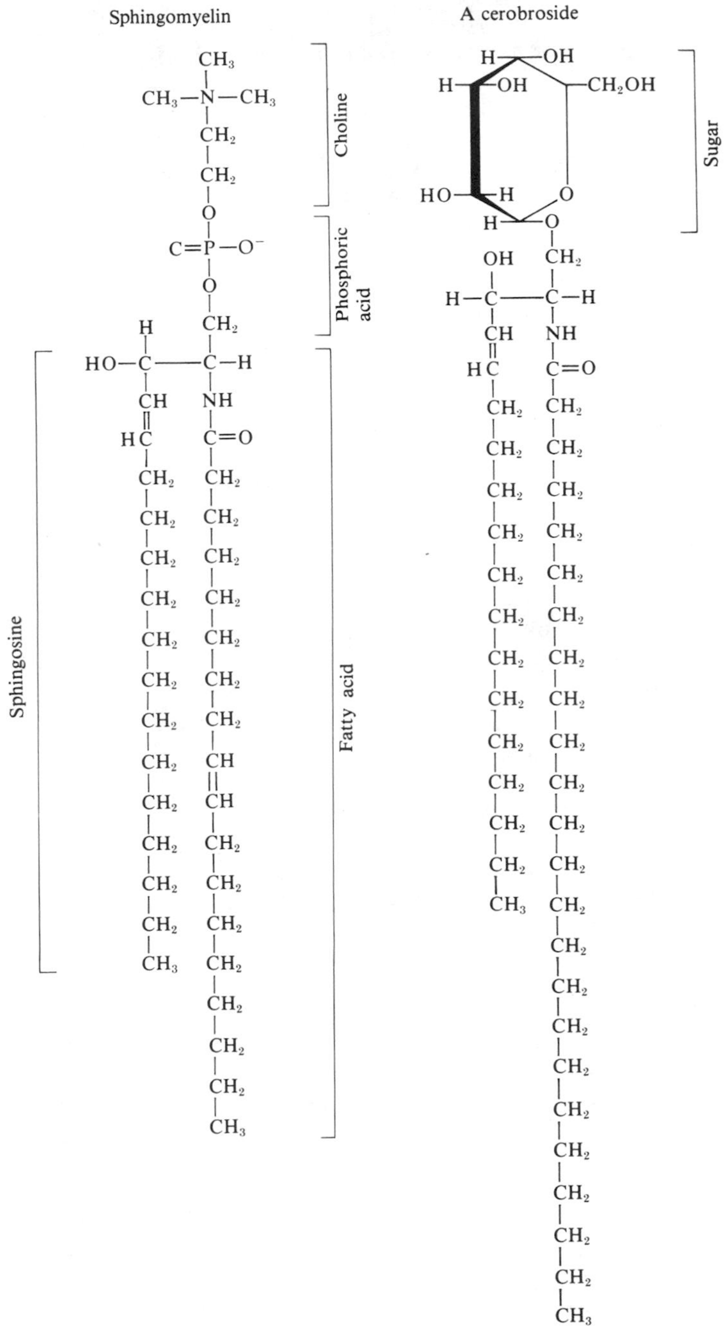

FIGURE 13. A SPHINGOLIPID AND A CEREBRO-SIDE. Sphingomyelin is the most common and the simplest sphingolipid. It contains one molecule of a fatty acid, one of sphingosine, one of phosphoric acid, and one of the alcohol choline. The cerebroside shown on the right is a sphingolipid that has a sugar molecule in addition to sphingosine and a fatty acid molecule.

An important feature of lipids is the water–soluble nature of the polar head, which is therefore designated as HYDROPHILIC. The fatty acid tails, on the other hand, are water insoluble and are designated as HYDROPHOBIC, a property that is exemplified by the insolubility of oils and waxes in water. Molecules with a hydrophilic end and a hydrophobic end are called AMPHIPATHIC: phospholipids and glycolipids are examples of amphipathic molecules. Because of the amphipathic nature of biological lipids, they naturally form a bilayer with the polar heads oriented toward the aqueous materials on the outside and the inside of the cell. The tails of the lipid molecules are oriented toward each other and are buried in the membrane interior (Figure 14). This lipid bilayer is about 4.5 nm thick and is the structural framework of the membrane as well as the anchoring structure for the proteins associated with the membrane.

The lipid bilayer has an additional function: It serves as an effective barrier to water-soluble (polar) substances such as metal ions, sugars, and amino acids. Yet, all of these substances are of importance in the viability and function of the cell. Therefore, in order for polar substances to be incorporated into nerve cells, some form of openings or "carriers" must be available to transport them through the lipid barrier. The "carrier" system consists of the proteins that are associated with the membranes. Moreover, each type of cell has its own typical protein carriers to transport those substances that are necessary for that cell's particular function. Where and how these proteins are synthesized and transported to the cell membrane is subject to considerable conjecture, but it is likely that the cytoplasmic ribosomes of each cell synthesizes its own appropriate membrane proteins (Bretscher, 1973).

Membrane Proteins. Proteins associated with membranes are of two types: extrinsic and intrinsic. The EXTRINSIC PROTEINS are located on the membrane surfaces (either on the inner or outer surface), whereas the INTRINSIC PROTEINS enter the lipid bilayer either partially or completely (i.e., spanning the membrane and protruding on both sides) (Figure 15). Such intrinsic proteins are amphipathic, as are the lipid molecules. Only part of an intrinsic protein molecule is exposed to the aqueous surface; the rest is submerged in an oily medium formed by the fatty acid chains. The stability of this molecule and its position in the membrane depends upon its amphipathic nature. Proteins are

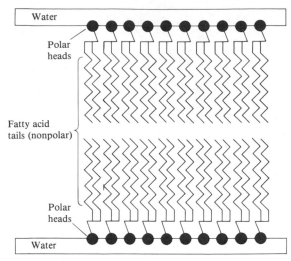

FIGURE 14.   CROSS-SECTION OF A LIPID MEMBRANE. The membrane is formed from two layers of lipid molecules. The polar heads of amphipathic lipids face the aqueous solution on each side of the membrane, whereas the nonpolar fatty acid tails face inward, toward each other.

made up of chains of amino acids, some of which are hydrophilic, others of which are hydrophobic. It turns out that intrinsic proteins have a large proportion of hydrophobic amino acids, whereas extrinsic membrane proteins have a large proportion of hydrophilic amino acids.

Cell membranes exhibit internal movement of proteins and lipids. It is probably very rare that lipids or proteins move from the inner to the outer layer or vice versa, as it would require much energy to force the hydrophilic end of a molecule down through the hydrophobic interior of the membrane. There is evidence, however, that lateral movement does occur. The factors that determine this movement are the extent of saturation of the lipid tails and the environmental temperature. SATURATION in this context means the degree to which hydrogen atoms are linked to every carbon atom. An unsaturated condition exits when carbon atoms are linked by double bonds to other carbon atoms. The lipid molecule of phosphatidylcholine shown in Figure 12 contains a saturated fatty acid tail on the left and an unsaturated tail on the right. When phospholipids are saturated, the fatty acid tails nest together and form a rigid structure (Figure 16). When double bonds are present, deformations interfere with orderly stacking and the fatty acid is more

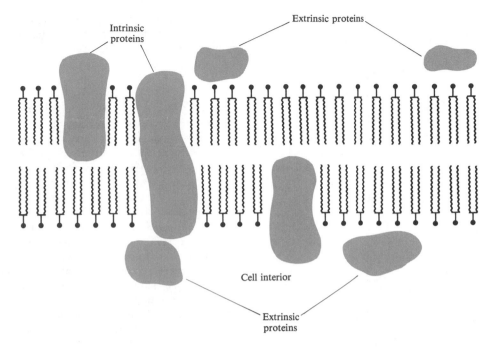

FIGURE 15.   A BIOLOGICAL MEMBRANE. The basic structure is formed of phospholipid molecules stacked side by side and tail to tail. The gray shapes represent protein molecules, seen in all possible positions with respect to the lipid layers: they can be entirely inside or outside the cell, they can penetrate one of the surfaces, or they can extend through the membrane.

fluid, especially at physiological temperatures around 37 °C. There is a relationship between the fluidity of the lipid layer and the rate of transfer of substances across the membrane. Experiments have shown that when the proportion of unsaturated fatty acids is high, transport across the membrane can be 20 times faster than when the membrane is low in unsaturated fatty acids (Capaldi, 1974). There is also a relationship between the environmental temperature and the amount of unsaturated fatty acids in membranes. The lower the temperature, the greater the proportion of unsaturated fatty acids in the membrane. It has been reported that there is a temperature gradient in the limbs of the reindeer: the temperature is highest near the body and lowest near the hooves. This has great functional significance. It can be appreciated that near the hooves the fatty acids could congeal because of low temperature, thus blocking adequate transfer of nutrients and other substances into cells. With an increased proportion of unsaturated fatty acids in the chilled parts of the leg, there is adequate compensation for the temperature differences and membrane function is equalized (Fox, 1972).

Transport Across Membranes

Living cells cannot exist for long without an influx of substances such as oxygen and nutrients and an excretion of waste products. Most cells have relatively short life spans and are replaced by cells that are newly formed by cell division. In warm-blooded species, however, nerve cells for the most part do not multiply after birth. Consequently, the continued vitality and function of nerve cells is dependent upon the flow of a variety of substances across their membranes. It should be especially noted that synaptic functioning depends upon rapid and efficient intake, release, and recapture of a variety of materials.

Many mechanisms control the transport of substances across membranes. These substances comprise small and large molecules, ionized and un-ionized molecules, and lipid-soluble molecules. Some substances simply flow down the concentration gradient

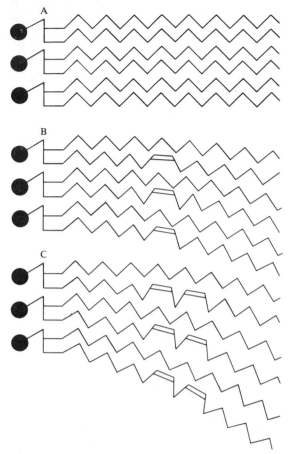

FIGURE 16.   EFFECTS OF VARIATION IN FATTY ACID COMPOSITION. (A) If a lipid layer is composed entirely of saturated fatty acids, the fatty acid chains nest together to form rigid structures. (B) In a lipid layer containing unsaturated fatty acids with one double bond, the double bond causes deformations that interfere with orderly stacking and makes the fatty acid region somewhat fluid. (C) When more double bonds are present, the deformations and resulting fluidity are greater still. (After Fox, 1972.)

(i.e., from a compartment with a high concentration to one with a low concentration); others must be transported against (up) a concentration gradient (i.e., from a compartment of low concentration to one of high concentration). In general, when substances flow across membranes and down a concentration gradient, there is no expenditure of energy by the cell. These forms of transport are designated as passive. In contrast, when substances are carried up a concentration,

a type of "pump" activity is necessary and requires energy to drive it. This energy–requiring process is known as active transport.

Passive Transport

Filtration

Small molecules that are dissolved in water easily penetrate the nerve cell membrane through small aqueous (water-filled) pores that are approximately 0.7 to 0.8 nm in diameter. This process is called FILTRATION.

These small pores are assumed to exist because studies have shown that water–soluble molecules pass freely through the cell membrane. The electron microscope has not revealed the presence of these pores because, first, their size is below the resolving power of the electron microscope, and, second, the pores are assumed to be relatively far apart (the total area of all the pores only accounts for 1/1600 of the total area of the membrane; Holter, 1961). The principal determinant of the direction of the flow of small molecules in or out of the cell depends for the most part on a PRESSURE GRADIENT across the membrane (i.e., a higher fluid pressure on one side of the membrane) and the size of the particles to be filtered in comparison to the size of the pores. Filtration is important for the movement of large molecules across membranes, the formation of urine in the kidneys, and the elimination of waste substances from the body (Levine, 1973).

Passive Diffusion

Some substances are soluble in the lipid part of the membrane. They can easily cross the lipid barrier, provided that they are for the most part un-ionized. This process is known as PASSIVE DIFFUSION. All that is needed for the transport of a lipid-soluble substance is a concentration gradient of the substance across the cell membrane.

Facilitated Diffusion

A third type of transport, FACILITATED DIFFUSION, accounts for some peculiarities in the way certain water-soluble and lipid-insoluble molecules pass through membranes. For example, optical isomers of molecules with similar lipid insolubilities have been found to have different rates of membrane penetration. Additionally, there are some molecules that show membrane penetration rates that initially are proportional to the gradient across the membrane. However, as the concentration in one compartment increases beyond a certain point, the penetration rate into the other compartment levels off, suggesting a limiting factor. To account for these effects, a hypothetical receptor or carrier has been proposed. The carrier binds with the molecule and "carries" the molecule through the membrane, down the concentration gradient (Figure 17A). It can be understood that if the proposed carriers (probably protein molecules) were more selec-

tive for one isomer than another it would account for differences in membrane penetration between isomers of the molecule. Also, if there were a limited number of "carriers," it would account for the limit imposed upon the penetration rate (Levine, 1973).

Within the CNS, some lipid-insoluble molecules (such as glucose) can readily penetrate the capillary walls and enter the brain, but in these cases transport

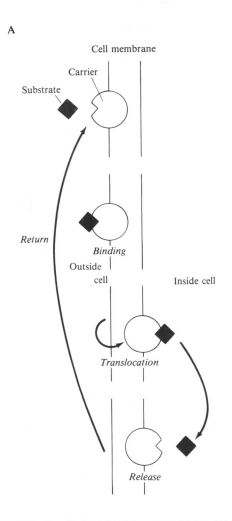
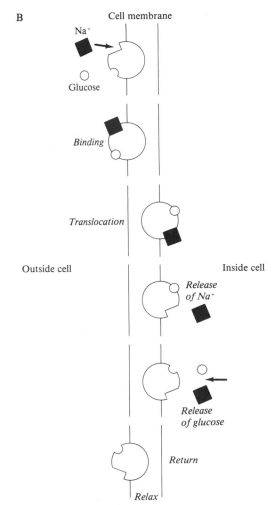

FIGURE 17. FACILITATED DIFFUSION. (A) The carrier, probably a protein, accepts the substrate and transports it into the cell. The driving force for the reaction is the concentration gradient of the substrate between the outside and the inside of the cell. (B) Glucose transport depends upon a high concentration of sodium ions outside the cell. In this model, the binding of Na$^+$ increases the affinity of the carrier protein for glucose. The Na$^+$ gradient thus contributes to the "recognition" of the glucose molecule and provides the driving force for the translocation of both Na$^+$ and glucose into the cell. (After Dyson, 1978.)

also depends on specialized proteins that are usually found on the endothelial cell membranes and that have a high affinity for the transported substance. The affinity here is also stereospecific, with the D form being preferred. In addition, the sodium ion assists in glucose transport. The high concentration of Na^+ outside the cell participates by altering the membrane protein so that it accepts the glucose molecule, and carries it into the cell where it is released (Figure 17B). Thus, the high extracellular Na^+ concentration provides the driving force for facilitated transport for this and other molecules, a condition called Na^+-DEPENDENT FACILITATED TRANSPORT. This form of transport affects the movement of certain amino acids, pyruvic acid, lactic acid, and some sugars.

The high specificity of the carrier proteins automatically excludes a wide range of useless or potentially harmful substances. Moreover, the finite number of specialized protein molecules limits the activity of this system, making it somewhat independent of the substrate concentration of most substances outside the cell. For example, sudden exertion could lead to a rapid elevation of blood lactic acid. An excessive flux of lactic acid into the brain could alter the brain acid–base balance. The limited amount of specialized protein carrier, however, reduces this possibility.

In summary, these three types of transport across the cell membrane—filtration (the transport of small molecules in solution through the hypothetical aqueous pores), passive diffusion of lipid-soluble substances, and facilitated diffusion—primarily require a concentration gradient across the membrane to provide the motive force for particle movement.

Active Transport

Membrane Pump

Membrane pumps are responsible for the movement of molecules up a concentration gradient, that is, from an area of low concentration to an area of high concentration. For example, many neurotransmitters are small water-soluble molecules that pass freely through membranes by filtration. However, these molecules are then carried back into the neuron and are used over and over again. This recycling may involve transport of molecules from an area of low concentration in the synaptic cleft back into the cell, where the concentration may be hundreds of times greater.

Consider another example. The concentration of potassium ions (K^+) is about 40 percent lower in the brain extracellular fluid (ECF) than in blood plasma, yet it is pumped from the ECF into the blood. Presumably this process requires a carrier mechanism and considerable energy expenditure, which is probably met by the action of the large number of mitochondria in the brain capillary endothelium (Oldendorf, 1975). The energy is required to alter the carrier molecule's shape, that is, to rotate it from one position and to enable it to rotate back to its original position. This process is known as the "pumping" action of cells. When cells are poisoned with DNP, thereby causing a decline in metabolic activity, the pumping action fails and substances flow only down their concentration gradients, either depleting the cell of vital materials or filling it with substances at concentrations incompatible with the cell's normal functions. The pumping action also accounts for the maintenance of the proper balance of Na^+ and K^+ within neurons.

Pinocytosis and Exocytosis

There are other mechanisms of active membrane transport. Pinocytosis was mentioned earlier as a mechanism for transporting large molecules through the membranes of the endothelial cells that make up blood capillary walls. PINOCYTOSIS refers to the capture of molecules for transport into a cell. This process involves the invagination of the outer surface of the cell membrane into which the transportable molecules migrate. The edges around the neck of the invagination fuse together, enveloping the molecules within the membrane. When the molecules reach the inner surface of the membrane, the membrane units presumably separate and lyse, permitting the release of the molecules into the cytoplasm.

EXOCYTOSIS refers to the transfer of a molecular product, which has been synthesized within a cell, across the cytoplasmic membrane to the extracellular or synaptic space or into ducts for storage and distribution. Exocytosis usually involves the transfer of molecules that have been taken up and sequestered in vesicles. These vesicles, which may be pinched-off terminal sections of neurotubules or may be synthesized in the perikaryon, are carried via axoplasmic flow in the cytoplasm to the axon terminals. There the vesicles join the cytoplasmic membrane and under certain conditions the combined membrane breaks, allowing the contents of the vesicles to spill out. Endocrine and exocrine glands release their products (hormones, enzymes, digestive secretions, milk) in this fashion.

Michaelis Constant

The transport of substances across membranes are sometimes designated as high- or low-affinity processes. Affinity in this context refers to the *rate of* membrane transport and is expressed as a MICHAELIS CONSTANT (K_m). It is applicable when the method of transport involves the binding of a SUBSTRATE (the substance to be transported) to a membrane receptor protein, which "carries" the substance across the membrane. In this instance, K_m refers to the extracellular concentration of the substrate that would yield one-half of the maximum velocity (V_{max}) for a given amount of the receptor protein. It can be seen graphically (Figure 18) that the velocity of the substrate, given an increase in its concentration, rises and reaches a plateau. This means that up to a point, transport is proportional to the amount of substrate. Ultimately, however, the rate of reaction cannot be increased by adding more substrate because the receptor protein becomes saturated. Stated another way, passage is already occurring at the maximum rate. It is also true that the steeper the slope of the curve, the smaller will be K_m. Thus, a more active receptor protein is associated with a low K_m and high affinity. Some cells will have both a high- and a low-affinity process for a given substrate. For example, the amino acids glycine and aspartic acid serve important physiological functions within most cells, but they serve as neurotransmitters for some nerve cells as well. In these cells, two distinct transport affinities for these substances have been found. The high affinity transport system associated with nerve terminals takes up the amino acids that are released as neurotransmitters; the low affinity system is most likely associated with the uptake of amino acids for metabolic purposes (Snyder et al., 1973).

Neuroglia

Even though neurons are the functional unit of the nervous system, neuroglia (or simply GLIA) vastly outnumber neurons. However, because of their small size compared to neurons, they constitute only about half the bulk of the human brain. Glia have cellular extensions but do not make synaptic contacts. However, adjacent glia have what appear to be fused membrane contacts or GAP JUNCTIONS. These are regions of high ionic conductance, meaning that ions pass across the membranes rather easily (see Chapter 5). Unlike neurons, glia continue to divide and multiply during

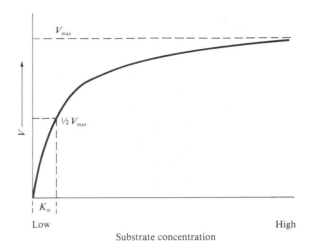

FIGURE 18. MICHAELIS CONSTANT (K_m). Substrate concentration affects the reaction rate. K_m is the substrate concentration that yields one-half the maximum velocity (V_{max}) for the reaction being studied.

the life of the organism. They also contain, like neurons, all of the structural elements of actively living cells, such as mitochondria, endoplasmic reticulum, and ribosomes.

There are three types of glial cells. ASTROGLIA, consisting of two subtypes (fibrous and protoplasmic), generally have star-shaped perikarya with many long cytoplasmic extensions which terminate in "end feet" (Figure 19A). These glia are interposed between neurons and blood capillaries, with their "end feet" making contact with both (see Figures 3 and 4 in Chapter 1). They fill in the space between neurons leaving gaps of approximately 15-20 nm. These gaps make up approximately 20-25 percent of the brain volume and constitute a true extracellular space, that is, the fluid-filled areas between cells (Davson, 1972). Astroglia also surround synapses, insulating one neuron from another and insuring independent functioning.

MICROGLIA are substantially smaller than astroglia and are always present in the vicinity of blood capillaries and neurons (Figure 19B). When neural tissue is injured, elongated microglia (Figure 19C) rapidly migrate in large numbers to the area of injury and serve a macrophagic function, that is, they digest damaged neural tissue. During phagocytosis they lose their celluar extensions and assume a globular form, and are laden with lipids and cell remnants (Figure 19D).

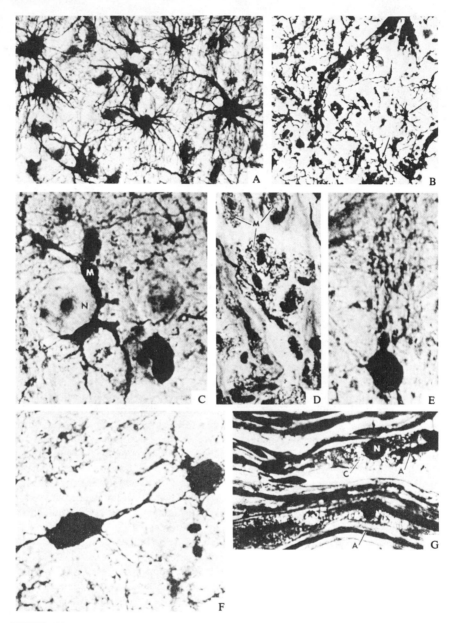

FIGURE 19.   TYPES OF NEUROGLIAL CELLS. (A) Astroglia of the fibrous type, illustrating the multiple cell extensions and variations in cell size. x500. (B) Typical microglia indicated by the arrows. At the same magnification they are significantly smaller than astroglia. x500. (C) Elongated microglia (M) in the process of migration to an injured area. It is in contact with a neuron (N). x1500. (D) Globular-shaped microglial cells (M) which have lost their processes and contain lipid droplets and cell debris. x1500. (E) Oligodendroglial cell with a characteristic round cell body and long beaded processes. x1500. (F) Oligodendroglial cell of the larger type. x1500. (G) Schwann cell in relation with a peripheral axon. (A, axon; C, cytoplasmic network of Schwann cell; N, nucleus of Schwann cell). x1500. (From Crosby et al., 1962.)

When examining stained brain tissue to find the track of a fine electrode that has penetrated the brain, a thin line of densely stained microglia lining a gap in the tissue is a good indication of the slight tissue damage caused by the electrode.

OLIGODENDROGLIA are found in four varieties, (1) small elements with numerous long beady processes (Figure 19E); (2) larger elements of similar type (Figure 19F); (3) transitional forms similar to Schwann cells; and (4) the Schwann cells themselves (Figure 19G). The first three types are abundant within the central nervous system maintaining a close relationship with neurons and their extensions while active in the process of myelin formation. The fourth type, the Schwann cells, are found primarily along peripheral nerves where they serve a myelinization function (see Figure 7).

It has been found that glia absorb surplus K^+ that may exist in the extracellular space. This is important because high levels of extracellullar K^+ increase the excitability of neurons. There is also evidence that glia take up a number of amino acids that serve either as precursors to neurotransmitters or as neurotransmitters themselves. Thus glia may serve to regulate the supply of these substances to nerve cells. In addition glia are thought to provide long-term metabolic support for neurons since neurons do not survive long in tissue cultures if they are separated from glial cells.

Summary

This chapter described the structure and internal activities of the functional unit of the nervous system, the nerve cell. Nerve cells function in many ways as all cells do except that they do not undergo cell division. Nerve cells metabolize fuels to maintain their own biological integrity and to carry out their unique functions—the transmission of messages from internal and external sense organs to different levels of coordination and integration, and the transmission of messages from the nervous system to muscles and glands for the execution of activities vital to the organism. Special emphasis has been made to point out the importance of cell membranes because drug molecules exert their initial effects in almost all cases on neuron membranes to set in motion the series of events that ultimately lead to behavioral effects.

Recommended Readings

Dyson, R.D. (1978). *Cell Biology*. Allyn & Bacon, Boston. A college text that is well written and profusely illustrated. It describes the structures of many kinds of cells, and the organelles within them and discusses the chemical reactions that are unique to living organisms.

Siegel, G.J., Albers, R.W., Agranoff, B.W., and Katzman, R. (Eds.) (1981). *Basic Neurochemistry*. Little, Brown, Boston. A fine collection of short essays on the chemistry of nerve cells in normal and pathological conditions.

Singer, S.J. and Nicolson, G.L. (1972). The fluid mosaic model of the structure of cell membranes. *Science*, 175, 720–731. A presentation of the generally accepted view of the structure of cell membranes.

Tower, D.B. (Ed. in Chief) (1975). *The Nervous System, Vol. 1, The Basic Neurosciences*. Raven Press, New York. A collection of short reviews on many aspects of nerve structure and function. Some areas that are considered are neuropharmacology, biochemistry of learning and memory, developmental neurobiology, neuroimmunology, and synthetic machinery.

CHAPTER FOUR

Neurophysiological Mechanisms

The foregoing account of nerve cell morphology now leads to a review of the physiological events that are responsible for neural functioning. Neurophysiology deals with the electrochemical events involved in the transmission of signals from one end of the nerve cell to the other and from cell to cell. This process is quite complicated; however, for our purposes a review of the basic principles can provide the basis for an understanding of drug actions on neural systems.

Contemporary knowledge of nerve physiology stems largely from work that was begun in the 1930s, was interrupted by World War II, and was resumed at an accelerated pace during the postwar years. In 1963, J.C. Eccles, A.L. Hodgkin, and A.F. Huxley were awarded the Nobel prize in physiology and medicine for their contributions to the understanding of nerve function. In 1970, J. Axelrod, B. Katz, and U.S. von Euler were also awarded the Nobel prize. These men and their associates were among the many scientists that laid the foundation of contemporary neurophysiology.

Neuron Excitability

Virtually all cells in biological systems are excitable in that they respond to external stimuli and perform functions appropriate to their morphology. Thus, glandular cells secrete, muscle cells contract, and nerve cells generate and conduct nerve impulses. Cell membranes play a major role in initiating and sustaining the activities for many kinds of cells. In the nerve cell, the membrane plays the principal role in generating and conducting nerve impulses. The membrane properties that are relevant to neuron excitability are *permeability* to some ions and *impermeability* to others and the

presence of carrier proteins for transport of substances through the membrane. The consequence of this selective permeability and transport is the development of a voltage difference between the inside and the outside of the cell. This voltage difference is known as the MEMBRANE POTENTIAL or RESTING POTENTIAL.

Resting Potential

Many of the important early experiments in neurophysiology were done on the giant axon of squid and related species. The giant axon conducts nerve impulses to the jetlike apparatus that propels these creatures through the water. The axons are 0.5–1.0 mm in diameter, which is approximately 100 times larger than the largest mammalian axons and is large enough to allow insertion of microelectrodes, used to stimulate and record internal neuroelectric events. If the electrode diameter is small enough (approximately 0.5 μm), the axon membrane will seal itself around the electrode, and the axon will function quite normally for many hours.

If two recording microelectrodes are in contact with the membrane of a squid axon placed in a seawater bath, no voltage is recorded (Figure 1A). When one electrode is inserted into the axoplasm, a voltage difference of approximately 70 millivolts (-70 mV) is recorded between the axoplasm and the axon exterior surface (Figure 1B). This voltage difference is defined as the RESTING POTENTIAL of an inactive neuron: the inside is negative with respect to the outside. Although the voltage difference is small, it must be remembered that the membrane is thin—about a millionth of a centimeter. Thus, the resting potential is equivalent to

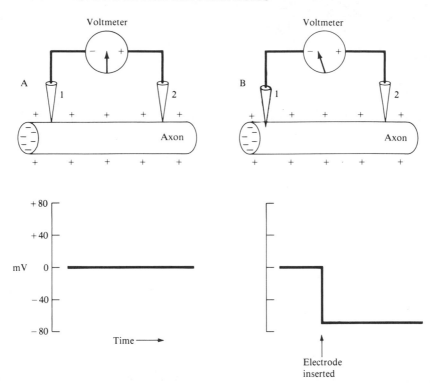

FIGURE 1 INTRACELLULAR RECORDING FROM A SQUID AXON. (A) Microelectrodes are applied to the membrane surface and detect no voltage change. (B) Microelec-trode 1 is inserted into the axoplasm, and a voltage change is recorded. The graphs chart the voltage changes over time.

100,000 volts across a membrane-like structure 1 cm thick. It should also be noted that -70 mV is only approximate and that the actual value for the resting potential differs for neurons of different animal species, for different neurons within the same organism, and, indeed, between membranes surrounding the cell body and the axon of the same neuron.

As mentioned earlier, resting potentials exist largely because of the differences in membrane permeability to different ion species. The differential permeability causes an unequal distribution of ions between the inside and the outside of the cell. Figure 2 schematically shows the relative concentrations of different ions on either side of the membrane of a squid axon in a seawater bath. The organic anions (A^-) are highly concentrated in the axoplasm but are absent in seawater. The concentration of K^+ is approximately 40 times greater inside than outside the membrane, whereas Na^+ is approximately 9 times and Cl^- is approximately 13.5 times greater outside than inside.

How does selective permeability lead to differen-tial ion concentrations and the resting potential? Specifically, the membrane is impermeable to organic anions (A^-) of aspartic, glutamic, and fumaric acids. The large size of the organic anions may prevent their passage through the aqueous pores of the axon membrane. They are also lipid insoluble. However, the membrane is quite permeable to K^+ but almost impermeable to Na^+. In fact, the permeability of K^+ is about 100 times the permeability of Na^+. This is due to the difference in size between hydrated K^+ and hydrated Na^+, whose diameters are 0.396 and 0.512 nm, respectively.* The difference in size affects the ease with which ions pass through the axon membrane. Cl^- are relatively small (0.386 nm), and the membrane is almost completely permeable to them.

The uneven distribution of ions occurs in the follow-

*Because of the electrical charge, ions attract water molecules, which form an envelope around them. Although Na^+ is smaller than K^+, it attracts more water and is larger in its hydrated form than hydrated K^+.

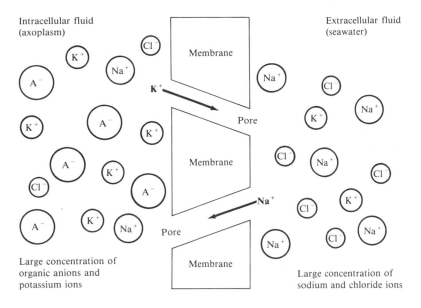

Intracellular fluid
(axoplasm)

Extracellular fluid
(seawater)

Membrane

Pore

Membrane

Pore

Membrane

Large concentration of
organic anions and
potassium ions

Large concentration of
sodium and chloride ions

| Ion | Concentration (mM) | |
	Axoplasm	Seawater
Organic anions (A⁻)	345	0
Potassium ions (K⁺)	400	10
Sodium ions (Na⁺)	50	460
Chloride ion (Cl⁻)	40	540

FIGURE 2 UNEQUAL ION CONCENTRATIONS. The shaded area represents a section of the membrane of a squid axon that divides the intracellular from the extracellular fluid (seawater). In the fluid of the two compartments, various ion species are suspended. The membrane pores are slanted to indicate the directions of the concentration gradients for K^+ and Na^+, that is, the higher intracellular concentration of K^+ induces it to flow out to the extracellular fluid, and the higher Na^+ concentration outside the cell induces it to flow inward. The membrane is impermeable to the organic anions (A^-), and the pores for Cl^- transport are not shown. The table shows the molar concentrations of the ion species in squid axoplasm and in seawater, which is similar to the extracellular fluid in animal tissue. (After Woodbury, 1966.)

ing way. As the organic acids dissociate in the cytoplasm, the organic anions (A^-) must remain within the cell, whereas the cations (+) are free to cross the membrane barrier. This causes a buildup of an electrostatic negative charge inside the axon that attracts cations into the cell. Thus, K^+ moves freely into the cell and is held there. However, as the internal concentration of K^+ increases, there is a tendency for K^+ to diffuse out of the cell down its concentration gradient (meaning that the ions flow from an area of high concentration toward an area of low concentration). Ultimately, an equilibrium is established in which the electrostatic force that attracts K^+ into the cell is balanced by the concentration force that causes K^+ to flow out of the cell. The electrostatic force that balances the concentration force for K^+ is -70 mV, which is the resting potential for the membrane. It can now be appreciated that the resting potential is essentially the result of the actions of K^+.

Cl^- flow easily through the membrane. Therefore, Cl^- concentration inside the cell also is approximately balanced by the resting potential and the external concentration. The high external concentration tends to push Cl^- into the cell, but the internal negative charge repels the negative charge of Cl^-.

Na^+ would also be attracted by the negative charge within the axon, but the membrane is not very permeable to this ion. The concentration of Na^+ increases outside the cell, and the concentration force adds to the tendency of Na^+ to flow into the axon.

But, again, because of the impermeability of the membrane, relatively few sodium ions enter the axon. The few that cross the membrane make the interior of the axon less negative, but this causes some K^+ to flow outward because the membrane is more permeable to K^+, restoring the resting potential to its usual value.

However, the exchange of Na^+ for K^+ leads to another problem. If K^+ are extruded to accommodate the presence of the incoming Na^+, it is possible that Na^+ would eventually replace almost all of the K^+. Another mechanism prevents this from occurring—a mechanism known as the sodium-potassium pump, or simply the sodium pump (Figure 3). The best evidence suggests that the sodium pump consists of an energy-requiring membrane-bound enzyme that exchanges Na^+ for K^+ across the membrane and thus maintains the proper internal and external concentrations of ions. The energy for the enzyme action (which is pushing ions against their concentration gradients) is supplied by ATP.

ATPase, an ATP splitting enzyme, is present in axon membranes and is activated by high internal concentrations of Na^+ and high external concentrations of K^+ (but interestingly, not by the reverse). It is inhibited by substances that interfere with sodium transport (Hodgkin, 1964a; Kuffler and Nicholls, 1976). When the ATP-dependent physiological activities of the neuron are interfered with by the toxic chemical 2,4-dinitrophenol, there is a marked reduction in K^+ influx and Na^+ efflux. Instead, there is increased influx of Na^+ and efflux of K^+. Thus, under conditions during which the sodium pump is inoperative, the ions move with their concentration gradients, a process that requires no energy from the cell.

In order to determine the number of sodium pump sites, peripheral nerves of rabbits were bathed in a solution containing OUABAIN, which is a drug that blocks the action of the sodium pump. The ouabain concentration used was just sufficient to block the pump. The amount of ouabain per unit weight of tissue was measured, and on the basis of the molecular weight of ouabain, the number of bound molecules was calculated. This led to an estimate of 750 pumping sites per square micrometer of tissue (Kuffler and Nicholls, 1976).

In summary, the resting potential of an axon membrane occurs because of its differential permeability to ionic species and because of the action of the sodium pump, which maintains the proper separation of the ions by driving them against their concentration gra-

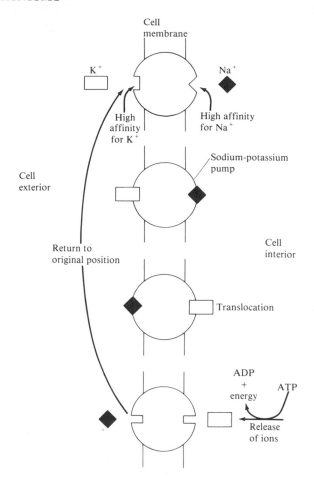

FIGURE 3   THE SODIUM PUMP. In this model, the carrier assumes two configurations. There is a high affinity for K^+ on the outside and a low affinity for K^+ on the inside. The reverse is true for Na^+—a high affinity on the inside and low on the outside. The transition of the carrier is fostered by the hydrolysis of ATP and lasts until the carrier has returned to its original position, that is, with its K^+ binding site on the outside and the Na^+ site on the inside. As a result, Na^+ is pumped out and K^+ is pumped in. (After Dyson, 1978).

dients—K^+ is carried into the cell and Na^+ is carried out. (It will be seen later that the sodium pump plays an additional vital role in maintaining the proper ion concentrations during neural activity.)

Passive Electrical Conduction by Neurons

It is generally known that nerve impulses are some type of electrochemical event. Thus, there is a tendency to think of nerve impulses as being in some ways

Ouabain

similar to the electrical signals carried by telephone wires. It is true that there is some passive* conduction of electrical currents in nerves, as in wires, because the inner contents are wet and contain salts in solution. However, in comparison to a copper wire, neurons are poor conductors because the strength of the currents is rapidly diminished over distance and any on–off pattern of the currents becomes distorted. Therefore, neurons are 1 million to 100 million times worse as conductors than metal wires for the following reasons:

1. In a wire, the charges are carried by a very large number of rapidly moving electrons, whereas in an axon the charge is carried in the axoplasm by much slower and many fewer ions.
2. Neurons are exceedingly thin, ranging from 0.1 to 10 μm in diameter, making them highly resistive.
3. The capacitive characteristics of the neuron membrane cause the positive and negative charges to be separated and stored as in a capacitor. Accordingly, before any current can proceed along the interior of the axon, the capacitive elements have to be filled up. This slows conduction and distorts the electrical signal. An analogous situation occurs during heating of an iron rod. If one end of the rod is placed in a fire, each part of the rod must be heated up before the next part becomes warmer. If the heat is applied in pulses, the pulsations are hardly detectable at the other end.
4. An axolemma (the membrane that surrounds the axon) is only 7.0 nm thick and is a poor insulator. Thus, there is considerable leakage, causing the current to rapidly dissipate with distance. It would be

*Passive in this context means that the neuron conducts current much as a metal wire would, with no expenditure of energy by the wire itself.

as though the iron rod in the previous example were covered with an insulator full of holes.

Hodgkin (1964b) compared electrical conduction in neurons and metal wires. He pointed out that a nerve fiber with a diameter of 1.0 μm has a resistance of 10 ohms/cm. Thus, an axon 1.0 meter in length would, have the same resistivity as a 22-gauge copper wire 10^{10} miles in length—the distance roughly 10 times that between the earth and the planet, Saturn.

The preceding characteristics make neurons poor passive conductors. Therefore, their superb ability as signal carriers must depend upon other features.

Signal Conduction within Neurons

The generation and the propagation of the nerve signal in a squid axon serves as an excellent model because these neural phenomena are virtually the same in every known animal species.

Local Potential

Although action potentials are the signals that are transmitted by neuraxons, there are other important membrane changes called LOCAL POTENTIALS that precede the action potential. In the laboratory, local potentials are generated by a stimulator, which produces electrical pulses that are delivered to the axoplasm through a stimulating electrode (Figure 4). This stimulation induces membrane changes that in turn stimulate the normal activities of the neuron. Oscilloscopes V_1 and V_2 record the resulting voltage changes through the recording electrodes R_1 and R_2 which are

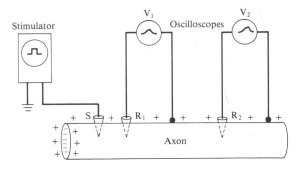

FIGURE 4 STIMULATION AND RECORDING FROM A SQUID AXON. The stimulator delivers a brief electric pulse via the stimulating electrode (S) inserted into the axoplasm. Recording microelectrodes R_1 and R_2 detect voltage changes occurring across the axon membrane. The changes are displayed upon the screens of the oscilloscopes that are acting as voltmeters—V_1 and V_2.

only a few millimeters apart. If the stimulus pulse is positive (+), the stimulus makes the axon interior less negative (say from −70 to −65 mV) and the membrane would be partially depolarized.* If the stimulus pulse is negative (−), then the internal negativity is increased perhaps from −70 to −75 mV, thus hyperpolarizing the membrane.

Figure 5 shows that when brief (1.0 msec) positive stimuli of increasing intensity are applied to the axoplasm, brief depolarizing changes occur at R_1 and R_2 and are recorded by V_1 and V_2. The voltage changes are proportional to the stimulus intensity and the voltage deflections recorded from V_2 have less amplitude than those recorded from V_1. This difference occurs because the distance between S and R_2 is greater than the distance between S and R_1. This suggests that even though the stimulus current travels down the axon almost as rapidly as in a metal wire, the intensity of the stimulus is markedly attenuated by distance, resulting in a smaller voltage change in the membrane. The figure also shows that, if the polarity of the stimulus is reversed from positive to negative,

*It is conventional to say that the membrane is depolarized, but if this were literally true there would be no potential across the membrane—the resting potential would be zero. Thus, "depolarized" only means less negative by 5–10 mV.

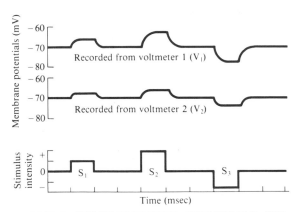

FIGURE 5 STIMULUS-EVOKED POTENTIALS. With positive stimuli to the axoplasm (upward deflections S_1 and S_2 shown on the bottom trace), a depolarizing local potential was recorded. The greater intensity of S_2 caused a greater local potential. The potentials recorded from V_2 are less than those recorded from V_1, indicating that the evoked response had diminished over distance. A negative stimulus (S_3, downward deflection) elicits hyperpolarization of the membrane.

the stimulus causes hyperpolarizations or an increase in the internal negativity of the axon.

Accordingly, these depolarizing and hyperpolarizing voltage changes are defined as "graded" because their amplitude is proportional to the stimulus intensity and as "decremental" because the amplitude of the membrane voltage declines in proportion to the distance between the stimulating and recording electrode. This latter phenomenon is, as mentioned earlier, attributable to the fewer charge carriers, the high resistance and capacity of the neuron, and its leaky insulation. Quantitatively, the factors that account for the voltage decrement determine the LENGTH CONSTANT of the nerve fiber, which is defined as the distance over which the stimulus-induced voltage falls to 37 percent of its original value (a 63 percent loss) (Katz, 1966). For very thin axons, the length constant value is approximately 0.2 mm; and for the thickest axons, it may be as much as 10.0 mm. Thus, because stimulus intensity declines quite rapidly, the membrane changes can only be detected close to the stimulus source. Therefore, they are designated as local potentials. However, despite their limitations, we shall see that local potentials play a significant role in generating the signal-bearing action potential.

Action Potential

Figure 6 illustrates the effect of depolarizing stimuli of greater intensity (note the change of scale from Figure 5). In this illustration, assume that the recording electrodes R_1 and R_2 are separated by a greater distance—about 20.0 mm. In this example the first stimulus (S_1) elicits a local potential recorded by V_1, but a trace from V_2 is absent. This absence is due to the length constant for the axon; and the potential change occurring at R_2 is too small to be detected.

The second stimulus (S_2) is stronger than S_1 and has a greater effect on the axon. First, at V_1 the membrane is depolarized to approximately −40 mV; then a sudden reversal of polarity occurs within the axon as the voltage jumps from −40 to +45 mV. The polarity then reverses again and declines to a level slightly below the resting potential before returning to it. These potential changes are the components of an action potential, the whole event occurring in approximately 1.0 msec in a squid axon and in half that time in mammalian neurons.

These observations indicate that if a depolarizing stimulus is strong enough a threshold is crossed, bring-

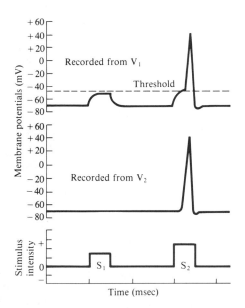

FIGURE 6 STIMULUS-EVOKED ACTION POTEN-
TIALS. The recordings from V_1 show that stimulus S_1 elicited a local potential. The suprathreshold stimulus S_2 evoked
an action potential. The recording from V_2 showed no
response from S_1, indicating that the response decayed before
it reached R_2 which was 20.0 mm from R_1. However, the action potential was recorded by V_2 even though the local potential component was absent. Note the slight "overshoot"
of the declining phase to -80 mV before returning to the
resting potential.

ing into play a new series of events that produce the action potential. Experiments have shown that the increase in stimulus intensity needed to convert a local
potential to an action potential must only be 1/5000
greater than the subthreshold stimulus, and according
to some calculations, the difference need only be 1×10^{-14} greater than the subthreshold (Brinley, 1974).

If the suprathreshold stimulus were increased significantly, the amplitude and duration of the action
potential would still be the same, except that the slope
of the local potential component would be steeper.
Thus, the action potential would occur somewhat
sooner after the onset of the stimulus.

V_2 also records the action potential; and even
though the local potential component is absent, the
amplitude of the action potential is undiminished.
Even when recording electrodes are placed a meter
away from the stimulus site (which is possible on a
neuron of a large animal), the amplitude of action

potentials is the same as those recorded near the
stimulus site. Accordingly, action potentials are said to
have an all-or-none quality (meaning that they appear
with their full effect or not at all); and they are
nondecremental.

The explanation for this is that an action potential
serves as the stimulus for the next action potential at
an adjacent site, and the potential energy for the succeeding action potential exists at that site and is independent of the original stimulus. A simple analogy
illustrates this mechanism. One can ignite a fuse with a
match. The burning fuse then ignites adjacent parts of
the fuse if there is enough combustible material in the
adjacent section. The burning match does not now
have anything to do with the propagation of the flame.
The potential energy is in the fuse itself and it will burn
with equal intensity throughout its length. But one
should not press this analogy too far; an action potential does not induce its own propagation by transfer-
ring heat to an adjacent site. How it does so requires
an understanding of events that occur during the action potential.

Briefly, the change in membrane polarity from -70
to $+45$ mV that characterizes the action potential occurs because the stimulus alters the permeability of the
axon membrane, causing Na^+ to move more freely
along the Na^+ concentration gradient. As Na^+ flows
into the axon, the internal negativity is reduced, for example, from -70 to -65 mV. If the stimulus is weak,
this effect of Na^+ influx is rapidly counteracted by K^+
efflux, which returns the axon membrane to its resting
potential (-70 mV). However, if the stimulus sur-
passes the threshold value, the Na^+ influx is significantly increased and this by itself depolarizes (or increases) the permeability of the membrane even more.
The net result is regenerative influx of Na^+: which
means that the more Na^+ influx there is, the more Na^+
influx is possible. This explains why the action potential is an all-or-none event; once it starts, it runs on to
completion.

It would be expected that Na^+ influx would continue until the internal concentration of Na^+ raises the
interior voltage to a degree that would repel further influx of Na^+. For Na^+, the necessary internal voltage is
about $+50$ mV. That voltage is known as the
EQUILIBRIUM POTENTIAL (EP). However, soon after
Na^+ influx causes the inside of the axon to be less
negative, K^+ efflux starts. This slows the rise of the
membrane voltage and ultimately reverses the polarity

back toward the resting potential. At this point, the membrane again becomes impermeable to Na^+, but because K^+ efflux lasts a little longer, there is a slight overshoot before the resting potential is restored. This is known as an AFTER POTENTIAL.

One result of all this is that there is a gain of a little Na^+ and a loss of some K^+ from the axon. This is of little importance because, although the increase in Na^+ influx is great, the duration of flow is short. Thus, a squid axon loses only about one millionth of its K^+ per nerve impulse, and this is quickly restored by the sodium pump. A very thin mammalian axon may lose as much as one-thousandth of its K^+ content per impulse; but, as mentioned previously, the action of the sodium pump is accelerated by high internal concentrations of Na^+ and high external concentrations of K^+. So even if a thin axon fires hundreds of times per second over a sustained period, the internal concentration of K^+ and Na^+ will remain constant.

Sodium and Potassium Channels *exclusive*

It is worthwhile to pose here the question of why ion flow seems to occur so efficiently. One would suppose that because Na^+ channels are large enough to accommodate K^+, collisions would occur as incoming Na^+ encountered outgoing K^+. However, evidence points to exclusive channels for each of these ions. First, Na^+ influx begins before K^+ efflux; and Na^+ influx rises rapidly and then declines rapidly, whereas K^+ efflux rises slowly to a lower peak and then gradually declines over a somewhat longer period. Figure 7 shows a comparison of the rate of flow of these two ions across a squid axon membrane. The mathematical derivations of these curves were worked out by Hodgkin and Hux-

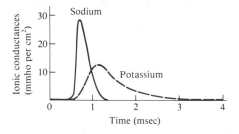

FIGURE 7   CONDUCTANCE OF Na^+ AND K^+ DURING AN ACTION POTENTIAL. The curves represent the flow of Na^+ into and K^+ out of a square centimeter of squid axolemma over 4 msec. The rate of flow is expressed as conductance in millimhos (mho is the reciprocal of ohm, the unit of resistance to electrical flow).

Tetraethylammonium ion (TEA)

ley (1952). Second, when a squid axon is poisoned by tetrodotoxin (TTX)* Na^+ permeability is blocked, but K^+ permeability is unaffected (Moore et al. 1967). On the other hand, Armstrong and Hille (1972) showed that tetraethylammonium (TEA) selectively blocked K^+ permeability, leaving Na^+ permeability intact. Moreover, TTX is effective only when it is applied to the outside of the axon, whereas TEA must be injected into the axon (Eccles, 1977). Tetrodotoxin seems to act by entering the mouth of the sodium channel where it sticks, plugging the channel. Interestingly, a third agent, pronase, which is a proteolytic (protein-destroying) enzyme, blocks the inactivation of Na^+ influx, but only when it is perfused through the inside of the squid axon. These findings square with the notion that specific channels exist for Na^+ and K^+ and that ion flow (and inactivation) are controlled by molecules (probably proteins) that are strategically situated to control the movement of specific ion species (Keynes, 1975; 1979).

It is of interest to note that local anesthetics, such as cocaine and procaine (Novocain) exert their anesthetic effect by blocking the transmission of action potentials along axons. This effect occurs presumably because

Procaine

the drugs alter the lipid layers of the cell membranes so that the ion channels for Na^+ and K^+ are blocked. It is also significant that fibers mediating pain impulses are generally blocked before fibers that mediate touch, kinesthetic impulses, and motor impulses. This would suggest that the drugs have a clinical specificity for "pain" fibers; but the effect is due to the complete

*TTX is a virulent poison found in the ovaries of the puffer fish *Spheroides porphyreus*, and in a few other species. Saxitoxin is another poison that acts similarly to TTX. Under favorable conditions saxitoxin is elaborated by the marine plankton *Gonyaulax*, and can multiply so rapidly that it forms a "red tide"; shellfish feeding in red tide waters concentrate the toxin in their tissues and become poisonous to man. Fatal paralysis can result from the ingestion of one milligram of saxitoxin.

lack of myelinization of the very thin "pain" fibers, or to the presence of many nodes of Ranvier in thinly myelinated fibers where the anesthetic gains access to the axolemma and exerts a maximum effect (Ritchie and Cohen, 1975).

Propagation of the Action Potential

Previous discussion emphasized the fact that stimuli can induce voltage changes in axonal membranes (depolarizations) but that these so-called local potentials diminish rapidly over distance and thus are ineffective for information propagation. However, an action potential can be propagated over long distances without decrement.

Now we can explain propagation without decrement as the spread of voltage changes caused by the action potentials themselves. For simplicity, assume that one end of an axon has been stimulated (depolarized), allowing Na^+ to flow into the axoplasm and causing an action potential. The positive charges (Na^+) flow through the axoplasm and spread to adjacent areas, attracted by the abundant negative charges on the inside of the axon membrane. This causes the negative charges at the adjacent areas to be neutralized, thus depolarizing these areas, which then causes a Na^+ influx at these new sites and a new action potential to occur; and so on to the next adjacent site, until the end terminals are reached. In other words, the voltage change caused by the action potential is sufficient to depolarize an adjacent site, causing an action potential to be initiated there. This continues to happen throughout the length of the neuraxon.

The next point to consider is the propagation velocity of the nerve impulse. This turns out to be between 1 and 100 meters per second, or between 2 and 224 miles per hour—a velocity that is considerably slower than the rate of passive spread of membrane currents. The major proportion of the delay is attributed to the time needed to initiate and complete the action potentials. The wide range in propagation velocity results from the fact that propagation velocity is proportional to the square root of the axon diameter. For example, increasing the diameter 16-fold increases the velocity only 4-fold. However, axon diameter cannot solely account for the wide range of propagation velocities; there are no axons in existence that can support the higher ranges of propagation velocities on the basis of axon diameter alone. It is interesting to note that a crab axon 30 μm in diameter conducts nerve impulses

at 5 m/sec. The axon would have to be 1.2 cm in diameter in order to conduct at 100 m/sec if axon diameter were the sole consideration. In this case, a 20-fold increase in conduction velocity would require a 400-fold increase in axon diameter.

The structure that accounts for the highest propagation velocities is the myelin sheath, which forms a segmented insulating cover around the axon. All fast-conducting axons are equipped with this structure. Functionally, the myelin sheath speeds propagation velocity in three ways. First, myelinization makes the axon membrane less leaky, so that there is less decrement of passive currents over distance. Second, and perhaps more important, the myelin sheath reduces the capacitive characteristics of the axon membrane to less than 1 percent of the expected value; this also prevents voltage decrements over distance. Third, the intersegmental areas of the myelin sheath (the nodes of Ranvier) are areas where the naked axon membrane is in contact with the extracellular fluid, and it is there that the transmembrane resistance is low enough to permit ion flow in and out of the axon.

Action potentials develop at the nodes and initiate passive currents that travel quickly and efficiently (without loss) to the next node, where depolarization of the axon membrane and an action potential can occur. Becauses the nodes are relatively far apart compared to the axon diameter (separated by about a millimeter or so), the action potentials appear to skip from node to node, a process called SALTATORY CONDUCTION. In contrast, the action potentials in nonmyelinated fibers are generated practically next to each other and proceed down the neuron like the flame of a burning fuse. Neural messages are transmitted much faster in the myelinated axon because there are fewer points at which action potentials are generated. A crude analogy for comparing speed of conduction of action potentials in unmyelinated and myelinated fibers is that of a "local" train stopping at every little station compared to an "express" that stops only at a few principal stations and therefore gets to the end of the line much sooner.

An ancillary benefit of myelinization is the need for a smaller expenditure of energy to get the signal from one end of the axon to the other. After an action potential, energy is expended to restore the ions to their respective places and proper concentrations. Thus, the fewer action potentials generated over the course of the axon, the less energy is spent. Consequently, a myelinated neuron can function efficiently even under conditions of great demand for a considerable period of time. In the human, myelinization saves energy by a factor of 5000 and saves packing volume by a factor of 1000 (Morell, 1978). This means that a human nervous system, to have the same capability without the benefit of myelin, would have to be 1000 times larger.

Determinants and Effects of Nerve Impulse Frequency

The nature of nervous systems is such that an essential part of the information transmitted by neurons is expressed in terms of nerve impulse frequency. Nerve impulse frequency can vary in a number of ways, depending upon the duration and intensity of the stimulus and the neural system involved. It is a common observation that a stimulus applied to the skin can be perceived as weak or strong. The determining factors are (1) the number of sense organs and neurons that are stimulated and (2) the frequency of nerve impulses that are generated. Both of these factors are proportional to the stimulus intensity (Figure 8). It is also known that when a watch is strapped to the wrist, a sensation is felt, but shortly thereafter no sensation is appreciated. This suggests that stimuli can elicit a burst of nerve impulses that then disappear even though the stimulating object is still in place. Thus, neural systems undergo adaptation, and responses to stimuli are diminished or cease altogether. There is also a rebound phenomenon—the return of a burst of impulses when the stimulus is removed.

Refractory Periods

Refractory periods are important determinants of impulse frequency and are of two types: absolute and relative. The ABSOLUTE REFRACTORY PERIOD is an interval of time during the course of an action potential when the voltage changes cannot be altered by the arrival of a second stimulus. The time interval coincides with the falling phase of the action potential and is caused by K^+ efflux. For example, suppose we were making an intracellular recording from an axon of a spinal motor neuron of a cat. If the neuron were given a suprathreshold stimulus, an action potential would occur. However, if the stimulus were followed by another stimulus (no matter how strong) within 0.7 msec of the first, there would be no noticeable effect on the action potential. If, on the other hand, the interval between stimuli were increased to 0.8 msec, a second action potential might immediately follow the

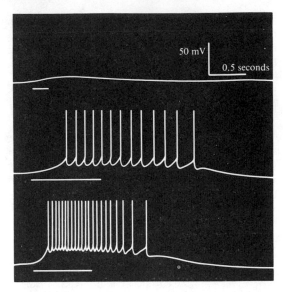

FIGURE 8 PARAMETERS OF ACTION POTENTIAL FREQUENCY. Duration and intensity of a stimulus affect the frequency of action potentials. The top trace shows the effect of a brief stimulus (a light) of low intensity; only a local depolarization occurs. The middle trace shows the effect of a longer stimulus of greater intensity; a burst of action potentials occurs. The bottom trace is the result of a stimulus of even greater intensity and of shorter duration than the second; the frequency of action potentials is greater, but the duration of each burst is shorter. The ratio of the intensities of the stimuli (top to bottom) was 0.05 to 0.2 to 2.0. (After Arvanitaki and Chalazonitis, 1961.)

first, but its amplitude might be slightly diminished. If the interval were increased to 2.3 msec, the successive action potential would be quite normal. Thus, after the onset of an action potential, there is a "silent" period during which the neuron is unresponsive to stimuli, and this limits the frequency of action potentials that can be elicited.

The "silent" period also prevents action potentials from oscillating between adjacent points. As mentioned earlier, when an action potential occurs, there is an influx of Na^+, and these ions can spread in both directions to initiate action potentials at neighboring sites. Indeed, if an axon is stimulated electrically somewhere near the middle of its length, action potentials will spread in both directions from the point of stimulation. Accordingly, an action potential could cause another action potential to occur back at the preceding site as well as at a site farther down the axon. This would result in action potentials oscillating between one site and another. However, under normal conditions, after an action potential occurs at the initial site and is propagated to an adjacent site, the propagated impulse does *not* return to the initial site because the initial site is in its absolute refractory phase and cannot be excited again so soon. Consequently, propagation occurs in one direction only.

The RELATIVE REFRACTORY PERIOD occurs shortly after the absolute refractory period and is accompanied by after potentials. After potentials follow the action potential and are transient depolarizations or hyperpolarizations that may occur in sequence, alone, or not at all, depending on the animal or type of neuron. During a depression (or "overshoot") as seen in Figure 6, the axon is in a subnormal state, that is, the threshold is elevated and a stimulus from the perikaryon must be stronger than normal to elicit an action potential in its axon. During an elevation (an "undershoot"), the axon is in a supernormal state with a lowered threshold. Thus, the relative refractory periods serve to modulate the threshold for action potentials, and thus serve to increase or decrease the probability of the occurrence of action potentials.

Other factors can determine the frequency of action potentials, for example, the rate of deactivation of the transmitters and the design of synaptic junctions (this determines the amount of membrane area that is exposed to the neurotransmitter). In general, the maximum rates for motoneurons are approximately 200-300 discharges/sec, whereas rates as high as 1600 discharges/sec have been recorded from Renshaw cells (the interneurons found in the ventral horn of the spinal cord).

Functional Effects of Action Potential Frequency

The frequency of nerve impulses is an important consideration of neural function because it plays a significant role in information transmission and in transmission of nerve impulses from one neuron to another.

Information Transmission. As a result of the all-or-none response, information about the intensity of a stimulus cannot and is not forwarded to the brain by amplitude modulation (AM) of membrane potentials. Rather remarkably, information about intensity differences between stimuli is transmitted by a frequency modulating (FM) system—the greater the stimulus intensity, the higher the nerve impulse frequency. The great advantage of this system lies in its high signal-to-noise ratio. The concept of signal-to-noise ratio is best understood by comparing AM to FM radio transmission during adverse conditions. In AM radio, the radio station transmits the signal (speech or music) by modulating the amplitude of a carrier wave of a given frequency to which the radio (receiver) is tuned. However, electrical storms and electric motors also cause changes in the amplitude of the signal, creating static. The signal is then unclear, because the signal and the static (noise) are close together in intensity—a condition having a low signal-to-noise ratio. Turning up the volume control does not help because the noise as well as the signal becomes louder. In FM radio (and television), the signal is transmitted by varying the frequency of a carrier wave and FM devices detect changes in the frequency but not in the amplitude of the wave. Consequently, changes in amplitude go unheard so that speech and music (as well as TV pictures) are not affected by the usual kinds of static. In this case, the ratio between the signal and noise is very high.

In the nervous system, there are metabolic changes in neurons that cause slight changes in the resting potential. If the change in intensity between slightly different stimuli caused slight changes in axon membrane potentials, this message would always be contaminated by the spontaneous changes occurring in the membrane. However, these spontaneous membrane changes would not seriously affect the message about a change in stimulus intensity if the message were conveyed by a change in nerve impulse frequency—say, from 60 to 62 impulses/sec. In this latter case, the metabolic changes in neurons (the noise) would have virtually no effect on the clarity of the signal because the signal is expressed as a frequency change.

Impulse Transmission between Neurons. The earlier discussion of squid axon physiology might lead us to draw the incorrect conclusion that if one neuron terminal adequately stimulates another neuron, an action potential is likely to occur in the second neuron. It is very unlikely that action potentials are normally generated in this way. Microscopic examination shows that the dendrites and soma of neurons are covered by thousands of axon terminals from other neurons and it is the interaction of the effects of all these terminals that determines whether or not action potentials will occur in the recipient neuron.

It is estimated that the magnitude of a depolarization at one synaptic junction is approximately 0.5 mV, whereas a depolarization of about 5.0 mV or more above the resting potential is necessary to elicit an action potential. A depolarization of 5.0 mV is easily accomplished by the processes of temporal and spatial summation. This means that a number of axon terminals are located close together on a recipient neuron, and if the action potentials arrive close together in time, the stimulus effects will summate to form a suprathreshold stimulus that can generate an action potential in the recipient neuron. Thus, nerve impulse frequency is a significant factor in determining whether summative effects are adequate for synaptic transmission.

Interactions between Excitatory and Inhibitory Effects

Neurons not only receive inputs that depolarize membranes (excitatory inputs), they also receive hyperpolarizing inputs (inhibitory inputs). For example, stimulation of motor neurons in the spinal cord of a cat may cause leg flexion, but in order for leg extension to occur, the flexor muscles must be inhibited (Figure 9). This type of inhibition occurs at the aforementioned motoneuron, usually by way of interneurons similar to Renshaw cells. An excitatory input

causes a depolarization or EXCITATORY POSTSYNAPTIC POTENTIAL (EPSP) on the membrane, whereas an inhibitory input causes a hyperpolarization or an INHIBITORY POSTSYNAPTIC POTENTIAL (IPSP). The interaction of EPSPs and IPSPs determine whether or not action potentials are generated in the postsynaptic neuron, and if they are generated, how long they will continue.

What determines whether a nerve impulse arriving at an axon terminal causes an EPSP or an IPSP on the postsynaptic membrane? In general, the determinants are (1) the difference in the transmitter substance that is released from the axon terminal and that serves to depolarize or hyperpolarize the postsynaptic membrane, and/or (2) the nature of the receptor site on the postsynaptic membrane; the motoneuron probably has different receptor sites for different transmitter substances. (The excitatory transmitter substance for a motoneuron is probably glutamic acid and the inhibitory transmitter is probably glycine; both substances are amino acids.) However, it has been well established (at least, in the autonomic nervous system) that a given neurotransmitter can have both excitatory and inhibitory effects, depending upon which organs are involved. For example, acetylcholine stimulates somatic muscles but lowers the force of the heart beat and

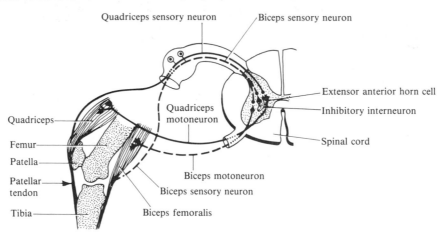

Quadriceps sensory neuron
Biceps sensory neuron
Quadriceps
Quadriceps motoneuron
Extensor anterior horn cell
Inhibitory interneuron
Femur
Spinal cord
Patella
Patellar tendon
Biceps motoneuron
Tibia
Biceps sensory neuron
Biceps femoralis

FIGURE 9 EXCITATION AND INHIBITION PATHWAYS IN THE SPINAL CORD. A brisk tap on the patellar tendon (arrow) briefly stretches the quadriceps muscle. The stretch stimulates the quadriceps sensory neuron which enters the spinal cord and stimulates the extensor anterior horn cell (quadriceps motoneuron) which contracts the quadriceps muscle and extends the lower leg. This reflex is shown by the solid lines. When the biceps femoralis is contracted to bend the knee, this also stretches the quadriceps, but reflex contraction of the quadriceps does not occur. The explanation is that whereas the receptors in the biceps muscle spindles send excitatory messages via the biceps sensory neuron to contract the biceps muscles (dashed lines), they also stimulate the inhibitory interneurons that inhibit the extensor anterior horn cell.

reduces the heart rate, whereas norepinephrine increases the force and rate of the heart beat but relaxes the gastrointestinal tract. The role of neurotransmitters will be examined in greater detail later, but here it is sufficient to emphasize that the type and number of nerve terminals and receptor sites that are activated determines the degree of excitatory and inhibitory influences that will affect a neuron or effector cell. If the excitatory influences dominate the inhibitory influences there is a likelihood that action potentials will occur in postsynaptic neurons, and effector organs will respond appropriately. If the inhibitory influences are dominant, the action potentials may be blocked, delayed, or reduced in frequency, and the effector organs will be less active.

Integration within a Neuron

Threshold differences for generating action potentials occur among motoneurons, as well as among other neuron types. Eccles (1964a) has shown by careful analysis of recorded action potentials in motoneurons that the algebraic sum of EPSPs and IPSPs first influences the initial segment (IS) of the motoneuron axon (Figure 4, Chapter 3). This area of the neuron has a lower threshold for generation of an action potential than the soma–dendritic (SD) parts of the cell. The threshold for IS discharge ranges from 6 to 18 mV, whereas that of the SD spike is between 20 and 40 mV. In motoneurons, the IS threshold is never less than half of the SD threshold, although for some neurons, the difference is barely detectable. The initial segment is the point at which the balance between excitation and inhibition is resolved. We can readily appreciate that this is a better arrangement than having determinations about action potentials simultaneously occurring at different parts of the cell. This arrangement has another consequence. After the occurrence of the SD spike, prolonged after potentials may develop that modulate the membrane resting potential in the SD region. Hyperpolarizations occurring after the SD spike delay the development of the next action potential and effectively control the frequency of neuron discharges. For example, motoneurons supplying the postural muscles have a much more prolonged SD hyperpolarizing after potential than motoneurons supplying the fast phasic muscles.

Also, within each neuron, the frequency of action potentials determines the rate of release of transmitter substances at the axon terminals. In this respect, the frequency-modulated action potentials lead to graded effects at the soma and dendrites of recipient neurons. Thus, in effect, each neuron in a neuron chain is a "decision-making" locus, where excitatory and inhibitory influences are integrated and where determinations are made with respect to the continuation of neural signals to further points and the frequency with which they are to proceed.

From the foregoing we have seen that nerve impulses are the coinage of nerve function, and we shall show that the frequency of nerve impulses is determined by neurotransmitter substances. This is of direct relevance to psychopharmacology as the availability, the rate of release, the rate of recapture, and the metabolism of neurotransmitters are directly influenced by psychoactive drugs. In this way psychoactive drugs can modify nerve impulse frequency and thereby alter the direction and vigor of behavior.

Recommended Readings

Axelrod, J. (1971). Noradrenaline: fate and control of its biosynthesis. *Science*, 173, 598–606. Axelrod's Nobel prize acceptance speech.

Eccles, J.C. (1964a). Ionic mechanisms of postsynaptic inhibition. *Science*, 145, 1140–1147. Eccles' Nobel prize acceptance speech.

Eccles, J.C. (1977). *The Understanding of the Brain,* 2nd Edition. McGraw-Hill, New York. This brief volume by Nobel Laureate Eccles surveys the important developments in neurophysiology in this century.

Hodgkin, A.L. (1964b). The ionic basis of nervous conduction. *Science,* 145, 1148–1153. Hodgkin's Nobel prize acceptance speech.

Huxley. A.F. (1964). Excitation and conduction in nerve: quantitative analysis. *Science*, 145, 1154–1159. Huxley's Nobel prize acceptance speech.

Katz, B. (1971). Quantal mechanism of neural transmitter release. *Science*, 173, 123–126. Katz' Nobel prize acceptance speech.

Kuffler, S.W. and Nicholls, J.G. (1976). *From Neuron to Brain*. Sinauer Associates, Sunderland, Massachusetts. A fine text of neurophysiology well within the grasp of the interested college student.

Noback, C.R. and Demarest, R.J. (1977). *The Nervous System, Introduction and Review*. McGraw-Hill, New York. Written by an anatomy professor and illustrated by the director of medical illustration at the

Columbia University Medical School, this small volume serves well as an introductory text in neuroanatomy.

Scientific American, September, 1979, Vol. 241, No. 3. This issue is devoted to the structure and function of the nervous system. There are eleven articles by outstanding researchers and writers in the field.

Von Euler, U.S. (1971). Adrenergic neurotransmitter function. *Science,* 173, 202–206. Von Euler's Nobel prize acceptance speech.

CHAPTER FIVE

Synaptic Structure and Function

At one time, neurotropic drugs were known as SYM-PATHOMIMETICS, indicating that the drugs mimicked the action of the sympathetic nerves of the autonomic nervous system, or CHOLINOMIMETICS, indicating mimicry of the action of acetylcholine. Later, some drugs were classified as ANALEPTICS, meaning a stimulant of the nervous system (e.g., caffeine and amphetamine), or as NEUROLEPTICS, meaning drugs that have overall beneficial effects upon patients with mental disease (e.g., chlorpromazine and haloperidol). Still later, as more precise anatomical and physiological information about the effects of drugs upon the nervous system was obtained, neurotropic drugs were described in terms of their effects upon synapses. Thus, amphetamine was described as a dopamine and norepinephrine agonist, and neuroleptic drugs used in the treatment of schizophrenia became known as dopamine receptor blockers.

Because virtually all neurotropic drugs exert their physiological and behavioral effects by altering the degree or duration of synaptic activity, it is important that synaptic structure and function be clearly understood, thereby enabling construction of models explaining the mode of action of drugs and their side effects. Moreover, the fact that synapses are the sites of action of these drugs suggests that psychopathological states and some neurological diseases can be traced to abnormal synaptic function. For example, the psychopathology of schizophrenia may be due to excessive amounts of dopamine in the brain or to postsynaptic receptors that are hypersensitive to it. Whether dopamine sensitivity is the primary or the secondary cause of schizophrenia is not known, but it is signif-

icant that drugs that block dopamine receptors do relieve the symptoms of this disease (Snyder et al., 1977). Also there is substantial evidence that the neurological ailment Parkinson's disease is related to deficits of the neurotransmitter dopamine (Hornykiewicz, 1974), and abnormal degeneration of acetylcholine receptors on muscle cells accounts for the extreme muscle weakness of myasthenia gravis (Kao and Drachman, 1977).

However, it should be mentioned that some neurotropic drugs do not act upon synapses. For example, the local anesthetic procaine (Novocain) acts upon the axonal membrane in a way that blocks the conduction of action potentials, especially in thinly or nonmyelinated axons (a property characteristic of axons mediating impulses denoting pain).

This chapter will present detailed descriptions of synapses and their mode of action. A number of examples describing the features of acetylcholine (cholinergic) synapses will be given. These synapses were among the earliest to be discovered and accurately identified, along with the identification of their neurotransmitter. Moreover, the structure and function of cholinergic synapses will, with a few exceptions, be found to be typical of all types of synapses and thus are good examples.

Morphology of Synapses

Methods of Analysis

The word "synapse" was coined in 1897 by Sir Charles Sherrington, a British neurophysiologist. He derived it from the Greek word "synapto," which means "to clasp." Sherrington's research was limited by the relatively low resolution of the light microscope, but he was able to observe the bulbous expansions at the axon terminals that were first described by Held in the same year. He later attributed the particular features of the reflex arc to the special structure of the opposing membranes of two neurons in close juxtaposition. For example, he tried to explain why a nerve impulse passed only in one direction and why there was a 1.0 to 3.0 msec delay when a nerve impulse traversed a synapse (Eccles, 1964b). An understanding of these phenomena developed slowly until the 1950s, when the process of subcellular fractionation made it possible to separate the various parts of neurons and synaptic junctions, visualize the cell fragments with the use of the electron microscope, and derive the chemical nature of the various parts by using advanced biochemical techniques.

The process of SUBCELLULAR FRACTIONATION consists of homogenizing and centrifuging neural tissue to separate its cellular components. For instance, centrifugation of whole-brain homogenates at high speeds (up to 100,000 g*) for 20 minutes will separate myelin

*g = force of gravity.

and other lightweight components from heavier components such as the synaptosomes and mitochondria (Figure 1).

Synaptosomes

Among tissue fragments found in sucrose gradient layers of intermediate densities are the SYNAPTOSOMES, which are torn-off axon terminals that are often attached to portions of the postsynaptic membrane (i.e., to parts of the dendritic spines). When separated from the axons, the axonal stumps of the synaptosomes become sealed off, thereby keeping the synaptosomal contents intact. The particle fraction containing synaptosomes (verified with the electron microscope as well as by other means) is drawn off and lysed (or broken up). Lysis is usually carried out by osmotic shock and involves treating the cell fraction with a hypotonic salt solution, causing the synaptosomes to burst. The lysed material is suspended and centrifuged again to separate the synaptosomal contents (e.g., the vesicles, synaptic membranes, and unspecified microsomes). The constituents of synaptosomes can be verified by electron microscopy or by the use of MARKER ENZYMES (enzymes that are especially active in particular cellular

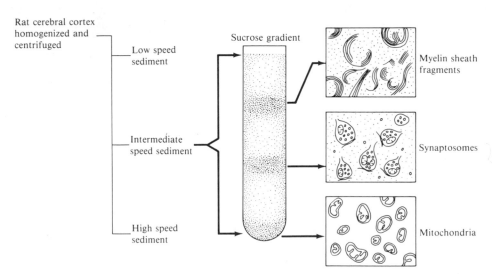

FIGURE 1   SUBCELLULAR FRACTIONATION OF BRAIN TISSUE. After tissue homogenization, the cell particles are centrifuged at intermediate speed. The sediment separated from the cytoplasm is then placed on layered sucrose solutions of increasing density (density increases from the top to the bottom of the tube). After high speed cen-

trifugation, the lightest subfraction containing myelin sheath fragments remains near the top, a heavier subfraction containing synaptosomes and vesicles is found near the middle, and the heaviest particles (the mitochondria) are found at the bottom.

organelles). For example, the presence of choline acetyltransferase (CAT) in synaptosomes would indicate the presence of acetylcholine synthesis as CAT is the enzyme necessary for the synthetic reaction. Thus, the synaptosomes could be correctly identified as cholinergic synapses.

Synaptic Vesicles

Generally an interneuronal synaptic junction consists of an axon terminal (bulb, knob, bouton), the presynaptic element, and a postsynaptic receptor area that can be the surface of a dendritic spine (Figure 2) or a site on the cytoplasmic membrane of the soma of an adjacent cell. An electron micrograph of a synapse

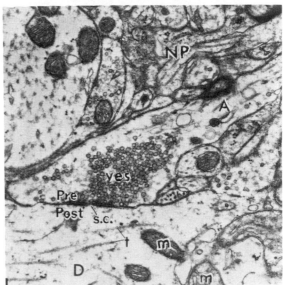

FIGURE 3 SYNAPSE IN THE OCCULOMOTOR NUCLEUS in the brain stem of a cat. An axon courses from the upper right-hand corner of the micrograph to the center, where it swells to form an axon terminal containing vesicles (ves). The vesicles are clustered near the presynaptic membrane (pre), which is separated from the postsynaptic membrane (post) by the synaptic cleft (sc). D, dendrite; m, mitochondrion; t, tubules; NP, adjacent neuropil (a network of fine unmyelinated axons). (From Pappas and Waxman, 1972.)

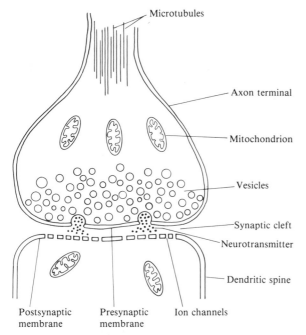

FIGURE 2 CROSS SECTION OF A SYNAPSE. Molecules of neurotransmitter are enclosed in the vesicles, two of which are shown fused to the presynaptic membrane. The neurotransmitter is released into the synaptic space by the arrival of an action potential and an influx of calcium ions (Ca^{2+}). The neurotransmitter initiates activities on the postsynaptic membrane (on the dendritic spine) that open ion channels, allowing the influx of sodium (Na^+) or chloride (Cl^-) ions. This constitutes the EPSP or IPSP on the postsynaptic membrane and facilitates or inhibits, respectively, the generation of an action potential in the postsynaptic neuron.

in a cat's brain (Figure 3) shows a presynaptic bulb in the center of the picture. The terminal can be as large as 5.0 μm, but most are between 1 and 2 μm in diameter and are surrounded by a thin membrane. A large number of mitochondria are usually seen within the cytoplasm, indicating a high level of metabolic activity. The mitochondrial membranes are also a source of special enzymes involved in the metabolism of some transmitters. In addition, there are large numbers of small spherical capsules or vesicles that are within the bulb and that range in size from approximately 40 to 200 nm in diameter. The size of a vesicle is largely related to the type of neurotransmitter substance that is enclosed within it. The vesicles seem to be congregated in the area where the presynaptic and postsynaptic membranes are separated only by the synaptic cleft, a space whose width varies from 10 to 50 nm, depending upon the material studied. At the mammalian motoneuron in the spinal cord, the average width of the synaptic cleft is about 20 to 30 nm (McLennan, 1970).

The synaptic vesicles were first described by De Robertis and Bennett (1954, 1955), Palade and Palay (1954), and Palay and Palade (1955). De Robertis and his colleagues (1962) showed that the cellular fraction containing the synaptic vesicles had the highest concentration of transmitter substance—in their case, acetylcholine. It is believed that the vesicles, at least in part, are formed in the perikaryon and rapidly transported (100 mm/day) to the axon terminals. In addition, some vesicles seem to be formed from detached ends of the smooth endoplasmic reticulum, which extends into the axon terminals. There is also evidence that new vesicles are formed by a process of endocytosis, whereby pieces of vesicular membranes that are attached to the presynaptic membrane are detached and recycled into newly filled vesicles—all of this taking place within the cytoplasm of the axon terminal.

The asymmetric presence of synaptic vesicles (i.e., they are only found near the presynaptic membrane) has become for all practical purposes an identifying marker for synaptic junctions. However, vesicles may be found in both the presynaptic and postsynaptic elements that form axoaxonic synapses (Figure 5); and RECIPROCAL JUNCTIONS have been described in which vesicles are found on both sides of the synaptic cleft, with vesicle clusters in one area on one side of the synaptic cleft and in another area on the other side.

Reciprocal junction

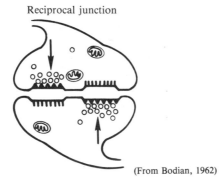

(From Bodian, 1962)

Thus, synaptic action can go in either direction; in some instances, the action is excitatory in one direction and inhibitory in the opposite direction (Mountcastle and Baldessarini, 1974). The vesicles are enclosed by a thin (8.0 nm) membrane that probably differs, at least in its protein constituents, from the cytoplasmic membrane. This conclusion is based in part on the fact that certain drugs (e.g., reserpine) can cause the selective release of the neurotransmitters norepinephrine, dopamine, and serotonin through the vesicle membrane but not through the cytoplasmic membrane. Calcium ions (Ca^{2+}) are necessary for the release of neurotransmitters from vesicles and act directly upon the membrane, judging by the fact that Ca^{2+} binding sites have been identified on the vesicle membranes.

Vesicles vary in size, shape, and contents. Relatively large, round vesicles that are 40 to 80 nm in diameter and are agranular (clear) in electron micrographs are presumed to contain acetylcholine. This assumption is

Spherical agranular vesicles   Spherical granular vesicles

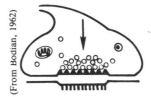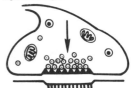

(From Bodian, 1962)

based on the fact that muscles which are innervated predominantly by acetylcholine, such as the sphincter muscle of the iris, contain such vesicles. A second type of vesicle has an electron-dense core that appears opaque when viewed in the electron microscope. These granular vesicles range in size from small (50 nm in diameter) to large (up to 200 nm) and contain norepinephrine and serotonin. It has been proposed that, because agranular and granular vesicles sometimes appear in the same axon terminal, there may be more than one transmitter in the terminal, or they may represent stages in the synthesis of the transmitter (Marshall, 1974).

Synaptic Cleft

The synaptic cleft lies between the presynaptic axon terminal and the postsynaptic membrane and has a width ranging from 10 to 50 nm. This space or gap has sometimes been characterized as having intersynaptic filaments that serve to attach the pre- and postsynaptic membranes and to perhaps guide transmitter molecules to their receptor sites (De Robertis, 1967). Pappas (1975) observed that the synaptic cleft contains some material of intermediate density that he designated as the SYNAPTIC GAP SUBSTANCE. This material is made up of alkaline proteins and carbohydrates in the form of mucopolysaccharides and glycoproteins. It has been suggested that this is the material that binds the membranes together and guides ions and neuro-transmitter molecules to their proper sites, as well as preventing the diffusion of these molecules away from the synaptic cleft. This suggestion is a reasonable one, as mucopolysaccharides form chemical bonds with water to produce mucilagenous and lubricating fluids such as those found in mucous secretions and in inter-cellular spaces. Furthermore, glycoproteins on mem-branes are known to be AUTOIMMUNOLOGICALLY AC-TIVE, meaning that they possess the ability to cause antibody production. Thus, the glycoproteins, serving as an antigen, trigger antibody production in other cells. These autoantibodies interact with the antigen to form autoimmune complexes and result in adhesions between cells. Therefore, within the CNS glyco-proteins may play a role in intercellular recognition and thereby be important during synaptogenesis, that is, when the developing CNS is forming genetically determined synaptic connections (Roseman, 1974; Quarles, 1975).

Quantitative Considerations

Synaptic junctions usually occur on the dendrites and somata of neurons. Somata and glial cell bodies make up only about 5 percent of the gray matter of the CNS; the rest consists of neuronal axons, dendrites, and associated blood capillaries. Consequently, effec-tive neural control of the organism is managed at synapses that constitute a small proportion of the bulk of the CNS. However, this is the area most in contact with the extracellular space through which most drugs diffuse and where drugs are retained in depot fashion.

The number of synaptic terminals terminating on a single receptor cell varies enormously, depending upon cellular features such as size, extent of the dendritic tree, function, and so on. In the case of sensory bi-polar neurons (such as those in the retina), a single axon of a bipolar cell may be the only input to the next cell (the ganglion cell). On the other hand, a single motoneuron in the spinal cord may receive many thou-sands of synaptic terminals (boutons). Judging by size alone, there may be five different terminal species rep-resented, for example, terminals that are excitatory or inhibitory, terminals from recurrent collaterals, some having one type of transmitter, and others having another (Figure 4). Presumably, each of these has its own specific function, for example, maintaining mus-cle tone, exerting postural control, effecting nocicep-tive responses, facilitating excitatory and inhibitory in-fluences upon intersegmental, crossed, and reciprocal

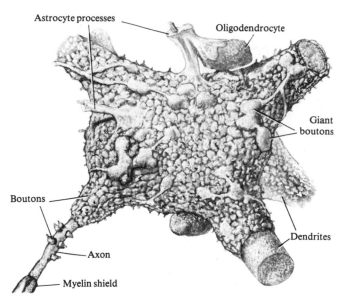

FIGURE 4 SYNAPSES ON THE SURFACE OF A MOTONEURON. The figure is a reconstruction based upon serial sections seen in electron micrographs. Note that the surface of the cell and dendrites are completely covered with synaptic knobs (boutons) of different sizes. (From Poritsky, 1969.)

reflexes for locomotion, cortical influence for fine skilled movements, modulations by the cerebellum and the corpus striatum, and automatic movements. It has been estimated that 20,000 terminals can influence a single PYRAMIDAL CELL in the cerebral cortex (cells that influence fine motor activity during skilled movements and are so named because of the pyramid-like shape of their cell bodies). There are also an estimated 200,000 synapses on the dendritic tree of each Purkinje cell of the human cerebellar cortex, cells that modulate the muscle tone and coordinate the somatic musculature. These facts emphasize the extreme variety and complexity of the input to these systems and the interactions within them.

Qualitative Considerations

Electron microscopic studies of synaptic junctions have revealed a wide variety of forms. An extensive description of even a small number of these would be beyond the scope of this book. However, a few examples of types of synapses are presented to illustrate their variety and to show possible structural and func-

tional relationships. Within the CNS there are generally three types of synaptic linkages: axon terminals that join dendritic trunks or spines (AXODENDRITIC); axon terminals that join the cytoplasmic membranes of cell bodies (AXOSOMATIC); and axon terminals that join other terminals (AXOAXONIC) (Figure 5).

Attempts have been made to relate certain morphological features of axodendritic and axosomatic synapses to specific functions. For example, some axon terminals in the cerebral cortex terminate upon dendritic spines and have been classed as type I synapses (which are excitatory). The synaptic cleft of these synapses is relatively wide (30 nm), and the presynaptic membranes have a continuous and especially thick dense area along the length of the cleft (Figure 6A). There are also dense projections that extend from the dense membrane areas back into the axon terminal cytoplasm and around which the vesicles congregate. The postsynaptic membrane has a corresponding continuous dense area that is somewhat thicker than that on the presynaptic side; hence these synapses are characterized as being asymmetric.

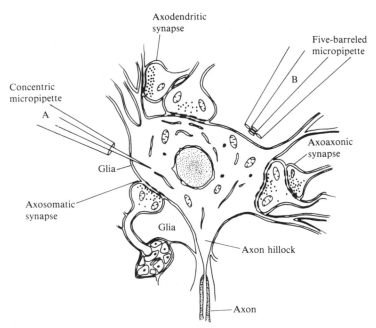

FIGURE 5 NEURON WITH THREE TYPES OF SYNAPSES. Axosomatic, axodendritic, and axoaxonic synapses are shown. Nonsynaptic areas of the cell membrane are covered by the end feet of glia. Subsynaptic patches are shown as thickenings of the subsynaptic membrane. The tips of the two main types of micropipette electrodes are shown: concentric (A) and five-barreled (B). These are used in microiontophoretic studies. Glial end feet form gap junctions with the cell membrane.

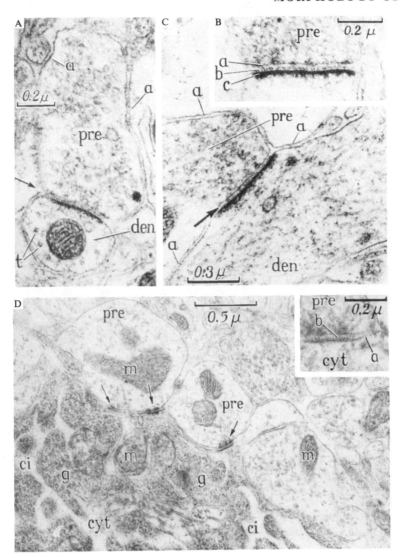

FIGURE 6   TYPE I AND TYPE II SYNAPSES FROM RAT CORTEX. (A) At (a) there are nonthickened membranes at nonsynaptic zones. The arrow points to an active synaptic zone having a much thicker postsynaptic dendritic (den) membrane. The synaptic zone is continuous and asymmetric. (B) Greater details of the pre- and postsynaptic membranes (a and c) with a band of extracellular material in the synaptic cleft. (C) Vesicles are seen congregated above the presynaptic (pre) membrane at the active synaptic zone (arrow). (D) Axosomatic type II synapse has discontinuous but symmetric pre- and postsynaptic dense areas (arrows). The cytoplasm (cyt), mitochondria (m), cisterns (ci), and granules (g) are seen in the soma. (From Gray, 1959.)

Other synapses, classed as type II, typically terminate on cell bodies and are inhibitory (Figure 6B). They have narrower clefts (20 nm), and the dense area of the presynaptic membrane is discontinuous, forming small spots around which cluster the synaptic vesicles. The postsynaptic membrane also has discrete thickenings that match the position of the dense areas on the opposite membrane: hence these are defined as symmetrical synapses (Whittaker and Gray, 1962; Gray, 1959; 1970; McLennan, 1970).

Uchizono (1965, 1967) reported that vesicles in the excitatory axodendritic knobs on cerebellar Purkinje cells retain their spherical shape when the tissue is treated with certain fixatives (chemicals used to prepare the tissue for microscopy), but the vesicles in the inhibitory axosomatic knobs change to a smaller flattened elliptical shape when treated with the same fixatives. Also, there is evidence that flattened vesicles are associated with inhibitory transmitters, such as

Flattened vesicles

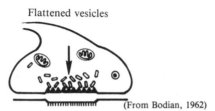

(From Bodian, 1962)

γ-aminobutyric acid (GABA) and serotonin, and with norepinephrine in some parts of the CNS (Bodian, 1962, 1972; McGeer et al., 1975).

The interpretation of the preceding data is rather general and rests upon the finding that certain vesicles are altered when treated with certain chemical fixatives. Moreover, the association of spherical vesicles with axodendritic synapses and flattened vesicles with axosomatic synapses is disputed by investigators who have found vesicles of each type lying adjacent to each other in the same electron micrograph. Furthermore, it is not necessary that morphological differences between excitatory and inhibitory synapses should reside on the presynaptic side of the junction because the same neurotransmitter can serve at both types of synapses. As mentioned earlier, acetylcholine in spherical vesicles is excitatory in sympathetic ganglia and inhibitory in the postganglionic terminations of the vagus nerve on the heart (McLennan, 1970).

Axoaxonic Synapses and Presynaptic Inhibition

This type of synaptic junction deserves special mention. As illustrated in Figure 7, one axon terminal forms a synaptic junction upon another axon terminal. The primary axon terminal (usually from a primary sensory neuron) normally produces EPSPs on the postsynaptic membrane of a secondary sensory neuron within the brain stem. Secondary neurons send their messages to motoneurons of the spinal cord for reflex responses or to higher centers in the brain stem or forebrain for sensory awareness and for fine motor control. From these higher centers, descending modulat-

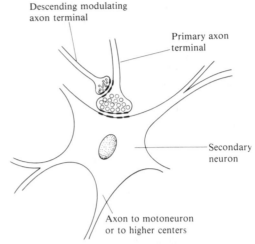

FIGURE 7 PRESYNAPTIC INHIBITION. The primary axon terminal is from an afferent branch of a spinal nerve. The secondary neuron is in the spinal cord, and its axon goes to spinal motoneurons or to higher centers for sensory awareness or fine motor control. The descending modulating axon descends from nuclei in the brain stem or cerebrum and modulates the sensory input to these higher centers. See text for the mechanism of action.

ing axons form axoaxonic synaptic junctions with the primary axon terminals.

The modulating axons serve to control the activity of the secondary neurons in the following way. The axoaxonic junction is excitatory, and if an action potential arrives at the modulating axon terminal, a neurotransmitter is released that slightly depolarizes the primary axon terminal by about 10 mV (from a resting potential of −70 mV to a new potential of −60 mV) (Eccles, 1964b). This is called a CONDITIONING STIMULUS. If an action potential arrives at the primary axon terminal shortly after the conditioning stimulus, the magnitude of the action potential is diminished because it starts from a lower resting potential. Thus, the amplitude range of the action potential is from −60 to +45 mV rather than from −70 to +45 mV. This causes a smaller output of neurotransmitter from the primary axon terminal and a smaller effect (i.e., a smaller EPSP) on the secondary neuron. Should a number of axoaxonic endings be activated on primary axon terminals, there can be a significant decrease in the number of action potentials generated by secondary neurons, thereby reducing the effect of sensory stimuli on the nervous system. This phenomenon is called PRESYNAPTIC INHIBITION because the modulating effect is exerted upon the presynaptic rather than the postsynaptic membrane. Muscle relaxant drugs such as diazepam exert significant effects on this mechanism, causing changes in muscle tension and coordination.

Neuroeffector Junctions

In a physiological sense, neuroeffector junctions are different from synapses because neuroeffector junctions are the last connection between the CNS and the muscles and glands, with behavior as the end result. Functionally, the effects served by these connections are muscular contractions and glandular secretions, either within the body (e.g., stomach contractions, increased strength of the heart beat, secretion of bile from the gall bladder) or on the body surface (e.g., jumping away from danger and increased perspiration). The degree to which these events occur is determined by the frequency of the nerve impulses directed to the respective effector organ.

One type of neuroeffector junction comprises the nerve terminals of autonomic nerves, which activate smooth muscles and glands (such as the muscles of the gastrointestinal tract, the smooth muscles of the iris for pupil dilation and constriction, and salivary and tear glands).

The axons of these nerves divide into fine branches (as many as a few thousand). Along the course of these fine branches are numerous swellings, or varicosities, serially arranged and separated by short lengths (2 to 3 μm) of the axon. The varicosities contain neurotransmitters: acetylcholine in parasympathetic fibers and norepinephrine in sympathetic fibers.

Electron micrographs of the sympathetic innervation of the mesenteric veins from the intestines of a sheep show typical smooth muscle innervation. The finely branched axons lie within 20 to 30 μm of the smooth muscle membrane, sometimes within indentations on the surface of the muscle cell. The varicosities are also within the indentations but are somewhat closer (15 μm) to the muscle cell membrane. These thin axons spread their effects to many different smooth muscle cells by releasing their neurotransmitter, norepinephrine, from many points along the axon, forming *synapses en passage* (Marshall, 1974) (Figure 8). The neurotransmitter is released when nerve impulses arrive at these sites and serves to initiate muscle contraction or glandular secretion. This synaptic arrange-

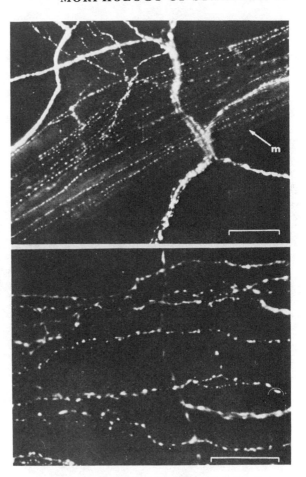

FIGURE 8 SYNAPSE "EN PASSAGE." Using fluorescent microscopic methods that cause norepinephrine-containing axons to glow when viewed in ultraviolet light, long fine strands of axon branches containing bead-like swellings or varicosities are seen on mesenteric veins of a sheep. Through these varicosities, one of the many axon strands from a single cell can form synaptic junctions with thousands of other cells. The bars represent 50 μm. (From Burnstock, 1970.)

ment results in a distribution of transmitter substance that causes widespread activation of muscular or glandular tissue.

This type of synaptic arrangement is also found in the CNS. It has been estimated that one cell body may give rise to 500,000 terminals of this type, thereby influencing activity in widespread areas of the viscera or brain.

Different features can be noted at neuromuscular

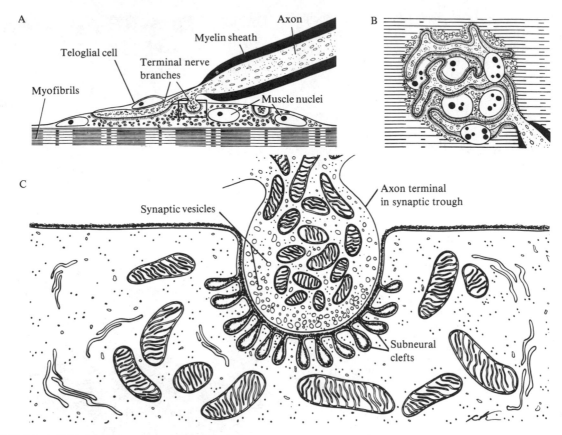

FIGURE 9 NEUROMUSCULAR JUNCTION. (A) An end plate lying on muscle cells. (B) End plates as seen in a surface view. (C) Enlarged view of the area outlined by the rectangle in A. (From Couteaux, 1958.)

junctions (i.e., the connection between axon terminals and striated muscle fibers). Figure 9 shows the motoneuron axon terminal lying next to the muscle membrane within the invagination known as the SYNAPTIC GUTTER on the surface of the muscle cells. The floor of the gutter is further invaginated by a series of SUBNEURAL CLEFTS or JUNCTIONAL FOLDS, which substantially increase the synaptic surface and widen the exposure to the transmitter, thereby increasing the efficiency of the transmission process. Also shown are the numerous mitochondria that are characteristically found in areas of intense metabolic activity.

Figure 10 shows a highly magnified three-dimensional model of a neuromuscular junction of a frog. The model was constructed after analysis of electron micrographs of material prepared by the FREEZE-FRACTURE TECHNIQUE. Freeze–fracture produces frag-

ments of frozen tissue (Akert et al., 1969). The fractures occur within the bilayers of the membranes themselves rather than between the pre- and postsynaptic membranes; thus, the membranes are shown as split apart. On the inner side of the presynaptic membrane, the vesicles are lined up along both sides of transverse bars of electron-dense material. This material may serve as recognition sites for vesicle binding (Heuser and Reese, 1977) and makes up the ACTIVE ZONES where neurotransmitters may be released. There are about 50 closely apposed vesicles per terminal bar and about 500 such bars in each neuromuscular junction (Heuser, 1976). The vesicles are fused to the presynaptic membrane over synaptopores, through which the neurotransmitter may be ejected into the synaptic cleft. The inner leaflet of the presynaptic membrane contains particles that protrude into pits of the outer leaflet of the presynaptic membrane that faces the synaptic cleft. These pits could be calcium channels (Heuser et al., 1974).

The postsynaptic membrane includes junctional folds that are opposite the active zones of the presynaptic membrane. The neurotransmitter flows into these invaginations, thus widening the area of neurotransmitter contact. The particles seen between the layers of the postsynaptic membrane are thought to be related to membrane proteins, but this has not yet been verified (Robertson, 1975).

A similar model has been constructed for interneuro-

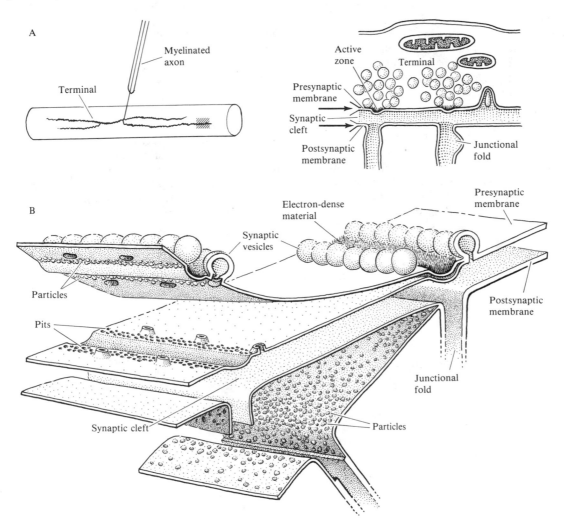

FIGURE 10 SYNAPTIC MEMBRANE STRUCTURE. (A) An entire frog neuromuscular junction (left) and a longitudinal section through a portion of the nerve terminal (shaded rectangle right). (B) Three-dimensional view of pre- and postsynaptic membranes with active zones and immediately adjacent rows of synaptic vesicles. The plasma membranes are split (at arrows in A) to illustrate structures observed upon freeze–fracture. The cytoplasmic half of the presynaptic membrane at the active zone shows on its fracture face protruding particles whose counterparts are seen as pits on the fracture face of the outer membrane leaflet. Vesicles that fuse with the presynaptic membrane give rise to characteristic protrusions and pores in the fracture faces. The fractured postsynaptic membrane in the region of the folds shows a high concentration of the particles on the cytoplasmic leaflet. The particles are probably ACh receptors. (From Kuffler and Nicholls, 1976.)

nal synapses using the freeze-fracture technique (Figure 11). The synaptic vesicles are arranged in a hexagonal array around dense structures. On the right of the figure, the vesicles and the dense structures have been removed, revealing small swellings that protrude into the synaptic knob from the synaptic cleft. The swellings seem to have pits through which the vesicles may discharge their contents into the synaptic cleft. The postsynaptic membrane beneath the synaptic knob appears to be encrusted with fine particles, which may be the postsynaptic receptor sites. Also shown is the subsynaptic web that De Robertis (1967) described. However, it is not seen in some preparations and may be an artifact of the drying process for electron micrography.

There are many drugs that can alter the activity of neuroeffector junctions and the effects can have psychological consequences. For example, curare can block neuromuscular transmission, which leads to paralysis (a condition that would be extremely frightening to anyone treated with this drug). But the fear is a secondary effect of the drug because curare has no known effect on the CNS. From a psychopharmacological point of view, neuroeffector drugs are important for two reasons: First, some of these drugs also stimulate neurons in the CNS with strong and predictable consequences; and second, the mechanisms of action of some of these drugs are in many instances similar to those that occur within the CNS.

Special Synaptic Junctions

The following examples of synaptic junctions illustrate the complexity of presynaptic terminals that virtually envelop dendrites and other receptor areas that have their own elaborate characteristics.

The pulvinar (a nucleus in the posterior thalamus) receives auditory and visual inputs from the medial and lateral geniculate nuclei of the thalamus, respectively, as well as somesthetic inputs from the ventral posterior nucleus (Figure 12). The pulvinar projects its axons to the posterior parietal and temporal lobes and to EXTRASTRIATE CORTEX (areas surrounding striate or optic cortex). Thus, this structure seems to integrate

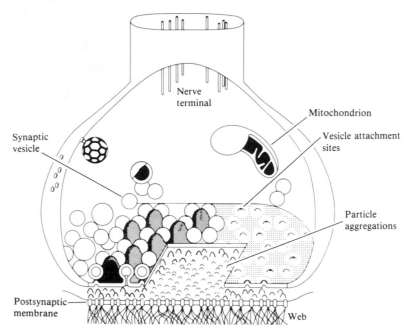

FIGURE 11   INTERNEURONAL SYNAPSE. The model was constructed after an examination of the internal and external aspects of a freeze-fracture preparation of a central (interneuronal) synapse. Vesicles surround the dense structures and discharge their contents through the pits of the vesicle attachment sites shown on the right. The particle aggregations on the postsynaptic membrane may be postsynaptic receptor sites. The connection between the subsynaptic web and the particles is hypothetical. (From Akert et al., 1975.)

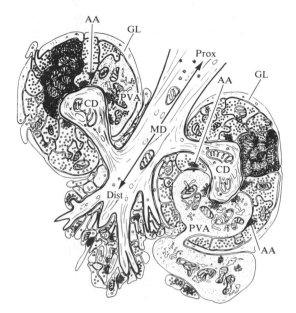

FIGURE 12 SYNAPSE IN THE PULVINAR. The main dendrites (MD) of these neurons have short, blunt terminating central dendrites (CD), which enter a cluster of closely packed terminals surrounding them. This cluster (a glomerulus) is made up of several types of axon terminals. Typical axodendritic contacts are seen as well as axoaxonic (AA) junctions. In the latter, the more usual appearing axon terminals form synapses upon poor vesicle axon (PVA) terminals, whereas the PVA terminals themselves attach to the central dendrites. Glial barriers (GL) surround the glomeruli. The distal part of the main dendrite (Dist) divides into numerous small branches, which also engage many axon terminals. (From Majorossy et al., 1965.)

auditory, visual, and somesthetic impulses for projection to the association areas of the brain. It can be seen that the dendrite receives many synaptic inputs, some of which are conditioned by axoaxonic endings that mediate presynaptic inhibition.

The terminals of basket cells form synapses at the bottom of the Purkinje cell body and along the initial segment of its axon (Figure 13). These junctions are inhibitory, and it appears that these endings are strategically placed to inhibit the generation of action potentials in the Purkinje cells of the cerebellum.

Gap Junctions

Gap junctions represent another type of synapse and differ from regular synaptic junctions by the close

apposition of their pre- and postsynaptic membranes—2 nm, compared to 20 nm in regular synapses (Kuffler and Nicholls, 1976). More importantly, local potentials are conducted across these junctions without the benefit of chemical transmitters. It is estimated that the threshold for passage for local signals is in the submillivolt range as compared to a range between 20 and 100 mV in chemically mediated synapses. Also, it seems that some of these junctions are not polarized, meaning that currents flow in either direction.

Gap junctions are found between neurons and between glia and neurons in the nervous systems of many

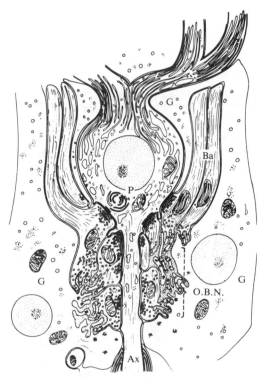

FIGURE 13 BASKET SYNAPSE ON A PURKINJE CELL. The inset at the top shows the arrangement of the basket cell (BC) to a cerebellar Purkinje cell (PC). The greater part of the Purkinje cell body (P) and dendrite surface is covered by glia (G). The terminal branches of the basket cell axon (Ba) make synaptic contacts with the bottom of the Purkinje cell body and the "preaxon." The real axon (Ax) begins about 30 μm below and becomes myelinated. Finger-shaped processes of basket axon endings and similar processes of the glia are entangled in a relatively loose outer basket neuropil (O.B.N.), which is devoid of synaptic contacts. (From Hamori and Szentagothai, 1965.)

species (e.g., annelids, mollusks, arthropods, birds, and mammals). Electrical transmission between cells is not modified by drugs such as curare (a drug that blocks neuromuscular junctions) or neostigmine (a drug that intensifies the action of acetylcholine). In some synapses, part of the interface between the pre- and postsynaptic membrane has a synaptic morphology suggesting chemical transmission, while adjacent to it is a gap junction. These synapses are known as MIXED JUNCTIONS. Gap junctions unquestionably play important roles in neural activity; however, their direct relevance to neuropharmacological effects is unknown.

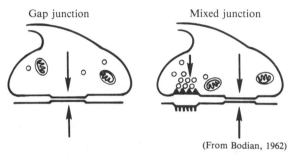

Gap junction　　　　Mixed junction

(From Bodian, 1962)

Microiontophoresis

ELECTROPHORESIS or MICROIONTOPHORESIS is an important procedure used in the study of synaptic functions. In Figure 5 there are two types of electrodes that are typically used to study synaptic activity. On the left is a concentric electrode with a central recording tip surrounded by a hollow tube through which molecules of drugs or neurotransmitters may be ejected upon the surface of a cell membrane. The recording tip, which is usually made of a noncorroding metal such as platinum, can be passed through the cell membrane into the cytoplasm. The membrane seems to fuse around the electrode so that there is no leakage around it. This preparation is able to indicate the degree to which the ejected material alters the electrical characteristics of the cell. However, the concentric electrode requires a pressure pulse to eject the material. Because the orifice of the pipette tip is so small (sometimes less than 1.0 μm in diameter), a comparatively high pressure is required, and this may be difficult to control. However, larger openings would allow leakage and small orifices could become blocked, thereby contributing to the errors of measurement.

The five-barreled micropipette shown on the right in Figure 5 was designed by Curtis and Eccles (1958) and is made by fusing five sections of fine glass tubing,

simply by putting them together and heating them until they are soft and stick together. After cooling, the five-tube array is heated near one end. When the glass is soft, the cold end on the other side of the flame is grasped and the hot end is quickly pulled away, causing the formation of a fine five-channeled thread. When cooled, the thread is cut and trimmed to a point where all the channels are open. The overall tip diameter of this multibarreled cluster is between 3 and 8 μm, small enough to stimulate and record from a single cell body without seriously damaging surrounding tissue. This micropipette assembly is used for electrophoresis and operates on principles different from those of the concentric electrode. The center barrel is filled with a conducting fluid (concentrated NaCl). A silver wire is inserted from the back into the fluid of the barrel and is connected to an amplifier and an oscilloscope to provide a visual display of the electrical events that occur on the cell membrane. The other barrels, all equidistant from the recording or center barrel, are used to eject neurotransmitters, drugs, and control substances (alone or in combination) upon the cell membrane. If the test materials are ionized, they can be ejected by applying a DC current of the appropriate polarity. For example, if positively charged cations are to be ejected, a positive charge is applied to the barrel to repel the cations, thereby pushing them from the pipette. To prevent leakage of the cations from the tip, a reversed (negative) polarity or "backing" current is applied to the barrel at all other times. The quantity of the material ejected conforms approximately to Faraday's Law according to which a nanoampere of current flow would eject a 1×10^{-14} gram-equivalent of drug ions per second (McLennan, 1970).

The results of this type of experiment can be photographed by positioning the electron beam of an oscilloscope so that the spot of light is in the center of a screen. While drugs are ejected from the pipettes, the center electrode records the change in membrane voltage and controls the movement of the light spot—down for negative and up for positive. Thus, a burst of action potentials would appear on the screen as a thin vertical line. If a photographic film is moved continuously past the vertical line and perpendicular to it, a tracing such as that seen in Figure 14 will appear. Figure 14A shows the effect of applying acetylcholine (ACh) from one pipette upon the cell membrane of a neuron in the cerebral cortex of a rabbit. The electrophoresis current was 130 nanoamperes (nA) and was

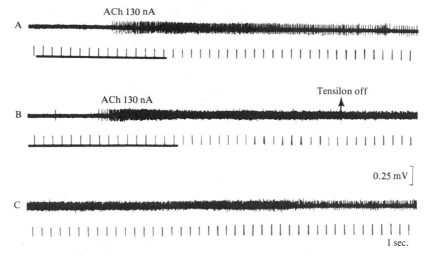

FIGURE 14   ELECTRICAL RESPONSE TO IONTO-PHORESIS applied to a cerebral cortex neuron of a rabbit. (A) The effect of iontophoretically applied ACh. The time of application of the ACh is indicated by the black lines under the time marks (1 second). After a short delay, ACh elicits a burst of action potentials. (B) and (C) are a continuous record and began 12 seconds after the start of the experiment, that is, after the release of Tensilon by a current of 80 nA. Tensilon by itself had no effect, but when ACh was applied, the action potentials were significantly prolonged. (From Krnjević and Phillis, 1963.)

applied for 14 seconds. The result was a burst of action potentials that began approximately 10 seconds after the start of electrophoresis and continued for approximately 40 seconds. Figures 14B and C are one continuous record of an experiment in which the drug Tensilon was applied from one barrel before the start of recording and was halted 34 seconds after ACh was applied from a second barrel (ACh was applied for 17 seconds). Tensilon is a drug that blocks the action of acetylcholine esterase (the enzyme that decomposes ACh molecules). Thus, in this case the action of the ACh was significantly prolonged. These methods have become so precise that it is possible to compare the effects of material ejected on the outside versus material injected into the inside of cells or the effect of material ejected near a synaptic junction versus ejection at a position a fraction of a millimeter away.

Neurochemistry of Synaptic Transmission

In 1877, Du Bois-Reymond reported that transmission from one neuron to the other could occur either chemically or electrically, and it is true that both mechanisms occur in nervous systems. However, much evidence clearly shows that the preponderance of synaptic action in warm-blooded animals is chemically mediated. The accumulation of this evidence was perhaps first of all dependent upon refinements in the design and construction of microelectrodes, electrical stimulators, amplifiers, and recording equipment such as the cathode ray oscilloscope (Minz, 1955).

The early experimenters sought to discover the characteristics of the electrical events that were observed during synaptic transmission. The following facts emerged.

1. After a presynaptic element was stimulated, there was a short delay (about 0.3 msec) before the postsynaptic element showed a response. This delay was too long to support the hypothesis that an electrical pulse passed directly from one cell to the next.
2. If the postsynaptic element was stimulated, a response was not recorded in the presynaptic element, indicating that the synapses were polarized, that is, the impulse could go in one direction only. This did not rule out electrical transmission, since a device that could act as a diode could also polarize a circuit; indeed, such polarized electrical synapses have been described. But this finding did suggest that some intervening mechanism existed between the cells that transmitted the pulse from one cell to the other.

3. Stimulation of the presynaptic element could result in an inhibitory influence rather than an excitatory one on the postsynaptic element. This would be difficult to explain in terms of a direct passage of the electrical event since nerve impulses are of only one kind and would not be likely to excite some neurons and inhibit others.

4. There was no relationship between the magnitude of the presynaptic electrical event and the postsynaptic one. That is, the presynaptic event might be smaller as well as larger than the postsynaptic event. From an electrical standpoint, it would be easy to explain a slight decrement, but more difficult to explain an increment, in the absence of some intervening process.

With respect to the chemical hypothesis, however, all of the facts listed above are in complete harmony.

1. The synaptic delay of 0.3 msec has been calculated to be an amount of time appropriate for the release and transport of the transmitter substance across a gap of 20 nm (the width of the synaptic space).

2. The fact that stimulating the postsynaptic element does not produce a response in the presynaptic element may simply mean that the release of the transmitter occurs only at the ends of axons and not the other way around (i.e., release at dendrites).

3. Excitation and inhibition caused by identical nerve impulses are compatible with the idea that nerve impulses occurring in one cell might cause it to release an inhibitory transmitter, whereas a nerve impulse in a different cell would lead to the release of an excitatory transmitter. It is also true that the same transmitter may be excitatory on some cells and inhibitory on others. This is due to differences in the receptors for the two types of affected cells.

4. Finally, the fact that there is no correlation between the magnitude of the pre- and postsynaptic electrical discharge speaks strongly for an intervening process whereby a small electrical signal may cause the release of enough chemical transmitter to produce a much larger electrical response in the postsynaptic element.

The Identity of Neurotransmitters

While the above discoveries were taking place, attempts were already being made to identify the chemical substances that might be the transmitters. Early in this century, Elliott (1904, 1905) suggested that nerves in the sympathetic nervous system (e.g., nerves that supply excitatory impulses to the heart and blood vessels) produce their effect by liberating adrenalin (epinephrine) on the effector organ. He came to this conclusion on the basis of his own and earlier observations made by Langley in 1901 that direct application of the hormone from the adrenal gland (adrenalin) to visceral muscles had the same effect as direct stimulation of the nerves to those muscles (Langley, 1921). Actually, the sympathetic transmitter was found some years later to be noradrenalin (or as it is known in the United States, norepinephrine). This discovery was made in 1946 by Ulf von Euler, who shared the 1970 Nobel prize for this and related work (von Euler, 1971).

In 1906 Dixon proposed that parasympathetic nerves released a substance that could be identified only as being equivalent to muscarine (a substance obtained from the mushroom *Amanita muscaria*). This substance caused the same effect as that obtained by stimulating parasympathetic nerves (e.g., the vagus nerve that stimulates the visceral organs of the gastrointestinal tract). It was 1921 when Otto Loewi did a simple, but effective, experiment that showed that Dixon was correct and that offered substantial proof of a neurotransmitter that was released from the vagus nerve.

Loewi was aware that stimulating the cardiac nerve (a branch of the vagus) arrested heart contractions and that these effects persisted for a short time after the electrical stimulation ceased. Loewi suspected that some substance was released by the stimulation that continued to affect the force of the heartbeat. Experiencing a flash of insight one night about 3:00 A.M., he conceived of an experiment that would test his hypothesis. He hurriedly arose and went to his laboratory to perform the experiment for which he justly became famous. He inserted a double cannula (two thin tubes side by side) into a frog's heart to permit Ringer's solution to flow into and out of the heart and into a second frog's heart from which the nerves were detached (Figure 15). Under these conditions, the hearts continued to beat. When the cardiac branch of the vagus nerve attached to the first heart was stimulated, there was an abrupt and persistent arrest of the heartbeat. When the nerve was stimulated while Ringer's solution flowed from the first to the second heart, the second heart, after a short delay (15 seconds) also showed an arrested heartbeat.

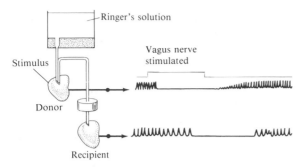

Ringer's solution

Vagus nerve
stimulated

Stimulus

Donor

Recipient

FIGURE 15 LOEWI'S EXPERIMENT. The cardiac branch of the vagus nerve attached to a frog's donor heart was electrically stimulated, causing arrest of the heartbeat. Ringer's solution perfusing the donor heart was transferred to the recipient heart. After 15 seconds, the beat in the second heart was also arrested.

In a second experiment, the sympathetic accelerator nerve of the first heart was stimulated, producing a tachycardia (increased heartbeat and rate). During the heart perfusions, the second heart also showed a tachycardia. Thus, there was little doubt that stimulation of the nerves of the heart caused a release of an inhibitory or excitatory substance that could mimic the action of the nerves. The inhibitory substance was called "Vagusstoff" or material from the vagus. This later turned out to be acetylcholine, and subsequent experiments showed that it was the transmitter substance that acted on glands, smooth muscles and striated muscles.

It was fortunate that Loewi used Ringer's solution as the transfer medium, because if he had used blood, the enzyme acetylcholine esterase would have neutralized the ACh in solution and Loewi's experiment would have led to another conclusion. In the case of the excitatory transmitter, Loewi first referred to an "Acceleranzstoff" but later correctly identified the substance as adrenalin. It was not known until 25 years later that the transmitter in a frog heart is unusual in nature, noradrenalin being the transmitter in most other species (von Euler, 1971).

Neurotransmitters within the Central Nervous System

From the foregoing we have seen that early knowledge of neurotransmitters came from experiments on synapses in the peripheral nervous system. For example, neurotransmitters were identified at neuromuscular junctions (including smooth, cardiac, and striated muscle) and at synapses in the para- and prevertebral ganglia (the loci of cell bodies whose axons innervate autonomic structures) (see Figure 1 in Chapter 6 and Figure 2 in Chapter 7). Analysis at these structures was relatively easy because the transmitter was almost always completely homogeneous. That is, in the paravertebral ganglia, the transmitter is almost solely ACh, which is also the neurotransmitter at the neuromuscular junction of the somatic musculature. It is also quite clear that the transmitter at the terminals of sympathetic nerves is in almost all instances norepinephrine (see Figure 2 in Chapter 7).

Within the central nervous system, however, a given cell may be acted upon by a wide variety of terminals having different transmitters. Electron micrographs show that a single motoneuron in a cat may have as many as 16,000 synaptic contacts. This makes identification of a particular transmitter acting on that cell rather difficult. Also, although samples of transmitter metabolites that help to identify the transmitter can easily be collected in peripheral synapses, this becomes more difficult in the CNS. Furthermore, if a suspected transmitter were tested as to its effectiveness by having it directly applied to a brain site, the transmitter might have an indirect effect on the brain site by causing a local vasoconstriction and ischemia (a limited blood supply) and thereby altering the function at that site. In this case, one could be misled into thinking that the suspected transmitter directly influenced behavior by modifying brain function.

Criteria for Neurotransmitters

For the above reasons, a series of proposed criteria must be met before a substance can be designated as a neurotransmitter (McLennan, 1970). However, in many instances all the criteria cannot be met; nevertheless, frequently there is enough evidence to support a transmitter role for a given substance. The proposed criteria are:

1. The presynaptic terminal should contain a store of the suspected transmitter material, preferably in a bound or sequestered form. However, in a high traffic terminal, a usually abundant transmitter may exist in a small but sufficient amount at a given time as a result of its rapid turnover. It is also possible that a nontransmitter might accumulate, leading to an incorrect determination of a transmitter.
2. The exogenous application of a suspected transmit-

ter to the region of the synapse itself should completely mimic the stimulation of the presynaptic terminal at that synapse. Here the technical problems are considerable. However, it is possible to couple intracellular recordings with extracellular applications of the suspected transmitter by iontophoresis and then compare these effects with the stimulation of known synaptic inputs to the same cell. If the two effects are the same, this can provide strong support for the natural existence of that transmitter.

3. If a drug is known to mimic a transmitter on the postsynaptic side of a synapse, the drug should have the same effect as the transmitter that becomes available by the electrical stimulation of the presynaptic element. If the drug blocks the transmitter, then the drug should block exogenous sources of the transmitter as well as transmitter that is released from the presynaptic terminal. The difficulty with this procedure is that in some cases it may not be known whether the drug is acting directly upon the receptor site or the presynaptic terminal to effect the release of the transmitter.

The way to settle this question is to try to detect an antidromic response in the presynaptic cell. An ANTIDROMIC RESPONSE is a response that occurs in a cell when an action potential is propagated in the reverse direction, that is, from the axon terminal back to the soma. The presence of an antidromic response in a cell following the application of a drug would indicate that the presynaptic terminal may have been stimulated, thus causing the release of the endogenous transmitter.

It is also true that detecting antidromic responses in the CNS is very difficult. In the case of a blocking drug, it may not be known whether the drug blocks the postsynaptic receptor site or the release of the transmitter. If the latter were true, then the antidromic test would not be of any help because the drug might prevent transmitter release even when the presynaptic element is stimulated. Thus, the identification of the transmitter would be indeterminate.

4. A mechanism must exist for the synthesis of the transmitter. Therefore, the precursors and the appropriate enzymes should be present in the synaptic terminal.

5. A mechanism must exist for inactivating the transmitter. This may be a catabolic enzyme system or an active reuptake system in the presynaptic terminal or possibly in adjacent glial elements.

With these criteria in mind, many transmitters have been identified with a fair degree of certainty. These include epinephrine, norepinephrine, dopamine, serotonin, γ-aminobutyric acid, glycine, aspartate, and glutamate. In addition, other compounds have been found that seem to influence synaptic events in perhaps less direct ways. These substances may be designated as neuromodulators, which act in a hormone-like manner (Barchas, Akil, et al., 1978). They are not responsible for direct transfer of nerve impulses from one neuron to another; rather, their release from neurons, glia, or other secretory cells may alter the action of neurotransmitters either by enhancing or reducing their effectiveness. They could do this by influencing neurotransmitter synthesis, release, receptor interactions, reuptake, and metabolism. For example, glucocorticoids (which are secreted by the adrenal gland) influence the rate of synthesis of norepinephrine by controlling the activity of its synthesizing enzyme, tyrosine hydroxylase. Thus it can be seen how stress—leading to steroid release—can influence the availability of a crucial neurotransmitter responsible for sympathetic activity associated with emergency reactions. A list of putative neurotransmitters is provided (Table I).

Chemical Characteristics of Neurotransmitters

The chemical structure of all known and suspected neurotransmitters is well established. Most of these are small, water-soluble molecules containing amine groups and are ionized at physiological pH. These diffuse easily through the aqueous pores of cell membranes, except those membranes that are responsible for the blood brain barrier (see Chapter 1). Some neurotransmitters and neuromodulators are amino acids that exist alone or in chains called PEPTIDES. These amino acids contain one or more CARBOLIC ACIDS (containing the carboxyl group, COOH) that also ionize at physiological pH and are water soluble. There is some evidence that the transmitters leak in small amounts from the synaptic terminals but that nerve impulses arriving at the terminals cause a many-fold increase in neurotransmitter release.

Neurotransmitter Synthesis

A considerable amount of research has gone into the questions of origin and synthesis of synaptic transmitters. Unquestionably these efforts are among the greatest achievements in the history of science. Most of the principal scientists became Nobel laureates, and

TABLE I Substances Found to Have Neurotransmitter or Neuroregulator Properties

Phenethylamines and derivatives
Dopamine
Norepinephrine
Epinephrine
Tyramine
Octopamine
Phenethylamine
Phenethanolamine
Dimethoxyphenylethylamine (DMPEA)
Tetrahydroisoquinalines

Indoleamines
Serotonin (5-hydroxytryptamine)
Melatonin
Tryptamine
Dimethyltryptamine (DMT)
5-Methoxytryptamine
5-Methoxydimethyltryptamine (bufotenine)
Tryptolines

Cholinergics
Acetylcholine
Choline

Amino acids, analogues, and nucleosides
Histamine
γ-Aminobutyric acid (GABA)
γ-Hydroxybutyrate (GHB)
Glycine
Taurine
Adenosine
Aspartate
Glutamate

Hormones
Prostaglandins
Corticosteroids
Estrogens
Testosterone
Thyroid hormone

Peptides
Enkephalins
β-Endorphin
Substance P
Somatostatin
Angiotensin
Luteinizing hormone releasing hormone (LHRH)
Vasoactive intestinal polypeptide (VIP)
Adrenocorticotropic hormone (ACTH)
Thyroid releasing hormone (TRH)
Delta sleep factor

they and their colleagues continue to elucidate what was once a formidable problem. Neurotransmitters are synthesized within the neuron perikarya and then enclosed in vesicles for transport to the axon terminals. In some instances, a stage of transmitter synthesis occurs within the vesicles or within the axon terminal. For example, after the release of acetylcholine into the synaptic cleft, the transmitter is broken down and one breakdown product (choline) is taken up by the presynaptic terminal and used to synthesize new acetylcholine. Some transmitters require a number of synthesizing enzymes, whereas others, such as amino acids, are regular cellular constituents and require no futher treatment.

Neurotransmitter synthesis is an important subject in psychopharmacology because drugs that are therapeutically useful and many that serve as research tools exert their effects by limiting or blocking synthesis. Therefore, the synthesis of the best-known transmitters will be described in detail in separate chapters.

Transmitter Release

The mechanism whereby nerve impulses lead to transmitter release is known as excitation–secretion coupling. Neurotransmitters to a considerable extent are found in a bound form within the terminal vesicles. In part this serves to prevent degradation of the transmitter by metabolizing enzymes. That vesicles play a role in synaptic transmission was shown in experiments in which black widow spider venom (BWSV) strongly stimulated frog neuromuscular junctions. After 10 to 15 minutes of stimulation, the muscle became quiet and could no longer be stimulated. If the tissue were fixed at that time, examination by electron microscopy revealed almost total vesicle depletion within the terminals. Also there were significant increases in the lengths of the presynaptic membranes that correlated with vesicle depletion. Thus, the venom stimulated the axon terminals at high rates, leading to vesicle depletion and to vesicle fusion with the presynaptic membrane (Clark et al., 1972). It was also shown that electrical stimulation of frog neuromuscular junctions for 6 to 8 hours depleted terminal stores of the transmitter and their vesicles (Figure 16). When spider venom was added to this prestimulated preparation, virtually no muscular activity was noted. But when venom was added to an unstimulated preparation, the muscle showed violent FIBRILLATION (uncoordinated contractions of muscle fibers). This was added proof that prolonged stimulation ultimately depletes the stores of

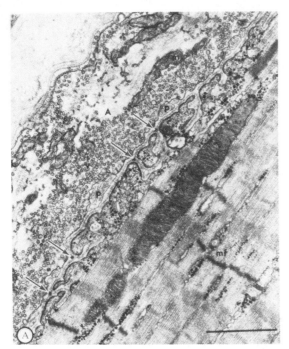

FIGURE 16 VESICLE DEPLETION FROM A FROG NEUROMUSCULAR JUNCTION. (A) An electron micrograph of a control preparation soaked in Ringer's solution and curare (3 x 10^{-6} gm/ml). The axonal ending contains many mitochondria and synaptic vesicles. Active zones (arrows) are seen as the dense areas on the presynaptic membranes opposite the openings of the junctional folds. Projections of glial cells are interposed between the terminal and the end plate membrane. The bar at the lower right represents 1 μm ($\times 34,000$). (B) A preparation that has been stimulated for 8 hours. Note that the axonal ending appears swollen, and few vesicles are evident. Bar represents 1 μm ($\times 30,000$). (From Ceccarelli et al., 1972.)

neurotransmitters and vesicles (Ceccarelli et al., 1972).

However, although these results strongly suggest that the source of the transmitter is vesicular, it does not explain how the substance is actually released. One possible mechanism involves the axon terminal protein NEUROSTENIN, which is composed of neurin (a protein abundant in the plasma membrane) and stenin (a protein abundant in the vesicle membrane). These substances combine in a manner similar to the combination of actin and myosin, which produces actomyosin, the contractile protein in muscles. Indeed, neurostenin has been referred to as brain or synaptosomal actomyosin. When a nerve impulse depolarizes a presynaptic membrane, there is a Ca^{2+} influx. Ca^{2+} is necessary for the contraction of actomyosin, and similarly it is necessary for transmitter release. In muscles, Ca^{2+} acts by blocking the activity of a protein complex, the troponin–tropomyosin system, which inhibits the interaction between actin and myosin. A similar process appears to occur in neural tissue, that is, Ca^{2+} serves a similar function for the muscle-like contraction of neurostenin, resulting in emptying of the synaptic vesicles after they have fused to the axon membrane (Berl et al., 1973; Berl, 1975).

Another possibility is that Ca^{2+} plays a role in the movement of the vesicles toward the presynaptic membrane. The movement results in the fusion of the two membranes and the expulsion of the transmitter into the synaptic cleft. Explusion is accomplished by the action of Ca^{2+}, which is a divalent cation that neutralizes negative charges existing on the vesicle membrane and the inside of the presynaptic membrane, thus canceling electrostatic repulsive forces between them (Heuser, 1977). However, when the distance between the vesicle and terminal membranes is closer than 300 nm, there is a repulsion that is independent of the electrostatic charges. These secondary repulsive forces depend upon water, which stabilizes the cellular membrane by clinging to water-soluble groups (such as the polar heads of lipids that make up the membranes). The polar groups may be removed by Ca^{2+}-dependent phospholipase activity, (i.e., the action of a phospholipid-metabolizing enzyme), or the stablizing polar groups may be pulled away from the site of membrane contact by Ca^{2+}-dependent contractile proteins. In either of these two ways there could be a merger of the two lipid membrane interiors, allowing them to fuse spontaneously to permit exocytosis of the transmitter (Parsegian, 1977). (See the section on calmodulin in this chapter).

The process of exocytosis has been studied using the electron microscope. First, frog neuromuscular junctions were pre-incubated in a bath containing 4-aminopyridine, which prolongs the duration of action potentials. This has the effect of increasing Ca^{2+} influx and the release of the neurotransmitter by 100-fold. The junctions were stimulated and within 5.1 msec were instantly frozen to preserve the vesicles in the process of exocytosis. Many examples of synaptic vesicles in the process of exocytosis can be seen in Figures 17 and 18. It appears that the fused membranes split, leaving a small opening through which vesicle contents can diffuse across the synaptic cleft and interact with the postsynaptic receptor sites. All of this is presumed to take place within 1 msec after the arrival of the nerve impulse to the axon terminal and continues from 1 to 100 msec thereafter (Heuser, 1977).

Vesicle Membrane Recycling

Empty vesicles appear to be recycled. Recycling is necessary to prevent a continuous growth of the plasma membrane resulting from fusion of vesicle membranes with it. Moreover, although many of the proteins and lipids are the same for the two types of membranes, some are not. Gangliosides are a form of glycolipids and are found in plasma membrane but not in vesicle membrane. Thus, these two types of membranes are not completely identical. If recycling does occur (i.e., if the plasma membrane is indeed the source of new vesicles), some mechanism must select some substances and reject others in the formation of new vesicles. Recycling of vesicular membranes has been observed in the neuromuscular junction of the frog (Heuser and Reese, 1973; Heuser, 1977). When the motor nerve was stimulated, there was a depletion

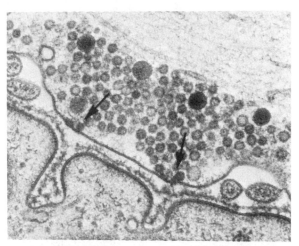

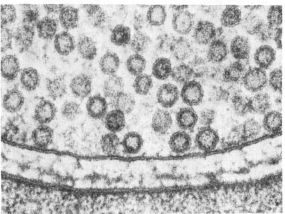

FIGURE 17 FROG NEUROMUSCULAR JUNCTION. Top photo shows synaptic vesicles collected just inside the presynaptic membrane at the active zones (arrows) above the junctional folds of the postjunctional membrane ($\times$ 40,000). Bottom: higher magnification ($\times$ 112,000). (After Heuser, 1977.)

of synaptic vesicles and an appearance of coated vesicles and cisternae. The longer the stimulation, the more pronounced were these effects. This suggested that the coated vesicles had been "pinched off" from invaginations of the synaptic membranes by endocytosis. The coated vesicles in turn were converted into the cisternae, from which new synaptic vesicles were formed. The "coats" were returned to the terminal membrane (Figure 19)

Evidence to support this model came from studies with horseradish peroxidase (HP), which is a com-

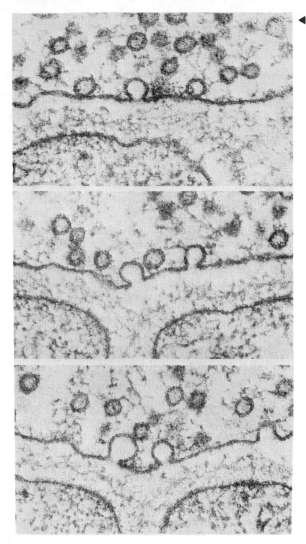

◀ FIGURE 18 FROG NEUROMUSCULAR JUNCTIONS. Three sections of frozen frog neuromuscular junctions shown at high magnification (×145,000). The muscle was frozen within 5.1 msec after a chemically induced, abnormally large burst of ACh release following a single nerve stimulus. Many synaptic vesicles are seen in the act of exocytosis. In all cases the open vesicles were found above the mouths of the junctional folds, hence at the site of the presynaptic active zones. (From Heuser, 1977.)

Questions about the Vesicle Hypothesis

The foregoing account of the role of synaptic vesicles in synaptic transmission represents the currently accepted view of a large majority of investigators in the fields of neurocytology and neurochemistry. However, certain questions about the generality of the vesicle hypothesis have arisen, and a brief review of these questions seems appropriate here. One aspect of the problem is whether vesicles play a role in synaptic transmission in all instances. A second problem involves the notion that the release of transmitters occurs in finite amounts, or QUANTA, and that vesicles determine the quantal size. Said another way: Is the amount

pound that will cross neuron membranes by an uptake process. This substance can be detected by a specific stain and its presence within a cell is direct evidence of membrane activity. When unstimulated muscle tissue was bathed in a solution containing HP, the HP did not penetrate synaptic membranes. However, after prolonged stimulation, HP was found in synaptic vesicles. It can be concluded that HP entered the cell by an endocytotic process and was later incorporated into cisternae and synaptic vesicles.

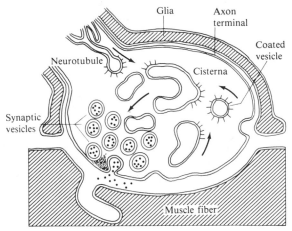

FIGURE 19 SYNAPTIC VESICLE RECYCLING. After exocytosis of the synaptic vesicles the fused vesicles cause the presynaptic membrane to buckle and invaginate. Endocytosis occurs by the pinching off of coated vesicles, which probably contain parts of the presynaptic membrane. The coated vesicles expand, forming cisternae that lead to the formation of new vesicles. New vesicles also appear to be formed from the ends of the neurotubules. (From Heuser, 1977.)

of neurotransmitter released equal to the number of molecules in one vesicle multiplied by the number of vesicles that are emptied? This second problem is discussed in detail in Chapter 6.

Vesicular Versus Cytoplasmic Acetylcholine

Many of the investigations on transmitter release have been done with the electric organ of the torpedo, a ray that stuns its prey by emitting electric shocks. This tissue has a high concentration of cholinergic cells (i.e., cells that synthesize and secrete acetylcholine). Fractionation studies of electric organ tissue showed that the vesicular fraction had the highest concentration of ACh, supporting the notion that ACh is sequestered within the vesicles. However, all tissue ACh was not found within the vesicles; a significant amount was found within the cytoplasm and was estimated to be as much as 50 percent of total. This finding could be explained by the fact that the enzyme that synthesizes ACh, CHOLINE ACETYLASE, is found only in the cytoplasm, suggesting that after synthesis the vesicles are filled with cytoplasmic ACh and a sizable fraction remains in the cytoplasm (Dunant and Israel, 1979).

Zimmermann (1979) questioned the size of the cytoplasmic pool of ACh proposed by Dunant and Israel and pointed out that it depends upon extracellular calcium (Ca^{2+}). It is known that factors in the disruption and homogenization of tissue in the presence of Ca^{2+} cause the release of ACh from vesicles. In the presence of Ca^{2+} CHELATING AGENTS (chemicals that bind Ca^{2+} and render it inactive), the harvesting of ACh from synaptosomal tissue is enhanced. Thus, Collier (1979) proposed that cytoplasmic ACh could merely be the result of tissue fractionation and therefore questioned whether there were significant amounts of cytoplasmic ACh in the living organism. On the other hand, there are studies that showed that newly synthesized ACh was preferentially released in sympathetic ganglia, and the presumption is that this store is not sequestered in vesicles (see Chapter 6).

Other studies showed that stimulating the nerves to the electric organ of the torpedo ray for 3 minutes led to a significant depletion of cytoplasmic ACh without any appreciable change in the number of vesicles or vesicular ACh. More tests showed that these results were not due to depletion and rapid refilling of vesicles. In still another experiment using aplysia (a large sea snail), the preparation was treated with ACh esterase, the enzyme that destroys ACh. This treat-

ment was supposed to abolish the cytoplasmic ACh while sparing the vesicular ACh. Before ACh esterase treatment, stimulation caused the release of ACh, but after the treatment there was no release. This showed that in this preparation cytoplasmic ACh was releasable but vesicular ACh was not (Collier, 1979).

Although the photomicrographs of Heuser (Figures 17–19) show vesicles that are presumably excreting neurotransmitters, there is no proof that they are actually doing so. It is quite possible that they are expelling calcium ions or other substances that are involved in neurotransmitter release.

Zimmermann (1979) suggests that, rather than vesicular and cytoplasmic pools of ACh, there are at least two types of vesicles, one of which is 25 percent smaller than the other and has a higher incorporation rate of newly synthesized ACh. These smaller vesicles appear in nerve terminals after stimulation, and they can be separated from the larger vesicles by centrifugation.

This discussion demonstrates that there is neither proof nor disproof of the vesicular hypothesis of ACh release. Even if a vesicular mechanism is at work in one tissue, it may not be present in other cholinergic systems, nor is it the only mechanism that can operate. The fact that most of these studies dealt with cholinergic synapses and used atypical tissues like electric organs readily raises the question about the generality of these findings for other neurotransmitter systems.

Neurotransmitter Action on Receptors

When transmitters diffuse across the synaptic cleft, they combine with specific sites on the postsynaptic membrane. The consequence of this combination is a change in the permeability of the membrane to Na^+, K^+, or Cl^-, which may be excitatory or inhibitory to the postsynaptic cell, depending upon the receptor site at a particular junction. For example, the cholinergic neuromuscular junctions between the vagus nerve and the heart are inhibitory because release of ACh causes an increased permeability to K^+. Because potassium inside the muscle cell has a greater concentration it flows out of the cell, thereby increasing the negativity of the cell interior and hyperpolarizing the cell membrane. This makes it more difficult for an action potential to be generated. In the case of somatic neuromuscular junctions, the effect of ACh release is to increase the permeability of the postsynaptic membrane to Na^+. Because sodium ions are in greater concentration outside the cell, there is an influx of Na^+, thereby decreasing internal negativity or depolarizing the post-synaptic membrane. If the depolarization is wide-spread and frequent, summation occurs and an action potential will be generated in the postsynaptic cell. Thus, although ACh is the transmitter in both cases, it has opposite physiological effects because of the nature of the receptor sites. γ-Aminobutyric acid (GABA) is a widely distributed inhibitory transmitter in the CNS. It increases membrane permeability to Cl^-. Because chloride ions occur in greater concentration outside the cell, there is a net influx into the cell, thereby hyperpolarizing it.

It is almost certain that transmitter receptor sites are located on the surface of the postsynaptic membrane, which is not surprising because it is there that they would be most accessible to the released transmitter. When ACh was applied via a micropipette to the surface of a muscle fiber, action potentials were recorded with an intracellular recording electrode. However, when the tip of the micropipette was inserted *into* the muscle fiber, no response was recorded, even when the amount of ACh inserted into the cell was increased 10-fold (Del Castillo and Katz, 1955).

One of the most perplexing problems was how the synaptic transmitter, in conjunction with the post-synaptic receptor, is able to effect changes that ultimately lead to the formation of action potentials in postsynaptic neurons. This is a problem of transduction. It is like the problem of explaining how pressure changes caused by vibrating air molecules enter the ear canal and cause vibration of membranes and the auditory ossicles, which then lead to vibrations in the cochlear fluid and so forth until nerve impulses that go to the brain are generated, to make hearing possible. To solve problems of transduction, there must be an understanding of the steps through which energy is transferred from one state to the next. The problem of determining transduction mechanisms in synapses has been greatly aided by the discovery within the last decade or so of two classes of substances that play a role in many physiological activities. They are the cyclic nucleotides and calmodulin.

Role of the Cyclic Nucleotides

The cyclic nucleotides are cyclic adenosine 3′,5′-monophosphate (cAMP) and cyclic guanosine 3′,5′-monophosphate (cGMP). In 1971, the late E.W. Sutherland was awarded the Nobel prize for his pioneering work on the discovery and identification of

these substances. Sutherland was interested in how epinephrine (adrenalin) stimulated the breakdown of glycogen in liver and muscle. Glycogen is a storage form of glucose, and the breakdown reaction is a crucial one for providing glucose for conversion to energy in stressful situations. Sutherland found that epineprhine increased the activity of the enzyme phosphorylase, which is responsible for the conversion of glycogen to glucose. In addition, he found an intermediate substance that converted an inactive form of phosphorylase to an active one. This substance was cAMP. Because epinephrine is unable to penetrate cell membranes, cAMP acts as an intermediary for the process of glycogenolysis (the conversion of glycogen to glucose) (Sutherland, 1972).

More specifically, epinephrine activates the enzyme adenylate cyclase, which freely circulates among the lipid molecules of membranes. Adenylate cyclase converts ATP to cAMP, which acts to convert the inactive phosphorylase to the active one. The cAMP is degraded by cyclic nucleotide phosphodiesterase (or just phosphodiesterase), an enzyme that converts cAMP to 5′-AMP (which is inert).* Thus, epinephrine is regarded as the "first messenger" and cAMP is regarded as the "second messenger" in the mobilization of glucose by the neurotransmitter epinephrine (Figures 20 and 21).

Cyclic Nucleotides in Neural Function

Following the discovery of cAMP, investigators found that the brain is an unusually rich source of adenylate cyclase and phosphodiesterase. It was also found that neurotransmitters and electrical stimulation caused an increase of cAMP synthesis in bovine sympathetic ganglia and brain slices (Kebabian and Greengard, 1971). Furthermore, it was shown that applying cAMP to the sympathetic ganglia of rabbits caused a hyperpolarization of the ganglia that delayed synaptic transmission through them (McAfee and Greengard, 1972). In investigations of the cerebellum, it was discovered that stimulation of noradrenergic nerves to the cerebellum or application of norepinephrine or cAMP on the surface of the Purkinje cells gave the same hyperpolarizing effect in the Purkinje cells (Bloom et al., 1973). It was also discovered that the methylxanthines (which include caffeine and theophylline—stim-

---

*A compound, dibutyryl cAMP (D-cAMP) is used experimentally to study the effects of cAMP because D-cAMP is less readily metabolized by phosphodiesterase.

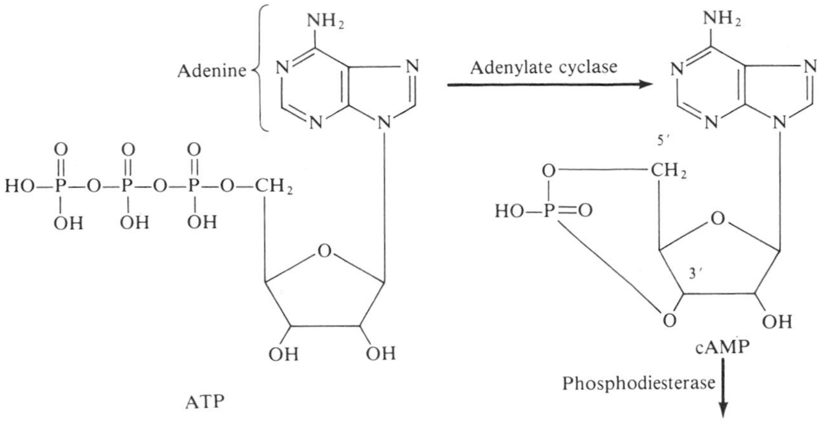

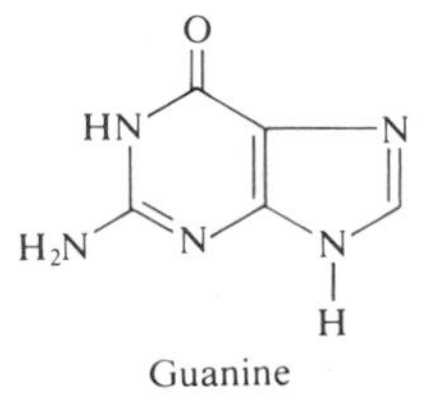

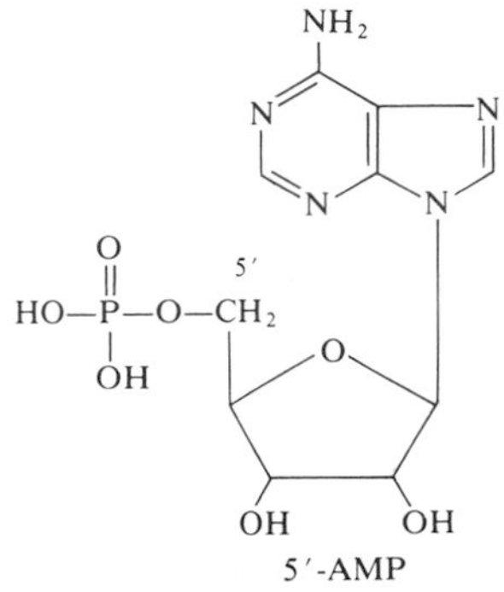

FIGURE 20 SYNTHESIS OF CYCLIC AMP. Adenylate cyclase converts adenosine triphosphate (ATP) into cAMP. Phosphodiesterase converts cAMP into the inert compound 5'-AMP. In cGMP, guanine is substituted for the adenine moiety.

ulants found in tea) were phosphodiesterase inhibitors. These potentiated the action of cAMP by blocking its metabolism by phosphodiestrase (Robison et al., 1971). The stimulating effects of coffee and tea are assumed to be linked to this mechanism.

Cyclic AMP exerts specific effects upon different biological systems through the action of a group of enzymes called protein kinases (which catalyze the transfer of phosphate groups from ATP to acceptor proteins). Cyclic AMP stimulates the protein kinases; the stimulation results in the PHOSPHORYLATION (addition of phosphates) of specific proteins. As each type of cell has its own specific kinases, cAMP is able to energize each system in a rather specific way whether the system is involved in glycogenolysis, fat metabolism (LIPOLYSIS), secretion of thyroid hormone, or synaptic transmission. In synaptic transmission, the phosphorylation of membrane proteins results in the alteration of the shape of the proteins, thus providing channels for the influx or efflux of the ions responsible for synaptic potentials.

Synaptic membranes also contain phosphoprotein phosphatase, an enzyme that removes phosphate groups from proteins. Dephosphorylation reverses the molecular changes of membrane protein and closes the channels of ion conductance (Greengard, 1976). These mechanisms are illustrated in Figure 22.

A different nucleotide plays a role in synaptic transmission across cholinergic synapses in nonstriated muscle. This nucleotide is cGMP (McAfee and Greengard, 1972). Guanylate cyclase converts guanosine triphosphate (GTP) to cGMP. Also, the phosphodiesterase that terminates the action of cGMP appears to be specific for cGMP.

Cyclic nucleotides do not seem to be directly involved in stimulating the postsynaptic membrane of cholinergic synapses on striated muscle. The interval required for synthesis and intervention of cyclic nucleotides is too long compared to the interval between neurotransmitter release and muscle contraction, an action that takes only a few milliseconds (Nathanson and Greengard, 1976, 1977). Nevertheless,

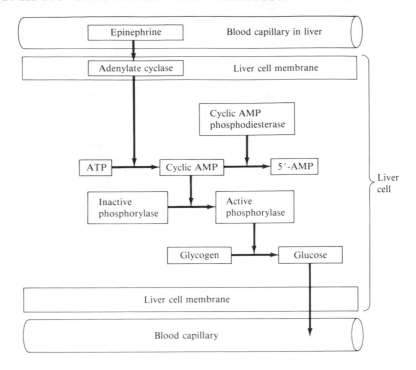

FIGURE 21 CYCLIC AMP ACTIVITY IN GLYCO-GENOLYSIS. In the liver, epinephrine leaves the capillaries and activates adenylate cyclase in the liver cell membranes. This converts ATP to cAMP. The cAMP activates the enzyme phosphorylase, which converts glycogen to glucose.

The glucose is transported out of the liver cells, reenters the capillaries, and is transported to muscles as a source of energy. Cyclic AMP is inactivated by phosphodiesterase to form 5'-AMP. Not all steps are shown.

at neuromyal junctions there is an enormous amplification of effect between ACh release and the depolarization of the sarcolemma (the muscle membrane) that leads to muscle contraction. It is estimated that one or two molecules of ACh can produce the translocation of 50,000 sodium and potassium ions at the neuromyal junction (Katz and Miledi, 1972). Perhaps the addition of high-energy phosphate bonds of the cyclic nucleotides supplying additional energy for chemical reactions in this case would be superfluous.

Finally, some pyramidal cells in the rat cerebral cortex are responsive to both NE and ACh, as well as to their respective second messengers, cAMP and cGMP. By microiontophoresis, small amounts of NE and cAMP caused an inhibition of the spontaneous discharge rate whereas application of ACh and cGMP on the same cell caused an increase in discharge rate. Thus, at least some pyramidal cells have a dual function and respond to different transmitters; these cells seem to be equipped with the appropriate cyclic nucleotides (Stone et al., 1975).

It seems that cAMP and cGMP antagonize each other while mediating the effects of neurotransmitters that have opposing actions on the same system. For example, acetylcholine causes muscle contractions of the gut, whereas epinephrine causes relaxation of the gut. ACh causes an increase of cGMP and a decrease in cAMP, whereas epinephrine causes the reverse. These effects seem to reflect modifications of adenylate and guanylate cyclase by the transmitters.

Greengard (1979) has described some other potentially important differences between cAMP and cGMP. The application of cAMP always seems to mimic the action of a neurotransmitter or hormone on a particular target cell. This suggests that cAMP mediates the action of the transmitter on the target cells. Cyclic GMP has similar effects; for example, cGMP mimics the action of acetylcholine on sympathetic ganglion cells and neurons in the cortex, as well as on autonomically innervated structures such as the pancreas and heart muscles. However, in other cases, cGMP does not mimic the action of the neurotransmitter or hormone in question. Thus, it is proposed that the increase in cGMP in these latter systems may serve merely to modulate the immediate response to the neurotransmitter.

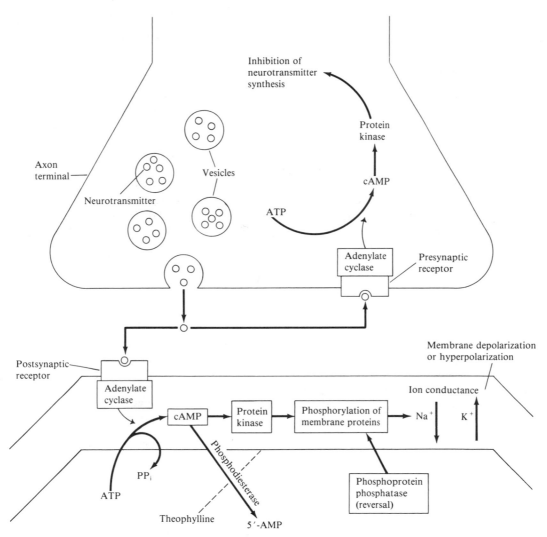

FIGURE 22. CYCLIC AMP IN SYNAPTIC TRANSMISSION. A presynaptic neurotransmitter activates adenylate cyclase in the postsynaptic receptor, which converts ATP to cAMP, giving off inorganic phosphates (PPi) as a byproduct. cAMP activates a protein kinase, which phosphorylates a receptor protein in the postsynaptic membrane. Phosphate addition alters the conformation of the receptor protein and allows increased ion conductance through the membrane. The ion conductance can result in either depolarization or hyperpolarization of the membrane. Membrane phosphorylation is reversed by the enzyme phosphoprotein phosphatase, and cAMP is deactivated by phosphodiesterase. A presynaptic receptor also utilizes cAMP to inhibit transmitter synthesis. Theophylline is a phosphodiesterase inhibitor and prolongs the action of cAMP.

Contrary Findings

Although the results of the studies cited above point to a significant role for the cyclic nucleotides in neural functioning, some later data raised questions about certain details. For example, the earlier studies showed that chemical or electrical stimulation of bovine sympathetic ganglia caused an increase in cAMP production (Cramer et al., 1973), and that exogenous cAMP could mimic the dopamine-induced hyperpolarizing effect in the rabbit sympathetic ganglion. These observations served as the basis for the role of cAMP in the CNS, namely, that the neurotransmitters cause a buildup of cAMP or cGMP, which leads to membrane depolarization or hyperpolarization. However, the biochemical data (the buildup of cAMP) were derived from bovine ganglia and the electrophysiological data (the hyperpolarization of the ganglia) were from rabbit ganglia. The combination of these two kinds of data from two different species to formulate the hypothetical role of cAMP in neural function was deemed by some investigators to be less than satisfactory. Consequently, there were attempts to make both types of observations in the same tissue and assess the generality of the findings across different species.

The design of the experiments was to apply various transmitters and chemical agents to rat isolated sympathetic ganglia and measure cAMP production. Following that, while using the same tissue and chemical agents, measurements were made of the electrical characteristics of the ganglia. In one experiment, it was found that dopamine hyperpolarized ganglia, but the effect was not enhanced by theophylline. Moreover, drugs such as phenylephrine and clonidine (which stimulate dopamine receptors) did not increase cAMP levels. In other experiments, exogenous cAMP hyperpolarized the ganglia, but the same effect was obtained by the ribonucleoside adenosine, suggesting that an adenosine receptor was involved. It was also observed that the metabolite 5'-AMP caused ganglion hyperpolarization and that the cAMP effect was antagonized by theophylline. Therefore, the conversion of cAMP to 5'-AMP was concluded to be a necessary condition for the hyperpolarizing effect. Finally, drugs that stimulated receptors different from dopamine receptors raised cAMP levels, and antagonistic drugs blocked this effect. However, there were no electrical changes in the ganglion tissues that were treated in this way (Brown et al., 1979). Thus, these studies showed that there is a dissociation between dopamine-induced hyperpolarization and elevation of cAMP levels in rat ganglia, suggesting that cAMP is not the mediator of the membrane changes. However, it is possible that cAMP may act upon external adenosine receptors, an action that may produce long-term changes in neuron excitability.

In another series of experiments, Quenzer et al. (1979) obtained data showing that isoproterenol hyperpolarized ganglion cells and blocked synaptic transmission in rats, just as had been demonstrated in rabbits by McAfee and Greengard (1972). However, in the rat experiments, Quenzer's group found discrepancies in the amount of isoproterenol required to stimulate cAMP production and the amount necessary to block ganglion transmission. Concentrations of isoproterenol that elevated cAMP levels 9-fold had no effect on ganglion transmission. Conversely, dopamine concentrations that depressed ganglion transmission by 45 percent had no effect on cAMP production.

It was also found that the effects of isoproterenol on rat ganglia could be depressed by two different receptor-blocking drugs, suggesting that the identity of the receptors in the ganglia may be ambiguous.

Possible explanations for these results might rest upon differences among species in the number of dopamine-sensitive neurons within the ganglion: an estimate for cattle is 1750; for rabbits, 80; for cats, 50. No estimate has been made for rats (Greengard et al., 1972). Because it is known that cAMP acts upon intracellular sites to activate enzymes or alter intracellular membranes, cAMP may be serving general metabolic functions in neurons rather than having a specific role in synaptic transmission (Weiss and Kidman, 1979). (For more discussion of dopamine receptors in sympathetic ganglia, see Chapter 7.)

Although there seem to be some inconsistencies in the results of studies of sympathetic ganglia, there is considerable evidence for a role for the cyclic nucleotides in synaptic transmission. The generality of this mechanism is attested to by the fact that transmitter-sensitive adenylate cyclases and cAMP have already been identified for β-adrenergic, dopaminergic, and serotonergic receptors, for the H_2 form of the histamine receptors, and for octopamine, opiate, and perhaps glutamate receptors (Mahler, 1977). Cyclic GMP has been associated with α-adrenergic, cholinergic, and the H_1 form of histamine synaptic receptors (Greengard, 1979).

Calmodulin, Another Second Messenger

Another development in synaptic physiology involves a protein called calmodulin, which seems to play a role in many other biological phenomena as well. This protein has been identified in virtually all nucleated cells—from one-celled organisms and plant cells to human brain cells. It is directly related to the activity of calcium (Ca^{2+}) in cell function. It was independently discovered by many researchers, who did not realize that they were all working on the same thing.

Calmodulin is a protein with a molecular weight of 16,700. It is a single polypeptide that has been chemically characterized and appears to have a similar if not identical amino acid sequence in widely divergent species. Ca^{2+} and calmodulin by themselves do not appear to be active; their activity depends upon the formation of a calmodulin–Ca^{2+} complex. This is the basis for Cheung's (1980) suggestion that the protein be called calmodulin, which is now the accepted name. The complex participates in kinase phosphorylation of membrane proteins. It is also active in neurotransmitter release and in Ca^{2+} transport in erythrocytes and striated muscle. In the latter, calmodulin is one of four subunits in the enzyme PHOSPHORYLASE KINASE, which participates in glycogenolysis to supply energy for muscle contraction. In muscle, it is also related chemically to TROPONIN C, which is involved in muscle contraction itself. Calmodulin plays a role in changes in cell shape, in the beating of flagella and cilia in unicellular organisms, in egg fertilization, and in cell division. It interacts with the cyclic nucleotides (cAMP and cGMP) to accentuate or attenuate their effects. Because adenylate cyclase and phosphodiesterase are Ca^{2+} dependent, the molecular link between these two intercellular regulators is now apparent (Cheung, 1980). The intricate details of the chemistry of the calmodulin–Ca^{2+} complex is described by Cheung (1980) and Means and Dedman (1980).

Investigations of the role of calmodulin on synaptic vesicle release of neurotransmitters have shown that there is a depolarization-dependent entry of Ca^{2+} into the presynaptic nerve terminal and that these Ca^{2+} fluxes are sufficient to activate the synaptic vesicle calmodulin–protein kinase system, leading to phosphorylation of vesicle and pre- and postsynaptic membrane proteins. Thus, calmodulin regulates the phosphoproteins that modulate synaptic transmission.

In another procedure, vesicles were extracted from synaptosomes and incubated in a calmodulin-free medium. Electron microscopy revealed vesicles that appeared rather dispersed, about 50 percent of them being classed as free vesicles (i.e., those that did not touch other vesicles). When calmodulin alone was added to the incubation mixture, there was no significant change; when Ca^{2+} alone was added, there was some reduction in free vesicles. But when Ca^{2+} and calmodulin were added together, there was a marked aggregation of vesicles into tight clusters, with apparent vesicle fusion, vesicle rupture, and decrease in vesicle diameter. Under these conditions, only about 13.5 percent were classed as free vesicles (DeLorenzo, 1980a).

When vesicles and synaptic membranes were studied under the preceding conditions, it was found that Ca^{2+} and calmodulin caused a significant increase in the number of synaptic vesicles that became attached to synaptic membranes. Ca^{2+} and calmodulin alone were not as effective as these agents together in causing these effects. These results suggest that calmodulin modulates the effects of Ca^{2+} on synaptic membranes and synaptic vesicles, possibly initiating exocytosis or other membrane-vesicle interactions (Figure 23). It has been shown that the Ca^{2+}-calmodulin system acts upon tubulin, a cytoskeletal protein that is found in high concentrations in nerve terminals and can polymerize (the molecules can join together into long chains) into microtubules. Whereas microtubules are absent in axon terminals, tubulin has been shown to be present in synaptic vesicle membranes, and vesicles have an endogenous tubulin-kinase system. It is possible that a Ca^{2+}-calmodulin-stimulated phosphorylation of tubulin can alter the physiochemical properties of tubulin in mediating membrane interactions.

Interestingly, during investigations into the mechanism of action of the antipsychotic drug trifluoperazine (Stelazine), and the anticonvulsive drugs (used in the treatment of epilepsy) diphenylhydantoin (Dilantin) and diazepam (Valium), it was found that the drugs block the phosphorylation of membrane proteins and norepinephrine release, suggesting the drugs block the action of the Ca^{2+}-calmodulin complex, thereby increasing the threshold of excitation of these neurons (DeLorenzo, 1980a; 1980b; 1981).

The role of calmodulin was investigated in the striatum (the basal ganglia), an area rich in dopamine axon terminals. In this region, dopamine activated

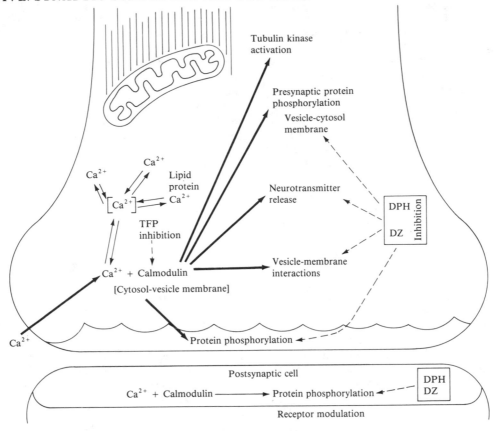

FIGURE 23 CALMODULIN EFFECTS WITHIN SYNAPSES. Calmodulin is bound to vesicle and pre- and postsynaptic membranes. It is also found in the cytosol (cytoplasm). After depolarization-dependent influx into the nerve terminal, Ca^{2+} is immediately bound to calmodulin. The Ca^{2+}-calmodulin complex then induces presynaptic protein phosphorylation of vesicle tubulin and terminal membranes that participate in neurotransmitter release, and modulates the activities of adenylate and guanylate cyclases and phosphodiesterase. Trifluoperazine, TFP; diphenylhydantoin, DPH; and diazepam, DZ presumably block the action of calmodulin. (After DeLorenzo, 1982.)

adenylate cyclase in the postsynaptic membrane in a reaction coupled to the activity of guanosine triphosphate (GTP). Calmodulin, which was bound to the inner leaflet of the membrane, was also involved in regulating the coupling of the membrane-bound adenylate cyclase to the dopamine recognition site. Stimulation of the dopamine receptors caused an accumulation of cAMP that activated a protein kinase, leading to the phosphorylation of membrane proteins in a manner described earlier. But with persistent stimulation of the dopamine receptors, calmodulin was released from the membranes into the cytoplasm, where it increased the affinity of phosphodiesterase for cAMP (Hanbauer et al., 1980).

When certain drugs such as *d*-amphetamine are used to cause a release of dopamine—thereby persistently stimulating dopamine receptors—there is only a transient increase in striatal cAMP. This is probably due to the fact that dopamine receptors trigger cytoplasmic calmodulin activation of phosphodiesterase, which degrades cAMP. This may account for the rapid tolerance that develops with persistent use of this drug.

When receptors are continuously deprived of normal transmitter inputs (e.g., by denervating the presynaptic terminals), the receptors develop a supersensitivity that is expressed when the transmitter is later supplied exogenously. One explanation of this phenomenon is that there is a compensatory multiplication of receptors. Another explanation derives from the finding that transmitter deprivation increases calmodulin binding to the synaptic membranes; therefore, less is released into the cytoplasm. High concentrations of membrane-bound calmodulin coincide with supersensitivity of striatal adenylate cyclase to stimulation by dopamine. Thus, receptor supersensitivity is related to calmodulin-mediated hyperactivity of cAMP (Hanbauer et al., 1980).

It is to be noted from the above discussion that in neurons membrane-bound calmodulin promotes the action of adenylate cyclase and cAMP production, whereas cytoplasmic calmodulin promotes the activity of phosphodiesterase and cAMP metabolism. Thus, it would appear that calmodulin could be working at cross purposes: Membrane-bound calmodulin initiates postsynaptic membrane activity, and cytoplasmic calmodulin terminates it. This arrangement serves as a mechanism to regulate neurotransmitter effects.

In summary, we have shown that synaptic action involves an intricate set of operations that begins with the arrival of an action potential at the axon terminal. This leads to an influx of calcium ions, which interact with intracellular calmodulin to mobilize synaptic vesicles and bind them to presynaptic terminal membranes for exocytosis (the discharge of the vesicle contents of neurotransmitter). The neurotransmitter is conveyed across the synaptic cleft to the postsynaptic membrane, where it is recognized and bound to membrane receptor proteins. The receptor proteins utilize the calmodulin–Ca^{2+} complex to initiate the synthesis of cyclic nucleotides that are instrumental in the phosphorylation of postsynaptic membrane proteins. Calmodulin also interacts with proteins and enzymes within the sequences constituting cAMP synthesis and kinase-mediated membrane protein phosphorylation. And finally, cytoplasmic calmodulin, which is released from membranes by transmitter action, facilitates the action of phosphodiesterase (to metabolize cAMP) while phosphoprotein phosphatase restores membrane proteins to their former status as controllers of membrane permeability. Normally, all of these events, and probably others, sensitively modulate synaptic transmission.

Autoreceptors

In describing the functions of synapses, we have pointed out that neurotransmitters exert their chemical effects on receptors that are situated on postsynaptic membranes. However, there is a growing body of evidence showing that receptors also exist on presynaptic terminals, on the cell's soma, and on dendrites. These receptors respond to the cell's own transmitter. Thus, they are called autoreceptors. The autoreceptors do not always respond to transmitter agonists and antagonists in the same ways as the postsynaptic receptors. It is also true that the autoreceptors may differ substantially in their sensitivity, which probably corresponds to their affinity for various substances. These differences in affinity may depend on special structural features of the autoreceptors and/or on their concentration. According to recent theories, the role of the autoreceptors may be in negative or positive feedback mechanisms controlling the release or synthesis of neurotransmitters (Carlsson, 1978; Iversen, 1978). Thus far there is rather substantial support for the existence of adrenergic, dopaminergic, and serotonergic autoreceptors, and it is likely that they will be found in other systems. It has also been found that cAMP is involved in their activity. The details of autoreceptor activity will be considered in more detail in the chapters dealing with each specific neurotransmitter.

Termination of Transmitter Action

How are transmitter effects terminated? How do postsynaptic membranes return to their resting state? As mentioned previously, acetylcholine is inactivated by acetylcholine esterase, which splits the ACh molecules to choline and acetic acid. However, such neurotransmitter metabolism is not the usual mechanism for terminating transmitter action. Much of the pioneer work on this and other problems was done by the Nobel laureate Julius Axelrod and his colleagues (1971). During studies of the metabolism of norepinephrine, they discovered that after the intravenous injection of tritiated norepinephrine ([^{3}H]NE), into cats, there was a rapid and unequal distribution of this substance in tissues. Relatively little was found in brain tissue, suggesting that there was a barrier preventing the transfer of NE from the bloodstream to brain tissue. (See the discussion of the blood brain barrier in Chapter 1). On the other hand, [^{3}H]NE was selectively taken up by tissues that were heavily innervated by sympathetic nerves, such as the heart and the spleen. Also, when these tissues were examined 2 hours after injection of [^{3}H]NE (i.e., long after the physiological effects such as tachycardia had disappeared), they were found to have almost the same levels of [^{3}H]NE as those found in subjects that had been sacrificed only 2 minutes after injection. This showed that NE is rapidly taken up and retained in a physiological inactive form by the sympathetic nerves. The uptake process is accomplished by an active sodium and potassium-dependent transport system that can take up NE against concentration gradients as high as 10,000 to 1.

To investigate this phenomenon further, the superior cervical sympathetic ganglion (the cell bodies of sympathetic nerves that go to the iris for pupil dilation, etc.) was surgically removed unilaterally in cats. After complete degeneration of the sympathetic nerve fibers had occurred, [^{3}H]NE was injected intravenously. One hour after the injection the animals were sacrificed. It was found that there was a sharp reduction in the uptake of [^{3}H]NE in the denervated structures as compared to uptake by the normal structures on the opposite side. This showed that sympathetic nerve endings take up and retain circulating noreprinephrine.

In an effort to localize precisely where within the cell the [^{3}H]NE was taken up, Axelrod and his colleagues (1971) used a technique involving electron microscopy and autoradiography. In this technique, a thin slice of tissue suspected of containing a radioactive substance is coated with a very thin film of photographic emulsion. The coated tissue is sandwiched between glass plates and refrigerated to prevent spoilage. After an interval long enough to let the radioactivity act on the film, the tissue–film specimen is developed and examined under the electron microscope. The microscopic details of the tissue are visible and are overlaid with dark photographic grains where the radioactive materials caused changes in the photographic emulsion.

In one of Axelrod's experiments, the pineal glands of rats were examined for the uptake of [^{3}H]NE because the pineal gland is rich in sympathetic nerve terminals. Thirty minutes after intravenous injection of [^{3}H]NE, the pineal glands were removed and prepared for autoradiography. It was found that dark grains overlaid the thin nonmyelinated axons innervating the pineal gland. These nerves contained vesicles that were approximately 50 nm in diameter. When rat heart tissue that had taken up [^{3}H]NE was homogenized and separated by differential centrifugation, the synaptosomal fraction was found to contain the most NE and radioactivity; this fraction also contained the vesicles. These observations were added proof that [^{3}H]NE was taken up by the vesicles. Moreover, this

NE was inactive unless the vesicles were lysed with dilute acid. It is now well established that the uptake process also occurs after synaptic release of other transmitters.

It should be emphasized, however, that reuptake or recapture is not the sole method of transmitter inactivation. Considerable evidence indicates that small amounts of transmitter simply diffuse out of the synaptic cleft and, after degradation, the metabolites enter the bloodstream and are eventually excreted in the urine.

A third way of terminating transmitter action is by way of immediate degradation within the synaptic cleft and the absorption of the metabolites into the bloodstream. For example, ACh is broken down into choline and acetate in the synaptic cleft by the enzyme ACh esterase. The choline is taken back up and used to synthesize new ACh, and the acetate enters other metabolic pathways. In other cases, the transmitter itself or its metabolites are taken up by glia that enclose or surround the synaptic junction.

Summary

It seems to be well established that synaptic transmission (the communication from one nerve cell to another) involves a series of chemical events. Nerve impulses (action potentials) occurring at axon terminals lead to an influx of calcium ions, which act in conjunction with calmodulin to mobilize synaptic vesicles and fuse them to the presynaptic membrane. Calmodulin participates in phosphorylation of membrane proteins that permits the release of neurotransmitters from the vesicles. The neurotransmitters then cross the synaptic cleft to interact with receptor zones on postsynaptic membranes.

The stimulation of the postsynaptic receptors leads to the production of the cyclic nucleotides cAMP or cGMP, which activate the protein kinases that exert specific effects by phosphorylating certain membrane proteins that open channels to sodium ions for depolarization or to potassium and chloride ions for hyperpolarization of the postsynaptic membrane. These electrical changes on the postsynaptic membrane summate either to produce action potentials or to inhibit them.

The transmitter (or at least part of the molecule, as in the case of acetylcholine) is then recaptured by the presynaptic terminal (possibly to be reinserted into the synaptic vesicles and to be used over and over again). The economy of this mechanism is self-evident—it results in a reduced need for precursors and for resynthesis. Some fraction of the transmitter diffuses out of the synaptic cleft, some is taken up by surrounding glia, and some is metabolized. But the principal mode of transmitter deactivation is the reuptake process.

Another class of transmitter receptors is found on the soma, dendrites, and presynaptic membranes of cells. These receptors are activated by the same transmitter that is released by the cell; hence, they are known as autoreceptors. The somatic and dendritic autoreceptors are activated by way of recurrent axon collaterals, whereas autoreceptors located on axon terminals are activated by the neurotransmitter that is released from the terminal. These autoreceptors are known to have a role in negative or positive feedback, depending upon the structure or upon the needs of the system.

Finally, it should be recalled that a number of substances called neuromodulators may significantly influence synaptic events in indirect ways. These compounds may be released within the brain or from sources quite distant from their sites of action, and their effects may be widespread and long lasting. It is believed, for instance, that individual differences in the response to stress may hinge upon genetically determined differences in the activation and deactivation of synaptic processes. In a similar way, stress may affect neuromodulators that contribute to the overall effect.

Recommended Readings

Appel, S.H. and Day, E.D. (1976). Cellular and subcellular fractionation. In *Basic Neurochemistry* (G.J. Siegel, R.W. Albers, R. Katzman and B.W. Agranoff, Eds.), pp. 34–59. Little, Brown & Co., Boston. Description of important techniques and other subjects in neurochemistry are covered in this popular volume.

Bennett, M.V.L. (Ed.) (1974) *Synaptic Transmission and Neuronal Interaction*. Raven Press, New York. Advanced research on the morphology and physiology of synapses.

Costa, E., Giacobini, E. and Paoletti, R. (Eds.) (1976). *Advances in Biochemical Psychopharmacology, Vol. 15. First and Second Messengers—New Vistas*. Raven Press, New York. A series of papers on neurotransmitters, neuromodulators and cyclic nucleotides.

Cotman, C.W., Poste, G. and Nicolson, G.L. (Eds.) (1980). *The Cell Surface and Neuronal Function*. Elsevier, New York. A recent collection of papers on membrane function, and receptors for neurotransmitters and drugs.

Hall, Z.W., Hildebrand, J.G. and Kravitz, E.A. (Eds.) (1974). *Chemistry of Synaptic Transmission*. Chiron Press, Newton, Massachusetts. A series of papers and commentaries on the historical development of synaptology.

Iverson, L.L. (1975). Uptake processes for biogenic amines. In *Handbook of Psychopharmacology, Vol. 3, Biochemistry of Biogenic Amines* (L.L. Iverson, S.D. Iverson and S.H. Snyder, Eds.), pp. 381–442. Plenum Press, New York. A review of the physiology of uptake processes.

Mahadik, S.P., Tamir, H. and Rapport, M. (1975). Molecular composition and functional organization of synaptic structures. In *Advances in Neurochemistry, Vol. 3* (B.W. Agranoff and M.H. Aprison, Eds.), pp. 99–163, Plenum Press, New York. An excellent review of synaptic processes and an extensive reference list.

Quarles, R.H. (1975). Glycoproteins in the nervous system. In *The Nervous System, Vol. 1* (D.B. Tower, Ed. in Chief), pp. 493–501, Raven Press, New York. One of several reviews of synaptic function.

Robison, G.A., Butcher, R.W. and Sutherland, E.W. (1971). *Cyclic AMP*. Academic Press, New York. The discovery of cAMP and its role in physiological processes is described well.

Roseman, S. (1974). Complex carbohydrates and intercellular adhesionns. In *The Cell Surface in Development* (A. Moscona, Ed.), pp. 255–271. Wiley, New York. A review of the ontogeny of synaptic connections.

Schmitt, F.O., Dev, P. and Smith, B.H. (1976). Electrotonic processing of information by brain cells. *Science,* 193, 114–120. An excellent discussion of specialized synaptic junctions.

Usdin, E. and Bunney, W.E. Jr. (Eds.) (1975). *Pre- and Postsynaptic Receptors*. Marcel Dekker, New York. A collection of research papers on synaptic function.

Watterson, D.M. and Vincenzi, F.F. (Eds.) (1980). *Calmodulin and Cell Function*. Annals of the New York Academy of Sciences, Vol. 356, New York. An outstanding series of research papers on aspects of calmodulin chemistry and physiology.

CHAPTER SIX

Acetylcholine

Acetylcholine (ACh) was first synthesized in 1867. However, its biological importance was not known for many years thereafter. Dale (1914) noted that applications of ACh mimicked stimulation of parasympathetic nerves; Loewi (1921) discovered its effect on the heartbeat. Dale et al. (1936) chemically identified ACh as the neurotransmitter at the skeletal neuromuscular junction. Despite these early beginnings, the difficulties encountered while studying this substance resulted in comparatively slow progress in understanding its effects (Minz, 1955).

In this chapter we will review ACh synthesis and its control, ACh binding within and ACh release from vesicles, ACh action on postsynaptic receptors, and ACh metabolism. We will also describe the distribution of cholinergic neurons in the peripheral and central nervous system and in doing so cover the distribution of cholinergic responses. Finally, we will describe the nature and action of drugs that affect cholinergic synapses and how these drug effects relate to ensuing behavioral changes.

Part I   Anatomy of Cholinergic Systems

Peripheral Distribution of Cholinergic Systems

Acetylcholine is synthesized in spinal and cranial motoneurons and is the transmitter at neuromuscular junctions affecting the skeletal musculature of the body and head. For example, motoneurons of the spinal cord are responsible for the movement of the limbs and the trunk, whereas cranial motoneurons cause the movement of the eye (the occulomotor nerve), the jaw (the trigeminal nerve), the muscles of facial expression (the facial nerve), the pharynx, larynx, and upper esophagus (the glossopharyngeal and the vagus nerve), and the tongue (the hypoglossal nerve). All of these motoneurons are influenced by reflex inputs, and are controlled by higher centers such as the cerebral cortex, the cerebellum, the hypothalamus, and so on.

In addition, ACh is the principal transmitter in the neural–neural synapses of the parasympathetic and the sympathetic divisions of the autonomic nervous sys-

tem. Figure 1 shows the general organization of the autonomic nervous system. The cranial group of parasympathetic preganglionic nerves (heavy lines) originate in nuclei (aggregations of cell bodies) in the brain stem and convey nerve impulses to the peripheral ganglia such as the ciliary, sphenopalatine and the otic. These ganglia are comprised of the cell bodies of postganglionic fibers (heavy dashed lines) that innervate the iris for pupil constriction, the tear glands, and the salivary glands respectively. The vagus nerve consists of long, preganglionic fibers that terminate upon ganglia that are situated near the organs of the chest and viscera. From these ganglia, short postganglionic fibers (short dashed heavy lines) convey nerve impulses to the cardiac and smooth muscles, and to the glands of the body cavity, such as the heart, trachea, stomach, intestines, pancreas, and so on. All of the neural–

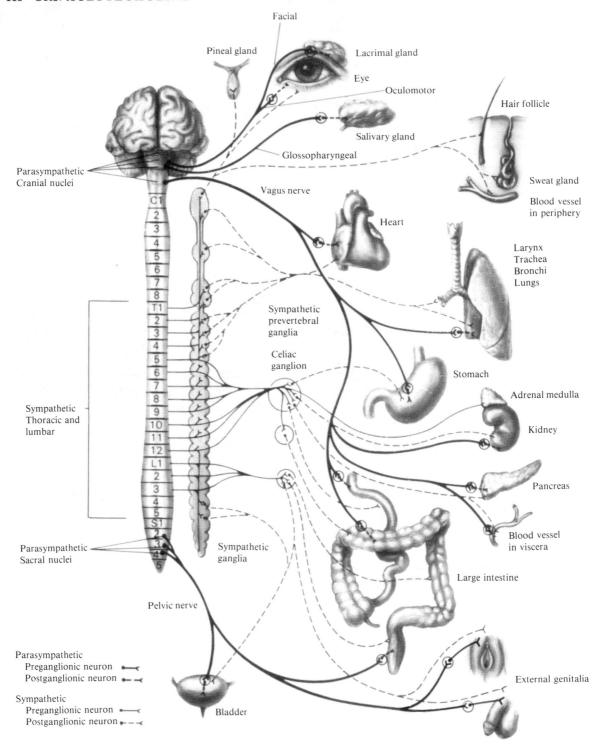

Facial

Pineal gland

Lacrimal gland

Eye

Oculomotor

Hair follicle

Salivary gland

Glossopharyngeal

Parasympathetic
Cranial nuclei

Vagus nerve

Sweat gland

Blood vessel
in periphery

Heart

Larynx
Trachea
Bronchi
Lungs

C1
2
3
4
5
6
7
8
T1
2
3
4
5
6
7
8
9
10
11
12
L1
2
3
4
5
S1
2
3
4
5

Sympathetic
prevertebral
ganglia

Celiac
ganglion

Stomach

Adrenal medulla

Kidney

Sympathetic
Thoracic and
lumbar

Pancreas

Blood vessel
in viscera

Parasympathetic
Sacral nuclei

Sympathetic
ganglia

Large intestine

Pelvic nerve

Parasympathetic
  Preganglionic neuron
  Postganglionic neuron

Sympathetic
  Preganglionic neuron
  Postganglionic neuron

External genitalia

Bladder

◄ FIGURE 1 AUTONOMIC NERVOUS SYSTEM. Preganglionic fibers (heavy solid lines) extend from parasympathetic cranial nuclei (such as the occulomotor, lacrimal, salivatory and vagal nuclei) and from nuclei in the sacral segment of the spinal cord. The cranial preganglionic fibers make neural-neural synapses in the peripheral ganglia, such as the ciliary, sphenopalatine and otic ganglia, which are situated near the innervated organs. These synapses are cholinergic. Short postganglionic fibers (dashed continuation of heavy lines) extend to the effectors (smooth muscles and glands) and form cholinergic neuroeffector junctions. The vagus nerve via many branches forms synapses with small ganglia situated on the organs of the chest and visceral cavity, and short postganglionic fibers innervate these organs and glands. The thin lines represent sympathetic nerves. The preganglionic fibers are cholinergic (ACh); the postganglionic neurons are noradrenergic (NE). (After Carlson, 1980.)

neural synapses and neuroeffector junctions of this system are cholinergic. The cells of origin in the brain stem of this system are also under the influence of higher centers in the brain; thus the thought of food can lead to salivation, scolding can lead to tears, and confrontation with danger can slow digestion.

The pre- and postganglionic axons of the sacral division of the parasympathetic system innervate the lower colon and some structures associated with the bladder and reproductive system (Figure 1, bottom). These neurons are activated reflexly by afferent signals arising from the organs themselves (such as the filling of the bladder) as well as by neural signals from higher centers as in the case of the cranial parasympathetic nerves. Thus the hypothalamus, the hippocampus, and the cerebral cortex exert control over some aspects of urination, defecation, and sexual behavior.

Other cholinergic interneuronal, neuromuscular, and neurosecretory synapses are associated with the sympathetic division of the autonomic system (see also Figure 2 in Chapter 7). In the sympathetic system, all preganglionic fibers (solid light lines) are cholinergic, whereas the postganglionic fibers (dashed light lines) are noradrenergic, except the postganglionic fibers that activate the sweat glands which are cholinergic. Thus, it is seen that acetylcholine is the neurotransmitter controlling all of the somatic musculature, and is the dominant transmitter in both divisions of the autonomic nervous system. Table I presents the neurons and the effector organs that are innervated via cholinergic (nicotinic and muscarinic) receptors. The

main concern here is peripheral ACh systems, but Table I also shows that there are cholinergic systems in the brain—in the cerebral cortex and in a number of subcortical structures.

Nicotinic and Muscarinic Receptors

An essential feature of cholinergic systems is the presence of at least two types of receptors that are responsive to ACh. They are designated as NICOTINIC RECEPTORS and MUSCARINIC RECEPTORS. The distinction between them is made on the basis of responses to certain drugs. One type of receptor is activated by muscarine (an alkaloid* found in the mushroom *Amanita muscaria*) and blocked by the drug scopolamine. The other type of receptor is activated by nicotine (an alkaloid found in the tobacco plant *Nicotiana tabacum*) and blocked by curare. Yet all types of cholinergic receptors are responsive to ACh. It should be especially noted that the differences between the receptors with respect to their drug response is not related to their excitatory or inhibitory nature. For ex-

*Alkaloids are organic compounds that contain nitrogen atoms, have a bitter taste, and are usually of plant origin.

TABLE I. Neurons and Effector Organs That Are Activated via Cholinergic (Nicotinic or Muscarinic) Receptors

Nicotinic	Muscarinic
1. All skeletal muscles and striated muscles of the head (muscles of facial expression, chewing, etc.)	1. Parasympathetically innervated cardiac and smooth muscles (heart, constrictors of the iris, stomach, bronchioles, intestines, etc.)
2. Postganglionic parasympathetic neurons*	2. Salivary, tear, and sweat glands
3. Postganglionic sympathetic neurons*	3. Cholinergic receptors in cortical and subcortical neurons
4. Some cholinergic receptors in the cortex and subcortical structures	4. Organs innervated by the parasympathetic sacral division (lower colon, bladder, urogenital organs)
5. Sacral postganglionic parasympathetic fibers	

*Some of these neurons also have a few muscarinic receptors.

ample, the postganglionic sections of the vagus nerve release ACh, which acts at only one type of receptor—muscarinic; yet ACh mediates inhibitory actions on the heart and excitatory actions on the gastrointestinal tract. The difference in action is probably due to secondary differences in the respective receptors.

The flexibility that exists because a single transmitter can have both excitatory and inhibitory effects obviously is a great advantage in that the number of transmitters can be small and still be able to affect a wide variety of physiological functions because of differences in receptor structure. From a pharmacological point of view, a second advantage lies in the possibility of being able to design drugs that will alter the activity of one part of the cholinergic system without affecting other parts.

Excitatory and Inhibitory Cholinergic Receptors

The nicotinic receptors found on skeletal muscle end plates and on postganglionic sympathetic and parasympathetic neurons are excitatory (i.e., stimulation of these receptors leads to muscle contraction or excitation of postganglionic nerve fibers). The muscarinic receptors are found at all parasympathetically innervated effector organs (such as the heart, the gastrointestinal tract, and various glands). The synapses on the heart and some parts of the genital system are inhibitory; the rest are excitatory. In addition, the sweat glands also have muscarinic receptors, even though they are innervated by postganglionic sympathetic neurons.

Mechanisms of Excitation and Inhibition of Cholinergic Synapses

Mechanistic distinctions can be made between nicotinic and muscarinic receptors. It is generally believed that ACh, acting upon excitatory nicotinic receptors, is directly involved in the membrane changes associated with depolarization because the onset of the reaction is rapid and its duration is short—in fact, so rapid and so short as to preclude much possibility of intervening "second messenger" devices. Evidence suggests that the ACh receptor may be directly coupled to the channel that allows Na^+ passage through the membrane (McGeer et al., 1978). Rapid depolarization can be seen after stimulation of motor axon collaterals to Renshaw cells (see Figure 8 in Chapter 3). The Renshaw cells respond with changes in membrane potential following extremely short

latencies, which can also be elicited by iontophoretic application of ACh or nicotine. Similar effects have been observed in the medulla, thalamus and hypothalamus, cerebellum, and some cortical cells (Phillis, 1976a).

Muscarinic receptors at excitatory junctions, however, respond to iontophoretic ACh by showing a slow onset and prolonged depolarization. This effect is due to a reduction of potassium conductance (or K^+ efflux), meaning that K^+ do not flow out of the stimulated cell to reverse the depolarizing effect of sodium influx as rapidly as usual. When inhibitory muscarinic receptors are stimulated, there is a slowly developing and prolonged hyperpolarization that is due to an increased K^+ efflux, such as that found with vagal stimulation of the heart. These effects are found in the cortex, hypothalamus, pons, medulla, and other areas. Parenthetically it can be noted that the thalamus and cerebellar cortex are regarded as having nicotinic receptors, whereas most of the other brain areas are predominantly muscarinic by a ratio of about 100 to 1.

Lee et al. (1972) found that slices of mammalian cerebral cortex, heart muscle, and intestine showed a 2- to 3-fold increase of cGMP during a 3-minute incubation in medium containing 1.0 μM (1 micromolar*) ACh. All of these tissues have muscarinic ACh receptors. Similar effects were obtained by adding drugs having muscarinic actions but not by those having nicotinic actions; and the effects of the drugs were blocked by muscarinic antagonists but not by nicotinic antagonists. No changes in the cGMP content in these preparations were observed. Thus, it appears that muscarinic actions may be mediated by metabolic processes such as the synthesis of cGMP (METABOTROPIC), whereas nicotinic actions are directly involved in the changes in ionic fluxes associated with membrane depolarization (IONOTROPIC) (McGeer et al., 1978).

Cholinergic Systems within the Central Nervous System

The existence of cholinergic neurons within the CNS has been established by several lines of evidence. (1) Synaptosomes from brain tissue have been found to contain ACh and the enzymes necessary for its synthesis [choline acetyltransferase (CAT) or choline acetylase (ChAc)] and degradation [acetylcholinesterase

---

*A 1 micromolar solution contains 1 micromole of solute per liter of solvent.

(AChE)]. (2) Both ACh synthesis and release have been demonstrated in cerebral cortical slices. (3) Direct application or intracarotid injection of ACh causes changes in neural activity as measured by the electroencephalogram (EEG). (4) Spinal reflexes were shown to be influenced by ACh infused into the spinal cord via its vascular supply. (5) ACh receptors have been demonstrated in the brain—in the cortex and in a number of subcortical structures. These are mostly muscarinic, although there are some nicotinic receptors. Pyramidal cells in the hippocampus have both muscarinic and nicotinic characteristics and thus appear to have a "hybrid" type of cholinergic receptor. It has been suggested that terms like nicotinic and muscarinic may not be applicable to all brain ACh receptors (Kuhar, 1978).

Finally, Krnjevic and Reinhardt (1979) reported that choline itself evoked action potentials in the sensorimotor cortex of cats. The choline was applied through one unit of a multibarrelled micropipette. Effective iontophoretic currents for choline were only eight times weaker than those for ACh through a different pipette unit. The choline effects were suppressed by atropine (a muscarinic blocker); but choline was not potentiated, whereas ACh was potentiated by physostigmine (an anticholinesterase). The atropine test suggested that muscarinic receptors were involved, and the physostigmine test indicated that choline was a unique transmitter and was not merely converted to ACh to produce the effect. Choline in large doses has been found to have therapeutic effects in cases of tardive dyskinesia (see Chapter 12), an effect that was thought to be due to increased ACh synthesis. These results suggest that choline may have this effect by acting as a direct transmitter.

Neurochemistry of Renshaw Cells

The first cholinergic synapses described in the CNS were those between collaterals of somatic motoneurons and Renshaw cells in the spinal cord (Figure 8 in Chapter 3). Because spinal motoneurons that activate somatic muscles are cholinergic, the axon collaterals that excite the Renshaw cells were presumed to be cholinergic as well. Using iontophoretic techniques, it was found that (1) ACh depolarized the Renshaw cell, (2) the effect was blocked by cholinergic receptor blocking agents such as curare and dihydro-β-erythroidine, and (3) excitation of these neurons was induced by the cholinomimetic drugs, such as nicotine.

In addition, the response of Renshaw cells differs upon application of nicotinic or muscarinic drugs. The nicotinic agent acetyl-β-methylcholine induced an abrupt increase in spike discharges that was blocked by a nicotinic blocking drug, whereas ACh induced a more gradual increase in firing rate that lasted for hundreds of milliseconds and was rapidly suppressed by the muscarinic blocking agent atropine (Krnjevic, 1975). Thus, Renshaw cells may have both types of receptors or the "hybrid" type suggested by Kuhar (1978), an arrangement different from that in the peripheral nerves.

Nicotinic and Muscarinic Effects in the Brain

It has been proposed that muscarinic receptors associated with excitatory effects that are slow in onset and long in duration serve to modulate the general level of cell excitability over periods of seconds or minutes rather than being involved in a system for rapid transfer (in milliseconds) of information. As will be described later, ACh is released at terminals of the ascending reticular arousal system (ARAS) that projects widely to areas of the forebrain, midbrain, and cerebellum. The function served by this system (namely, to regulate levels of arousal and attention) is consistent with a modulating role for ACh on the excitability of neurons in this system. Within the cortex itself, ACh can initiate slow depolarization of cortical neurons, which may or may not lead to the generation of action potentials, but which potentiates the effects of other excitatory inputs. However, it must be pointed out that ACh also depressed other cortical neurons. These neurons have been located in the more superficial layers of all primary projection (sensory) areas as well as in association areas. The receptors on these cells are also predominantly muscarinic.

In summary, evidence indicates that in the brain, as elsewhere in the nervous system, nicotinic receptors are associated with rapid conduction across the synapse, that is, for rapid information transfer such as that at neuromuscular junctions. Muscarinic receptor properties, however, are more consistent with a modulatory function associated with the "second messenger" cGMP. Some of the neuronal activities are not easily categorized as either nicotinic or muscarinic. Thus, some activities require the presence of both types of receptors, or alternatively, a third type is present with properties intermediate between the other two (Phillis, 1976a; Krnjevic, 1975).

Methods of Identification of Cholinergic Systems in the Central Nervous System

Attempts to establish the presence of cholinergic pathways in the CNS have proved to be quite complicated. Techniques developed in the 1960s by a group of Swedish investigators made it possible to identify aminergic neurotransmitter-bearing neurons in brain tissues, but such techniques for cholinergic systems were lacking or unreliable until more recently. Furthermore, those techniques that were developed were complicated and expensive to use. Also, it was not feasible to identify cholinergic neurons by the presence of ACh because the ACh molecule is quite unstable. Although an alternative method of identifying cholinergic neurons is to measure the amount of ACh precursor choline, until recently there were no accurate chemical methods to do so. To complicate matters further, choline rapidly increases in postmortem brain tissue. This latter problem was largely overcome by sacrificing the animals with a focused microwave beam, which kills the animal within seconds by heating the brain tissue and inactivates the enzymes that synthesize and degrade ACh. Because ACh is stable at the temperatures generated by the microwave treatment, it is unaffected by the treatment (Stavinoha and Weintraub, 1974). Although it is possible to identify the enzyme that degrades ACh (AChE), the enzyme is found not only in ACh neurons but also in cell membranes of neurons that receive a cholinergic input but clearly are not cholinergic themselves. Moreover, there is more than one ACh degrading enzyme, and this complicates matters even more. Nevertheless, AChE is present in large amounts along the whole length of cholinergic motoneurons, suggesting that tracts in the CNS that contain AChE in high concentration are likely to constitute cholinergic pathways (Lewis and Shute, 1978: Krnjevic, 1975; Marchbanks, 1975; Cheney and Costa, 1978; and Karczmar and Dun, 1978).

Major Cholinergic Pathways in the Central Nervous System

Figure 2 illustrates some of the major cholinergic pathways of the rat brain. It shows three pathways emanating from the midbrain reticular formation. One proceeds dorsally to innervate the inferior colliculi and (not shown) the adjoining geniculate bodies and the pretectal area. The superficial layer of the superior colliculi is largely supplied by an underlying layer of AChE-containing cells. A second pathway, the dorsal

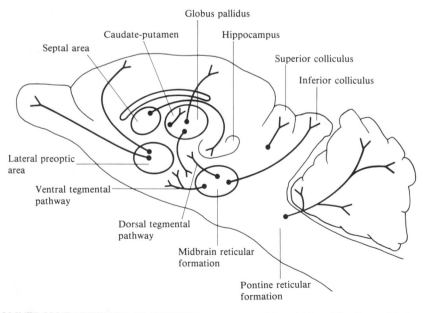

FIGURE 2   CHOLINERGIC PATHWAYS OF THE RAT BRAIN. These pathways have been identified by a histochemical technique for detecting acetylcholinesterase which is presumed to exist in cell bodies and in large amounts along the whole length of cholinergic axons.

tegmental pathway, proceeds rostrally to the nonspecific and intralaminar thalamic nuclei, including the centromedian nucleus. The third, or ventral tegmental pathway, innervates the basal forebrain areas such as the lateral preoptic area and the globus pallidus. From the lateral preoptic area there are projections to the olfactory bulbs and the cortex. The two rostrally directed pathways are considered to be part of the ascending reticular formation that is involved in arousal. The existence of these pathways is supported by strong evidence that ACh is released in the cortex by reticular stimulation and that some of the effects of this phenomenon are blocked by muscarinic antagonists (Krnjevic, 1975).

From the septal nuclei, cholinergic fibers project to the hippocampus. The hypothesis that this pathway is cholinergic was supported by findings that (1) stimulation of the medial septal nucleus results in the release of ACh from the dorsal hippocampus (Dudar, 1975; Smith, 1972); (2) microiontophoretic applications of ACh elicit responses from the hippocampus (Biscoe and Straughan, 1966); and (3) septal lesions cause a decrease in hippocampal ACh as well as in its synthesizing and metabolizing enzymes (Kuhar et al., 1973b).

Within the striatum (the caudate–putamen and the globus pallidus) are numerous cholinergic neurons. Lesions of the afferent pathways to the striatum do not diminish its choline acetyltransferase activity, indicating that the cholinergic cells are intrinsic interneurons of the striatum (McGeer et al., 1971). Striatum interneurons are inhibited by a dopaminergic input that arises from the substantia nigra. This circuit is disrupted when the dopaminergic cell bodies in the substantia nigra are damaged. Degeneration of this dopaminergic pathway is typically found in the brains of patients that had Parkinson's disease, suggesting that the tremors, rigidity, and other symptoms of Parkinson's disease reflect the release of the cholinergic activity in the striatum. As long ago as the latter part of the nineteenth century, it was known that atropine (an ACh receptor blocker) temporarily relieved the symptoms of parkinsonism, but at that time there was no rational explanation for the effect.

Cholinergic projections to the cerebellum arise from the pontine reticular formation as well as from other sources, but all connections to the cerebellum are not exclusively cholinergic. It is noteworthy that areas involved in motor function, such as the reticular formation, the cerebellum, the striatum, the intralaminar nuclei of the thalamus, and the cranial and spinal nerves that activate the somatic musculature are cholinergically innervated. This suggests a chemical integration of these structures; however, an elaboration of this matter is beyond the scope of this chapter.

The proposed cholinergic pathways described above have been verified to some extent by many studies using microapplications of cholinergic agonists and antagonists. Thus far, responses that are presumably from cholinergic cells have been recorded from the cerebral cortex, olfactory bulbs, caudate nucleus, hippocampus (Bird and Aghajanian, 1975), thalamus, midbrain structures, the medulla, cerebellar cortex, and the spinal cord (Krnjevic, 1975). Other supporting observations include specific physiologic effects: (1) EEG changes and seizures result from cholinergic agonist drug treatments. (2) Sleep changes are induced by ACh antagonists. (3) Learning and memory are said to be improved in experimental animals by ACh agonists. (4) ACh is involved in motor dysfunctions traced to pathology of the striatum and substantia nigra (Parkinson's disease and possibly Huntington's chorea). (5) Morphine and alcohol addiction are said to be accompanied by changes in ACh synthesis, release and utilization. (6) There is evidence that senile dementia (Alzheimer's disease) is related to a deficit of choline acetyltransferase which in turn is related to the degree of degeneration of nerve endings in the brain (Kolata, 1981b). Furthermore, ACh systems are implicated in aggression, sensory effects, biorhythms, ingestive behavior, temperature control, nociception, and sexual behavior. Therefore, it is quite clear that ACh is the probable transmitter or neuromodulator for a wide assortment of neural systems. It should be emphasized, however, that ACh is not the only, nor perhaps the principal, neurotransmitter that is involved in these behavioral phenomena; all have multiple determinants (Karczmar and Dun, 1978; Lewis and Shute, 1978).

Part II   Neurochemistry of Acetylcholine and Receptors

Within the dashed rectangle of the ACh diagram is a structure having a positively charged nitrogen atom with four attached organic groups. The + charge makes the nitrogen quadrivalent. The nitrogen is termed a QUATERNARY NITROGEN, and the compound is called a QUATERNARY AMINE. Many neurotransmitters are also amines, but not necessarily of this type.

Figure 3 is a schematic diagram of a cholinergic

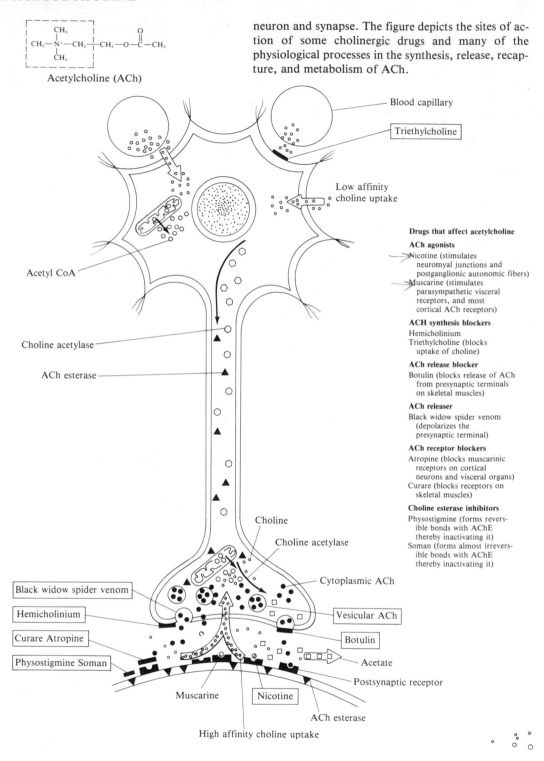

Acetylcholine (ACh)

neuron and synapse. The figure depicts the sites of action of some cholinergic drugs and many of the physiological processes in the synthesis, release, recapture, and metabolism of ACh.

Blood capillary

Triethylcholine

Low affinity choline uptake

Acetyl CoA

Choline acetylase

ACh esterase

Choline

Choline acetylase

Cytoplasmic ACh

Black widow spider venom

Hemicholinium

Vesicular ACh

Curare Atropine

Botulin

Physostigmine Soman

Acetate

Muscarine

Nicotine

Postsynaptic receptor

ACh esterase

High affinity choline uptake

Drugs that affect acetylcholine

ACh agonists
Nicotine (stimulates
  neuromyal junctions and
  postganglionic autonomic fibers)
Muscarine (stimulates
  parasympathetic visceral
  receptors, and most
  cortical ACh receptors)

ACH synthesis blockers
Hemicholinium
Triethylcholine (blocks
  uptake of choline)

ACh release blocker
Botulin (blocks release of ACh
  from presynaptic terminals
  on skeletal muscles)

ACh releaser
Black widow spider venom
  (depolarizes the
  presynaptic terminal)

ACh receptor blockers
Atropine (blocks muscarinic
  receptors on cortical
  neurons and visceral organs)
Curare (blocks receptors on
  skeletal muscles)

Choline esterase inhibitors
Physostigmine (forms reversible bonds with AChE
  thereby inactivating it)
Soman (forms almost irreversible bonds with AChE
  thereby inactivating it)

Acetylcholine Synthesis

The synthesis of ACh is the result of the reaction between acetyl coenzyme A (acetyl CoA) and choline. The reaction is catalyzed by the enzyme choline acetyltransferase (CAT) [sometimes called choline acetylase (ChAc)].

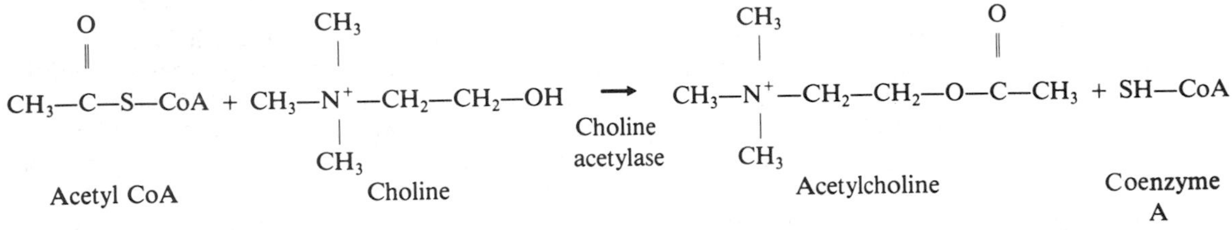

$$CH_3-\overset{\overset{\displaystyle O}{\|}}{C}-S-CoA + CH_3-\overset{\overset{\displaystyle CH_3}{|}}{\underset{\underset{\displaystyle CH_3}{|}}{N^+}}-CH_2-CH_2-OH \xrightarrow{\text{Choline acetylase}} CH_3-\overset{\overset{\displaystyle CH_3}{|}}{\underset{\underset{\displaystyle CH_3}{|}}{N^+}}-CH_2-CH_2-O-\overset{\overset{\displaystyle O}{\|}}{C}-CH_3 + SH-CoA$$

Acetyl CoA   Choline   Acetylcholine   Coenzyme A

The Sources of Acetylcholine Precursors

1. Coenzyme A is found within mitochondria and contains the purine nucleotide base adenine, the vitamin pantothenic acid, and other chemical groups (Figure 4). The sulfhydral group at the bottom of the hydrocarbon chain is the site of attachment of the acetyl group found in acetyl CoA.

2. Acetyl CoA is synthesized within mitochondria in virtually all cells. It participates in many acetylating metabolic reactions, one of which initiates the tricarboxylic acid cycle (the Krebs cycle), the principal pathway for the aerobic oxidation of carbohydrates. Acetyl CoA itself is synthesized by a number of pathways, but the most important one involves pyruvic acid, which is derived from glucose by anaerobic gly-

◄ FIGURE 3   CHOLINERGIC NEURON AND SYNAPSE. The figure illustrates the cytoplasmic presence of choline acetylase, acetylcholinesterase, and the mitochondrial source of acetyl coenzyme A (Acetyl CoA) (open circles). Acetyl CoA combines with choline (small spheres) to form ACh (large solid spheres). The large arrows represent the high affinity choline uptake system; the small arrows represent the low affinity system for choline absorbed from the bloodstream. This source of choline is derived from phosphatidylcholine catabolism and dietary sources. The loosely bound stores of ACh are shown adhering to the vesicles containing the stable stores of ACh. In the postsynaptic region, the ACh receptors are separated from the acetylcholinesterase (AChE) molecules. AChE is also found in small amounts in the axoplasm and serves to regulate the concentration of loosely bound ACh. Drugs and toxins (boxes) such as triethylcholine and hemicholinium block choline uptake; black widow spider venom causes the release of ACh, curare and atropine block ACh receptors, botulin blocks the release of ACh, muscarine and nicotine stimulate ACh receptors, and physostigmine and soman block the action of acetylcholinesterase.

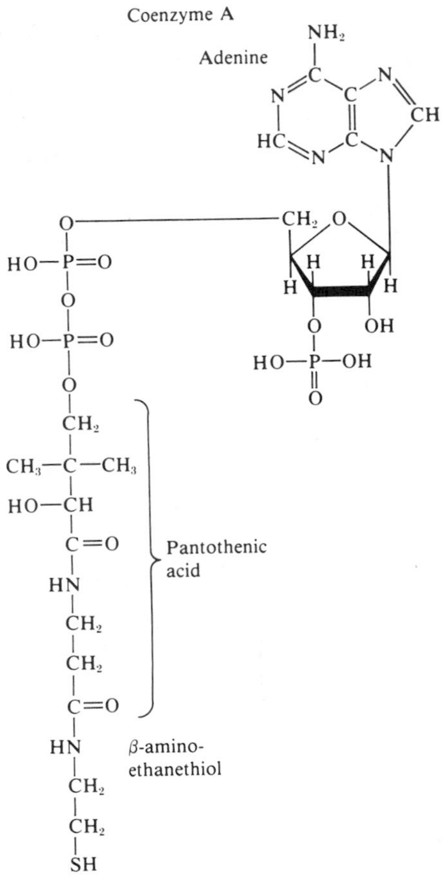

FIGURE 4   CHEMICAL STRUCTURES of pantothenic acid and coenzyme A.

colysis. Pyruvic acid is altered by three different en-zymes and five different coenzymes and combined with the sulfur-containing CoA to form acetyl CoA. Acetyl CoA participates in the formation of ACh in the presence of choline and choline acetylase. It is not known precisely how acetyl CoA is transported through the mitochondrial membrane to participate in ACh synthesis. However, there is evidence that there is a calcium-dependent transport of acetyl CoA across the membrane into the cholinergic synaptoplasm. This process is mediated by the enzyme phospholipase A which catalyzes the breakdown of membrane phospholipids by hydrolysis (Benjamin and Quastel, 1981).

3. Choline is a common base material (i.e. having OH groups) found in foods such as vegetables, egg yolk, kidney, liver, seeds, and legumes. It is also produced in the liver. Synaptic choline is absorbed from the bloodstream and is derived at least in part from the hydrolysis of phospholipids such as phosphatidylcholine (lecithin). However, a major source of choline for synthesis of ACh comes from ACh that is hydrolyzed by the enzyme acetylcholinesterase (AChE). By the process of recapture, the choline reenters the presynaptic terminal from the extracellular fluid. It is estimated that 35–50 percent of the liberated choline is reutilized as a result of the recapture process. The rest is either degraded or reincorporated into phospholipids. Choline is recaptured either specifically in the synaptic zone or more generally at other sites along the axon or perikaryon membrane. At the synaptic zone uptake is a high-affinity process that is sodium (Na^+) dependent. This means that choline will be taken up rapidly even when its concentration is low as long as Na^+ ions are available. In contrast, low affinity uptake occurs only if the concentration of choline is high, and the availability of Na^+ ions is not so crucial. Choline that is taken up by the high-affinity system goes directly into ACh synthesis, whereas choline that is taken up by the low-affinity system presumably goes into the synthesis of phospholipids. Data support the hypothesis that the amount of choline taken up by the cell determines the amount of ACh that will be available for transmitter action. Thus, choline uptake is the rate-limiting step in ACh synthesis.

4. Following homogenization and differential centrifugation of cholinergic tissue, choline acetylase is found in the cytoplasm of synaptosomes. Some of the enzyme exists freely in the cytoplasm, and some seems to adhere to vesicles. The concentration of this enzyme in any particular region of the nervous system parallels the concentration of ACh neurons in that region. Thus, there is a large concentration of the enzyme in the caudate nucleus and virtually none in the cerebellum. The enzyme is abundant in ventral spinal roots which is in keeping with the cholinergic nature of neuromuscular transmission, but there is very little in the dorsal sensory roots which are not cholinergic. The ventral spinal roots can synthesize 10.8 milligrams (mg) of ACh per gram of tissue per hour, whereas dorsal spinal roots can synthesize only 0.025 mg, almost a 450-fold difference. Choline acetylase is almost certainly synthesized in the perikaryon and transported via axoplasmic flow to the axon terminals. Some experiments revealed a rather sluggish axoplasmic flow in the vagus and hypoglossal nerves of the rabbit (5–20 mm/24h), whereas others found that only 5–20 percent of the enzyme was mobile and moved at a fast rate (50–200 mm/24h). In addition, a retrograde flow (from axon terminals to the perikaryon) was found for a small fraction of the enzyme. In common with other transported proteins, the flow of choline acetylase was inhibited by local injections of colchicine (Marchbanks, 1975).

Regulation of Acetylcholine Synthesis

What turns the acetylcholine synthesizing system on and what turns it off? It is quite obvious that low levels of the transmitter should be linked to the onset of synthesis and the elimination of the deficit should terminate synthesis. It stands to reason that any viable biological system must have initiating and terminating mechanisms, because the lack of the former would lead to the demise of the system when essential cell constituents are exhausted. In the absence of terminating mechanisms, uncontrolled synthesis would be uneconomical and at the very worst would lead to imbalances that might be incompatible with normal cell function.

The important controlling mechanism in the synthesis of ACh and other neurotransmitters is a process called end-product inhibition or feedback inhibition. That is, the quantity of the end product of the synthesizing process (the neurotransmitter) controls the on–off switch. Thus, when there is (within certain limits) enough transmitter available for its usual task, synthesis slows; when the transmitter is being utilized at a rapid rate, synthesis rates increase.

The ACh synthesizing enzyme ChAc is sensitive to

the substrates (acetyl CoA and/or choline) as well as to the end product (acetylcholine). The enzyme has different binding sites for the substrates and the end product. When the end product is present in high concentration, it becomes attached to the enzyme. End-product binding causes the structure of the enzyme to change, reducing its ability to bind to the substrates and blocking or slowing the ACh synthesis rate.

The regulation of ACh synthesis has been demonstrated by a number of investigators using different tissues. For example, Birks and MacIntosh (1961) found that when superior cervical ganglia of cats (which have cholinergic synapses) were perfused with normal saline containing choline, the amount of ACh remained normal for 2 hours or more. When they electrically stimulated a ganglion at 20 pulses per second for the same period, the ACh content still remained constant even though there was a considerable liberation of ACh during the stimulation period.

The same experiment was repeated in the presence of eserine (physostigmine), which inhibits AChE. As mentioned earlier, AChE has been identified in cholinergic neurons, where it probably plays a role in controlling cellular levels of ACh. With no stimulation, the level of ACh in the ganglia doubled within an hour and then remained at that level for another hour. Thus, without the degradative effects of AChE, the steady rate of synthesis led to a buildup of ACh that was maintained at the new level. When the ganglia were stimulated in the presence of eserine, the ganglionic content of ACh still only doubled, showing the role of feedback inhibition in controlling ACh levels. When the output of ACh was carefully monitored during the stimulation experiment, there was a slight fall in output rate during the first few minutes; thereafter it was constant for the remainder of the experiment. The total amount of ACh that was released was five times the intracellular amount before stimulation, suggesting that synthesis was still closely regulated by the feedback mechanism.

Another observation of interest was that while the ACh level was doubling, the release of ACh was constant. Had these events occurred *in vivo*, there would have been no physiological effect because the ACh release rate would have remained the same despite the rising intracellular ACh level. This finding also serves as a warning against trying to relate transmitter levels in neural tissue with behavioral changes without a direct measure of the activity of the physiological system

to be sure that its function has changed (Kravitz, 1967). In other words, using our example above, if eserine had caused a behavioral change, one might come to the conclusion that the superior cervical ganglion must be involved because its level of ACh doubled. But because the ACh output remained unchanged, the ganglion would not have been involved in the behavior change.

In another experiment, eserine was combined with hemicholinium, a drug that blocks the uptake of choline. With no stimulation, there was a slight increase in the ACh level of the ganglion for 5–10 minutes, followed by no further change in level. This was interpreted to mean that eserine was responsible for the slight rise in ACh level by preventing ACh degradation; and hemicholinium, limited the extent to which ACh levels could increase by blocking the uptake of the substrate choline. With stimulation, the ganglion level of ACh fell rapidly to a low level and the output of ACh followed the same time course. Thus, it appears that the uptake of extracellular choline is necessary to maintain adequate output levels of ACh during prolonged stimulation. Once the level of ACh is doubled, however, it seems that end-product inhibition serves to limit synthetic activity.

Acetylcholine Release

Miniature End Plate Potentials

Fatt and Katz (1952) suggested that the axon terminal at a neuromuscular junction releases ACh even in the absence of nerve impulses. When they inserted a microelectrode into the muscle fiber of a frog near the neuromuscular junction, they recorded small random spontaneous depolarizations of the muscle cell membrane. The amplitudes of the depolarizations were between 0.5 and 1.0 millivolts (mV). When they moved the electrode approximately 2 mm away from the junction, the depolarization did not appear. They called the depolarization MINIATURE END PLATE POTENTIALS (MEPPs) (Figure 5) to distinguish them from END PLATE POTENTIALS (EPPs), which have a much higher amplitude (around 5.0 mV; similar to EPSPs) and which are the result of a presynaptic action potential acting at a neuromuscular junction.

Katz and his colleagues also found that the discharge rate of the MEPPs was increased by depolarization and decreased by hyperpolarization of the presynaptic membrane. These data led to the conclusion that the

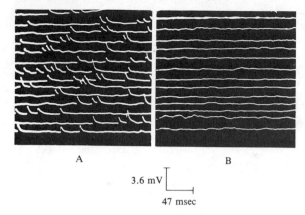

3.6 mV

47 msec

FIGURE 5   MINIATURE END PLATE POTENTIALS (MEPPS). Recordings are shown of the electrical events that occur (A) when a microelectrode was placed inside a frog muscle fiber at a neuromuscular junction; and (B) when the electrode was placed 2 mm away. (A) shows randomly occurring, spontaneous potential changes that sometimes superimpose and sum. (B) shows amplifier "noise" but no MEPPS. (From Fatt and Katz, 1952.)

MEPP represented a response of the muscle membrane to a spontaneously released packet of ACh of a specific quantal size. Shortly after the discovery of MEPPs, synaptic vesicles were observed with the electron microscope. Consequently it was surmised that one quantum of the molecules comprised the contents of one ACh vesicle. Although the amplitude of MEPPs varied between 0.5 and 1.0 mV, it was assumed that the quanta were of equal size and that amplitude differences of the MEPPs were the result of local differences in muscle membrane sensitivity.

On the basis of further studies, it was estimated that the MEPP is produced by 10,000 to 40,000 ACh ions. These figures were based on the amount of iontophoretically applied ACh needed to produce the same effect. However, these figures are subject to a large margin of error because the sensitivity of the muscle end plate was not exactly known, and the recording apparatus may not have been sensitive enough to record the very minimum number of molecules necessary for the effect. It has since been ascertained that there are differences in vesicle content: 10,000 molecules is the upper limit, 5,000 the lower

(Kuffler and Yoshikami, 1975). Also, it is probable that MEPPs are not confined to cholinergic synapses. Rather, they may occur at diverse types of synapses and are probably characteristic of all chemically mediated synapses.

Chemical Effects on Miniature End Plate Potentials

Black widow spider venom causes a marked rise and then a fall in MEPP frequency (Nastuk, 1974). The rise in frequency is consonant with the stimulating effect of the venom, and the fall is in agreement with the resulting depletion of synaptic vesicles. We have also mentioned that calcium ions (Ca^{2+}) are necessary for transmitter release. Katz and Miledi (1970) showed that Ca^{2+} was also necessary for the appearance of MEPPs. They applied Ca^{2+} iontophoretically to a neuromuscular junction of a frog sartorius muscle. By adjusting the stimulating current through the micropipette filled with calcium chloride ($CaCl_2$) they could control the number of calcium ions deposited on the neuromuscular junction. They found a direct relationship between the number of Ca^{2+} applied and the frequency of MEPPs.

Presumably, calcium ions go to the internal surface of the axon membrane and initiate quantal release, perhaps by effecting the contraction of the vesicles fused to the terminal membrane or by forming calcium-calmodulin complexes that lead to the presynaptic membrane changes permitting transmitter release. It has been concluded from other experiments that it takes four calcium ions to effect the release of one quantum of transmitter (Nastuk, 1974). Magnesium ions (Mg^{2+}) also have an affinity for the terminal processes, and if the Mg^{2+} concentration is high enough, they will actually block the influx of Ca^{2+}. Because Mg^{2+} are incapable of effecting the release of ACh, they will block cholinergic transmission at the synapse.

In contrast to the MEPP, the EPP is the muscle membrane response to ACh release following a nerve discharge in the presynaptic membrane. It has been calculated that approximately 100–300 quanta are released under that circumstance. Considering the fact that approximately 300,000 quanta are stored in a neuron terminal and as many as a few hundred nerve discharges may occur within a second, it is readily seen that sustained neural activity could quickly deplete available stores of ACh. Consequently, there is a need for an ACh synthesizing mechanism that is sensitive to the rate of depletion. We have already discussed evidence that suggests that such a mechanism exists in cholinergic terminals.

Vesicular versus Cytoplasmic Acetylcholine

One final point should be made with respect to ACh storage and release. Earlier it was indicated that ACh is found in several subfractions of homogenized neural tissue. There is evidence that ACh exists in the perikaryon, the synaptosomal cytoplasm, and the synaptic vesicles (MacIntosh, 1976). The existence of these different pools of ACh has been established by infusing cholinergic neurons with radioactive choline and then electrically stimulating them. In one experiment, the superior cervical ganglion was perfused with radioactive choline until the ACh was fully labeled. Then the nerve was stimulated in the presence of normal (unlabeled) choline. The released ACh had lower levels of radioactivity than the ACh remaining in the ganglia. Thus, during stimulation the unlabeled choline rapidly entered the terminals, took part in synthesis of ACh, and was the first to be released. In another experiment, the reverse was done. Unlabeled rabbit brain tissue was stimulated in the presence of radioactive choline. In this case, the released ACh was more radioactive than the tissue ACh. Thus, the released ACh must have been recently synthesized from the radioactive choline.

In a third experiment, the electric organ of a torpedo fish was used. These organs have been extensively studied because they have cholinergic synapses in both high and uncontaminated concentrations. During stimulation of the electric organ, there was a rapid fall in the free ACh that existed in the cytoplasm, and only after prolonged stimulation did the vesicular ACh decline. Thus, it appeared that under these conditions stimulation caused the release of the most recently synthesized ACh (that loosely bound to the cytoplasmic membrane) and not vesicular ACh. Perhaps these findings can be generalized and applied to other cholinergic systems. It then becomes difficult to reconcile these results with the concept of the synaptic vesicle as the exclusive repository for transmitter substances, as well as with the concept of the vesicle as the exclusive agent in exocytosis (MacIntosh and Collier, 1976). It is therefore possible that some revision in our present concepts will have to take place.

Acetylcholine Catabolism and the Termination of Acetylcholine Action

The catabolism of ACh has already been mentioned briefly in connection with the source of choline for ACh synthesis. There is no evidence showing significant uptake of ACh into any part of nerve cells. Thus, ACh degradation and diffusion out of the synaptic cleft are probably the principal mechanisms for terminating transmitter action and for allowing the presynaptic terminal to return at least briefly (1–2 msec) to its resting state. As previously mentioned, ACh is degraded by acetylcholinesterase (AChE) to yield choline and acetic acid. This process occurs in two steps as follows.

The enzyme molecule (E) has a negatively charged region that becomes attached to the positively charged quaternary nitrogen, $(CH_3)_3N^+$—R of ACh. The enzyme also contains a positively charged ESTERATIC SITE to which acetate (CH_3—CO^-; an ESTER) can be attached. In this way the ACh molecule is split, liberating the choline, which is recaptured by the presynaptic membrane.

$$E \cdot ACh \rightarrow E \cdot A + Ch$$

where $E \cdot A$ = acetylated enzyme.

The acetylated enzyme is hydrolyzed to regenerate the enzyme and release acetic acid, which then enters other metabolic processes.

$$E \cdot A + H_2O \rightarrow E + A$$

The total chemical reaction is illustrated in Figure 6.

AChE is one of a number of esterases found in cells, some of which can hydrolyze ACh, but not as efficiently as AChE. One of the other esterases, butyrylcholinesterase, is found in glia and may be important in the inactivation of the ACh that diffuses in appreciable amounts from the synaptic cleft. It has been estimated that the ACh release in neuromuscular transmission is hydrolyzed within 2 msec, and the turnover time for AChE is less than 100 μsec (Nastuk, 1974). The concentration of AChE parallels that of ACh and choline acetylase. This is reasonable as they are all involved in the synaptic transmission mediated by ACh. For instance, there is a high concentration of AChE at neuromuscular junctions, especially at the end plate regions of the muscle. The high concentration is partially explained by the convolutions of the postjunctional membrane, which obviously increases the recep-

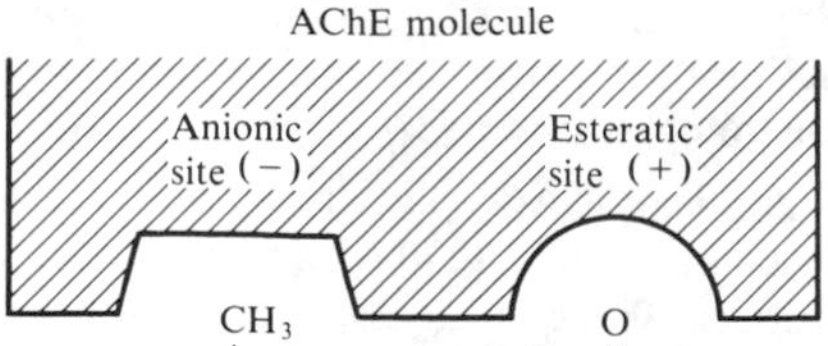

AChE molecule

FIGURE 6 CATABOLISM OF ACETYLCHOLINE. Acetylcholine binds to the AChE molecule and is hydrolyzed (combined with an H_2O molecule) to form choline and acetic acid.

tive surface in that region (see Figures 9 and 10 in Chapter 5).

At some receptor sites, high concentrations of ACh can inhibit the action of AChE. The inhibition occurs when a second molecule of ACh attaches itself to the negatively charged region of the acetylated enzyme complex just prior to the hydrolysis that releases acetate. Under these conditions, the hydrolysis that splits the acetate from the enzyme surface is slowed down. This is a positive feedback system; the higher the concentration of ACh near the receptors, the slower the breakdown. The positive feedback may appear to be self-defeating except in cases where long, protracted stimulation by the transmitter is called for. On the other hand, it is also true that when some receptor areas are continuously exposed to ACh, the receptors undergo a process of desensitization and no longer respond to the transmitter (Katz and Thesleff, 1957). It may seem paradoxical that there are mechanisms for both accentuation and attenuation of the action of ACh at the synapse. This paradox is resolved if it is appreciated that the demands of the particular synaptic junction, whether it be on heart muscle or on skeletal muscle, control the choice of mechanism that is appropriate.

Identity of the Cholinergic Receptor

The chemical identification of the cholinergic receptor has been a difficult problem to solve. It was believed earlier that AChE was the receptor protein as well as the degrading enzyme. However, chemical studies showed that this is unlikely even though the number of active sites of AChE was very similar to the number of receptor sites. When the receptor sites were blocked by curare (at the skeletal neuromuscular junction) or by atropine (in the heart), AChE still functioned and quickly degraded ACh. Although these results suggest there is a difference between the recep-

tor and AChE, they do not tell us how far apart they are, or whether they are on the same molecule. It is now believed that the receptor is a membrane-bound protein molecule that forms an IONOPHORE,* whose conformation is altered by the attachment of ACh. In this way channels are created that permit the passage of Na^+ and K^+ through the cell membrane. Standard protein analyses of isolated receptor protein indicate that it has a high molecule weight (about 300,000) and is made up of three or more subunits—properties that are typical of other membrane receptors.

A technique used by Molinoff (1974) and Molinoff and Potter (1972) involved the use of α-bungarotoxin as a tag for nicotinic receptors. (This material is one of the neurotoxins in the venom of a poisonous snake, *Bungarus multicinctus*, found in Taiwan.) The rationale for using bungarotoxin as a tagging agent is based on studies by Lee et al. (1967). They found that the toxin rapidly and irreversibly blocked cholinergic transmission at the neuromuscular junction. The toxin acted by binding to nicotinic receptors and did not alter action potentials in nerves, prevent the release of ACh, or change cholinesterase activity. Therefore, the toxin provided a selective tool with which to study the receptor. Because the toxin acts by occupying cholinergic receptor sites, it prevents ACh-induced depolarizing end plate potentials (EPPs) on the postsynaptic membrane. (Blocking cholinergic transmission leads ultimately to asphyxiation because of paralysis of the respiratory apparatus.) It has been shown that if cell fractions containing ACh receptors are bathed in a solution containing labeled toxin, the toxin will attach itself to the cholinergic receptor sites, thus making a

*An ionophore is a group of molecules imbedded in a membrane. The shape of the molecules can be altered by the action of neurotransmitters to form openings—pores—in the membrane that increase the permeability of specific ion species.

radioactive complex (Changeux, 1975). Moreover, by carefully adjusting the concentrations, it was found that the amount of the toxin binding to the protein could be reduced by other drugs that competed for the binding sites. The competing drugs are nicotinic agonists and antagonists such as *d*-tubocurarine (the active ingredient in curare, blocks ACh receptor sites), nicotine, and atropine. This labeling technique has enabled identification of cholinergic receptors in the postsynaptic membranes of neural tissue (Eterovic and Bennett, 1974) and on muscle membranes.

Examinations of neuromuscular junctions showed that labeled toxin was concentrated at the MUSCLE END PLATE (that part of the muscle that receives innervation by the motoneuron and develops EPPs) (Miledi and Potter, 1971; Hartzell and Fambrough, 1972). In mammals, bungarotoxin receptors (toxin sites) were not present where ACh sensitivity was absent. Furthermore, if the nerve to the muscle was cut, the binding sites spread all over the muscle, increasing the number of sites by 20-fold for a period of about 3 weeks. Sensitivity to acetylcholine increased with a similar time course (Potter, 1973). The phenomenon is called DENERVATION SUPERSENSITIVITY and demonstrates that receptor protein can be modified by chronic events involving nerve terminals. Changes of this type in receptors may provide a model for the phenomenon of drug tolerance. It is not unreasonable to consider some drug action as a "pharmacological denervation," in which case altered receptor sensitivity may diminish the effects of the drug after repeated administration.

De Robertis' Receptor Model

De Robertis (1971) studied the properties of ACh receptors by extracting a proteolipid (macromolecule containing protein and lipid) from the electric organ of *Electrophorus electrica* (an Amazonian electric eel). He separated two solutions with an artificial lipid membrane having an area about 1 mm². Into the artificial membrane he inserted the putative receptor proteolipid. The proportion of protein to lipid was 1:10,000. By applying different voltages across the membrane,

the conductivity of the membrane could be measured. When the proteolipid was inserted, the resistance across the membrane dropped and the conductivity increased. Also when ACh was applied to the membrane, there was a considerable, but transient, increase in conductivity that was blocked by *d*-tubocurarine (the drug that blocks ACh receptor sites). When these membranes were examined under the electron microscope, a transient structural modification of the membrane was found that paralleled the duration of the ACh-induced conductance change. The membrane also showed a corrugated appearance with spots that could "actually represent openings of a potential pore, the ionophoric portion of the postulated receptor."

De Robertis formulated a model of a lipid membrane containing ACh receptors (Figure 7). The membrane is assumed to be about 7 nm thick and contains the usual bilayer of lipid molecules arranged so that the hydrophilic polar heads are oriented toward the internal and external aqueous surfaces. On the surfaces are structural proteins that are arranged to contribute to the rigidity of the membrane. Embedded in the membrane are four proteolipid molecules in a tetrameric arrangement that form a tube-like pore in the membrane connecting the inside to the outside. The proteolipids are surrounded and tightly bound to a lipoid (fat-like) coat of phosphatidylinositol. The combination of these elements make up the ionophore, the center of which (the pore) allows the passage of the metallic ions of sodium or potassium through the membrane during the development of an excitatory or inhibitory membrane potential.

The molecules of phosphatidylinositol are implicated in the action of ACh because brain slices that are stimulated electrically or by ACh show an increase in turnover of this substance. It has been suggested that they may modulate synaptic function. The receptor sites for ACh are situated at the outer ends of the proteolipids making up the "pore," and binding sites for AChE are separately located on neighboring protein molecules (De Robertis, 1971; De Robertis et al., 1978).

Part III   Pharmacology of Cholinergic Systems

Substances That Affect Cholinergic Systems

So far we have discussed acetylcholine in terms of synthesis, storage, release, interaction with receptor sites, and degradation. We have mentioned the effects

of drugs on some of these phases of cholinergic activity. In this section, we will show that drugs that affect neural systems and behavior are, for the most part, substances that alter the availability of the transmitter (acetylcholine) during synaptic events.

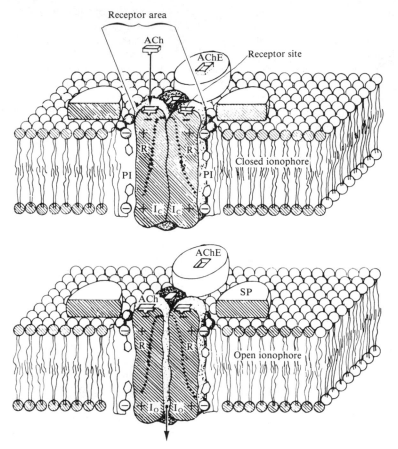

FIGURE 7 DE ROBERTIS MODEL OF AN ACh RE-CEPTOR COMPLEX. The receptor complex, an ionophore, consists of ACh receptor sites on the end surface of receptor protein molecules (R) that are arranged in a tetramere to form a pore in a lipid membrane. Upper figure shows the ionophore closed (I_c), bottom figure shows it open (I_o). The ACh receptor sites control the opening and closing of the pore. Phosphatidylinositol (PI) molecules surround the receptor proteins (proteolipids) and modulate their activity. Structural proteins (SP) contribute to the rigidity of the membrane. AChE receptor sites are seen on neighboring protein molecules. (From De Robertis et al., 1978.)

Before proceeding, we want to make our terminology clear. Drugs are chemical compounds that affect living organisms and are usually intended for the prevention, cure, or diagnosis of disease. However, there are a number of pharmacologically active substances that are used by individuals that are free of disease. For example, tons of caffeine (found in coffee and other beverages) are consumed every day; nicotine is ingested via tobacco use by millions of people the world over, and the amount of alcohol ingested every day is almost incalculable. Moreover, plant substances such as Δ9-tetrahydrocannabinol found in marijuana have pharmacological properties, as do toxins from microorganisms; these substances are not always called drugs. To avoid confusion, we will refer to all chemicals that affect biological systems as "substances" or "agents" and restrict the use of the word "drug" to mean a substance that is used experimentally or clinically to study or treat disease. To be sure, some substances that would not be called drugs today may be so designated in the future, which suggests that any distinction that we propose is, in the last analysis, arbitrary and only used for convenience.

Table II contains the substances and drugs discussed

TABLE II. Substances and Drugs That Interact with Cholinergic Systems

Compound	Central effects*	Mechanism of action
4-1 Napthylvinyl pyridine	?	Blocks choline acetylase
Hemicholinium (HC-3)	?	Choline uptake inhibitor
Triethylcholine	?	
Botulinus toxin (Botulin)	−	Inhibits ACh release
Black widow spider venom	−	Facilitates ACh release
Nicotine	+	Ganglionic and neuromuscular agonist
α-Bungarotoxin	−	Neuromuscular receptor blocker
Curare	−	
d-Tubocurarine	−	
Gallamine (Flaxedil)	−	
Succinylcholine	−	Neuromuscular depolarizer
Decamethonium	−	
Hexamethonium	−	Ganglionic blocker
Mecamylamine	+	
Muscarine	+	Muscarinic agonist
Carbachol	−	
Methacholine	−	
Pilocarpine	+	
Arecoline	+	
Oxotremorine	+	
Atropine	+	Muscarinic blocker
Methylatropine	−	
Scopolamine	+	
Methylscopolamine	−	
Benztropine	+	
Benactyzine	−	
Physostigmine	+	Competitive cholinesterase inhibitor
Neostigmine	−	
Edrophonium (Tensilon)	−	
Malathion	+	Irreversible cholinesterase inhibitor
Parathion	+	
Sarin	+	
Soman	+	
Tabun	+	
Diisopropylfluorophosphate (DFP)	+	
Echothiophate (Phospholine)	−	
Pyrimidine-2-aldoxime methiodide	+	Regenerator of cholinesterase
Trimedoxime	+	

*Substances marked "+" affect the CNS; those marked "−" do not. CNS effects of the first 3 substances are unclear.

in this section and briefly mentions their mechanisms of action. Also, Figure 3 shows the locus of action of some of these drugs.

Drugs That Block Acetylcholine Synthesis

Although there are many drugs that affect cholinergic synapses, there are only a few that block ACh synthesis. One of these is hemicholinium (HC-3). HC-3

Hemicholinium (HC-3)

exerts its effect by blocking both the high- and low-affinity uptake of choline, regardless of whether the choline is the metabolic byproduct of choline-containing lipids (phosphatidylcholine) or of ACh. Triethylcholine (TEC) probably blocks synthesis in the same

Triethylcholine (TEC)

way. There are other compounds that block the activity of the synthesizing enzyme choline acetylase *in vitro* but are ineffective *in vivo*, probably because they cannot obtain access to the enzyme *in vivo*. With respect to central effects of HC-3, there are reports of physiological effects (DeFeudis, 1974) but negative findings for behavioral effects (Schecter and Rosecrans, 1971).

Substances That Affect Acetylcholine Release

As mentioned previously, calcium ions are required for the release of ACh from presynaptic membranes. The uptake of calcium can be blocked by the presence of magnesium ions (Mg^{2+}), thereby blocking ACh release. However, this effect is not specific for ACh release; Mg^{2+} blocks release of virtually all neurotransmitters.

We have also mentioned that black widow spider venom causes a marked increase of ACh release. This effect is indirect because the venom depolarizes the axon terminal. In any case, the venom is only used *in vitro* because its toxicity precludes accurate analysis of behavioral effects.

Among the few substances that are selectively taken up by cholinergic nerve terminals and that block the release of ACh is botulinus toxin (botulin), which is well known for its extraordinary toxicity. Botulin is

one of the most potent poisons known, with the lethal dose estimated to be 0.3 μg in man. Said in another way, 1.0 gram (the equivalent of three aspirin tablets in weight) is enough to kill 350,000 individuals, a total equal to the population of a city the size of Rochester, New York.

The toxin is given off by the bacterium *Clostridium botulinum* in an anaerobic environment, which can occur in a sealed food can. Fortunately the bacterium, although common, cannot produce the toxin in the presence of oxygen, so the incidence of botulism is rare. Kao et al. (1976) investigated the mechanism by which botulin interferes with ACh release. They treated phrenic nerve–hemidiaphragm neuromuscular junctions from mice with botulin (0.1 μg/ml) while they monitored miniature end plate potentials (MEPPs) with microelectrodes. In 2–3 hours, the frequency of MEPPs was reduced to less than 1.0 percent of the normal value of 1.0/sec and the amplitude was reduced as well. After 5 hours, neuromuscular transmission could no longer be elicited by nerve stimulation.

In order to test the hypothesis that botulin might interfere with Ca^{2+} influx and thus inhibit ACh release, other neuromuscular preparations were treated with the antibiotic X537A. The antibiotic increases quantal release of ACh by serving as an ionophore for the calcium ion. In control experiments, with Ca^{2+} in the bathing medium, X537A caused a 5- to 10-fold increase in MEPP frequency within 30 minutes. However, neuromuscular preparations treated with botulin failed to respond to the ionophore. Thus, because Ca^{2+} influx did not reverse the action of botulin, it is unlikely that the toxin has its effect by blocking Ca^{2+} entry.

A second experiment examined the effect of black widow spider venom (BWSV) on botulin-treated neuromuscular junctions. Normally BWSV causes a calcium-independent release of ACh vesicles from nerve terminals. In a control test, BWSV caused a sharp increase of MEPPs from the control rate of 1/sec to more than 350/sec, followed by a quick decline, signifying the exhaustion of vesicles in the terminal. When BWSV was added to a botulin-treated preparation, the massive increase in MEPPs still occurred. Thus, the toxin probably does not interfere with the vesicular storage of ACh because BWSV-induced release was not inhibited. However, electron microscopic examination of the terminals treated with botulin showed a residual clumping of vesicles, a kind of logjam of vesicles opposite the junctional folds.

Clumping was absent from normal terminals or terminals treated with BWSV alone.

Kao et al. (1976) concluded that botulin probably does not block entry of Ca^{2+} because Ca^{2+} ionophores failed to induce release of ACh from botulin treated tissue. Second, it is unlikely that the toxin interferes with ACh storage in vesicles because there was a BWSV-induced barrage of vesicles from botulin-treated terminals. Finally, they suggested, on the basis of the observed clumping of vesicles, that botulin interferes in some fashion with a membrane component of vesicle release, but the change can be visualized only when there is forced exocytosis induced by BWSV.

Cholinomimetic Agents: Drugs That Mimic the Action of Acetylcholine

Nicotinic Agents and Drugs

Nicotine is an alkaloid that was first isolated from the tobacco plant *Nicotiana tabacum* in 1828. It is very toxic; only 60 mg can be fatal to an adult. It may be surprising to learn that an ordinary cigar contains enough nicotine to provide about two lethal doses. However, the burning of tobacco destroys much of the nicotine, so that the amount absorbed by a smoker is dependent upon the quantity of nicotine that is bound to the smoke as it is drawn through the unburned portion of the tobacco product.

Nicotine

Small doses of nicotine have an excitatory effect upon the nicotinic receptors in the neuromuscular junctions and in the receptors of the autonomic ganglia. The latter effect is more pronounced than the former. At higher doses, nicotine produces blockade at nicotinic junctions; and if the dose is high enough, asphyxia can occur as a result of paralysis of the muscles of respiration. Nicotine exemplifies how a drug that stimulates autonomic ganglia can have a wide variety of physiological and behavioral manifestations. For example, nicotine, even in the small amounts absorbed when smoking tobacco, can increase heart rate by stimulating sympathetic ganglia or by stimulating the adrenal gland to release epinephrine, which also increases heart rate. Also, the heart rate can be indirectly increased by nicotine following

the increase in blood pressure caused by the constriction of blood vessels resulting from the stimulation of autonomic ganglia. The nicotinic action on autonomic ganglia also increases hydrochloric acid secretion in the stomach (which exacerbates or contributes to the formation of stomach ulcers) and increases motor activity in the bowel (sometimes leading to chronic diarrhea which is especially harmful to individuals with colitis, a chronic irritability of the colon). These and other nicotine-induced effects produce the unhealthful consequences of heavy and prolonged use of tobacco products.

Acute Nicotine Poisoning

Most cases of acute nicotine poisoning are the result of accidental ingestion of insecticides in which nicotine is the effective agent. When swallowed in the form of tobacco, nicotine is less toxic than would be expected. Children who swallow cigarettes, which may contain 20–30 mg of nicotine, show minor effects, probably because nicotine absorption from tobacco in the stomach is slow. In addition, the low levels absorbed are sufficient to stimulate the chemical trigger zone (vomiting center) in the area postrema of the medulla and cause the expulsion of much of the tobacco remaining in the stomach. On the other hand, beginning smokers who inhale tobacco smoke even slightly frequently show signs of nicotine toxicity, including nausea, vomiting, pallor, abdominal pain, headache, dizziness, and weakness (Volle and Koelle, 1975). Continued smoking usually leads to tolerance and the absence of these signs, but the serious diseases associated with chronic tobacco use, such as lung cancer, respiratory diseases, coronary artery disease, tobacco amblyopia (dimness of vision), and complications of pregnancy, testify to the fact that tolerance to some of the effects of nicotine and other ingredients of tobacco does not occur (Gritz and Jarvik, 1978).

In acute toxicity associated with ingestion of insecticides, death may occur within a few minutes. The symptoms are grossly exaggerated autonomic effects that quickly lead to prostration, convulsions, and respiratory failure.

Physiological Effects of Nicotine in the Central Nervous System

Nicotine passes the blood brain barrier and exerts effects on the CNS. It acts as a stimulant to produce tremors and convulsions at high doses; it increases respiration rates; it acts upon vasomotor centers in the medulla to induce cardiovascular changes; and it causes the release of antidiuretic hormone from the pituitary gland (Volle and Koelle, 1975). Topically applied nicotine blocked a light response in cells of the optic tectum in frogs, and infusion of nicotine into the blood supply of the spinal cord inhibited motoneural reflex discharges (DeFeudis, 1974).

A number of studies have investigated the effects of tobacco-derived nicotine on cortical activity. Nicotine induced an activated neocortical EEG (a 13–30 Hz low-voltage pattern) and increased theta wave activity in the hippocampus (a 4–7 Hz high-voltage pattern). Simultaneous occurrence of both patterns is associated with heightened attention. However, both effects can be blocked by atropine (a muscarinic blocker), suggesting that the involved receptors are not purely nicotinic. In man and animals, the activation of the EEG caused by nicotine derived from tobacco smoke was thought to be due to a direct effect upon the brain stem reticular activating system. (Stimulation of this structure increases levels of arousal.) When chronic cigarette smokers were deprived of cigarettes for 24 hours, there was an increase in slow EEG activity, a rebound that may be analogous to a drug withdrawal effect. However, more recently investigations have shown that the brain stem activation was not in the reticular formation nor related to the cortical EEG changes. Neither did the EEG changes correlate with arousal and sleep as they normally do.

Muscarinic Agents

Methacholine, carbachol, muscarine, and pilocarpine are among the cholinomimetic drugs that affect muscarinic receptors. Because these substances have strong effects on structures innervated by postganglionic parasympathetic neurons, they are known as parasympathomimetic agents. Methacholine and carbachol are synthetic choline derivatives that do not cross the blood brain barrier; consequently, they have

Methacholine

Carbachol

no central effects unless they are directly applied to the tissue of the CNS. Methacholine has a prolonged inhibitory action on the heart rate resulting from stimulation of the muscarinic receptors on the heart. Methacholine is hydrolyzed by AChE at 1/3 the rate of

ACh and is almost totally resistant to hydrolysis of nonspecific cholinesterases. Carbachol has a greater affinity for muscarinic receptors of the viscera; hence, it is used for prolonged stimulation of the GI tract and the urinary bladder. This compound is almost totally resistant to hydrolysis by AChE.

Muscarine is a toxic alkaloid that was first extracted from the mushroom *Amanita muscaria* in 1869. Other mushrooms of the genera *Clitocybe* and *Inocybe* have even greater concentrations of this toxin. Muscarine

Muscarine

has no therapeutic use; it is mainly used as a pharmacological tool. In cases of accidental ingestion of muscarine-bearing mushrooms, the symptoms consist of marked lacrimation (tearing), salivation, sweating, pinpoint pupils, severe abdominal pain due to strong contractions of the smooth muscles of the viscera, painful diarrhea, cardiovascular collapse, coma, convulsions, and death. Fortunately, atropine (which is a parasympathetic blocking agent) displaces muscarine from its receptor sites and can reverse the effects of muscarine even in severe cases of intoxication, provided that the cause of intoxication is recognized early enough.*

Pilocarpine is a naturally occurring alkaloid first isolated in 1875. It is extracted from the leaves of the South American shrub *Pilocarpus jaborandi*. The

Pilocarpine

natives knew that chewing the leaves of the shrub stimulated salivation, and in 1874 a Brazilian physician found that an extract from the leaves produced sweating. A dose of 10–15 mg administered intramuscularly can induce the secretion of 2–3 liters of sweat, but not without the unpleasant side effects of excessive salivation (as much as 350 ml in 2 hours), nausea, vomiting

---

*Ingestion of *Amanita muscaria* leads to other effects caused by the presence of muscimol and ibotenic acid, substances that are GABA agonists (see Chapter 9). These substances are very toxic. *Amanita phalloides* contains fatal toxins that destroy liver and kidney tissues (Litten, 1975).

Arecoline   Oxotremorine

weakness, and occasionally collapse (Koelle, 1975b).

Arecoline is an alkaloid derived from the betel nut. It has effects like those of pilocarpine and passes the blood brain barrier, as does oxotremorine, which is a synthetic muscarinic agonist.

Anticholinesterase Substances

Anticholinesterase agents increase the duration of the effect of endogenous ACh at cholinergic receptor sites by blocking the hydrolysis of ACh by AChE. They accomplish this effect by competing with ACh for binding sites on the AChE molecule. Some of the anticholinesterase drugs form loose (reversible) bonds with AChE and thus are competitive with ACh molecules, whereas others form irreversible attachments to the enzyme and can have fatal effects at high doses.

Some anticholinesterases have a short duration of action because, although they have a high affinity for the enzyme, they form weak attachments only at the anionic sites of the AChE molecule, even when the drug is present in a relatively high concentration. As the drug concentration falls because of degradation, diffusion, and excretion, drug-enzyme complexes dissociate and normal ACh catabolism returns. Edrophonium (Tensilon) is such a drug. Because of its short duration of action, it is used diagnostically for detecting MYASTHENIA GRAVIS, a disorder characterized by muscular weakness and resulting from an abnormality or paucity of ACh receptor sites on the muscle membrane (Kao and Drachman, 1977; Satyamurti et al., 1975). Injection of edrophonium causes a sudden increase in muscle action potentials and muscle strength upon exertion. This activity would not occur if the muscle weakness were due to damage of the motoneuron rather than to some malfunction of the muscle membrane.

One of the earliest known anticholinesterase substances is physostigmine or Eserine. It is obtained from the Calabar bean, the seed of *Physostigma venenosum* Balfour, a climbing woody plant found in West Africa. In 1864 the pure alkaloid was isolated and given the name physostigmine, and in 1865 another group of investigators isolated the alkaloid and gave it the name eserine, after the French name of the Calabar bean, the Esére nut. In 1877 it was first used in the treatment of glaucoma by direct application to the eye, and it still is used for this purpose today. GLAUCOMA is a disease of the eye characterized by abnormally high intraocular pressure. By stimulating the muscarinic receptors of the iris to form a small pupil, the drug facilitates the drainage of the aqueous humor and lowers the intraocular pressure. This drug passes the blood brain barrier and has CNS effects.

Another drug in this class is neostigmine (Prostigmin). This drug was introduced in 1931 and is a synthetic agent having a quaternary nitrogen with a positive charge. Thus, like ACh itself, it does not pass the blood brain barrier and has no central effects. Moreover, this compound forms bonds at both the anionic and esteratic sites of the AChE molecule.

Neostigmine

However, although the acetylated enzyme formed by physostigmine is readily hydrolyzed, neostigmine forms a *carbamylated** enzyme complex that is hydrolyzed a million times more slowly, thus regenerating the enzyme at a much slower rate. The drug, therefore, has a more prolonged duration of action with about the same potency of physostigmine. Neostigmine is useful for stimulating the gastrointestinal tract and is also effective in treating myasthenia gravis. It is also an antidote for curare poisoning. All of these beneficial effects occur without psychotropic side effects since neostigmine has no CNS effects. Moreover, neostigmine has a slight cholinomimetic action, thereby augmenting its effects.

Another group among the anticholinesterase drugs is the ORGANOPHOSPHOROUS COMPOUNDS, one of which interestingly enough was synthesized in 1854, 10

*Carbamylation is the formation of a compound with a carbamate group. A carbamate group is an ester of carbamic acid NH_2—COOH.

Edrophonium   Physostigmine

years before the isolation of physostigmine. However, their commercial potential dates from a 1932 German publication that described the effect of inhalation of vapor from these compounds (Koelle, 1975a). The German authors, Lange and Krueger, described persistent choking sensations and blurred vision. Other German investigators then began looking into these compounds as possible insecticides. After examining about 2000 compounds, they found what was required for good anticholinesterase insecticidal activity. Parathion became the most widely used product of this class. In many situations malathion replaced parathion because it is metabolized to inactive metabolites in man and is therefore much safer.

During World War II, anticholinesterase properties were incorporated into chemical warfare agents. Agents of much greater toxicity than parathion (such as sarin, soman, and tabun) were developed in Germany. Over 10,000 tons of tabun were manufactured in that country but were never used. In the Allied countries there was also a search for chemical warfare agents, and diisopropylfluorophosphate (DFP) was studied intensively.

Organophosphorus compounds are un-ionizable, very lipid soluble, and thus pass readily into the CNS tissue. In cholinergic tissue, these compounds form highly stable phosphorylated complexes with enzymes such as AChE at the esteratic site. The complexes are resistant to hydrolytic cleavage for many hours. For those anticholinesterase agents with isopropyl groups (C_3H_7), the phosphorylated complex is so stable that there is no hydrolysis. Therefore, the return of AChE activity requires the synthesis of new enzyme, a process requiring days or weeks (Koelle, 1975a; Marx, 1980).

These so-called war gases (sarin, tabun, and soman) are stored as liquids and can be released as a vapor cloud or spray. They enter the body by inhalation or by absorption through the skin. As they bind to AChE and inactivate it, a rapid accumulation of ACh occurs in autonomic ganglia and parasympathetically innervated effectors, at neuromuscular junctions, and at the cholinergic synapses of the CNS. The ACh accumulation causes a wide variety of symptoms such as intense sweating, filling of bronchial passages with mucus, bronchial constriction, dimmed vision, uncontrollable vomiting and defecation, convulsions, and ultimately paralysis and asphyxiation from respiratory failure. The effect of acute poisoning is asphyxia within a few minutes. However, if the agent is received through the

Parathion   Malathion

Sarin   Soman   Tabun

Diisopropyl fluorophosphate (DFP)

skin, it may take several hours for the victim to die. Even when the dose is sublethal, there is evidence of long-lasting neurological and psychiatric disorders. It is estimated that 1.0 mg of sarin or 0.7 mg of soman is a lethal dose (Meselson and Robinson, 1980).

After World War II, DFP was studied for possible therapeutic effects. It was found that solutions of DFP, containing between 0.005 and 0.2 percent of the active agent, could be used for the treatment of glaucoma. Its main therapeutic advantage is that it need be applied only once daily or weekly in cases resistant to physostigmine. Better compounds, which are related to DFP, have been developed for this purpose. One of these is echothiophate (Phospholine). Echothiophate resembles DFP and in addition has a quaternary nitrogen that enables the compound to bind at the anionic as well as at the esteratic site of AChE. This feature contributes to the potency of the drug and the duration of action in the treatment of glaucoma. Echothiophate has other advantages for ophthalmic use; it is water soluble and becomes ionized, which contributes to low lipid solubility. Thus, the drug remains localized, with little systemic absorption (Gringauz, 1978).

Anticholinesterase agents have the potential for great toxicity because uncontrolled action of ACh can

Echothiophate (Phospholine)

seriously disrupt vital biological functions. Not only are autonomic and neuromuscular systems affected, but the cholinergic systems within the CNS also become involved. It is unfortunate that the wide availability and use of agricultural organophosphorous insecticides lead not only to accidental poisoning by these chemicals but also to their use in suicide and homocide. Consequently, there has been a search for effective antidotes for these agents.

To counteract the unrestrained activity of ACh at muscarinic sites, atropine is given in large doses. However, atropine has no effect upon the nicotinic neuromuscular receptor sites. Consequently, artificial respiration is necessary to overcome paralysis of the respiratory muscles. Also, paralysis of the muscles involved with swallowing results in the danger of aspiration of drug-induced excessive oral secretions. Finally, antidotes are given to reactivate AChE.

Using considerable ingenuity, Kewitz et al. (1956) developed AChE-reactivating antidotes by applying their understanding of how organophosphorous compounds cause the irreversible formation of the phosphorylated enzyme. A group of compounds called oximes were found to reactivate cholinesterase enzymes by breaking the phosphate–enzyme bond. This discovery led to the development of pyridine-2-aldoxime methiodide (PAM or pralidoxime), which is especially effective as an antidote to DFP. This compound was fashioned to fit the DFP–enzyme complex exactly and to break the bonds of attachment of the poison, thus removing it from the AChE molecule and restoring AChE activity. When animals were injected with a lethal dose of DFP, followed by an injection of PAM, there was 100 percent survival among the animals.

Pralidoxime (PAM)

A special combination of drugs has been formulated to protect military personnel from the effects of organophosphorus war gases. The combination comprises trimedoxime,* atropine, and an ACh antagonist benactyzine. Referred to as TAB, it is supplied in an

*Trimedoxime is another compound that reverses the effects of organophosphate anticholinesterase compounds.

autoinjector to be used on the battlefield (i.e., the soldier can quickly self-administer the drug). The dosage can save the life of a person receiving somewhat more than the median lethal dose of gas, and it can reduce the severity of symptoms due to sublethal doses of gas (Meselson and Robinson, 1980).

Nicotinic Receptor Blocking Agents

Nicotinic receptor blocking agents make up a group of ANTICHOLINERGIC SUBSTANCES (or CHOLINOLYTIC SUBSTANCES) that block the effects of acetylcholine on nicotinic receptors. Two of the best known blockers of nicotinic receptors at the neuromyal junction are curare and its purified alkaloid form, *d*-tubocurarine.

d-Tubocurarine

The famous physiologist Claude Bernard first described in 1856 what is now the classic experiment for demonstrating the site action of this drug. Bernard showed that if one leg of a frog is ligated to cut off circulation to that limb, an injection of curare into the body will paralyze all of the limbs except the ligated one. He also showed that stimulating the afferent nerve of one limb resulted in a crossed reflex from the ligated limb but no reflex from the stimulated limb. This demonstrated that the drug did not act centrally (i.e., within the spinal cord), but rather had to get to the neuromuscular junction to exert its effect. He also showed that if the sciatic nerve were soaked in a curare solution, it still conducted nerve impulses to the muscle; and if the muscle were curarized, it could be depolarized by an increase of extracellular K^+ or excited by direct electrical stimulation. These results confirmed the neuromuscular junction as the site of action. *d*-Tubocurarine acts by competitively blocking the nicotinic neuromuscular receptor sites, but the mechanism of blockade is not known. The competitive nature of the blocking action means that curare can be displaced from its blocking position by increasing the concentration of available ACh. This can be done with an anticholinesterase such as neostigmine, which is the drug of choice in cases of curare overdose.

Curare and curare-like drugs are not likely to have any effect within the central nervous system because they do not pass the blood brain barrier. Consequently, these drugs were found to have no influence on brain activity as measured by the electroencephalograph, on pain threshold, on sensory processes such as hearing, vision, and smell, and on mentation, consciousness, or memory. Because animal studies could never be conclusive on this point, one had to wait for an experiment with a human subject. In 1947, S.M. Smith (an anesthetist) and his associates published an account of an experiment in which Smith was given a dose of *d*-tubocurarine 2.5 times greater than that which produces complete muscle paralysis (Myers, 1974). His respiration was maintained artificially. At no time did Smith note any absence of consciousness or any other change in sensory or other mental function, but along with total peripheral paralysis, he could not swallow or speak. Smith was very fortunate, because later experiments showed that when tubocurarine was injected into the lateral ventricle of the cat, generalized convulsions occurred that apparently had their origin in the hippocampus. It was possible that some of the drug might have entered Smith's brain; if it had, a serious accident could have ensued.

A number of synthetic curare-type drugs have been developed, for example, gallamine (Flaxedil), succinylcholine, and decamethonium. They also act on nicotinic receptors at neuromuscular junctions. They are used in medicine to obtain muscular relaxation during surgery (especially during abdominal surgery) and during resetting of dislocated joints and aligning of broken bones. Succinylcholine is especially useful for relaxing the muscles of the throat to prevent gagging during examination of the esophagus and trachea. It has the advantage of a short duration of action as a result of its rapid breakdown by pseudocholinesterases. All of these drugs, including *d*-tubocurarine, have little effect on autonomic ganglia. Succinylcholine and decamethonium differ from curare and gallamine in that, instead of blocking the receptors, they depolarize the muscle membranes, making them unresponsive to ACh (Koelle, 1975c).

Another group of nicotinic receptor blockers includes hexamethonium and mecamylamine. These are synthetic agents that block nicotinic receptors at autonomic ganglia. They can pass the blood brain barrier and can block the action of centrally acting nicotinic drugs. They were designed for controlling autonomic dysfunction such as gastrointestinal hypermotility or cardiovascular hypertension. However, the side effects of these drugs are quite pronounced. For example, when hexamethonium was used for duodenal ulcers, postural hypotension (feeling faint when rising from a supine position) was particularly bothersome; and when the drug was used to control high blood pressure, there was dry mouth, difficulties in voiding urine, constipation, nausea, anorexia, and other gastrointestinal symptoms. As a result, newer, more specific compounds have superceded them. Hexamethonium and mecamyline are described here because they were used in many behavioral studies, and the side effects must be considered in evaluating the studies.

Muscarinic Receptor Blocking Agents

This class of drugs is known as ANTIMUSCARINIC AGENTS or PARASYMPATHOLYTIC AGENTS. Although antimuscarinic drugs have a high specificity for peripheral muscarinic receptor sites, they slightly block transmission at nicotinic sites in autonomic ganglia at high doses. As muscarinic receptors may be either excitatory or inhibitory, the action of these antagonists will block the activity that is appropriate for given receptors. Antimuscarinic drugs easily pass the blood brain barrier and affect synapses within the CNS.

Antimuscarinic drugs have been used for a century or more to control dysfunctions of parasympathetically innervated structures, and dozens of synthetic analogs have been prepared to improve the specificity

Gallamine (Flaxedil)

Succinylcholine

Decamethonium

Hexamethonium

Mecamylamine

of action on selected organs (Innes and Nickerson, 1975). The atropine-like drugs have been used to block the sphincter muscles of the iris and ciliary body (to produce dilitation of the pupil and far fixation), to inhibit secretions from the nose, throat, and bronchi, to reduce heart rate and blood pressure, and to reduce salivation, gastric secretions, and motility of the GI tract. It is readily appreciated that this approach to the control of a particular parasympathetic function often results in undesirable changes in other systems. Fortunately, atropine in particular has a wide margin of safety, so that side effects are unlikely to reach dangerous levels. However, in the past, children have been seriously poisoned when atropine was given at bedtime to control enuresis—a practice that has been discontinued (Innes and Nickerson, 1970).

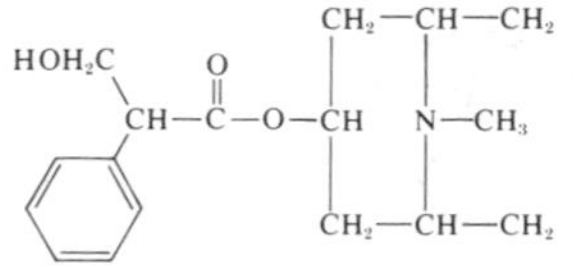

Atropine

The most important and well-known drug in this class, atropine, has already been mentioned. Atropine is the naturally occurring alkaloid of *Atropa belladonna* (deadly nightshade), a plant found in many parts of the world. During the Middle Ages, this substance was used as a poison to settle matters in many political and family intrigues. The name *Atropa belladonna* was given to the plant by Linné to reflect both its poisonous character as well as a cosmetic use of the juice of the plant. Atropos was the eldest of the Three Fates in Greek mythology, whose duty it was to cut the thread of life at the appropriate time. *Bella donna* in Latin means "beautiful woman." Women instilled the juice of the deadly nightshade berries into their eyes to cause pupil dilation (by blocking the muscarinic effects on the constrictor muscles of the iris). It was regarded then, and still is to some extent, that women with large pupils are more beautiful, or at least they command more attention.

Another widely used antimuscarinic drug is scopolamine (hyoscine), an alkaloid found in *Hyoscyamus niger* (henbane). Antimuscarinic drugs are competitive blockers of muscarinic receptor sites. Consequently, the antagonism to ACh characteristic of these drugs can be overcome by increasing the concentration of

ACh at the receptor sites by injecting an anticholinesterase or a cholinomimetic drug such as carbachol or pilocarpine. Therefore, overdoses of atropine can be corrected by anticholinesterases and overdoses of the reversible anticholinesterases can be corrected by atropine.

Atropine and scopolamine can be compared in terms of their pharmacological actions. Atropine has stronger effects on the heart, intestine, and bronchial muscles, whereas scopolamine has stronger action on the iris and ciliary body and the salivary and sweat glands. Scopolamine has a shorter duration of action: and it depresses the CNS, whereas atropine does so only in relatively large doses. Scopolamine in therapeutic doses produces drowsiness, euphoria, amnesia, fatigue, and dreamless sleep. It is frequently used along with narcotics as a preanesthetic medication prior to surgery or alone prior to childbirth to produce "twilight sleep"—a condition characterized by drowsiness and amnesia for events occurring during the duration of the drug action.

Two related compounds (congeners), methylatropine and methylscopolamine, have effects that are similar to those of the parent compounds, except they do not pass the blood brain barrier. These methylated compounds are used, therefore, when peripheral muscarinic blockade is desirable without central ef-

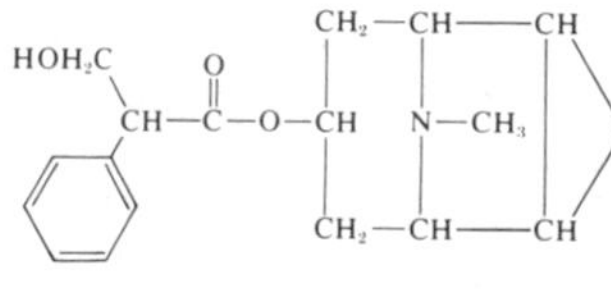

Scopolamine

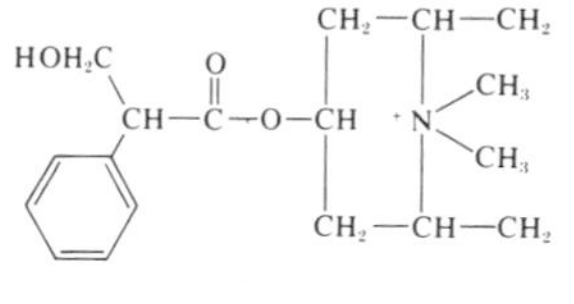

Methylatropine

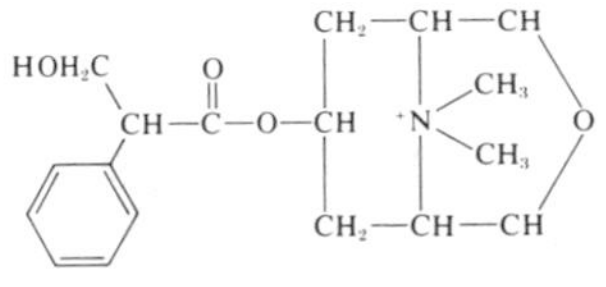

Methylscopolamine

fects. When anesthetic gases are to be inhaled, the methylated compounds are used in small doses to reduce saliva or mucus (which might enter the trachea) and to dilate the bronchial tubes. Also, in experiments that examine the behavioral effects of atropine or scopolamine, the methylated compounds are administered to control animals to see if the peripheral autonomic effects of these drugs are in any way responsible for the behavioral effects.

The drugs described in this section are only representative of the types that can influence cholinergic synaptic events *in vivo*. Some of these drugs are discussed in the next section, which deals with the behavioral effects of cholinergic drugs.

Part IV   Effects of Cholinergic Drugs on Behavior

General Principles

The widespread distribution of cholinergic systems in the CNS indicates that these systems play a significant role in brain function and behavior. Cholinergic drugs might reveal what that role is. However, there are some inherent difficulties that need to be overcome when one studies CNS effects of ACh or any other neurotransmitter.

First, it is clear that ACh is a major transmitter in the autonomic nervous system (ANS) and that cholinergic drugs can exert strong effects on this system, with marked behavioral consequences. For example, chemical warfare agents and related organophosphorous insecticides can exert powerful ANS effects (such as uncontrollable vomiting and diarrhea) that can markedly change the fighting capabilities of soldiers—without regard to the effects these chemicals can have within the CNS. This duality of effect is not peculiar to cholinergic drugs, because other transmitter systems also have receptors that can be influenced by drugs in the peripheral as well as in the central nervous system.

From one point of view, this duality of effect is an advantage because peripheral effects usually provide opportunities for simple experiments to verify a drug's mode of action. On the other hand, when central effects are being evaluated, methods must be found either to eliminate the peripheral effects or to evaluate them separately. This can be done in some instances by altering a drug so that it cannot pass the blood brain barrier, as in the case of methylatropine and methylscopolamine. In that case, the effects of the drug are confined primarily to peripheral systems. Comparing the effect of a drug that can enter the ANS and the CNS with the effect of another compound that can act only on the ANS enables evaluation of the relative contributions of the central and peripheral nervous systems.

Some drugs do not pass the blood brain barrier. Their central effects can be observed by injecting the drug directly into brain tissue or into the cerebrospinal fluid; from there the drug will be taken up by the target tissue. By comparing the drug effect after an intraventricular drug dose with the effect following systemic administration, it is possible to evaluate the drug effect in each compartment.

Second, it is quite unlikely that a given behavior is solely determined by a single neurotransmitter system. For example, simple spinal reflexes involve different neurotransmitters at synapses mediating the sensory input, the interneuronal mechanisms concerned with excitation and inhibition, intersegmental and crossed reflex effects, and the final motor output. Clearly, although a cholinergic drug could disrupt a reflex, the fact of the disruption does not permit the conclusion that ACh is the only, or even the crucial, transmitter in the system. Because spinal neurons are relatively accessible and because techniques have been available to assess the location and physiological effect of a drug application to spinal neurons, the role of each transmitter in spinal reflexes is firmly established. However, when one attempts to study the effects of a cholinergic drug on sleep, sexual activity, or eating and drinking, the difficulties of determining what physiological events are responsible for a change in behavior are increased many fold. For example, there have been experiments showing that carbachol applied to the hypothalamus elicits increased drinking behavior. The effect occurs when the drug is applied to some CNS structures but not to others. Also, the effect does not occur with noncholinergic drugs, and the carbachol effect can be blocked with atropine (a muscarinic blocker) but not with mecamylamine (a nicotinic blocker). It would thus be reasonable to conclude that muscarinic receptors in the hypothalamus are involved with drinking behavior.

However, the above argument would be more convincing if it could be shown that the drug application was accompanied by change in cholinergic activity in the stimulated tissue, namely, by measuring ACh turnover (i.e., the rate at which the precursor choline was incorporated into newly synthesized ACh during the drug-induced behavior). Complicating this approach is the fact that some drugs given systemically cause ACh turnover changes in some parts of the brain but not in others. However, modern methods permit the measurement of neurotransmitter turnover in discrete areas of the brain. In one procedure, a radioactive choline derivative is infused into a rat for a fixed period of time before the rat is killed by microwave radiation focused on the skull. The animal is killed in a second or two and enzymatic action in the tissue is halted. After the brain is removed, it is sliced into 400-μm sections. The nuclei that are of interest in these sections are removed by stainless steel punches and the amount of radioactivity in these small samples is measured. It is assumed that the radioactivity level correlates with the activity of the nuclei in response to a drug or in response to the activity of another system that impinges upon it (Cheney and Costa, 1978).

Unfortunately, radiotracer techniques are relatively new and were not available for behavioral studies done in the last two decades. For that reason, there is some inconsistency in the findings and some uncertainty about the mechanism of action of some drugs. As neurochemical and physiological techniques continue to develop and improve, answers to our questions will continually be reevaluated.

Effects of Cholinergic Drugs on Schedule-Controlled Behavior

There are many reports of experiments on the effects of cholinergic drugs on behavior tested under the rubric of operant conditioning. In these procedures, animals are trained with specified schedules of reinforcement. The result is behavior patterns that are highly consistent from day to day and between species and that provide stable and sensitive baselines for observing drug effects upon behavior. (See Chapter 2 on the techniques of behavioral pharmacology.)

Nicotine Effects

The general effect of nicotine administration on positive reinforcement paradigms (e.g., bar pressing for water or food) is an initial suppression of response, which appears immediately following the drug injection in rats; the suppression is followed by a response

rate increase. In many instances, nicotine produced effects similar to those caused by the stimulant drug amphetamine. Except for the initial depression caused by nicotine, both drugs in low doses caused increased rates of responding, and higher doses produced smaller rate increases and even rate *decreases*.

Nicotine effects also resemble the effects of amphetamine in that both drugs increase bar-press responses during fixed interval (FI) schedules and decrease them during fixed ratio (FR) schedules. Under the FI schedule, reinforcements (rewards) occur after the first response following a fixed interval of time. This conditioning schedule normally produces a pause immediately after the reinforcement, followed by a gradually accelerating response rate until the next reinforcement. The FR schedule usually produces a high, uniform response rate. Nicotine increases the response rate in the FI-schedule experiment during the postreinforcement pause, when the response rate is normally low, thus increasing the overall rate for the schedule. On the other hand, nicotine reduces the uniformly high FR response rate. This is an example of behavior explained by the "rate dependency hypothesis" attributed to Dews (1958), which stresses the importance of the control rate of responding as a factor in determining drug effects (McMillan and Leander, 1976).

Anticholinesterase and Muscarinic Drug Effects

When the anticholinesterase drug physostigmine (0.25 mg/kg) was tested on pigeons that pecked for positive reinforcement on a multiple FR–FI schedule, there was an initial cessation of responding for 1–3 hr, followed by normal responding on both components of the schedule. If the dose was increased, the interval of no responding also increased. When the peripherally acting anticholinesterase drug neostigmine was tested, it also produced a cessation of responding. These results indicate that the drug effect was probably due to peripheral actions of the drugs. When the muscarinic cholinomimetic drug arecoline was tested on rats in a FR–20 schedule for positive reinforcement, there was an increase in the duration of the usually slight postreinforcement pause, followed by an overall decrease in response rate. When arecoline (0.5 mg/kg) tests were given under a FI–2 minute schedule, there was a rate increase by 50 percent of the rats, but larger doses decreased the effect. The same effect was seen in arecoline tests using a DRL schedule: Low doses (0.25, 0.5, and 1.0 mg/kg) increased responding, thereby decreasing the number of reinforcements; whereas the opposite effect occurred with a 2.0 mg/kg dose. Thus, under the FI schedule, the drug had little effect on the number of reinforcements, but under the DRL schedule, the increased response rate had a negative effect on the number of reinforcements, showing that under the influence of the drug responding was under diminished control of the reinforcements (Vaillant, 1964; 1967; Pradhan and Dutta, 1970).

Schedules of negative reinforcement are those in which animals learn to make responses to avoid an impending noxious stimulus such as shock. These paradigms are often coupled with escape learning, that is, if the animal fails to respond to avoid the shock, the apparatus is designed to enable the animal to respond and turn off the shock. In tests with the anticholinesterase drug physostigmine and the cholinergic agonists pilocarpine and arecoline, it was found that all three drugs reduced responding in a dose-related fashion, causing an increase in shock rates. However, the doses rarely suppressed escape responding (McMillan and Leander, 1976). In another study it was found that the dose of anticholinesterase drug that reduced avoidance behavior by 50 percent of control rates (ED 50) was three times less than the ED 50 for reducing escape behavior. It was also shown that the degree of reduction of avoidance behavior correlated highly with the actual degree of cholinesterase inhibition. Behavior suppression occurred when AChE was inhibited by at least 50 percent; thereafter, behavior suppression was directly proportional to AChE inhibition. It was pointed out that the correlation did not establish a causal connection between AChE inhibition and behavior suppression, but the absence of the correlation would raise doubts about the role of ACh in these effects.

The suppressive effects of ACh agonists could be blocked by atropine (an ACh receptor blocker), which did not affect avoidance behavior when given alone. However, when methylatropine (the drug that does not cross the blood brain barrier) was given, the suppressive effect was not blocked. Thus, the effects of the anticholinesterase drugs depended upon central rather than peripheral effects. It was also found that drugs that blocked the action of norepinephrine and dopamine also interfered with avoidance responding, but interestingly, these effects were also blocked by atropine and scopolamine, indicating that cholinergic neurons are part of an important link in the chain of neurons that maintains avoidance behavior.

The observation that a reduction of brain levels of ACh increases avoidance behavior is consistent with the results of the preceding experiments. The animals (rats) were trained on a continuous avoidance schedule, that is, the rat must respond by lever pressing to postpone the onset of shock. Each lever press resets the clock that times the shock onset. There are no external cues that warn the rat of the shock onset; only the cues from the rat's "internal clock" elicit the response. Once a baseline response rate was achieved the animals were given the drug combination iproniazid and tetrabenazine. The treatment reduced brain ACh to a degree that correlated with the increased rate of lever pressing and reduced shock incidence. However, the drugs also caused a release of norepinephrine and serotonin, although to a degree that did not correlate with the behavioral effect. This experiment suggested that the reduction of ACh was the important factor in response increase. It was also found that the drug-induced enhancement of responding in this study could be attenuated with atropine, if it were given 1 hour before the tetrabenazine (Seiden and Dykstra, 1977). This result suggested that the depletion of brain ACh was due to a potent release of synaptic ACh that was uncompensated by a suitable increase in ACh synthesis. It would thus be quite reasonable to expect that the effects of tetrabenazine would be blocked by the muscarinic receptor blocker atropine.

But this interpretation does not correlate with the results of other experiments described earlier that showed that anticholinesterase drugs *suppressed* avoidance responding and that this effect was also blocked by atropine. So it appears in one case that enhanced ACh activity enhanced avoidance behavior and in the other case that it suppressed avoidance behavior. Thus, the results of these experiments are difficult to explain because of the many inconsistencies. Without any ready explanation at hand, it may be that other transmitters are involved.

In summary, the results of these experiments indicate that a cholinergic mechanism is involved in the maintenance of avoidance behavior. Cholinomimetic drugs seem to reduce avoidance responding, and reduction of brain levels of ACh seem to enhance it. But paradoxically, both effects are blocked by atropine. How these findings can be reconciled is not clear.

Anticholinergic Drug Effects

Drugs used in studies on the effects of anticholinergic drugs on *positively* reinforced behavior were atropine, scopolamine, benztropine, and benactyzine. For the most part, the effects of these drugs are quite similar. They tend to increase low rates of responding and decrease high rates of responding. For example, animals responding in FI schedules generally show an increase in response rates, with the increase occurring during the postreinforcement pause. In pigeons, the increase in pecking occurred consistently in FI schedules. Scopolamine tended to decrease FI response rates, in particular during the terminal portion of the interval when response rates were usually high. Atropine and scopolamine also decreased responding under VI schedules, which also generate high response rates. Unlike nicotine, which depressed FR rates of responding and increased FI responding, anticholinergic drugs depressed responding equally in FR and FI components of a multiple schedule. That the effects of these drugs were not solely the result of nonspecific effects on arousal is indicated by the finding that anticholinergic drugs can increase response rates maintained by DRL schedules at doses that markedly decrease FR responding (McMillan and Leander, 1976).

With respect to the effects of anticholinergic drugs on *negative* reinforcement paradigms, the general effect is the opposite of that found with cholinomimetic drugs (physostigmine, pilocarpine, and arecoline). For example, physostigmine disrupted well-practiced avoidance behavior in a shuttle box (the rat had to run from one compartment to another during a warning signal to avoid foot shock), whereas atropine and scopolamine improved this conditioned avoidance behavior in rats that had been performing poorly (Rech, 1968). In other studies, the cholinomimetics disrupted continuous avoidance responding (Sidman, 1953; see Chapter 2), sometimes without changing the shock rate and sometimes with an increased shock rate. In the former case, the animal presses more than the baseline rate; in the latter case, the animal fails to lever-press to postpone and avoid the shock but then makes a burst of responses following the shock. The burst of responses raises the overall response rate, but only one response within the response–shock interval is necessary to reset the clock to postpone the next shock. Thus the effect of the shock may be to confuse the animal so that it no longer responds according to the contingencies of the situation. Instead of responding once or twice near the end of the response–shock interval to avoid shocks it inefficiently makes a burst of responses *following* a shock. Also, high doses of anticholinergics produced consistently decreasing response

rates with increasing shock rates. This was not due to overall depression because escape responding was not affected, that is, the animals quickly terminated the shock if it was not avoided.

With respect to shock-suppressed behavior, anticholinergic drugs suppressed the ability of rats to withhold a response that formerly had had aversive consequences (passive avoidance). Rats that were trained to avoid a shock grill had that learning suppressed by scopolamine, although a drug-caused hyperactivity may have effected these results. Also, the drugs did not restore responding for food to rats that ceased to barpress because they had been formerly shocked when they bar-pressed for food.

It has been concluded that anticholinergic drugs at low doses increase low baseline rates of responding, as in DRL and in early segments of an FI. Also, low doses of anticholinergic drugs increase avoidance responding, whereas higher doses decrease response rates. But when low response rates were the result of punishment, the drugs did not increase the response rate (McMillan and Leander, 1976).

Cholinergic Drug Effects on Arousal and Vigilance Task Performance

Effects on Arousal

The experiments testing the effects of cholinergic drugs on schedule-controlled behavior revealed that the drugs increased or decreased the rate of responding according to the schedules of reinforcement, baseline response rates, and positive or negative reinforcement contingencies. Because a significant component of the cholinergic neural system seems to be related to the ascending reticular formation which is important in arousal, the possibility exists that the drug effects on performance are due to changes in the arousal level. Thus, high arousal could be responsible for increased response rates when baseline rates are low, whereas hyperarousal could suppress response rates that are high and more dependent on efficiently integrated motor control. Therefore, it is of interest to look for correlations between drug-induced changes in arousal and behavior changes.

Studies of cholinergic drug effects on arousal and the electrical activity of the brain have suggested that nicotine, muscarinic agonists, and anticholinesterases induce activation of the reticular formation. Reticular activation produces a low-voltage, desynchronized cortical EEG, which is a pattern that can also be induced by strong sensory stimulation and which indicates a high state of arousal. Anticholinergic agents such as atropine can reverse the effects of cholinergic agonists and can induce a high-voltage slow wave EEG, which is characteristic of a stage of sleep. It seems (as with amphetamine) that heightened arousal caused by cholinergic agonists accounts for the increases in low baseline response rates and in the suppression of high baseline response rates.

However, further investigations have shown that the increased reticular activity caused by the cholinergic agonists differs from that caused by amphetamine and sensory stimulation in that the cholinergic and anticholinergic drug effects are not concomitant with behavioral arousal and sleep, respectively. Rather, cholinergic drugs, even in low doses, tend to suppress ongoing behavior, and high doses of atropine-like compounds cause excitement, confusion, and disinhibition instead of sleep. Physiologically, the cholinergic pathways in the brain stem are different from those in the reticular formation that are associated with arousal. They are not even dependent upon the reticular formation, as the desynchronized EEG pattern caused by cholinergic drugs can occur when the reticular pathways are blocked by adrenergic and other blocking drugs. Also, cholinergic agonists may desynchronize the cortical EEG by acting directly on cholinergic synapses in cortical cell populations (Karczmar and Dun, 1978). Therefore, a proposed role for ACh in arousal systems is tenuous at best and does not easily lend itself to explaining the cholinergic effects on schedule-controlled behavior.

Effects on Vigilance Task Performance

A number of studies on the effect of acute and chronic administration of nicotine on vigilance task performance in rats have included monitoring of the electrical activity of the reticular activating system, the limbic system, and the cerebral cortex. The VIGILANCE TASK involved the presentation of a weak stimulus light that signaled a limited period of access to a lever in an operant conditioning chamber. Pressing the lever yielded a food reward to a food–deprived animal. Animals that were well trained at this task showed a behavior deficit after an initial dose of nicotine. However, by the fourth week of chronic nicotine treatments, performance was facilitated by nicotine when compared to the performance of saline–treated controls. Appropriate controls for this experiment showed

that the facilitation of this behavior was independent of practice effects and was not due to tolerance to the initial suppression of behavior.

The EEG records showed a change with acute and chronic nicotine use. An activation–sedation pattern was seen after an acute nicotine administration (100 μg/kg s.c.), whereas after chronic administration (100 μg/kg) three times per day for three weeks, both phases of the nicotine effect were markedly diminished. However, there were no changes in the electrical activity of the reticular formation over time, but there were correlated changes in the cortical and hippocampal records.

In another study, nicotine impaired the acquisition of a vigilance task but facilitated task performance over saline-treated controls after the task was learned (Nelsen and Goldstein, 1972, 1973; and Nelsen et al., 1973). Nicotine increased performance that is maintained by schedules of positive reinforcement, for example bar-pressing for food rewards (Macmillan and Leander, 1976); and nicotine facilitated acquisition of an avoidance response by mice in a shuttle box (Oliverio, 1966). However, it has not been clearly established that arousal is a significant factor in these effects.

Behavioral Effects of Nicotine in Humans

The preceding studies are related in interesting ways to the effects of smoking in humans. Subjectively, some cigarette smokers report a calming effect from smoking, whereas other smokers report a stimulating effect. On the basis of answers to a questionnaire about smoking habits, two groups of light smokers (less than 15 cigarettes a day) were selected. One group reported that they smoked mostly during boring, monotonous situations (the low arousal group) and the other group smoked mostly during tense, stressful situations (the high arousal group). All subjects were given one of two vigilance-type sensorimotor tasks. One task was far more demanding and complex than the other, eliciting high and low levels of arousal, respectively. Half of each group of smokers was assigned to the low arousal task and half to the high arousal task. The results showed that smoking during the task facilitated the performance of the low arousal smokers in the low arousal task, and smoking had the same effect on the high arousal smokers in the high arousal task. However, for low arousal smokers with the high arousal task and high arousal smokers with the low arousal task, smoking impaired performance. In a nonsmoking situation, there were no differences in performance for either group in either task. Thus, smoking appeared to facilitate task performance depending upon the concordance between the arousal level of the task and the arousal level that elicited smoking (Myrsten et al., 1975).

In another study designed to relate nicotine intake by cigarette smoking to arousal level, the amount of nicotine intake was estimated by counting puffs and examining the butts of heavy and light smokers while they were watching a stressful film (high arousal) or lying down (low arousal). While watching the film, the heavy smokers reduced their smoking rate, suggesting an attempt to self-regulate the arousal level. However, although smoking rate decreased, the estimates of the nicotine intake were the same for the high and low arousal conditions. Complicating these results was the fact that both the heavy and light smokers increased their smoking rate in the low arousal condition (Fuller and Forrest, 1973). Thus, this study did not show a consistent relationship between smoking and arousal. Moreover, it is found that smoking behavior of given individuals occurs in situations that differ widely in arousal value, for example, when relaxing after a meal versus preparing to make a contentious telephone call or when feeling uncomfortable in the presence of business superiors. In general, when considering the relationship between smoking and arousal, the experimental evidence does not consistently tell us whether one smokes to maintain a given arousal level or to change that level. Thus, it would appear difficult to relate smoking behavior or nicotine intake to one selected variable such as arousal.

The evidence is convincing that smoking can facilitate concentration and work in humans. Also, smoking in humans, which was accompanied by higher heart rate (and possibly increased arousal), interfered with the learning of nonsense syllable lists. However, recall 45 minutes later, when the effects of a single cigarette had worn off, was better than that following a nonsmoking condition during the learning session (Andersson, 1975). Thus in this study, learning may have been reduced, but memory seems to have been facilitated by nicotine.

Addictive Nature of Nicotine

Smoking can quickly supply nicotine to the brain. When the smoke is inhaled deeply into the lungs, the ni-

cotine quickly enters the bloodstream and is rapidly absorbed into brain tissue. Moreover, smokers seem to be able to regulate their nicotine intake according to their perceived requirements. Some of the early studies that investigated this ability were methodologically flawed, but the overall results were supported by later studies with better controls and methods of measurement.

Studies (reviewed by Brecher, 1972), as long ago as 1942 showed that small injections of nicotine provided pleasant sensations to smokers, who were disinclined to smoke shortly thereafter. Repeated injections of nicotine became preferable to cigarettes, and when injections were discontinued, craving arose.

In one experiment, cigarettes with either low or high nicotine content were given to smokers (designated nonaddicted). Some smokers were not aware of a change when the experimental cigarettes were low in nicotine content; some sensed a vague lack in satisfaction from their smoking; and some definitely missed the nicotine and experienced heightened irritability, decreased ability to concentrate during mental tasks, and feelings of inner hunger and emptiness. These symptoms are frequently reported by individuals who have stopped smoking.

In 1967, a study by Lucchesi et al. was conducted at the University of Michigan Medical School, where under carefully controlled conditions subjects spent 6 hours per day for 15 consecutive days with an intravenous needle that supplied either saline or a nicotine solution. These subjects could do whatever they liked in the way of quiet activities and could smoke if they chose to. When nicotine was injected, the subjects smoked fewer cigarettes and left longer butts.

In 1971 at the London University (England) Institute of Psychiatry, a group of smokers was supplied with cigarettes having high, medium, or low nicotine concentrations. The more nicotine, the longer the interval between puffs and the longer it took to finish the cigarettes. This and other studies suggest that people smoke to maintain an optimum level of nicotine in the brain (Brecher, 1972; Lader, 1978a).

A number of clinical studies involved in breaking the smoking habit experimented with nicotine-containing chewing gum to be used in place of cigarettes with the hope that weaning away from the gum habit could be accomplished over time. At first, chewing nicotine-containing gum reduced smoking. However, the placebo effect was very strong (i.e., after chewing gum with no nicotine, the smokers also reduced their smoking). When gum was supplied on a continuous basis, 50 percent of the subjects dropped out of the experiment, whereas those remaining showed a decline of gum chewing and tobacco use over time. After 26 weeks, 25 percent of the subjects who completed the program were abstinent (i.e., were not smoking); 59 percent had relapsed entirely (i.e., they had gone back to their previous level of tobacco use); and 18 percent fell in between. Another study showed initial declines in tobacco use while using nicotine gum (compared to placebo group), but again, placebo subjects who tried to stop smoking did almost as well as the nicotine-gum groups. In the long run (after a year) only 26 percent of the subjects who completed the treatment were totally abstinent. These studies suggest that nicotine substitutes are not sufficient by themselves to eliminate tobacco use in most individuals. It is also likely that brain nicotine is only one of several reinforcers of smoking behavior.

In a third study, nicotine-gum chewing was combined with hypnotherapy (employing hypnosis). Again there was a 40–65 percent reduction of tobacco use over all groups, including placebo groups. But surprisingly, 10 subjects who claimed to be abstinent after 4 weeks of treatment showed high concentrations of nicotine in their urine, even though they knew that their urine samples could be analyzed for nicotine content. Thus, there is reason to seriously question the reliability of experiments that depend on self-reports of reduction in or abstinence from tobacco use.

From the foregoing it would appear that tobacco use in most instances is related to a craving for and an addiction to nicotine. Although there are questions arising from the term "addiction" with its connotations of abnormality, the facts of tobacco use would be consistent with Jaffe's (1975) definition of addiction.

It is a behavioral pattern of compulsive drug use characterized by overwhelming involvement with the use of a drug, the securing of its supply, and a high tendency to relapse after withdrawal.

The Diagnostic and Statistical Manual of Mental Disorders (DSM III, Third Edition, 1980) of the American Psychiatric Association provides us with a rather conservative definition of tobacco dependence while apparently discarding the term "addiction" altogether.

A. Continuous use of tobacco for at least one month.

B. At least one of the following:
   1. Serious attempts to stop or significantly reduce the amount of tobacco use on a permanent basis have been unsuccessful.
   2. Attempts to stop smoking have led to the development of Tobacco Withdrawal; i.e., craving for tobacco, irritability, anxiety, difficulty concentrating, restlessness, headache, drowsiness, gastrointestinal disturbances.
   3. The individual continues to use tobacco despite a serious physical disorder (e.g., respiratory or cardiovascular disease) that he or she knows is exacerbated by tobacco use.

From a physiological viewpoint, addiction is characterized by tolerance and withdrawal effects (see Chapters 1 and 13), and the experiments described above support the idea that nicotine ingestion via tobacco is compulsive, difficult to give up, and involves tolerance and withdrawal effects. Thus, by any criterion, there is considerable support for the idea that tobacco use can lead to dependence for its use, and that nicotine plays a significant role in establishing and maintaining that dependence (Health Consequences of Smoking. A report of the Surgeon General, 1980).

Dependence upon drugs is frequently associated with illegality in use and source of supply, but the almost universal availability of tobacco usually obviates those considerations. However, the antisocial and illegal aspects of an addiction in the case of nicotine become apparent when supplies of tobacco are restricted. After World War II, cigarettes became a means of exchange, with people trading them in illegal black markets. People were willing to work, trade priceless possessions, prostitute themselves, and do without food to obtain cigarettes. In defeated Germany, after World War II, the frequent observation of highly respected individuals following a smoker for considerable distances hoping to retrieve a discarded butt illustrates the energy they expended and the degree to which they abandoned their self-esteem to satisfy this craving—in most ways little different from the behavior of narcotic addicts in the present day (Brecher, 1972).

Summary

Cholinergic systems are a fertile ground for psychopharmacological investigations of memory and learning, sleep and arousal, consuming behavior, i.e. eating and drinking, sensory awareness, aggression, sexual behavior, and associated pathological conditions. In preceding sections we presented the principal anatomical and histological details of cholinergic systems, the chemistry and the actions of the transmitter acetylcholine, and the means of manipulating that chemistry and action with cholinergic drugs. Also, examples of the behavioral effects of some of these drugs have been provided.

The discussion of cholinergic drug effects on schedule-controlled behavior utilizing the strict controls of operant conditioning serves to illustrate an important contemporary approach to psychopharmacological research. It has shown that (1) the schedule of reinforcement, (2) the nature of the reinforcer (positive or negative), (3) baseline rates of responding, and (4) the drug and its dose, all influence the changes in behavior that occurred. (It is noted that intervening variables such as arousal, fear, hunger, sex drive and the like are not part of the hypotheses and explanations of drug effects on schedule-controlled behavior. By and large, psychopharmacologists who employ operant conditioning hold that these variables require their own special data, usually physiological in nature, to elucidate their role.) The effects of other drugs on schedule-controlled behavior will be illustrated in subsequent chapters with the aim of demonstrating the utility of this approach in addition to others.

Investigation of a possible connection between the action of cholinergic drugs and physiological measures of arousal were undertaken to provide some basis for the behavioral effects of these drugs. However, the results were not supportive of the hypothesized role of a cholinergic system in the reticular formation that influences cortical activity and arousal.

Nicotine causes a temporary deficit in performance of a vigilance task that is already learned, but later doses facilitate performance. However, another study showed that nicotine only impaired the *acquisition* of the vigilance task and facilitated the performance, if the task was learned, without an initial decrement of performance. These effects could not be traced to practice effects or to drug tolerance. Temporal effects of nicotine were also seen in EEG records. There was an activation-sedation pattern after chronic administration, but these EEG effects were markedly diminished as doses continued. There were no drug related changes recorded from the reticular formation.

Tobacco use by men and women, in pharmacological terms, is the self-administration of nicotine. The reasons why people smoke even when they express a desire to stop are consistent with the evidence for addiction or dependence on nicotine. Nicotine is capable of improving concentration and inducing feelings of relaxation and well being (perhaps by forestalling withdrawal effects) in the habitual user. As with many instances of drug self-administration, associated behaviors acquire the characteristics of secondary reinforcers and maintain the smoking habit or reinstate it when the desire for the primary reinforcer (nicotine) is no longer providing the motivation for smoking. Thus, most tobacco users who quit the smoking habit easily succumb to the distractions afforded by manipulating smoking paraphernalia, the smell and taste of tobacco and its smoke, the association between smoking and concentration, conversation, the cocktail hour and the coffee break, telephone calls, television, getting up in the morning and going to bed at night.

The Surgeon General of the United States warns of the perils of cigarette smoking on every pack of cigarettes and in every advertisement for them, and has stated that "Smoking will kill more Americans every year than died in our major wars combined, while smoking related disabilities continue to be the major personal and public health problem of U.S. citizens" (see Brecher, 1972). The tobacco industry has refused to acknowledge the danger of habitual cigarette smoking, and makes the self-serving assertion that the data are merely "statistical" (as though there were any other kind), thus not providing sufficient proof of hazardous consequences. Its most recent approach is to extol "freedom of choice" for those who want to smoke, while ignoring the fact that promoting the use of drugs that lead to dependence and addiction severely weakens even that option. In recent years the industry has supplied the market with cigarettes with low levels of nicotine and tar. (Tar has been strongly implicated as a carcinogen.) However, there is evidence that low nicotine levels in cigarettes usually result in faster puffing and deeper inhaling to maximize nicotine intake, thus defeating the intended purpose of the change. More injurious, perhaps, is the implicit encouragement to the young to begin smoking under the mistaken belief that cigarettes are now safe.

Recommended Readings

Bignami, G. and Michalek, H. (1978). Cholinergic mechanisms and aversely motivated behaviors. In *Psychopharmacology of Aversely Motivated Behavior*

(H. Anisman and G. Bignami, Eds.), pp. 173–255. Plenum Press, New York. A review of cholinergic mechanisms and drugs as they relate to behavior elicited by fear and aversive stimuli.

Changeux, J-P. (1975). The cholinergic receptor protein from fish electric organ. In *Handbook of Psychopharmacology, Vol. 6* (L.L. Iversen, S.D. Iversen and S.H. Snyder, Eds.), pp. 235–301. Plenum Press, New York. A review of ACh receptors with respect to chemistry and function.

Cheney, D.L. and Costa, E. (1978). Biochemical pharmacology of cholinergic neurons. In *Psychopharmacology: A Generation of Progress* (M.A. Lipton, A. DiMascio and K.F. Killam, Eds.), pp. 283–292. Raven Press, New York. An excellent survey of the discovery and physiology of cholinergic mechanisms.

Drachman, D.A. (1978). Central cholinergic system and memory. In *Psychopharmacology: A Generation of Progress* (M.A. Lipton, A. DiMascio and K.F. Killam, Eds.), pp. 651–662. Raven Press, New York. A review of studies on the possible role of ACh in memory.

Jaffe, J.H. and Jarvik, M.E. (1978). Tobacco use and tobacco use disorder. In *Psychopharmacology: A Generation of Progress* (M.A. Lipton, A. DiMascio and K.F. Killam, Eds.), pp. 1665–1676. Raven Press, New York. A review on the origins of smoking, why people smoke, and the possibilities that nicotine is an addictive drug.

Jarvik, M.E., Cullen, J.W., Gritz, E.R., Vogt, T.M. and West, L.J. (Eds.) (1977). *Research on Smoking Behavior. NIDA Research Monograph 17.* Supt. of Documents, U.S. Govt Printing Office, Washington, D.C. A comprehensive study of the epidemiology of tobacco use.

Karczmar, A.G. and Dun, N.J. (1978). Cholinergic synapses: physiological, pharmacological and behavioral considerations. In *Psychopharmacology: A Generation of Progress* (M.A. Lipton, A. DiMascio and K.F. Killam, Eds.), pp. 293–305. Raven Press, New York. A review of the cholinergic mechanisms implicated in sleep, memory and learning, motor behavior, aggression, nociception, and sexual behavior.

Litten, W. (1975). The most poisonous mushrooms. *Scientific American* 232, 3, 90–101. An interesting account of the varieties of poisonous mushrooms and the biochemistry of their toxic effects.

Marchbanks, R.M. (1975). Biochemistry of cholinergic neurons. In *Handbook of Psychopharmacology, Vol. 3* (L. L. Iversen, S.D. Iversen and S.H. Snyder, Eds.), pp. 247–326. Plenum Press, New York. A comprehensive review of the chemistry of ACh.

Meselson, M. and Robinson, J. P. (1980). Chemical warfare and chemical disarmament. *Scientific American*, 242, 4, 38–47. A compelling examination of the subject of chemical warfare and the need for disarmament.

Tucek, S. (Ed.) (1979). *The Cholinergic Synapse. Progress in Brain Research, Vol. 49*, Elsevier Scientific Publ. Co. New York. A collection of research papers covering many facets of this subject.

Zornetzer, S.F. (1978). Neurotransmitter modulation and memory: a new neuropharmacological phrenology? In *Psychopharmacology: A Generation of Progress* (M.A. Lipton, A. DiMascio and K.F. Killam, Eds), pp. 637–649. Raven Press, New York. A critique of chemical models of memory.

The Health Consequences of Smoking. A report of the Surgeon General. (1980). DHEW Publ. No. (PHS) 79-50066, U.S. Govt. Printing Office, Washington, D.C. Research papers on all aspects of smoking—physiology, epidemiology, economics, dangers to health, mortality statistics, prevention programs, and ways of breaking the habit.

CHAPTER SEVEN

Catecholamines

Part I   The Identity and Distribution of Catecholamine Systems

The group of neurotransmitters known as the catecholamines (CAs) includes dopamine (DA), norepinephrine (NE), and epinephrine (EPI). The terms *norepinephrine* and *noradrenaline* are synonymous, as are *epinephrine* and *adrenaline*. The term adrenaline came into use because the substance was thought to be produced solely by the adrenal gland (the gland located above the kidney); the name is derived from the Latin *ad ren*, which means "near kidney." Epinephrine is derived from the Greek *epi nephros* for "upon the kidney." In the United States these transmitters are called *epinephrine* and *norepinephrine*, although the adjective forms used are *adrenergic* and *noradrenergic*— probably because they are easier to pronounce than epinephrinergic and so on (Carlson, 1981). The reader should also be aware that in the pharmacological literature "adrenergic" is frequently used in a general sense to denote noradrenergic subjects as well. Thus α- and β-adrenergic drugs or receptors also include noradrenergic subjects. In this volume, we will try to avoid this confusion between adrenergic and noradrenergic by using the appropriate terms in each case.

The CAs play highly significant roles in the activities of the peripheral and central nervous systems. In this chapter they shall be described in terms of their chemistry and their distribution among the neurons of the nervous system. The activity of these systems is important in health and disease, and there have been many drugs discovered or created to modify catecholamine functions. There is a large body of evidence for direct catecholamine involvement in a variety of behaviors (such as sleep, reward, feeding, and drinking) and in the functional illnesses (such as schizophrenia and depression). Catecholamines are also implicated in organic diseases such as Parkinson's disease, cardiovascular hypertension, and paroxysmal tachycardia (sudden increases in heart rate). Advances in biochemistry and pharmacology have contributed greatly to our understanding of these phenomena.

Chemical Identity of Catecholamines

The catecholamines are monoamines, that is, compounds having only one amine group (NH_2). Each compound (dopamine, norepinephrine, and epinephrine) contains the catechol nucleus (a benzene ring with two attached hydroxyl groups, OH) and ethylamine or one of its derivatives (Figure 1).

During the 1960s, a group of Swedish investigators (prominent among them Dahlström and Fuxe, 1964) perfected a histofluorescence technique that had been discovered by Eränkö in 1955. The histofluorescence technique made it possible to identify the presence of monoamine-containing neurons within the CNS, and further refinements permitted the tracing of pathways and the connections made by these neurons. The technique consisted of treating monoamine-containing tissue with formaldehyde vapor to produce condensation products called ISOQUINOLINES. These products emit a fluorescent glow when illuminated by ultraviolet light.

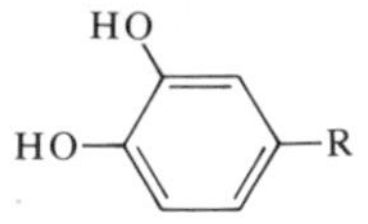

Catechol nucleus

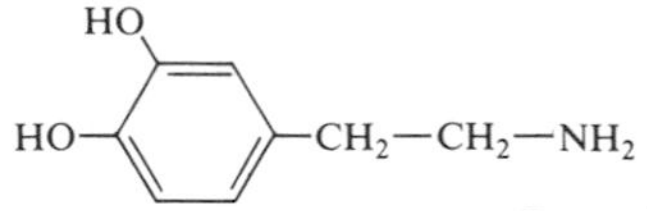

Dopamine
(3,4-dihydroxyphenylethylamine)

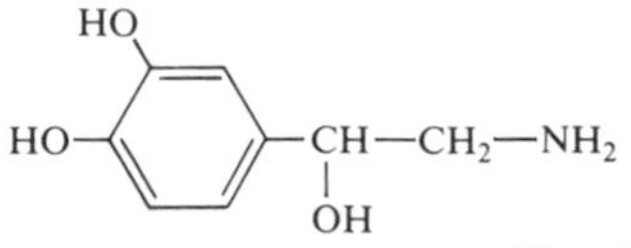

Norepinephrine (Noradrenaline)
(3,4-dihydroxyphenylethanolamine)

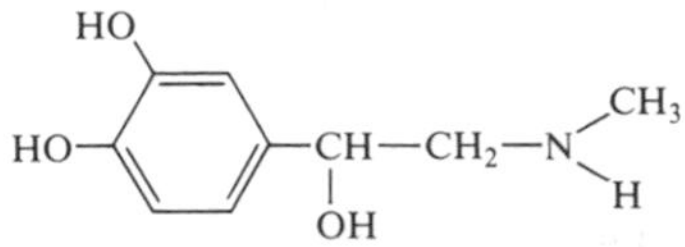

Epinephrine (Adrenaline)
(3,4-dihydroxyphenyl-N-methylethanolamine)

FIGURE 1   CATECHOL NUCLEUS AND CATECHOL-AMINE NEUROTRANSMITTERS. These relatively simple molecules differ from one another in the composition of their side chains.

The catecholamine products appear bright green and the serotonin product appears bright yellow. It is also possible by chemical means to shift the emission peak for NE to allow for discrimination between the presence of NE and DA. With fluorescence photomicrography, the pathways of monoaminergic neurons could be followed. Later a method for producing different greens to distinguish between norepinephrine and epinephrine was found (Eränkö, 1976). A further development showed that treatment of neural tissue with glyoxylic acid rather than formaldehyde formed

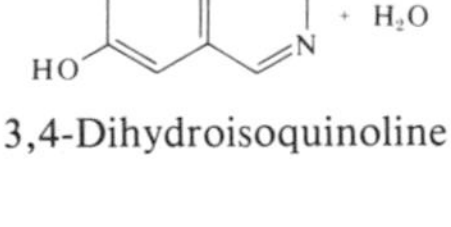

3,4-Dihydroisoquinoline

condensation products that provided even greater sensitivity in detecting CA systems (Lindvall and Björklund, 1974; 1978).

Using these methods, Dahlström et al. (1965a) showed that fluorescence of cells and terminals disappeared from animal tissue treated with reserpine (a drug that blocks the storage of monoamines, leading to their exposure to catabolizing enzymes). Carlsson et al. (1964) showed that the fluorescence disappeared from axons and terminals beyond the point at which the axons had been severed from their cell bodies. The same investigators also found that fluorescent material accumulated on the proximal side (the side nearest the cell body) of a compression of a peripheral aminergic nerve and on the proximal side of a transection of the spinal cord (Dahlström, 1965; Dahlström and Fuxe, 1965). This indicated that newly synthesized monoaminergic material was being conveyed down the axon and could not pass the block or transection. Finally, prolonged electrical stimulation caused a marked depletion of catecholamine stores, especially when synthesis-preventing drugs were also used (Fuxe and Gunne, 1964; Dahlström et al., 1965b).

Von Euler (1946a, 1946b, 1948) correctly identified the presence of norepinephrine in sympathetic nerves, and he predicted that this substance would be concentrated in the nerve terminals from which it would be released and act as a neurotransmitter. His predictions were confirmed with the development of the fluorescence technique. Shortly after von Euler's predictions, Holtz (1950) identified NE as a constituent of the mammalian brain. At that time, it was believed that NE served as a neurotransmitter at nerve terminals that innervated the smooth muscles of the blood vessels of the brain. However, later studies showed that NE concentration was not correlated with blood vessel distribution. Consequently, Vogt (1954) suggested that NE serves as a neurotransmitter in a specialized system in the brain. There is now abundant evidence showing the correctness of that suggestion.

Distribution of Noradrenergic Pathways

The histochemical methods used to identify the location of monoaminergic cell bodies and their axon projections in the CNS is a relatively recent development. Thus, there continues to be some ambiguity about the precise distribution of these systems. Also, the analysis of the monoamines in the human brain is difficult because of the breakdown of the fluorophores in the period between the death of the person and the chemical treatment of the neural tissue. Thus, virtually all of our information comes from animal studies. However, there is an additional advantage in animal studies in that electrolytic lesions, knife cuts, and other manipulations with neural tissue can be performed as aids in the investigations. That the findings in animal brains are applicable to the human is to a considerable extent borne out by studies of catecholaminergic pathways in human fetal brains (Nobin and Björklund, 1973). They concluded that the organization of the pathways in rat and human are quite similar.

The major proportion of noradrenergic neurons is found in the autonomic nervous system. These neurons are innervated by preganglionic cholinergic neurons whose cell bodies are in the intermediate horn of the thoracic and first two lumbar segments of the spinal cord (Figure 2). The axons of these cholinergic neurons leave the spinal cord by way of the ventral roots and enter the sympathetic ganglia via the *white* rami to form synapses with noradrenergic neurons in the sympathetic ganglia. The postganglionic sympathetic neurons are noradrenergic and their axons join the spinal nerves via the *gray* rami to be distributed to the surface of the body. These nerves innervate the smooth muscles of the blood vessels to control blood pressure, and innervate the follicles on the skin to fluff feathers or fur to conserve body heat (or to raise "goose bumps" in the human). Other fibers innervate the sweat glands but these nerves are cholinergic. From the upper thoracic segments, postganglionic NE fibers innervate the cardiac and pulmonary apparatus.

Some of the cholinergic preganglionic neurons pass through the sympathetic ganglia without synapse, and instead, form synapses in the prevertebral ganglia such as the celiac, and the superior and inferior mesenteric ganglia. From these ganglia, noradrenergic postganglionic fibers pass to the organs and glands of the viscera (stomach, intestines, pancreas, etc.) and to those of the pelvic region (bladder, colon, and genital structures). The sympathetic neurons exert the opposite effects of the cholinergic parasympathetic neurons, thereby balancing the activity of the internal organs of the body.

Another small group of cholinergic preganglionic neurons pass directly to the adrenal glands. There they form neuroeffector junctions with chromaffin cells of the adrenal medulla which synthesizes and releases epinephrine and norepinephrine into the blood stream. These circulating catecholamines augment the activities of the sympathetic system.

Within the CNS noradrenergic systems have been more difficult to trace because they are interspersed among other systems to a perplexing degree. However, histofluorescence and immunohistochemical techniques have now given us a fairly good understanding of the distribution of these pathways. Studies by Ungerstedt (1971a; Lindvall and Björklund, 1974, 1978), and others on the rat brain have revealed the details of monoaminergic systems. Figure 3 shows generalized horizontal projections of the noradrenergic and the dopaminergic systems, as well as the serotonergic system of the rat brain. Figure 4 shows the noradrenergic system from a medial view. By comparing these two views, some idea of the distribution and the major terminals of the catecholamine systems in the CNS can be grasped. The cell body aggregations are labeled according to the convention described by Dahlström and Fuxe (1964) and are located in the pons and medulla. Their schema has undergone some modification since it was first enunciated, because the populations of some cell groupings, such as A3, have been deemed too small to be designated as nuclear groups.

The A1 cell bodies (Figure 4) project their axons caudally to the spinal cord and rostrally as far as the forebrain. The rostrally projecting axons are joined by projections from A5 and A7 to form the ventral noradrenergic bundle. This bundle extends through the medullary reticular formation, through the pons and mesencephalon, and after at least part of it joins the medial forebrain bundle, terminates in the paraventricular nucleus of the hypothalamus, the preoptic area, the septal area, the pituitary, the mammillary bodies, and the substantia nigra.

The dorsal noradrenergic bundle has a wider distribution. It emanates from the locus caeruleus (A6) and, after coursing ventrolaterally, enters the zona incerta and the medial forebrain bundle. It innervates the cerebral cortex, the hippocampus, amygdala, the thalamus, geniculate bodies, colliculi, habenula, and some hypothalamic nuclei. The locus caeruleus is the largest of the noradrenergic nuclei, and in the cat and monkey, small numbers of fibers from it have been found to extend into the spinal cord. A caudal extension of the nucleus A4 projects to the cerebellum.

From A2, fibers project to the nucleus of tractus solitarius (a center receiving gustatory and visceral af-

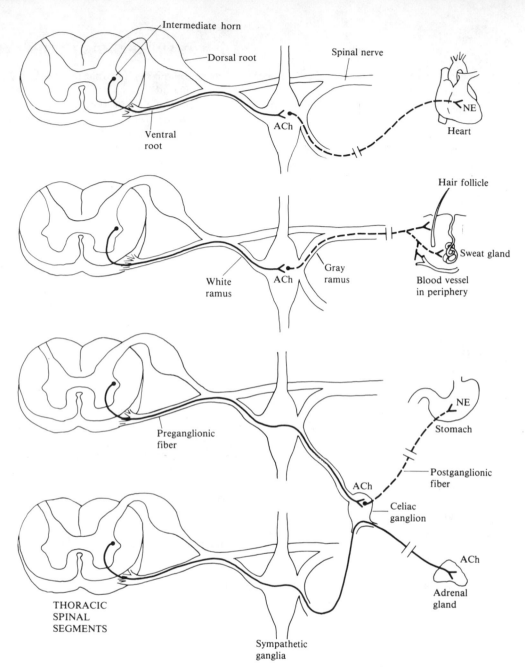

Intermediate horn

Dorsal root

Spinal nerve

NE

Heart

ACh

Ventral root

Hair follicle

Sweat gland

White ramus

ACh

Gray ramus

Blood vessel in periphery

NE

Stomach

Preganglionic fiber

Postganglionic fiber

ACh

Celiac ganglion

ACh

Adrenal gland

THORACIC SPINAL SEGMENTS

Sympathetic ganglia

FIGURE 2 SYMPATHETIC DIVISION OF THE AUTONOMIC NERVOUS SYSTEM. The preganglionic fibers (solid lines) emerge from cell bodies in the intermediate horn, and exit via the ventral roots of the thoracic and first two lumbar segments of the spinal cord. These fibers either synapse in the sympathetic ganglia or the prevertebral ganglia such as the celiac and are cholinergic. The postganglionic fibers (dashed lines) emerge from all of the sympathetic ganglia and the prevertebral ganglia. The former, in addition to innervating the cardiac and pulmonary systems, innervate the smooth muscles of the blood vessels and hair follicles, and the sweat glands on the surface of the body. The latter form neuroeffector junctions with the organs of the viscera. All of these fibers are noradrenergic with the exception of the innervation of the sweat glands which is cholinergic. No postganglionic fibers emerge from the adrenal gland. The medulla (inner core) of the gland secretes norepinephrine and epinephrine into the bloodstream, thus augmenting the activity of the sympathetic system.

154

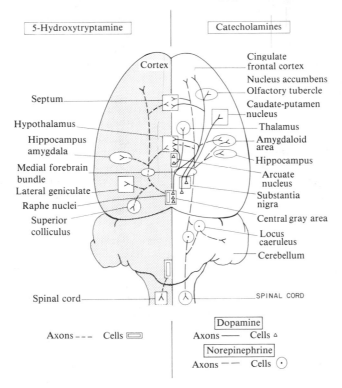

FIGURE 3 MONOAMINERGIC PATHWAYS IN THE RAT BRAIN. The indoleamine (serotonin) system is on the left; the catecholamine (norepinephrine and dopamine) systems are on the right. (From Elliott et al., 1977.)

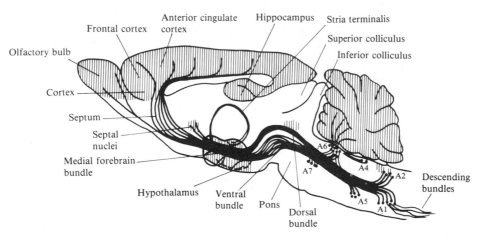

FIGURE 4 ASCENDING NORADRENERGIC PATHWAYS. This sagittal view of the rat brain shows the major NE pathways that emanate from nuclei A1, A2, etc. in the brain stem. The shaded parts of the brain show the principal areas of innervation from this system. (After Ungerstedt, 1971a.)

ferents), the motor nucleus of the vagus nerve, and the nucleus of the hypoglossal nerve.

Dopamine and Its Distribution

For a considerable time it was believed that dopamine was merely a precursor in the synthesis of NE. However, the histofluorescence technique of catecholamine identification revealed that DA was present in relatively large amounts in localized areas of the brain and was unaccompanied by similar concentrations of NE. This finding suggested that DA might have a specific role as a neurotransmitter in the brain. It is now believed that dopamine constitutes more than 50 percent of brain catecholamines.

Small Intensely Fluorescent Cells

An identification of dopaminergic neurons in the autonomic nervous system was reported by Greengard et al. (1972), Kebabian and Greengard (1971), and McAfee and Greengard (1972), who found evidence for dopaminergic interneurons [known as small intensely fluorescent (SIF) cells] in the superior cervical sympathetic ganglion of the rabbit. They found that stimulating the preganglionic fibers leading to the gan-

glion caused a fast depolarization (f-EPSP) of the postganglionic neurons. They believed that this action was the result of the release of ACh upon the nicotinic receptors of the postganglionic cells, because the effect could be blocked by the nicotinic receptor blocker hexamethonium. In addition, the excitation of the postganglionic cells was followed by a slow and long-lasting hyperpolarization (s-IPSP) that served to inhibit the postganglionic neurons. Because this latter effect could be blocked by atropine and not by hexamethonium, the inhibitory action was thought to be due to the muscarinic excitation of the dopaminergic SIF cells that inhibited the postganglionic neurons by hyperpolarizing them.

These effects are summarized in Figure 5, which shows the postganglionic cells with three types of receptors. One is a nicotinic ACh receptor, which when stimulated causes the f-EPSP that depolarizes the membrane and which is blocked by hexamethonium. A second receptor responds to dopamine from the SIF cells and is responsible for the s-IPSP that hyperpolarizes the postganglionic cell membranes. It is blocked by phentolamine and is stimulated by exogenous dopamine. A third receptor is muscarinic and

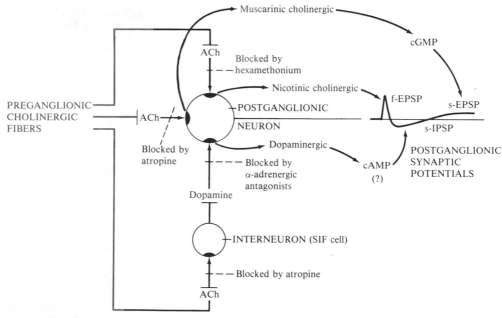

FIGURE 5   PROPOSED SYNAPTIC CONNECTIONS in the superior cervical ganglion. This proposed scheme shows how neurotransmitters and drugs may interact to generate the postganglionic synaptic potentials. (From Greengard, 1976.)

is responsible for the s-EPSP. It is blocked by atropine. Finally, the cholinergic receptor upon the SIF cell is also muscarinic because the action on the interneuron is blocked by atropine but not by hexamethonium (Kebabian and Greengard, 1971; Greengard, 1976).

Although a role for cAMP and cGMP in the s-IPSP and s-EPSP respectively has been suggested (Greengard, 1976) more recent research that was discussed in Chapter 4 calls some of the conclusions into question. First, the new evidence does not support earlier findings that cAMP is involved in the hyperpolarizing of postganglionic membranes (i.e., the s-IPSP). Rather, it is more likely that cAMP is instrumental in modulating the ACh receptor responsible for the s-EPSP. Also, the potentiation of the IPSP by a phosphodiesterase inhibitor (theophylline) is not replicated by the more specific phosphodiesterase inhibitor Ro-20-1724, which fails to augment the IPSP. It is believed that theophylline has an effect independent of its phosphodiesterase activity because the effect occurs even in the presence of prior phosphodiesterase inhibition with Ro-20-1724. It appears then that cAMP does not mediate the s-IPSP response but rather modulates the action of the muscarinic receptors on the ganglion cells that act via cGMP to induce the s-EPSP. Thus, these findings raise questions about the role of dopamine-

sensitive adenylate cyclase and cAMP in ganglionic transmission (Libet, 1979).

Dopaminergic Pathways in the Central Nervous System

Contemporary studies of the neuroanatomy of the rat brain have shown that there are at least four dopaminergic (DA) pathways within the CNS (Ungerstedt, 1971a; Thierry et al., 1973; Lindvall and Björklund, 1974; Berger et al., 1976; Jacobowitz, 1978). Figure 6 presents a comparison between the noradrenergic and dopaminergic pathways in the rat brain; and Figure 7 presents sagittal and transverse sections showing dopaminergic pathways. Cells from A8 in the ventrolateral midbrain tegmentum give rise to axons that continue rostrally through the cerebral peduncles of the midbrain and join axons emanating from cells in A9 that are located mostly in the zona compacta of the substantia nigra. The combined axons form the nigrostriatal pathway and innervate the caudate–putamen and the central nucleus of the amygdala. The nigrostriatal pathway plays an inhibitory role upon cholinergic neurons in the caudate–putamen. In humans, degeneration of the DA cells in the substantia nigra results in the tremors, spasticity, and poverty of movement in patients with Parkinson's disease.

Cell bodies from A10 are found almost along the

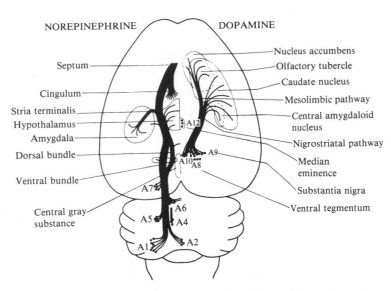

FIGURE 6 HORIZONTAL PROJECTIONS OF CATECHOLAMINE PATHWAYS. A comparison of ascending norepinephrine and dopamine pathways in the rat brain. (From Ungerstedt, 1971a.)

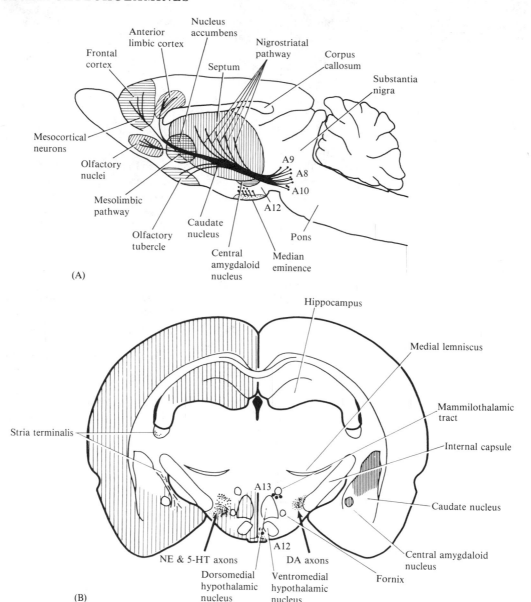

(A)

(B)

FIGURE 7   DOPAMINE PATHWAYS. (A) From the zona compacta of the substantia nigra (A9), nigrostriatal fibers project to the caudate nucleus. From the ventral tegmentum (A10), mesolimbocortical dopamine axons project to forebrain structures such as the nucleus accumbens, the olfactory tubercles, and cortical areas. (After Ungerstedt, 1974b; and Lindvall and Björklund, 1974.) (B) Frontal mid-hypothalamic section of rat brain. Nuclear groups A12 (ventral) and A13 (dorsal) are shown as large black dots. Arising from midbrain nuclear groups A8, 9 and 10, mesolimbocortical and nigrostriatal dopamine axons are seen as a bundle (small dots) lateral to the hypothalamus (right). Occupying a similar but more medial position are the ascending axons from the noradrenergic and serotonergic nuclei of the brain stem (left). Lightly shaded areas receive noradrenergic innervation; darkly shaded areas receive dopaminergic innervation. (After Ungerstedt, 1974b.)

midline of the tegmentum just above the interpeduncular nucleus and within the decussation of the superior cerebellar peduncle. Axons of these cells also course rostrally and join the medial forebrain bundle forming the mesolimbic projection pathway. These fibers terminate in forebrain areas (not all of which are shown) such as the nucleus accumbens, olfactory tubercle, the interstitial nucleus of the stria terminalis, the septum, and the nucleus of the diagonal band of Broca—all areas presumed to mediate primitive reactions to olfactory stimuli. More recently fibers have been found by more sensitive histofluorescence methods to extend in this pathway (along with some fibers in A9) to the frontal cortex (Lindvall and Björklund, 1974). These fibers are designated as mesocortical neurons. The mesolimbic and the mesocortical systems have been implicated as the source of the symptoms of schizophrenia, that is, they become too active or their target cells seem to be too sensitive to the transmitter dopamine (Bunney and Aghajanian, 1978). The mesolimbic system with its mesocortical extensions, now referred to as the mesolimbocortical DA pathway, is shown in Figure 7A.

Additional dopamine pathways emanate from cells in A11 (not shown), which is a nuclear group dorsolateral and more rostal to A10 and is found in the posterior hypothalamus. A13 shown in Figure 7B seems to be a rostral extension of A11 and seems to give rise to an incertohypothalamic system that projects to the dorsomedial nucleus of the thalamus as well as to the dorsal and anterior hypothalamic areas (Björklund et al., 1975). Making up another part of the incertohypothalamic tract are fibers from A14 (not shown), a covered cluster of cells found along the midline as part of the rostral portion of the paraventricular nucleus of the hypothalamus. A14 fibers project into the diencephalon to such structures as the paraventricular nucleus, preoptic areas, suprachiasmatic nucleus, anterior hypothalamic area, and caudal portions of the lateral septal nuclei. Finally, an A12 group found in the arcuate nucleus of the hypothalamus forms the tuberoinfundibular tract that projects to the median eminence and the pituitary gland. These latter systems probably are all involved in the control of secretion of pituitary hormones and provide a strong and significant linkage between neural and hormonal systems (Lindvall and Björklund, 1974).

Distribution of Adrenergic Pathways

As mentioned earlier, the histofluorescence technique when first developed was unable to discriminate between the presence of epinephrine and norepinephrine in the CNS. Consequently, the distribution of epinephrine within the CNS could not be established. Somewhat more recently, Hökfelt et al. (1973), using immunohistochemical techniques, were able to establish the presence of phenylethanolamine-N-methyltransferase (PNMT) in the CNS (PNMT converts NE to EPI).

The immunohistochemical technique required antibodies; these were supplied by injecting rat PNMT into a cow. The cow developed antibodies to the foreign protein, and the antibodies against PNMT were isolated and bound to a compound that caused them to fluoresce under ultraviolet light. The fluorophorebound antibodies were added to rat tissue suspected of containing PNMT. The antibodies bound to PNMT-containing cells, and were then detected by fluorescence microscopy.

Cells containing the highest PNMT activity were localized in two areas in the reticular formation in the medulla of rat brain. Group C1 was found in the ventrolateral reticular formation in rostral medulla lateral to the olivary complex. Group C2 was also located in the rostral medulla along the medial part of the ventral surface of the fourth ventricle (Figure 8). Terminals of the PNMT-containing cells were found in the dorsal motor nucleus of the vagus nerve (the principal cranial parasympathetic innervator of the visceral organs) and in the nucleus of tractus solitarius. [Cells of the n. tractus solitarius receive gustatory and visceral sensory inputs and project taste impulses to the thalamus; to other cranial nerve nuclei involved with salivation, mastication, and swallowing (the glossopharyngeal, facial, and trigeminal nerves); and via internuncial reticulospinal pathways to the spinal cord. These latter fibers terminate upon the phrenic nucleus in the cervical spinal cord to innervate the diaphragm, and upon the cells of the spinal cord that innervate the intercostal muscles for respiration, coughing, and vomiting.] Other adrenergic terminals were found in the paraventricular nuclei of the dorsal thalamus (cell groups that are believed to be associated with visceral activities) (Carpenter, 1976) and among the cells of the lateral horn of the spinal cord, which give rise to the sympathetic nerves of the autonomic nervous system.

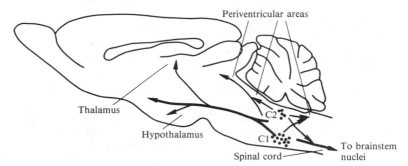

FIGURE 8 HYPOTHETICAL ADRENERGIC CON-
NECTIONS in the rat brain. The cell groups (C1 and C2) as
well as the ascending and descending axons that are positive
for PNMT are shown as giving rise to axon terminals in the
brain stem and spinal cord. The descending fibers ennervate
the nuclei of the vagus, glossopharyngeal, facial and trigeminal nerves and the spinal cord. (From Goldstein et al., 1978.)

Thus, it appears that there is a synaptic role for EPI in the CNS.

Adrenergic nerve terminals were also found in the locus caeruleus, which contain cells whose axons make up the dorsal noradrenergic bundle and fibers that ascend into the cerebellum. Other areas that may have PNMT-containing terminals are the prefornical area, the dorsomedial nucleus of the hypothalamus, the periventricular gray of the midbrain, the diencephalon, and the spinal cord. Postmortem human and monkey brains showed high PNMT activity in the reticular formation (which is equivalent to the C1 region of the rat brain) and in nucleus solitarius, the dorsal vagal nucleus, and the hypoglossal nucleus (which are equivalent to the C2 region of the rat brain). High enzyme activity was also found in the anterior and posterior hypothalamus, except for the mammillary bodies, where the activity was low. There were intermediate levels of enzyme activity in the locus caeruleus, some regions of the basal ganglia, the amygdala, the nucleus accumbens, and the habenula. In the postmorten human brain, intermediate activity was found in the dentate nucleus of the cerebellum and low activity was found in the olfactory tubercle and frontal cortex.

It is interesting to note that epinephrine-sensitive adenylate cyclase activity is present in the regions that surround PNMT activity, suggesting a synaptic role for central sources of EPI. It has also been shown that receptors that surround areas C1 and C2 are not typical α- and β-receptors (Goldstein et al., 1978) suggesting that there are unique receptors for central EPI.

Finally, it should be noted that epinephrine is synthesized in chromaffin cells of the adrenal medulla and is released into the bloodstream by stimulation of cholinergic preganglionic sympathetic nerves that innervate the adrenal gland (see Figure 2, and Figure 1 in Chapter 6). This circulating EPI stimulates the noradrenergic receptors on cardiac, and smooth muscles of the blood vessesls and visceral organs. These effects are particularly important during stress. EPI also has a hormone-like action that facilitates glucose mobilization and other functions. Circulating EPI from the adrenal glands does not pass the blood brain barrier and thus has no direct effect upon the CNS. In mammals EPI is the principal secretion of the adrenal medulla. However, in frogs EPI is found in sympathetic nerve endings as well as in the adrenal gland. In some species, such as the dogfish, which lack an adrenal cortex, only norepinephrine is secreted. Glucocorticoids, which are synthesized in the adrenal cortex and are under the influence of the pituitary gland, are instrumental in the synthesis of PNMT at the level of RNA transcription from DNA. Thus in the absence of PNMT, only NE is synthesized (Kopin, 1980).

Catecholaminergic Receptors

Noradrenergic Receptors

Little is known about the precise structure of noradrenergic receptors. On the basis of studies of peripheral organs innervated by sympathetic nerves, two types of noradrenergic receptors have been identified. Ahlquist (1948, 1979) designated them as alpha (α) and beta (β) and differentiated the two types on the basis of their responses to various sympathomimetic drugs and noradrenergic blocking agents such as isoproterenol, phentolamine, and propranolol. Thus, for example, the α-receptors are stimulated most by epinephrine and norepinephrine and least by isoproterenol (NE = EPI > ISOPR); whereas the β-receptors are affected in just the opposite way (ISOPR > EPI = NE). In response to noradrenergic receptor blockers, the α-receptors are blocked by phentolamine, whereas the β-receptors are blocked by propranolol.

In general, α-receptors are excitatory, whereas β-receptors are inhibitory, but not exclusively so. For example, epinephrine and drugs that mimic its action (e.g., ephedrine) are used in the treatment of bronchial asthma. They stimulate both α- and β-receptors. Stimulating the α-receptors causes the constriction of the blood vessels in the bronchial lining, thus reducing congestion and edema (a condition of tissue swelling), whereas stimulation of the β-receptor leads to relaxation of the bronchial muscles, providing a wider airway. On the other hand, it is known that stimulating both α- and β-receptors causes relaxation of the gut, whereas stimulation of the β-receptor stimulates the heart.

There is also a special type of α-receptor on the presynaptic membrane of some noradrenergic synapses. The presynaptic receptors are known as autoreceptors and probably have a lower affinity for the neurotransmitter than have the postsynaptic receptors. However, when relatively high levels of NE are released into the synaptic cleft, the NE stimulates the α-noradrenergic autoreceptors, which shut off NE release. This reaction was demonstrated in an experiment in which phenoxybenzamine (a α-noradrenergic blocking agent) was shown to increase the release of NE when the sympathetic nerve to the vas deferens was stimulated. Phenoxybenzamine alone had no effect upon an unstimulated preparation. Thus, these receptors may act as part of a negative feedback system to control transmitter release (Axelrod, 1974a).

Studies have also identified α-autoreceptors on the noradrenergic cell bodies in the locus caeruleus of the brain stem (A6 in Figure 4). On the basis of their different function (when the receptors are stimulated, the spontaneous firing of the cells is inhibited) and different sensitivity to certain drugs, they have been designated as α_2-receptors in contrast to regular α-receptors in the nervous system which have been designated as α_1-receptors (Cedarbaum and Aghajanian, 1977).

β-Receptors are also divided into two subtypes—β_1 and β_2—and the distinction between the two, like that between the α_1- and α_2-receptor, is based on the relative potency of agonists and antagonists. For example, for the β_1-receptor, isoproterenol is the most potent agonist followed by the equally potent NE and EPI (ISOPR > EPI = NE), and practolol is a selective antagonist. Isoproterenol is also the most potent agonist for the β_2-receptor; but EPI is significantly more potent then NE (ISOPR > EPI $\gg$ NE), and butoxamine is a more potent antagonist than practolol.

In the natural state the major physiological difference between β_1- and β_2-receptors is their differential sensitivity to NE. β_1-receptors have about the same affinity for EPI and NE, whereas β_2-receptors have a much higher affinity for EPI than for NE. Thus, β_1-receptors can be stimulated by the NE that is released by sympathetic nerves as well as by circulating EPI from the adrenal glands. On the other hand, β_2-receptors respond to EPI as though it were their natural agonist (Minneman et al., 1981).

β-Receptors appear alone or in different proportions in peripheral tissues or on postsynaptic neurons in the CNS. β_1-Receptors are in greater proportion than β_2-receptors in heart muscle and fat tissue and in mammalian neural tissue, whereas β_2-receptors are proportionately more numerous in the uterus and the smooth muscle of the trachea and bronchi and in the neural tissue of birds and frogs. All four types of receptors (α_1, α_2, β_1, and β_2) are found in the mammalian brain in different proportions in various brain areas, with species differences also being evident.

β-Receptors are distributed rather homogeneously in the rat brain, not as one would expect to find them, i.e., in association with NE neuron terminals and catecholamine-containing brain regions. It was suggested that β-receptors are associated with glial elements or with the smooth muscles of cerebral blood vessels. However, further scrutiny revealed that β_2-receptor density varied among brain regions by only two- or threefold, whereas β_1-receptor density varied by as much as 100 to 1. Thus, β_1-receptors may be related to the distribution of NE neurons and be more directly involved with brain function, whereas β_2-receptors may be associated with glia or blood vessels. The fact that β_2-receptors have a relatively low affinity for NE, the major CA neurotransmitter in the brain, supports this proposal.

In the rat cerebellum, there are proportionately few β_1-receptors compared to the large number of β_2-receptors, but evidence indicates that β_1-receptors (located upon the Purkinje cells) are the ones that are innervated by the NE inputs from the locus caeruleus. In the rat caudate nucleus, the β-receptor density is about equal to that in the cerebral cortex; however, the caudate contains little or no EPI or NE, whereas the cortex contains a dense NE innervation. What role these receptors play in the caudate is still an open question (Minneman et al. 1981). Further study is needed to specify the distribution and role of β-receptors and its subtypes in the CNS. Finally, it is important to note that the response of brain neurons to NE is predominantly inhibitory, an effect that is blocked by β-antagonists, which suggests that β-receptors are the predominant receptor type in mammalian brains (Haber and Wrenn, 1976; Clark, 1976).

For the most part, epinephrine receptors are the usual noradrenergic receptors in peripheral organs such as the heart, trachea, blood vessels, and intestines. However, the action of EPI and NE depends, to a significant extent, upon the distribution of α- and β-receptors because NE and EPI have an equal effect upon α-receptors, but the NE-induced inhibitory action on β-receptors is somewhat less than that of EPI. EPI receptors in the brain stem, as already pointed out, seem to be a special type that will have to be investigated further. All of these receptors will be considered again in another section that deals with the drugs that affect them.

Dopaminergic Receptors

These receptors seem to have some noradrenergic characteristics because at least some of them are blocked by the α-noradrenergic blocking drug phentolamine. However, α- and β-noradrenergic blocking agents are regarded as relatively ineffective as antagonists of dopamine (Kebabian et al. 1972). Groves et al. (1975) showed that there are receptors on the dendrites of dopaminergic neurons in the substantia nigra that can be activated by drugs such as amphetamine to release dopamine, which then blocks the firing of the dopaminergic neurons. Thus, the dopamine receptors also function as autoreceptors. This model is supported by the evidence of Aghajanian and Bunney (1973), who showed that iontophoretic application of dopamine to dopaminergic neurons in the substantia nigra produced inhibition of neuronal discharges. The inhibition was blocked by the systemic administration of the dopamine receptor blocker haloperidol. Also, Björklund and Lindvall (1975) re-

ported that these neurons have on their numerous small swellings dendrites with high concentrations of DA.

One of the characteristics of antipsychotic drugs such as chlorpromazine and haloperidol is that they lead to an increase of release and turnover of dopamine. This effect was believed to be the result of dopamine receptor blockade, leading to a compensatory increase in dopaminergic activity by a neuronal feedback circuit—the details of which have never been specified. It appears that the dopamine autoreceptors on the axon terminals that function to inhibit the DA release are being blocked by the drugs, thus allowing for the increased release of the transmitter from the terminals (Bunney and Aghajanian, 1975a).

Another type of dopamine receptor, designated as D-1, stimulates the activity of a dopamine-sensitive adenylate cyclase to form cAMP when activated by dopamine whereas a second type (D-2) does not. This designation was proposed by Kebabian and Calne (1979) after reviewing studies of dopamine receptor areas of the brain that had been treated with dopamine agonists and antagonists and comparing their potencies and ability to elicit an adenylate cyclase response. For example, they reported results showing that apomorphine, usually designated as a dopamine receptor agonist, has a potency nearly equal to that of dopamine at autoreceptors on terminals of nigro-striatal neurons. These receptors are of the D-2 type and are not associated with adenylate cyclase activity. However, apomorphine antagonizes the dopamine-stimulated accumulation of cAMP in bovine parathyroid glands via D-1 receptors and has no agonistic activity on these cells.

Bromocriptine is a potent antagonist at D-1 receptors but a potent agonist at D-2 receptors at the same concentration (in the nmolar range). This drug is being used at present as an experimental treatment of Parkinson's disease which is presumably caused by abnormally low dopamine inputs from the substantia nigra to the D-2 receptors in the striatum. Furthermore, the dopaminergic tuberoinfundibular tract acts upon cells in the median eminence or the pituitary gland having D-2 receptors. These cells inhibit the release of the hormone prolactin which regulates milk production and release in mammals (Sedvall, 1975). Bromocriptine was found to be a most satisfactory drug for stopping lactation in normal postpartum women and for treating pathological lactation in men and women. This abnormal lactation can occur in patients being treated with antipsychotic drugs which are dopamine receptor blockers. The antipsychotic drugs in the phenothiazine class such as chlorpromazine do not discriminate between the receptor types, but the butyrophenones such as haloperidol are less potent on D-1 receptors than D-2 even though their clinical potency is similar to that of the phenothiazines. (See Part III for further characterization of these drugs.)

Cools and van Rossum (1976) after reviewing electrophysiological, pharmacological, and functional studies, have proposed a different dual receptor concept for DA-sensitive neurons. They located a DA-excitatory receptor (DA_e) that occurs in high density in the neostriatum. DA_e receptors are identified by a diffuse green DA fluorescence and are more sensitive to the antagonist haloperidol and the agonist apomorphine than to peribedil (ET 495) and the ergot alkaloid ergometrine. The second receptor is an inhibitory

HO—CH_2—CH—NH—C ... NH
            |
            CH_3
            N
            |
            CH_3

Ergometrine

receptor (DA_i) found in the nucleus accumbens. DA_i receptors are characterized by a high density of dotted DA fluorescence and are more sensitive to ergometrine and unaffected by apomorphine and haloperidol. The distributions of these receptors seem to be similar in the rat, cat, and monkey. The DA_e receptors in the caudate of the rhesus monkey seem to be involved in the elicitation of skilled manipulation movements and spasmodic neck movements, whereas the DA_i receptors are involved in the elicitation of orolingual–facial dyskinesias and dyskinetic activities of the extremities. However, despite its thoroughness this proposal has not been correlated with other dual receptor concepts.

Receptor Supersensitivity

A feature of DA receptors that is probably common to all types of receptors is the development of supersensitivity following the loss of presynaptic input. This effect was demonstrated by Ungerstedt (1971b), who made unilateral lesions with intracranial injections of 6-hydroxydopamine (6-OHDA) in the nigrostriatal system of rats. 6-OHDA is taken up and destroys catecholamine-containing neurons, thereby depleting the

OH
OH— ... —CH_2—CH_2—NH_2
OH

6-Hydroxydopamine (6-OHDA)

dopamine and norepinephrine in any part of the brain so treated (Iversen, 1974). Injected unilaterally in the nigrostriatal pathway of the rat and other species, the behavioral effect of this treatment was the induction of postural asymmetries, which consist of leaning and moving in a direction toward the treated side and indicate the dominance of the untreated side. The rotational movement was quantified by a device called a rotometer, which measured the effects of drugs on the lesion-induced rotation (Figure 9). Systemic injections of amphetamine, which induce CA release, caused the animals to significantly increase their rotational movement toward the treated side, because of the drug-induced release of more DA on the normal side. However, when the animals were systemically treated with apomorphine (a DA agonist), the animals rotated in the opposite direction (i.e., toward the normal side). The dose of apomorphine needed to reverse the rotation direction was markedly lower (by a factor of 10-to 100-fold) than the dose needed to induce hyperactivity in normal animals (Figure 10). The same effect was obtained with the DA precursor L-dopa indicating that sufficient dopa decarboxylase was available for its con-

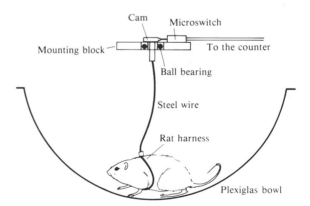

FIGURE 9 THE ROTOMETER. A wire connected to the recorder extends from a harness fitted around the rat's chest. This device records circling behavior in rats. The hemisphere-shaped bowl tends to encourage the circling behavior of treated rats. (After Ungerstedt, 1971c.)

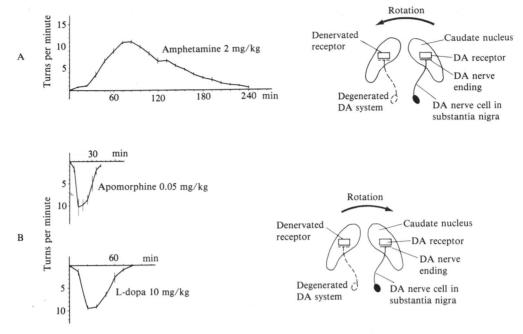

FIGURE 10   DRUG-INDUCED ROTATIONAL BEHAV-IOR. (A) Amphetamine (which releases dopamine) causes the animal to rotate toward the side with the lesion. (B) Apomor-phine or L-dopa, both of which stimulate more DA receptors on the denervated side, cause the animal to rotate toward the opposite (normal) side. (After Ungerstedt, 1974a.)

version to dopamine. This suggested that the treated side was more sensitive to the DA agonist than the nor-mal side. Supersensitivity was evident 24 hours after creation of the lesion, increased rapidly during the first week, and slowly reached its maximum during the next 3 to 4 weeks.

Rotational measures have also been used to estimate the time course of degeneration of 6-OHDA–treated pathways. Figure 11 shows the behavior of a rat that received a unilateral 6-OHDA lesion of the nigro-striatal bundle and 12 hours later received the first of a series of six rotational tests following six amphetamine injections, each 12 hours apart. During the first three tests, the rat rotated toward the normal side, appar-ently because the treated side was dominant. During the last three tests, the rat rotated toward the treated side. This suggested that shortly after treatment there was a greater amphetamine-induced DA spillage from the degenerating DA terminals on the treated side. But later, presumably after DA depletion from the degen-erating terminals, the greater drug-induced spillage oc-curred on the intact side.

Creece et al., (1977) used Ungerstedt's procedure and compared rotational scores with the binding prop-erties of the dopamine receptors in rats with unilateral 6-OHDA-induced nigrostriatal lesions. Two to seven months after 6-OHDA treatment, the animals were given subcutaneous doses of apomorphine and rota-tion was measured. One to ten weeks after apomor-phine treatment, the rats were sacrificed and the rats' striata were assayed for binding to [³H] haloperidol (a DA receptor blocker). For each rat the binding on the 6-OHDA-treated side was compared to binding on the normal side, and the difference was compared to the rat's rotation score. Twenty-seven rats that showed drug-induced rotation showed a mean of 50 percent in-crease in [³H]haloperidol binding on the treated as compared to the normal side. In some cases the bind-ing was doubled on the treated side. Meanwhile, ten rats that showed no appreciable increase in rotation scores showed a mean increase in binding of only 7.6 percent on the treated side. Further tests showed that the increased binding was not due to increase affinity for the radioactive ligand, but rather was due to a 40 percent increase in receptor sites on the treated striata.

From the foregoing it is clear that the direction of

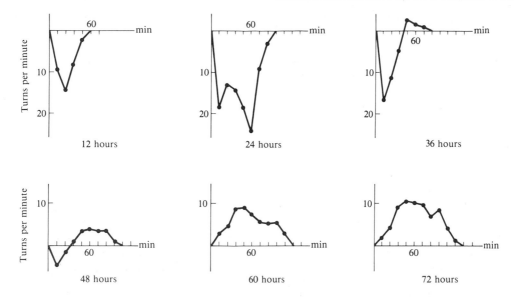

FIGURE 11 AMPHETAMINE-INDUCED ROTATION-AL BEHAVIOR. A dose of amphetamine (2 mg/kg) was given at various intervals after a 6-OHDA lesion of the nigrostriatal dopamine system. The record is from one animal that received amphetamine repeatedly at 12 hour intervals. Negative y values (12, 24, and 36 hr) indicate a dominance of the side with the lesion of the dopamine system, whereas positive y values (48, 60, and 72 hr) indicate dominance of the side with the intact dopamine system. (After Ungerstedt, 1971c.)

rotation is dependent upon which side of the striatum is being energized by nigrostriatal fibers. If these fibers are unilaterally lost, rotation is exerted toward the side of the lesion. But here an interesting question arises. It is known that the dopaminergic nigrostriatal input to the striatum is inhibitory, yet when this system is activated it appears to stimulate rotation rather than inhibit it. This apparent paradox can be resolved if it is assumed that the DA acts by inhibiting a "brake" and thereby releases rotational movement. If the DA input is unilaterally lost, the "brake" remains on and the affected side remains inactive. However, whereas this explanation is logical enough to explain the results of the rotation experiments on rats, it does not hold for the effects of nigrostriatal lesions in man, the condition in Parkinson's disease. In that case, a loss of DA input to the striatum from the substantia nigra results not in the persistence of a braking action, but rather in the release of cholinergic activity that accounts for the symptoms of the disease such as akinesia and muscle spasticity, symptoms that can be mitigated, at least temporarily, by anticholinergic drugs. These observations, the reports that bilateral lesions of the nigrostriatal bundles do not produce Parkinsonian symptoms in animals (Iversen and Iversen, 1981), and reports of opposite results (Ungerstedt, 1974a) point to the complexity of the striatal system.

Drug-Induced Receptor Supersensitivity

Creese and Snyder (1978) report that supersensitivity may also be the result of drug-induced transmitter blockade. This can occur in humans as well as in animals either by direct receptor blockade or by depletion of presynaptic transmitter stores. For example, long-term treatment of human schizophrenic patients with neuroleptic drugs (such as the phenothiazines) may result in TARDIVE DYSKINESIA (a disorder characterized by involuntary movement of facial muscles and the extremities). This symptom is frequently made worse by dose reduction or drug termination, whereas increasing the dose may temporarily relieve the symptom. Rats chronically treated with neuroleptic drugs also show increased sensitivity to apomorphine after the cessation of neuroleptic drug treatment. Increased sensitivity to apomorphine was also found after treatments with drugs that inhibited DA synthesis, and with drugs that depleted vesicular stores of DA in axon terminals. That these effects are due to drug-induced receptor supersensitivity is supported by the findings that treating rats for 3 weeks with effective DA receptor blocking neuroleptic drugs causes a significant increase in drug binding; and transmitter depletion from presynaptic terminals had the same effect. On the other hand, pretreatment with the clinically ineffective phenothiazine promethazine or the stimulant amphetamine failed to do so.

Two-State Model for the Dopaminergic Receptor

Another feature of DA receptors that may also be generally true for all neuroreceptors is their quantitative differences with respect to the potency of agonists and antagonists in competitive binding experiments (Creese and Snyder, 1978). That is to say, agonists are quite potent in displacing other agonists but weak for antagonists; and antagonists are more potent in displacing other antagonists than agonists. The displacement from a receptor of one ligand by another ligand depends on the concentration and the receptor's affinity for the displacing ligand. If the concentrations of the displacing ligands are held constant, the above observations obviously mean that receptors have different affinities for agonists and antagonists. It is also possible that there are two different receptors: one that binds agonists and another that binds antagonists; but the evidence does not support that possibility. Rather, the receptors seems to exist in either of two interconvertible states. Studies on the opiate receptor have shown that sodium and manganese ions control the proportion of receptors that will be in one state or another, with sodium favoring the antagonist state and manganese the agonist state. However, it has been suggested that the coupling of the dopamine receptor with its appropriate adenylate cyclase is what underlies its differential affinities. There is also some evidence that supports a two-state model for the muscarinic cholinergic, glycinergic, serotonergic, and α-adrenergic receptors.

Part II Catecholamine Synthesis and Catabolism

The catecholamines serve as important neurotransmitters and hormones in the central and peripheral nervous systems. Norepinephrine is synthesized in peripheral sympathetic nerves and within the brain. Dopamine is found only to a small extent in the peripheral nervous system, but it is synthesized in the central nervous system, where it plays an important biobehavioral role. Epinephrine is largely synthesized in the adrenal gland, but the existence of EPI-synthesizing enzymes within the CNS also suggests a significant role for this transmitter in central neural activity. Epinephrine also plays a significant role in fat metabolism and thyroid activity and acts as a trigger for the mobilization of glucose. Thus, it will be valuable to examine in considerable detail the mechanisms of CA synthesis and catabolism, and to study a number of the compounds that affect these and related processes.

Catecholamine Synthesis

The synthesis of catecholamine neurotransmitters appears to be very involved compared to acetylcholine synthesis. At least six enzymes and a number of cofactors*

*A cofactor is a chemical component or a metal that is tightly bound to an enzyme and is necesssary for the activity of the enzyme.

are involved. The final elucidation of the synthetic process as well as the catabolism of these transmitters has been one of the bright spots in the history of biochemistry. These discoveries are important not only for their own sake but because they provide rational answers to questions about nerve function, mental illness, and drug effects.

In 1939 the steps of NE synthesis were first proposed by Blaschko (1939), even though all of the enzymes and cofactors were unknown. Remarkably, his proposals turned out to be correct despite the fact that one of the most important enzymes, tyrosine hydroxylase, was not discovered until 25 years later by Nagatsu and his co-workers (1964).

Phenylalanine Hydroxylation

The steps of CA synthesis are now well understood (Figure 12). The immediate precurser for CA synthesis is tyrosine, a dietary amino acid that is found in the bloodstream and is readily taken up by brain tissue and sympathetic nerves by an active uptake process. Tyrosine can also be derived from dietary phenylalanine, an amino acid that can be converted to tyrosine by the enzyme phenylalanine hydroxylase and its cofactor tetrahydropteridine, both of which are found primarily in

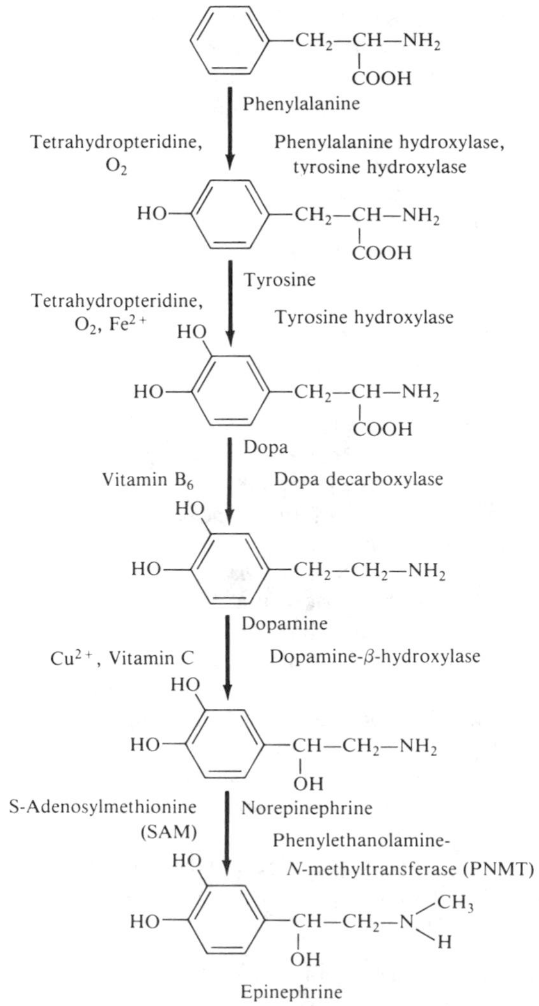

Phenylalanine

Tetrahydropteridine, O_2 — Phenylalanine hydroxylase, tyrosine hydroxylase

Tyrosine

Tetrahydropteridine, O_2, Fe^{2+} — Tyrosine hydroxylase

Dopa

Vitamin B_6 — Dopa decarboxylase

Dopamine

Cu^{2+}, Vitamin C — Dopamine-β-hydroxylase

Norepinephrine

S-Adenosylmethionine (SAM) — Phenylethanolamine-N-methyltransferase (PNMT)

Epinephrine

FIGURE 12 SYNTHESIS OF THE CATECHOLAMINE TRANSMITTERS. The synthesizing enzymes are shown to the right of the arrows; the cofactors and the methyl donor (SAM) are shown on the left.

the liver. This enzymatic process also requires the presence of oxygen. The brain does not have a supply of phenylalanine hydroxylase. Therefore, it depends upon the liver and the diet for its tyrosine supply. Although tyrosine hydroxylase will also hydroxylate phenylalanine, its activity is too low to satisfy the needs of the brain for tyrosine.

The hydroxylation of phenylalanine is an oxidation process that results in the substitution of an hydroxyl group (OH) for a hydrogen atom on the benzene ring at the para, or fourth position, opposite the side chain. Consequently, the chemical name for tyrosine is 4-hydroxyphenylalanine.

Phenylketonuria

We will digress briefly to discuss phenylketonuria (PKU) or PHENYLPYRUVIC OLIGOPHRENIA. This disability results when a recessive genetic defect leads to an almost total deficiency of phenylalanine hydroxylase and phenylalanine metabolism, that is, the loss of tyrosine synthesis. When both parents carry the recessive gene, an infant is expected to inherit the deficiency. The frequency of occurrence is about 1 in 20,000 infants born (Hsia, 1976). The syndrome is physically characterized by high levels of phenylalanine in the blood and brain and the presence of a phenylalanine metabolite in the urine (phenylpyruvic acid, a ketone compound; Figure 13): hence the name for the disorder—phenylketonuria.

It is believed that the phenylalanine competes for tyrosine hydroxylase and interferes with the metabolism of tyrosine in protein synthesis. Phenylalanine also interferes with the uptake of tyrosine and other amino acids into the brain because the same carrier is responsible for membrane transport of all of them. Phenylketonuria can be discovered early by using a simple chemical test on an infant's urine and testing for the presence of phenylpyruvic acid. If the defect is discovered early and a diet low in phenylalanine and high in tyrosine is quickly instituted, the consequences of the defect can be averted. Without appropriate treatment, there can be microcephaly, retarded development of myelinization of nerve fibers, and other changes in brain tissue leading to epileptic attacks,

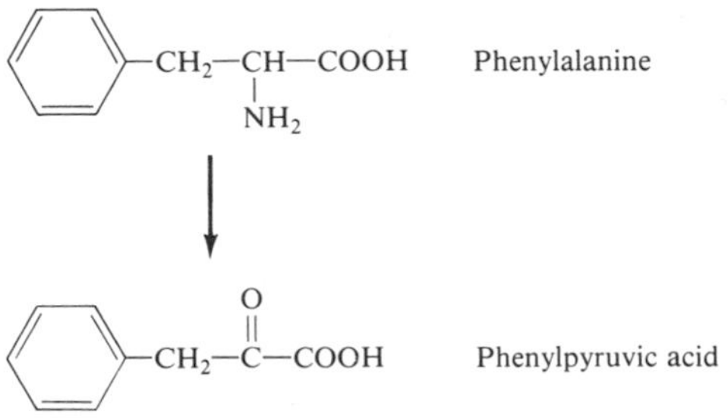

Phenylalanine

Phenylpyruvic acid

FIGURE 13 METABOLISM OF PHENYLALANINE TO FORM PHENYLPYRUVIC ACID. This reaction includes deamination and oxidation of phenylalanine.

psychotic episodes, hypertonicity and hyperactivity, destructiveness, self-mutilation, impulsiveness, rage, and hallucinations—all of which usually leads to permanent institutionalization (Berman and Hsia, 1970; Hsia, 1976).

Tyrosine Hydroxylation

The next stage in NE synthesis is the conversion by hydroxylation of tyrosine to DOPA (3,4-dihydroxyphenylalanine) (Figure 12). This conversion involves the addition of a second hydroxyl group to the benzene ring of tyrosine and requires the enzymatic action of tyrosine hydroxylase (TH) along with tetrahydropteridine, O_2, and Fe^{2+} as cofactors. Comparatively speaking, only a small amount of tyrosine is converted to catecholamines. Most of it enters into the synthesis of other important proteins, such as thyroid hormone, via iodotyrosine.

Tyrosine hydroxylase exists in either an oxidized (TH) or a reduced form (TH-H_2). It is only active in the reduced form; and during the conversion of tyrosine to DOPA, the enzyme is oxidized—thus becoming inactive. Tetrahydropteridine (pteridine-H_4) contributes hydrogen atoms to tyrosine hydroxylase, reducing TH to its active form and becoming dihydropteridine in the process. Another enzyme, pteridine reductase, donates hydrogens to dihydropteridine, thereby converting it back to tetrahydropteridine (Guroff, 1975). There have been reports of a few cases of PKU that were unresponsive to dietary control of phenylalanine and that manifested epileptic seizures and mental retardation despite normal liver phenylalanine hydroxylase activity. In these patients, enzyme assays revealed that dihydropteridine reductase activity was less than 1 percent of normal in liver, brain, and other tissue. Thus, the absence of this enzyme prevented the regeneration of tetrahydropteridine, thereby preventing the hydroxylation of tyrosine and the biosynthesis of catecholamines (Hsia, 1976).

One very important feature of the tyrosine hydroxylase reaction is that it serves as the rate-limiting step for all catecholamine synthesis. Experiments have shown that tissue stimulation, which causes the release of NE, causes an increase in TH activity and faster synthesis of DOPA. On the other hand, high levels of NE inhibit the activity of the tyrosine hydroxylase and limit synthesis. This latter process is called end-product inhibition and serves to maintain control of the synthetic process. The actual mechanism of the in-

hibitory process involves the action of dopamine upon pteridine-H_4, oxidizing it to pteridine-H_2 (McGeer et al., 1978). Without the reduced cofactor, TH remains inactive, thus blocking dopamine and NE synthesis.

Other enzymes are necessary for further stages of catecholamine synthesis, but they are far more active—100 to 1000 times—than TH. Consequently, if one were to attempt to limit catecholamine synthesis, it would be easier to do so by limiting TH activity. Experiments have borne this out.

DOPA Decarboxylation

The next step in catecholamine synthesis is the conversion of DOPA to dopamine (3,4-dihydroxyphenethylamine) (Figure 12). This step requires the activity of the enzyme DOPA decarboxylase and the cofactor pyridoxal phosphate (vitamin B_6). Decarboxylation involves the removal of the carboxyl group (COOH) from the side chain.

Actually DOPA decarboxylase is nonspecific and is also called AROMATIC AMINO ACID DECARBOXYLASE (AAAD). It will decarboxylate many aromatic amino acids (i.e., those containing a benzene ring). For example, tyrosine can be decarboxylated to form tyramine, a substance that can be taken up by CA terminals and released, thereby mimicking norepinephrine. Released in excessive amounts, it can cause cardiovascular excitation (Figure 14). AAAD is found in the cytoplasm of many tissues, including liver, stomach, brain, and kidney. Its wide distribution indicates that its metabolic significance is not limited to catecholamine synthesis.

Dopamine Hydroxylation

In addition to its role as a neurotransmitter, dopamine also serves as the precursor of NE and EPI. It is converted to NE by the enzyme dopamine-β-hydroxylase (DBH) and the cofactors oxygen and ascorbic acid (vitamin C). In this step, the β-carbon (the second to the left of the amine group) is hydroxylated, that is, a hydroxyl group is substituted for the hydrogen atom. A covalent bond is formed between an oxygen atom and the β-carbon, thus the carbon atom is oxidized. Thus, the enzyme is sometimes referred to as dopamine-β-oxidase. This enzyme is absent in neurons for which dopamine is the neurotransmitter. Thus, in these neurons the neurotransmitter is not metabolized further. The chemical name for NE is 3,4-dihydroxyphenylethanolamine. DBH is a copper (Cu^{2+})-contain-

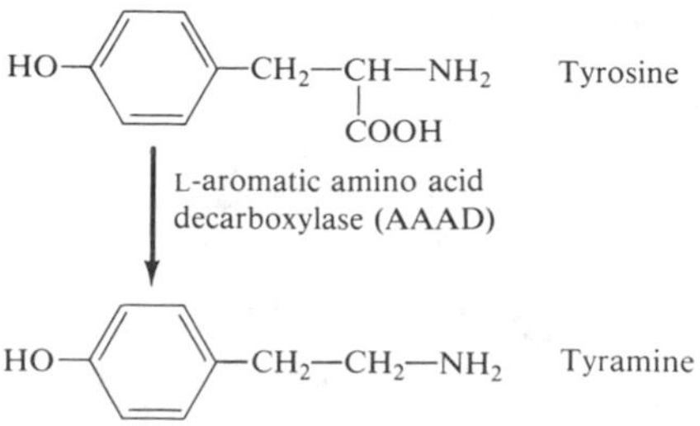

FIGURE 14. DECARBOXYLATION OF TYROSINE TO FORM TYRAMINE.

ing protein. Thus, chelating agents can bind with the copper and inhibit the enzyme action to a certain extent, thereby limiting NE synthesis.

On the basis of studies on peripheral noradrenergic nerves, DBH is believed to be located within the membrane of storage vesicles that are formed in the perikaryon in the vicinity of the cell nucleus and its associated organelles, the ergastoplasm and the Golgi apparatus. After uptake of DA, the vesicles migrate by axoplasmic flow to the axon terminals, where NE synthesis is completed and the vesicles are stored to provide available transmitter substance. When the vesicles discharge their contents into the synaptic cleft, DBH is also released along with ATP and other protein substances. There is evidence that there is little transmitter synthesis in the axon terminals, even though newly synthesized NE seems to be preferentially released, just as newly synthesized ACh is released. Also, as in ACh release, NE release depends upon the influx of Ca^{2+}, which with calmodulin is responsible for exocytosis.

Epinephrine Synthesis

In the adrenal medulla and to a slight degree in neural tissue of the heart, NE is further metabolized by the enzyme phenylethanolamine-N-methyltransferase (PNMT) to form epinephrine, a transmitter that must enter the bloodstream to reach noradrenergic receptor cells in the cardiovascular, respiratory, gastrointestinal, and other systems. EPI emanating from the adrenal gland and the heart does not pass the blood brain barrier, and its action is largely confined to peripheral organs. PNMT transfers a methyl group (CH_3) to the amine nitrogen of NE (Figure 12). The donor of the methyl group is S-adenosylmethionine (SAM), and the chemical name for epinephrine is 3,4-dihydroxyphenyl-N-methylethanolamine. As men-

tioned earlier, there may be some EPI synthesis in the reticular formation of the medulla.

Control of Catecholamine Synthesis

Regulation of Norepinephrine Synthesis

The catecholamines are continuously being released, metabolized, and synthesized, yet the tissue levels of these substances are remarkably constant. This fact by itself suggests that there must be synthesizing controls at work. Studies have shown that the maximum release of NE from sympathetic nerve terminals on the spleen occurs when the nerve is stimulated with 30 impulses per second. It was estimated that 0.01 percent of the amount of NE present was released during each impulse, or about 18 percent per minute of stimulation. If synthesis were inhibited completely, the store of NE would be depleted by 50 percent in a few minutes (Axelrod, 1974a).

During NE synthesis dopamine is formed in the cytoplasm and then taken up by vesicles to be converted to NE. An enzyme, monoamine oxidase (MAO), that is bound to mitochrondrial membranes can degrade cytoplasmic dopamine to inert metabolites that can diffuse from the axon terminals and thereby lower the availability of DA for NE synthesis. It appears that this action plays a role in the control of NE synthesis. There are drugs that can inhibit the action of MAO, thus increasing cytoplasmic levels of DA, but it is not known whether there are endogenous feedback controls on intracellular MAO-related metabolism.

It has already been mentioned that end-product inhibition plays a principal role in controlling catecholamine synthesis, just as it did in the case of ACh. For NE synthesis, high concentrations of NE cause competition for the pteridine cofactor, without which TH cannot function. A study by Dairman and Udenfriend (1971) illustrates this principle. When they gave large doses of L-dopa to rats, a significant increase in NE synthesis occurred in the heart and adrenal gland. This is to be expected, as L-dopa would be transformed to NE by the plentiful stores of dopa decarboxylase and DBH. When treatment continued for 4–7 days, they also found a decline in TH activity in the adrenal gland. A probable explanation for this finding is that the increase in NE synthesis led to end-product inhibition of TH activity.

Adrenocorticotropic hormone (ACTH) is instrumental in regulating synthesis of EPI in the adrenal gland. Removal of the pituitary gland caused a marked reduction of PNMT, which was restored to normal levels by administering ACTH, which is the hormone that is released from the pituitary gland in response to stress (Wurtman and Axelrod, 1966). The mechanism of action of ACTH also involves changes in the concentrations of the synthesizing enzymes TH, DBH, and PNMT. Axelrod (1971) found that after hypophysectomy in rats, there was an 80 percent drop in adrenal levels of PNMT; there was also a 50 percent drop in TH levels and a 30 percent drop in DBH levels. The administration of ACTH to these animals caused a return of TH and PNMT to normal levels and a partial rise of DBH. Administering ACTH to normal rats caused no increase in the levels of these enzymes.

The control of EPI synthesis by ACTH is obviously very useful as ACTH is liberated in times of stress and probably contributes to a speedup of EPI synthesis. The substance is thus more available for action in the respiratory and circulatory system at a time of great exertion (e.g., during pursuit, fighting, or escape behaviors).

It has also been shown that after prolonged stimulation of a sympathetic nerve, the amount of transmitter released plus the amount that remained was greater than the amount that was initially present. Thus, nerve impulses themselves increase biosynthesis of catecholamines. In other experiments, the stimulation of an isolated sympathetic nerve caused an increase of NE synthesis, but adding NE to the preparation blocked the increased synthesis. This indicated that there was a rapid feedback inhibition of synthesis by NE, and the effect was traced to an interference in TH activity. It would now seem obvious that increased activity of sympathetic neurons leads to the depletion of a strategic pool of NE that is responsible for end-product inhibition of NE synthesis, thus permitting increased TH activity and increased NE synthesis.

Roth and his associates (1975) proposed another mechanism by which high rates of stimulation of noradrenergic (NA) nerves can result in an increase of NE synthesis. They showed that TH activity in both peripheral and central NA neurons can be activated by Ca^{2+} or by cAMP. Activation by these substances seems to be due in part to an increased affinity of TH for the substrate tyrosine as well as for the pteridine cofactors and a decreased affinity for the natural end-product inhibitor norepinephrine. More precisely, as illustrated in the model shown in Figure 15, high levels

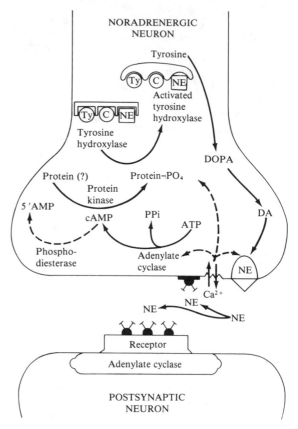

FIGURE 15 IMPULSE FLOW IN NA NEURONS CONTROLS NE SYNTHESIS. Increased impulse flow in NA neurons causes synaptic NE to activate presynaptic receptors that increase Ca^{2+} influx into the nerve terminals. The increased Ca^{2+} activates a presynaptic adenylate cyclase to form cAMP in the nerve terminal. The cAMP acts via a protein kinase to phosphorylate some unknown protein that activates TH; or possibly the TH itself is directly phosphorylated to a more active form. In the more active form, TH has a higher affinity for tyrosine (Ty) and the pteridine cofactor (C), and less affinity for the end-product inhibitor NE. Thus, increased activity in the neuron increases the production of its neurotransmitter. (After Roth et al., 1978.)

of neural activity and depolarization in the presynaptic membranes first cause an increase of Ca^{2+} influx. The increased volume of calcium ion is responsible for activating a *presynaptic receptor* adenylate cyclase, resulting in an increase in *presynaptic cAMP*. The cAMP, via a protein kinase, phosphorylates an acceptor protein that activates TH. Or cAMP may phosphorylate

TH itself, converting TH to a more active form and giving it a higher affinity for its substrate and cofactors and a lower affinity for its end product. This mechanism is a positive feedback process that increases NE production to keep up with the increased activity of the neuron. This is the opposite of the negative feedback process that inhibits the release of NE.

A similar mechanism has been proposed for the inhibition of DA synthesis and release. In this case, activation of presynaptic receptors by dopamine or dopamine agonists result in a damping effect on presynaptic DA activity. Conversely, the antipsychotic drugs such as chlorpromazine and haloperidol, that block postsynaptic DA receptors may also block the presynaptic inhibitory receptors, resulting in an increased synthesis and release of synaptic dopamine. This model may explain the marked increase in DA turnover when these drugs are used for the relief of schizophrenic symptoms (Roth et al., 1978).

Another of Axelrod's (1971) experiments was done using 6-hydroxydopamine (6-OHDA), a drug that destroys noradrenergic sympathetic terminals. As expected, synthesizing enzymes disappeared from the terminals within 2 days after application of 6-OHDA. However, when the adrenal gland was examined, there was an increase in TH activity. Furthermore, study showed that 6-OHDA caused a drop in blood pressure, and the increase in TH activity in the adrenal gland might have been due to the reflex increase in adrenal activity to restore blood pressure to normal levels. This hypothesis was verified when blood pressure was reduced by reserpine and phenoxybenzamine (an α-adrenergic blocking agent). Again, there was an elevation of TH activity in the adrenal gland and in the sympathetic nerves innervating the heart. It was also found that the actual effect was due to an increase in synthesis of TH. When a protein synthesis inhibitor such as cycloheximide was also administered, the reserpine-induced drop in blood pressure failed to yield increased TH activity.

Was the increased synthesis of TH in the adrenal gland caused by blood-borne factors like the induction of PNMT activity by ACTH or by increased activity of the nerves that innervate the adrenal gland? To answer this question the splanchnic nerve (sympathetic preganglionic) that innervates the adrenal gland was cut unilaterally and reserpine was administered to cause a lowered blood pressure. As expected, there was an increase in the TH activity in the adrenal gland on the

normal side but not on the denervated side. Thus, the increase in TH activity on the intact side was due to transynaptic induction.

Further studies showed that reserpine caused an induction of DBH synthesis in sympathetic nerves. This effect was also blocked when the presynaptic inputs to these nerves were blocked by denervation. Similar effects were found with PNMT: reserpine increased its synthesis and activity levels in the adrenal gland, and denervation of the gland blocked the increase.

Over the long term, animals subjected to stress develop different rates of catecholamine synthesis, depending on the nature of the stress. A group of mice were divided so that some of them were reared in complete isolation from one another while the other group was subjected to increased social stimulation. After 6 months, the adrenals of the socially deprived mice had a marked decrease in TH and PNMT content, whereas there was an increase in the amounts of these enzymes in the stimulated mice. On the other hand, rats that were subjected to prolonged forced immobilization showed higher content of TH and PNMT in the adrenals. This effect was abolished by interrupting the nerve innervating the adrenal gland. All these studies show that the stress-induced increases in enzyme activity can be neuronally mediated. They also show that the regulation of catecholamine synthesis is finely adjusted to the needs of the organism and that the control can be mediated by blood-borne factors such as ACTH or by transynaptic induction.

One other mechanism controlling catecholamine synthesis should be mentioned. Wurtman and his associates (1974) reported that catecholamine synthesis can be controlled to some degree by the level of brain tyrosine. These experimenters injected rats with R04-4602, a DOPA decarboxylase inhibitor. Fifteen minutes later, the rats were injected with various amino acids. Forty-five minutes after the second injection, the animals were sacrificed and the brains were removed and assayed for tyrosine and DOPA concentrations. Rats that had been given a low dose of tyrosine showed an increase of brain tyrosine that was 81 percent above normal and an increase of brain DOPA that was 13 percent above normal. Injection of a similar dose of tryptophan (the amino acid precursor of serotonin), which competes with tyrosine for uptake into the central nervous system, caused an 18 percent drop in brain tyrosine and a 32 percent drop in DOPA. Thus, the level of TH is not the sole determiner of CA synthesis;

the brain levels of the amino acid precursors are also important. In other tests, Wurtman found that a low dose of phenylalanine (50 mg/kg) elevated brain levels of tyrosine and accelerated DOPA synthesis, whereas a high dose of phenylalanine failed to modify brain levels of tyrosine, yet it slowed the accumulation of DOPA. This suggested that high doses of phenylalanine competed with tyrosine for TH activity. Here again we see a complex interaction between the levels of catecholamine precursors and the activity of enzymes involved in the synthesis of DOPA, dopamine, and NE. Apparently dietary levels of the amino acid precursors also have significant effects on transmitter levels in the brain.

Regulation of Dopamine Synthesis

Specifying the mechanisms that control DA synthesis is made especially difficult because there are two DA metabolic pathways. In one, DA serves as the precursor to NE; in the other, DA serves as a transmitter. Possibly the DA synthesis rate in one is different from that in the other (Costa and Trabucchi, 1975). This problem can be bypassed to some extent by examining brain nuclei having cells exclusively noradrenergic or dopaminergic. Studies have shown that an increase in nerve impulse flow in the nigrostriatal or mesolimbic dopaminergic systems causes an increase in the synthesis rate of dopamine (Cooper et al., 1978; Roth et al., 1978). However, if impulse flow is interrupted in these systems, the nerve terminals also show an increase in synthesis rate. This raises the question about the effectiveness of end-product inhibition in dopamine systems, as synthesis rate is increased either by increased or by decreased impulse flow. Normally with decreased flow, end-product inhibition of TH activity should occur. A possible resolution of this paradox lies in the assertion that in the case of increased synthesis with decreased impulse flow, the newly synthesized DA is in a bound form and is unable to influence the synthesis mechanism. Supporting evidence for this idea comes from the finding that if "free" soluble endogenous dopamine levels are raised by monoamine oxidase inhibitors, dopamine synthesis inhibition does occur.

Another model dealing with this problem postulates two types of dopaminergic receptors (Costa and Trabucchi, 1975). One type of receptor appears on the presynaptic terminal and the other on postsynaptic membranes, with the latter having a higher affinity for DA than the former. The postsynaptic receptor serves the usual role—it initiates cAMP formation and postsynaptic potentials. The other receptor is an autoreceptor for negative feedback of DA synthesis and release. However, it becomes active only when there is a relatively high concentration of DA in the synaptic cleft (Figure 16). In the case of low impulse traffic in the presynaptic neuron, the level of DA in the synaptic cleft would be too low to activate the presynaptic autoreceptor, with the consequence that dopamine synthesis would not be inhibited. Thus, increased DA synthesis would be compatible with interrupted impulse flow.

Roth et al. (1978) investigated this problem by blocking impulse flow in DA systems in rats by surgical and chemical means, that is, by making lesions in the neostriatum or by injecting γ-butyrolactone (GBL), a precursor of γ-hydroxybutyrate, which blocks impulse flow in DA neurons. These treatments caused a marked increase in the affinity of TH for tyrosine and the pteridine cofactor and a dramatic decrease in its affinity for the end-product inhibitor DA. Furthermore,

γ-Butyrolactone (GBL)   γ-Hydroxybutyrate

these changes in TH activity were reproduced by removing the calcium ion from DA tissue preparations with the calcium chelating agent EGTA. This led to the conclusion that reduced impulse flow and reduced depolarization of DA nerve terminals would reduce Ca^{2+} influx and thus alter the kinetic properties of TH.

The blockade of DA receptors by neuroleptic drugs such as haloperidol causes (by way of a neuronal feedback system) an increase in firing rates of DA neurons in the substantia nigra and an increase in DA synthesis. The increased DA synthesis has been traced to an increased affinity in TH for the pteridine cofactor. Moreover, animals receiving long-term treatment with haloperidol showed a greater stimulus-induced increase in TH activity than that found in nondrugged animals. Roth et al. (1978) suggested that this increase in TH activity might be due to the blockade of the presynaptic autoreceptors by haloperidol, thus removing the inhibiting effect of this negative feedback system.

Lerner et al. (1977) examined the short- and long-term aspects of these effects. TH activity was exam-

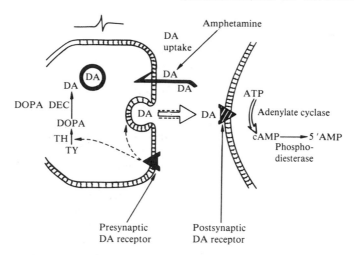

FIGURE 16   BRAIN DOPAMINERGIC SYNAPSE. The postsynaptic receptor has a higher affinity for DA than the presynaptic receptor. The postsynaptic receptor initiates the formation of cAMP and membrane postsynaptic potentials. The presynaptic receptors (autoreceptors) are only activated when synaptic levels of DA are high, and they serve to block DA synthesis and release. Amphetamine facilitates release and blocks reuptake of DA, initially producing a higher turnover rate of DA. But after an hour, synaptic DA activates the autoreceptors resulting in decreased DA turnover. (After Costa and Trabucci, 1975.)

ined after single or multiple daily doses of haloperidol. A definite increase in TH activity was detected 1 hour after a single haloperidol dose, but TH activity returned to normal 23 hours later. After four daily injections, the enzyme response to haloperidol was the same as after one dose. However, after 8 to 14 daily injections, the enzyme after 1 hour showed a higher V_{max} (see Figure 18 in Chapter 3), indicating that enzyme induction had occurred (i.e., there were now more enzyme molecules). However, after 23 hours, the TH activity was actually below control levels. Thus, it seems that long-term haloperidol treatment leads to enzyme induction that causes an increase in enzyme activity immediately after a haloperidol injection. Later the enzyme seems to become deactivated, serving to compensate for the former heightened activity of the system. The nature of the deactivated enzyme is not known at present. It is of interest to note that with short-term haloperidol treatment, extrapyramidal symptoms occur (Chapter 10), but that with continued treatment, the symptoms subside and the antipsychotic effects emerge. The changes in DA synthesis in the striatum may be related to these effects.

Support for this hypothesis was found earlier in a study by Goodwin and Post (1974), who examined the cerebrospinal fluid (CSF) levels of homovanillic acid (HVA; a dopamine metabolite) in psychiatric patients receiving phenothiazine neuroleptic drugs. The patients were treated with probenecid to block the transport of HVA out of the CSF. They found that at first

$$CH_3-CH_2-CH_2 \diagdown$$
$$N-SO_2-\!\!\!\!\!\!\bigcirc\!\!\!\!\!\!-COOH$$
$$CH_3-CH_2-CH_2 \diagup$$

Probenecid

the patients showed significantly elevated CSF levels of HVA compared to predrug levels. However, after extended treatment (25–77 days), the HVA levels returned to normal. These investigators suggested that although early stages of treatment did produce some remission of symptoms in acutely ill patients, maximum clinical effectiveness of the drugs was reached only after extended drug administration when adaptation occurred to the drug-induced increase in dopamine turnover. How extensively the various mechanisms that control DA synthesis act or interact and the importance to be ascribed to each of them are topics that require additional research.

Catabolism of Catecholamines

Except for acetylcholine, the principal process involved in the termination of transmitter function is the reuptake process (Chapter 4). This is especially true for NE and DA. Nevertheless, small but significant amounts of these transmitters simply diffuse out of the synaptic cleft, enter the blood stream, and ultimately pass out of the body in the urine. In addition, portions of NE and DA undergo metabolic breakdown. We will consider those metabolic processes in peripheral sympathetic neurons.

Norepinephrine Catabolism in Sympathetic Neurons

The catabolism of catecholamines primarily involves the enzymes monoamine oxidase (MAO) and catechol-O-methyltransferase (COMT). In addition, some intermediate steps require the enzymes aldehyde dehydrogenase and aldehyde reductase (Figure 17). MAO refers to one of a group of deaminating enzymes (i.e., those that remove the side chain amine group while oxidizing the residue to form an aldehyde). MAO is found on the outer mitochondrial membranes within the nerve terminals as well as on the mitochondria found in almost every cellular type in the body, including glia. The exceptions are skeletal muscle and red blood cells. However, MAO is found in the blood platelets (structures that are involved in blood clotting). Because NE is constantly leaking from storage vesicles within the nerve terminal, it becomes deaminated by the cytoplasmic MAO, which may in this way control the amine level within the cell. Moreover, because of its ubiquitousness, the deaminating action of MAO on catecholamines and their derivatives can occur outside of the cell as well.

When NE leaks from vesicles within nerve terminals, it is converted by MAO to the aldehyde 3,4-dihydroxyphenylglycoaldehyde (DOPGA)* (Figure 17, left pathway). DOPGA is almost immediately oxidized further by the enzyme aldehyde dehydrogenase to form 3,4-dihydroxymandelic acid (DOMA). This intermediate is also short-lived because DOMA, which is inert, leaks from the terminal and is O-methylated by catechol-O-methyltransferase (COMT). The process of O-methylation involves the transfer of a methyl group (CH_3) to the oxygen (O) at the third position of the benzene ring. The product of O-methylation is 3-methoxy-4-hydroxymandelic acid or VANILLY-MANDELIC ACID (VMA), which ultimately diffuses into the bloodstream and urine.

*When an aldehyde is associated with a hydroxyl group, it is called a glycoaldehyde because such combinations are characteristic of sugar molecules.

COMT, which was discovered by Axelrod in 1957, requires the presence of a divalent ion. Mg^{2+} is the ion that is usually present, but others such as Zn^{2+}, Fe^{2+}, and Ni^{2+} can be substituted. The enzyme also requires the presence of the methyl donor S-adenosylmethionine (SAM). COMT is nonspecific, meaning that, in addition to NE, it will methylate epinephrine, dopamine, DOPA, many NE metabolites, and catechols that are built upon drug bases such as ephedrine and amphetamine.

When NE is released from the synaptic terminals of sympathetic nerves, most of it is taken up by the presynaptic terminal and recycled. The small amounts remaining are metabolized, but the steps of the process are somewhat different from those within the axon terminals. Synaptic NE is first methylated by COMT, which is presumed to be present on the postsynaptic membranes. The product of this step is normetanephrine (3-methoxy-4-hydroxyphenylethanolamine) (Figure 17). This product is deaminated by MAO to form MHPGA (3-methoxy-4-hydroxyphenylglycoaldehyde), which in turn is oxidized by aldehyde dehydrogenase to form VMA, which is ultimately excreted in the urine. Of some significance is the ability of neurochemists to detect abnormal amounts of deaminated products in the blood (e.g., DOPGA which could indicate abnormal metabolism of NE within axon terminals) or methylated products (e.g., normetanephrine, which could indicate the occurrence of excessive synaptic NE activity).

Norepinephrine Catabolism in the Central Nervous System

The catabolic pathway for NE is slightly different in the central nervous system because VMA is not found to any great extent in CNS tissue. The major difference is that DOPGA is reduced by aldehyde reductase rather than oxidized to form 3,4-dihydroxyphenylglycol (DOPEG), which is then O-methylated by COMT to form 3-methoxy-4-hydroxyphenylglycol (MHPG). When noradrenergic synaptic transmission takes place in the CNS, the small amounts of NE that are metabolized are first acted upon by COMT and MAO to form MPHGA, just as occurred in peripheral nerves. However, because of the favored activity of aldehyde reductase, more MHPGA is reduced to MHPG, the end product. In addition, MHPG may be further metabolized to MHPG-sulfate (MHPG-S) by the action of the brain enzyme sulfotransferase.

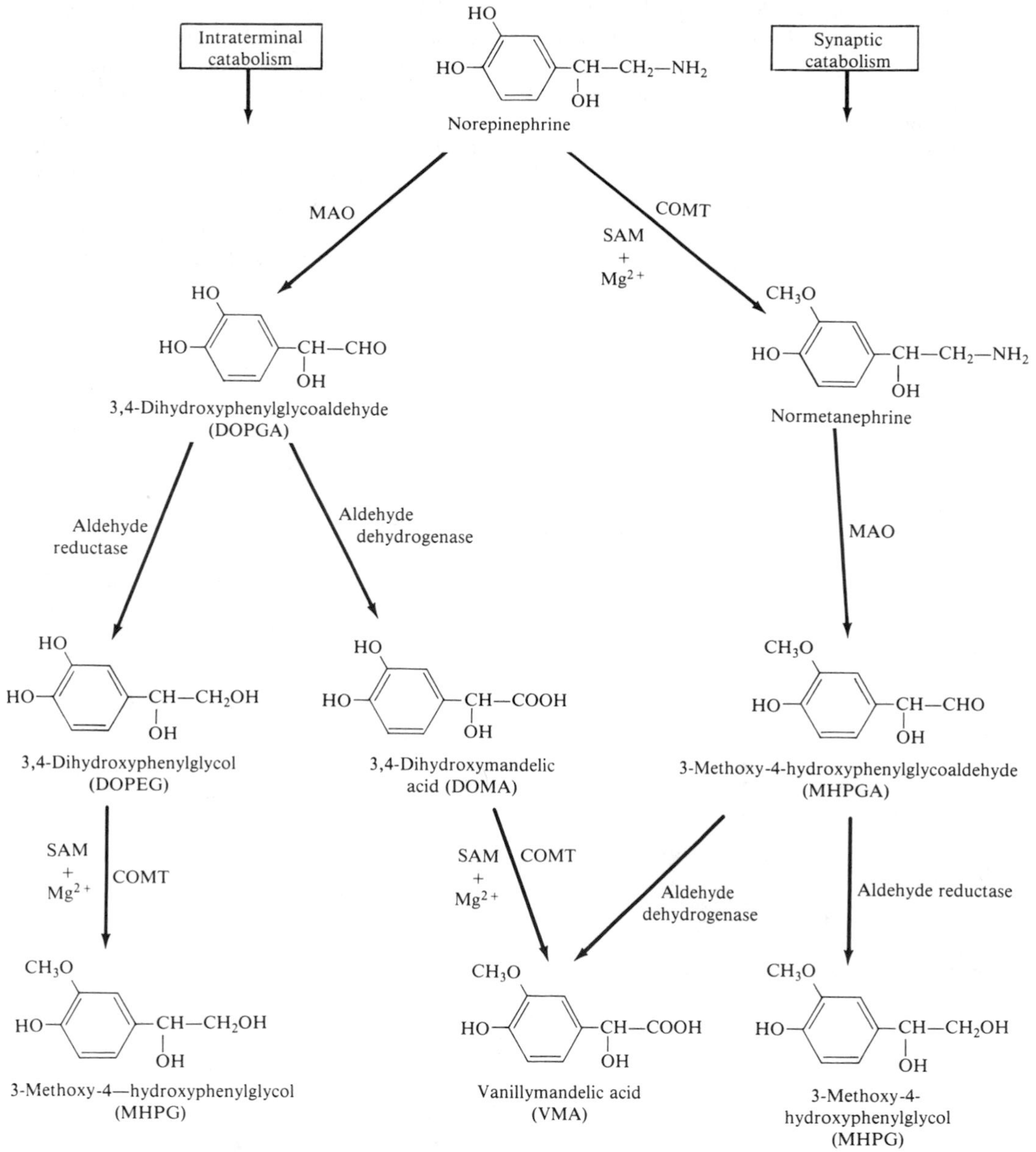

Intraterminal catabolism

Synaptic catabolism

HO

HO—⟨ ⟩—CH—CH_2—NH_2
  |
  OH

Norepinephrine

MAO

COMT

SAM + Mg^{2+}

HO

HO—⟨ ⟩—CH—CHO
  |
  OH

3,4-Dihydroxyphenylglycoaldehyde (DOPGA)

CH_3O

HO—⟨ ⟩—CH—CH_2—NH_2
  |
  OH

Normetanephrine

Aldehyde reductase

Aldehyde dehydrogenase

MAO

HO

HO—⟨ ⟩—CH—CH_2OH
  |
  OH

3,4-Dihydroxyphenylglycol (DOPEG)

HO

HO—⟨ ⟩—CH—$COOH$
  |
  OH

3,4-Dihydroxymandelic acid (DOMA)

CH_3O

HO—⟨ ⟩—CH—CHO
  |
  OH

3-Methoxy-4-hydroxyphenylglycoaldehyde (MHPGA)

SAM + Mg^{2+}

COMT

SAM + Mg^{2+}

COMT

Aldehyde dehydrogenase

Aldehyde reductase

CH_3O

HO—⟨ ⟩—CH—CH_2OH
  |
  OH

3-Methoxy-4—hydroxyphenylglycol (MHPG)

CH_3O

HO—⟨ ⟩—CH—$COOH$
  |
  OH

Vanillymandelic acid (VMA)

CH_3O

HO—⟨ ⟩—CH—CH_2OH
  |
  OH

3-Methoxy-4-hydroxyphenylglycol (MHPG)

FIGURE 17   CATABOLISM OF NE. When NE leaks from vesicles within axon terminals it is catabolized by the pathway shown on the left. Within peripheral sympathetic nerve terminals NE is first deaminated and oxidized by MAO and aldehyde dehydrogenase, respectively, to form DOMA. DOMA, which is inactive, leaks from the nerve terminal and is methylated by COMT to form VMA. During synaptic release the order of catabolism is somewhat reversed. NE is first methylated by COMT, then deaminated and oxidized to form VMA as shown in the pathway on the right. Within the CNS NE catabolism differs from that in sympathetic peripheral nerves in that more DOPGA (within the nerve terminal) is *reduced* by aldehyde reductase to form DOPEG and then MHPG rather than oxidized to form DOMA and VMA. Similarly, more MHPGA is *reduced* during synaptic release to form the final metabolite MHPG.

MHPG is also formed during the metabolism of NE from peripheral sympathetic nerves, although in smaller proportion to VMA. However, because there is so much more NE activity and metabolism in peripheral nerves than in the CNS, 80 percent of urinary MHPG is contributed by these nerves. Because most MHPG is eventually found in the urine, it, like VMA, may reflect the amount of activity in central and peripheral noradrenergic nerves. Even though most MHPG is contributed from peripheral NE activity,

Schildkraut and Keeler (1973) reported that urinary excretion levels of MHPG are significantly lower during the depressed phase in patients with manic–depressive psychosis. It could be argued that a lower MHPG level during depression would be expected because these patients are likely to be less active, less agitated, and less anxious during the depressed phase. However, the drop in MHPG levels was not related to the degree of retardation, agitation, or anxiety. This suggested that there were lower levels of central noradrenergic activ-

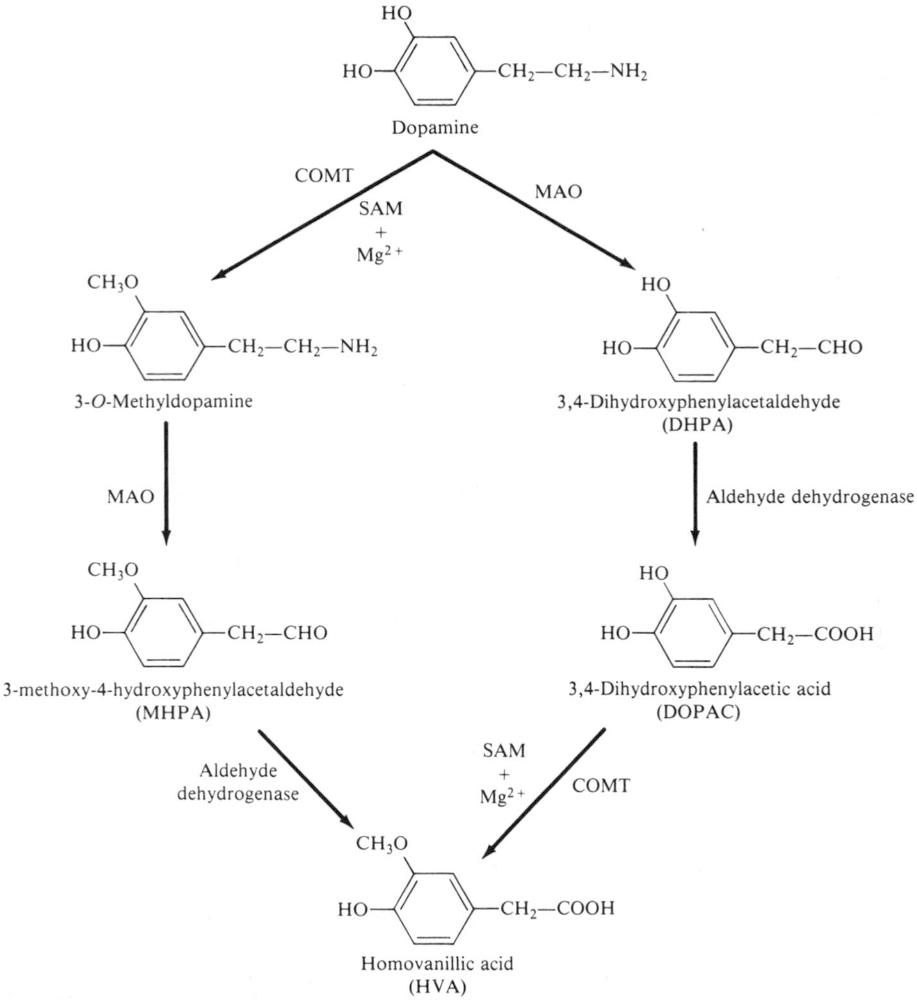

FIGURE 18   CATABOLISM OF DOPAMINE. Within the terminal, free dopamine is first deaminated and oxidized, then after leaving the terminal it is methylated to form HVA (right pathway). During synaptic release, the order is reversed (left pathway).

ity during the depressed phase for these patients and that the levels of noradrenergic activity were independent of the patient's activity.

Catabolism of Epinephrine

Virtually the same steps are followed for the catabolism of EPI as for NE. The end metabolite is VMA. EPI differs chemically from NE only in that its amine group is methylated to form —$NHCH_3$ (Figure 12). During EPI catabolism, this amine group is removed by MAO, and aldehyde dehydrogenase and COMT act on the residues to form VMA as in NE degradation.

VMA can be detected and quantified in the urine. A marked increase of VMA in the urine along with other symptoms such as paroxysmal tachycardia is diagnostic for the presence of pheochromocytoma, which is a tumor of the adrenal gland that causes an abnormally high output of epinephrine.

Catabolism of Dopamine

The termination of dopamine transmitter action is similar to that thought to occur with NE except that it is almost exclusively within the CNS. Most synaptically released dopamine is recaptured by the presynaptic terminal membrane, and the rest is catabolized by MAO, COMT and aldehyde dehydrogenase or aldehyde reductase. Some dopamine in the cytoplasm may be de-

aminated by MAO before gaining access to the vesicles where it is converted to NE. Therefore the cytoplasmic deamination process plus the additional metabolic steps may be a substantial source of urinary dopamine metabolites. The details of these processes are shown in Figure 18.

If the first step is intraneuronal deamination, dopamine is converted by MAO to 3,4-dihydroxyphenylacetaldehyde (DHPA) which leaves the cell. This is rapidly acted on by aldehyde dehydrogenase to form 3,4-dihydroxyphenylacetic acid (DOPAC). Small amounts of DOPAC are found in brain tissue, and some is excreted in the urine. The rest is O-methylated by COMT to form homovanillic acid (HVA), which enters the cerebrospinal fluid, the bloodstream, and ultimately the urine.

An alternate catabolic route starts with a synaptic release of dopamine. The first step in the alternate route involves O-methylation to form 3-O-methyl-dopamine* (3-methoxy-4-hydroxyphenethylamine). This product is deaminated to form 3-methoxy-4-hydroxyphenylacetaldehyde (MHPA). A similarity may again be noted between this deaminated product and deaminated dopamine (DHPA). Finally, the aldehyde is acted upon by aldehyde dehydrogenase to form HVA, which enters the bloodstream and urine (Figure 18).

Part III   Neuropharmacology of Catecholaminergic Synapses

Drugs That Affect Catecholaminergic Synapses: Overview

Thus far we have emphasized the biochemical aspects of CA systems in brain function with the hope that this may improve our attempts to relate the facts of brain function to behavior. We have frequently mentioned a number of drugs that affect the CA systems. The drugs have served two purposes. First, they are powerful tools for describing certain neurophysiological phenomena; and second, in cases where the drugs are therapeutically useful, we have found a rational basis for choosing drugs for whatever purposes we seek.

Thus, drugs are viewed here as tools to reach higher levels of understanding of CNS function and as agents that can be useful in alleviating illness and altering behavior that is unproductive or not conducive to pro-

moting one's welfare. With these goals in mind, we will discuss drugs that affect the synthesis, the release, the reuptake, and the metabolic processes of the CA neurotransmitters that are instrumental in the functioning of noradrenergic and dopaminergic systems (Table I).

Drugs That Inhibit Catecholamine Synthesis

Tyrosine Hydroxylase Inhibitors

As previously mentioned, the precursor in catecholamine synthesis is dietary tyrosine; the next step is the conversion of tyrosine to DOPA by the enzyme tyro-

---

*The removal of the CH_3O group from the ring structure results in the formation of tyramine. Thus, 3-O-methyl-dopamine is sometimes called 3-methoxytyramine.

TABLE I   Drugs That Affect Norepinephrine Synapses

Drug	Mechanism of action	Major effects
AGONISTS		
Clonidine	α_2-receptor agonist	Antihypertensive
Ephedrine	α- and β-receptor agonist	Relieves bronchospasm and nasal congestion
Isoproterenol	β-receptor agonist	Bronchiodilator, hypertensive
Phenethylamine	General receptor agonist	Weak sympathomimetic
Phenylephrine	α-receptor agonist	Hypertensive
Salbutamol	β_2-receptor agonist	Bronchial relaxation
Tazolol	β_1-receptor agonist	Stimulates the heart
ANTAGONISTS		
Phenoxybenzamine Phentolamine Piperoxane	α-receptor blockers	Antihypertensive
Propranolol Sotalol	β-receptor blockers	Antihypertensive
Practolol	β_1-receptor blocker	Blocks CA effects on heart
Butoxamine IPS 339	β_2-receptor blockers	Block vasodilation, uterine relaxation, and tracheal relaxation
RELEASERS		
Amphetamine Methamphetamine Tyramine Methylphenidate	Facilitate synaptic release	Sympathomimetic, euphoriant
STORAGE INHIBITORS		
Reserpine Tetrabenazine	Vesicle depletion	Antihypertensive, tranquilizer
PUMP INHIBITORS		
Cocaine	Inhibits NE reuptake	Euphoriant, stimulant
Amitriptyline Desipramine Imipramine	Inhibit NE reuptake	Antidepressant

sine hydroxylase (TH) (Figure 19). This latter synthetic step appears to be rate-limiting. Therefore, a drug that blocks the activity of TH can be very effective in reducing brain catecholamine levels. α-Methyl-p-tyrosine (AMPT) is such a drug. AMPT is used therapeutically to reduce catecholamine levels that are elevated

α-Methyl-p-tyrosine (AMPT)

TABLE I   (continued)

Drug	Mechanism of action	Major effects
SYNTHESIS INHIBITORS		
α-Methyl-*p*-tyrosine	Inhibits tyrosine hydroxylase	Depressant, cardiac inhibitor
α-Methyldopa	Forms false transmitter	Antihypertensive
α-Methyldopa-hydrazine	Inhibits dopa decarboxylase	Inhibits peripheral dopamine synthesis
Fusaric acid	Inhibit dopamine-β-hydroxylase	Antihypertensive
Disulfiram		
Diethyldithio-carbamate	Inhibit dopamine-β-hydroxylase	Experimental
FLA 63		
Phenylalanine	Competes with tyrosine uptake	Decreases NE synthesis
MONOAMINE OXIDASE INHIBITORS		
Iproniazid	Block action of MAO	Antidepressant
Nialamide		
Phenelzine		
Tranylcypromine		
Clorgyline	Blocks type A MAO	Experimental
Deprenyl	Blocks type B MAO	
COMT INHIBITORS		
Tropolone	Not known	Inhibits NE catabolism
Pyrogallol		
TOXIN		
6-Hydroxy-dopamine	Destroys NE neurons	Selective depletion of NE neurons

by pheochromocytoma (a tumor of the adrenal glands responsible for excessive synthesis and release of EPI causing distressing paroxysmal tachycardia). It should also be clear that a blockade of synthesis at the tyrosine–DOPA level would reduce levels of dopamine as well as of NE.

DOPA Decarboxylase Inhibitors

The enzyme DOPA decarboxylase (or AAAD) is highly abundant and active and accounts for the inability to detect endogenous DOPA in sympathetically innervated tissue and brain. Parkinson's disease, which is characterized by spasticity, tremors, and an inability to initiate movements, is caused by a degeneration of the nigrostriatal dopamine pathway,

resulting in a deficiency of dopamine in the striatum. These symptoms can be relieved by administering the dopamine precursor L-dopa,* which can cross the blood brain barrier, whereas dopamine cannot. L-dopa enters the brain and is decarboxylated to form dopamine, thus relieving the symptoms caused by the dopamine shortage (Hornykiewicz, 1963, 1966; Cotzias et al., 1967, 1969, 1975).

However, in order to achieve an adequate brain level of DOPA, a high dose has to be administered. The reason for this is that decarboxylase activity within the

---

*L-dopa is a pharmaceutical compound sold as Levodopa or Laradopa. It is used to control the symptoms of Parkinson's disease and as a research tool to supply the brain with added dopamine.

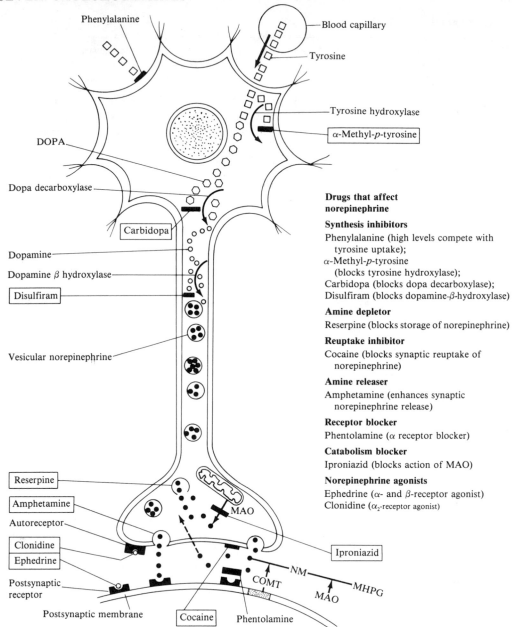

Phenylalanine

Blood capillary

Tyrosine

Tyrosine hydroxylase

α-Methyl-*p*-tyrosine

DOPA

Dopa decarboxylase

Carbidopa

Dopamine

Dopamine β hydroxylase

Disulfiram

Vesicular norepinephrine

**Drugs that affect
norepinephrine**

Synthesis inhibitors
Phenylalanine (high levels compete with
  tyrosine uptake);
α-Methyl-*p*-tyrosine
  (blocks tyrosine hydroxylase);
Carbidopa (blocks dopa decarboxylase);
Disulfiram (blocks dopamine-β-hydroxylase)

Amine depletor
Reserpine (blocks storage of norepinephrine)

Reuptake inhibitor
Cocaine (blocks synaptic reuptake of
  norepinephrine)

Amine releaser
Amphetamine (enhances synaptic
  norepinephrine release)

Receptor blocker
Phentolamine (α receptor blocker)

Catabolism blocker
Iproniazid (blocks action of MAO)

Norepinephrine agonists
Ephedrine (α- and β-receptor agonist)
Clonidine (α₂-receptor agonist)

Reserpine

Amphetamine

Autoreceptor

Clonidine

Ephedrine

Postsynaptic
receptor

MAO

Iproniazid

NM

COMT

MHPG

MAO

Postsynaptic membrane

Cocaine

Phentolamine

FIGURE 19 NORADRENERGIC SYNAPSES IN THE
CNS. NE synthesis, storage, and release is shown in the
neuron; and NA receptors are shown on the presynaptic as
well as on the postsynaptic membrane. Some noradrenergic
drugs are listed on the right, and their sites of action are
shown in the figure.

blood vessels converts the L-dopa to dopamine, thus
preventing a large portion of the dose from crossing
the blood brain barrier to brain tissue where it is
needed. Fortunately, drugs are available to compensate for this condition. For example, α-methyldopa
hydrazine (Carbidopa) competes with DOPA for
DOPA decarboxylase, thus reducing the synthesis of
dopamine in the bloodstream. Carbidopa does not

pass the blood brain barrier; therefore, it does not interfere with the necessary decarboxylation of DOPA in the brain.

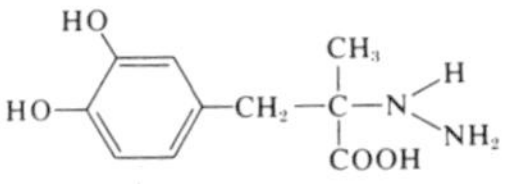

α-Methyldopa hydrazine (Carbidopa)

An analog of Carbidopa is Aldomet (α-methyldopa, α-MD). (The drug is so named because the methyl group is attached to the α-carbon, which is the first carbon next to the amine group in the side chain.) This drug also competes with DOPA for DOPA decarboxylase. The effect of this competition is also a reduction in the level of synthesis of dopamine and NE, but there are other consequences as well. First, α-MD undergoes decarboxylation to form α-methyldopamine, which is acted upon by dopamine-β-hydroxylase to form α-methylnorepinephrine (α-MNE) (Figure 20). α-MNE is taken up preferentially in synaptic vesicles and displaces NE. Upon nerve stimulation, α-MNE is released as a false transmitter. Consequently, α-methyldopa is used as an antihypertensive agent because in sympathetic nerves α-MNE does not activate the circulatory system as much as NE. Unfortunately, the same displacement of NE occurs within the CNS. This results in some instances in a severe depression similar to that caused by reserpine.

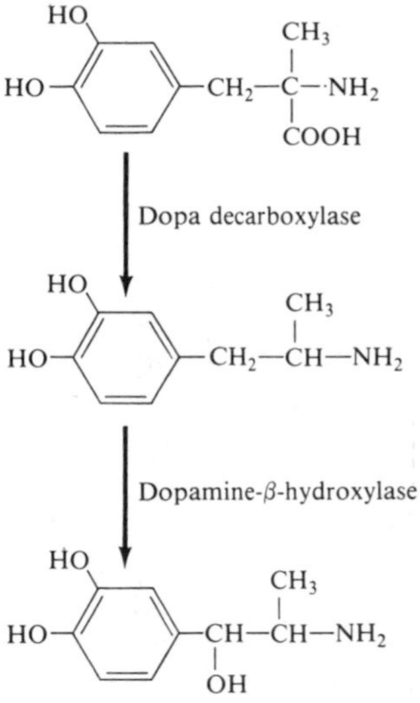

α-Methyldopa (Aldomet)

α-Methyldopamine

α-Methylnorepinephrine (α-MNE)

FIGURE 20 α-METHYLDOPA CONVERSION TO α-METHYLNOREPINEPHRINE.

Dopamine-β-Hydroxylase Inhibitors

There are drugs that block, at least to some extent, the activity of dopamine-β-hydroxylase (DBH). Recall that this enzyme is a copper-containing protein; thus, Cu^{2+} chelating compounds can effectively block the action of DBH. (CHELATING AGENTS are chemicals that bind with metals and carry them into the urine.) Diethyldithiocarbamate (DDC), FLA 63 [bis-(1-methyl-4-homopiperazinylthiocarbonyl)disulfide], fusaric acid, and disulfiram (Antabuse) are DBH inhibitors. In reasonable doses these drugs do not markedly reduce brain catecholamine levels and are used primarily as experimental tools to study the effects of other drugs on catecholamine levels. One such study used FLA 63 to identify DA terminals in the rat cortex (Hökfelt et al., 1974c). After repeatedly treating rats with this drug, the animals were sacrificed and their brains were examined. It was found that rats treated with FLA 63 had the same intensity of fluorescence in the limbic cortex as untreated control rats. FLA 63 at the doses used would have reduced the synthesis of NE from dopamine to 5 percent of normal. Therefore, if the dopamine were a precursor and the neurons were noradrenergic, there should have been a marked increase in dopamine fluorescence. There was no increase, indicating that the terminals were dopaminergic.

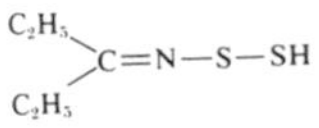

Diethyldithiocarbamate (DDC)

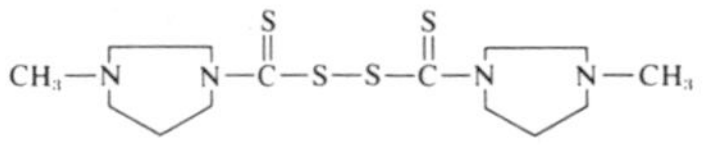

FLA 63

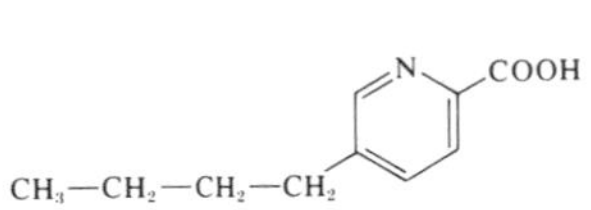

Fusaric acid

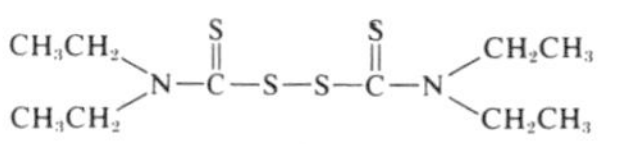

Tetraethylthiuram disulfide (Disulfiram)

DOPAMINE-β-hydroxylase inhibitors

Disulfiram has a therapeutic use. It was accidentally discovered that disulfiram (which is used to kill parasitic flat worms in the intestines) caused a distressing reaction when individuals taking the drug also drank alcoholic beverages. This effect is not related to the chelating properties of disulfiram but rather to its ability to block one stage in alcohol metabolism. Individuals who strongly desire to abstain from alcohol may be advised by their physician to take disulfiram, which has no effect by itself. However, the patients are instructed that any subsequent alcohol intake will be followed by extremely unpleasant physiological effects. The mechanism of action of disulfiram is shown in Figure 21. Ethanol is oxidized by the enzyme alcohol dehydrogenase to acetaldehyde. Acetaldehyde is immediately converted (oxidized) by aldehyde dehydrogenase to acetic acid, which then enters normal metabolic pathways. Disulfiram blocks the action of aldehyde dehydrogenase, allowing a buildup of acetaldehyde in the blood to five to ten times higher than normal. This substance in even small amounts is quite toxic, causing a hot flushing of the face, sweating, thirst, headache, nausea, vomiting, throbbing in the head and neck, breathing difficulties, chest pain, weakness, dizziness, blurred vision, and confusion. As little as 7 ml of alcohol can produce mild symptoms in a sensitive person. The drug metabolizes slowly in the liver. Therefore, a patient must wait several days before drinking alcohol, or the toxic symptoms will ensue (Ritchie, 1975a).

Drugs That Inhibit Catecholamine Storage

The most widely known drug in this category is reserpine (Figures 19 and 25). This drug is an alkaloid derived from the root of *Rauwolfia serpentina* (snake root), a plant known for centuries in the orient for its pharmacological properties. It was used as a sedative and to treat epilepsy, snake bite (because the roots of

Reserpine

the plant resembled a snake), and other ailments. In the 1930s it was used to calm agitated and excited mental patients, and there were many informal reports of its tranquilizing action without somnolence. In 1949 Dr. Rustom Jal Vakil in Bombay reported that reserpine was very effective in reducing high blood pressure in patients that were unresponsive to other forms of therapy. The drug unfortunately also caused in some patients severe mental depression that occasionally led to suicide. Similarly, when the drug was used to tranquilize agitated mental patients, a significant drop in blood pressure also appeared as an unwanted side effect.

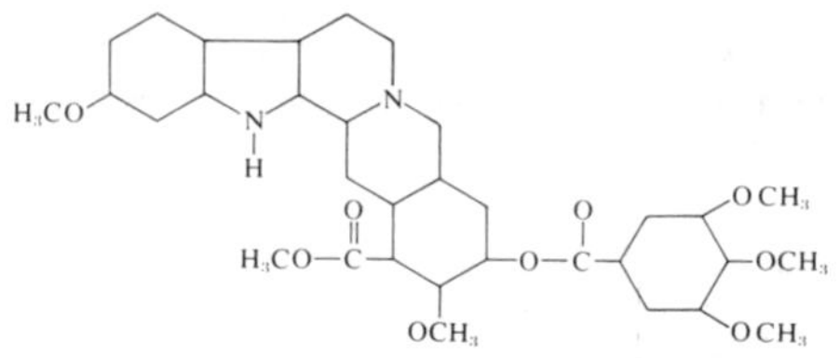

By the 1950s many mental patients had been treated with reserpine, and it seemed to be useful in calming disturbed individuals without making them unresponsive to their environment. By this time the phenothiazines had been discovered and were found to be more effective. Although phenothiazines ultimately displaced reserpine as a principal mode of treatment, reserpine is still used for patients who either require a reduction of hypertension or possess an idiosyncratic sensitivity to the phenothiazines.

Many studies have indicated that reserpine interferes with the vesicular uptake and causes release of brain amines from the storage vesicles of the noradrenergic axon terminals both centrally and peripherally. The action is not specific as this effect occurs in dopaminergic and serotonergic neurons as well. The hypothesis of inhibition of catecholamine storage by reserpine was derived from the observation that after animals were

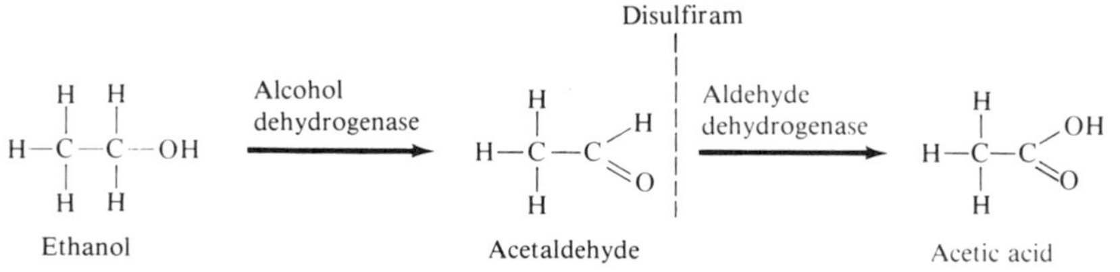

FIGURE 21   DISULFIRAM BLOCKADE OF ETHANOL METABOLISM. Disulfiram blocks the action of aldehyde dehydrogenase, causing a buildup of toxic levels of acetaldehyde.

treated with reserpine, there was a drop in O-methyl-ated metabolites of NE and an increase in deaminated metabolites. This indicates that DA and NE were being released from vesicles intraneuronally and being deaminated by MAO, thus reducing the availability of DA and NE for synaptic action. A large dose of reserpine rapidly administered to an animal caused a brief period of excitement prior to profound tranquilization and hypotension. The brief period of excitement was probably due to leakage of NE from the terminal vesicles at a faster rate than it could be deaminated. Consequently, NE also leaked across the synaptic cleft and stimulated receptors. It has also been demonstrated that if a drug that inhibits deamination by MAO (e.g., iproniazid) is given prior to reserpine administration, the result is prolonged excitement rather than sedation. One can conclude that reserpine has its tranquilizing and sympatholytic effects because there is depletion of NE in adrenergic terminals.

The action of reserpine is so marked that there is a significant depletion of brain catecholamines for several days after a single dose. However, reserpine also causes a marked increase in catecholamine synthesis in peripheral sympathetic nerves. This apparently comes about by a mechanism that compensates for a drop in blood pressure caused by the sympatholytic action of the drug. Increasing peripheral NE synthesis tends to correct somewhat for the lowered blood pressure.

As previously mentioned, reserpine also causes the release of serotonin from terminal vesicles. Consequently, there has been some doubt as to which transmitter system was involved in the tranquilizing action of the drug. The classic study by Carlsson and his colleagues (1957) seemed to resolve this issue. They found that DOPA (the precursor of NE) could antagonize reserpine-induced depression whereas 5-hydroxytryptophan (the precursor of serotonin) could not. This seemed to rule out any role for serotonin. However, it was also found that administering DOPA raised brain levels of dopamine but did not raise brain levels of NE. Therefore, it is possible that the depletion of dopamine rather than of NE is related to the tranquilizing effect of reserpine. This idea is supported by the finding that antipsychotic agents such as chlorpromazine block DA receptors and also cause tranquilization.

One more point is of interest. Reserpine effects illustrate an important concept in membrane physiology. The drug is able to block the uptake and storage of vesicular brain amines although it does not interfere with uptake by the cytoplasmic membrane. This strongly suggests that these two membranes are different in some way and that the vesicle membranes are not solely bits of pinched-off cytoplasmic membrane.

Another drug that has an action similar to that of reserpine is tetrabenazine (Nitoman). However, its action is shorter-lived, for reasons that are not clear. Nevertheless, it is a useful research tool for lowering brain amine levels for short periods of time.

Tetrabenazine

Drugs That Stimulate Catecholamine Release

Drugs in this category are often referred to as sympathomimetic agents. They are of considerable interest because of their potent physiological and psychological effects, and they are widely used therapeutically and experimentally. It is also true, unfortunately, that some of them have been abused and have led to effects that are harmful and dangerous. We will describe the mode of action of a representative sample of drugs in the group.

Perhaps the most widely known sympathomimetic drug is amphetamine. The resemblance of the chemical structure of this monoamine to the structure of the catecholamines is quite obvious, suggesting why it can combine with presynaptic membrane proteins to exert

Amphetamine

its effects. Amphetamine causes a leakage of NE and DA from presynaptic terminals and enhances the release of CAs when the synaptic terminals are stimulated (Burgen and Iversen, 1965; Glowinski and Axelrod, 1965). Amphetamine also blocks the reuptake of CAs, thus potentiating their transmitter action even more. Amphetamine is deaminated by MAO and competes with catecholamines for this enzyme. Therefore, the CAs are metabolized at a slower rate resulting in an additional enhancement of catecholamine action.

Experiments have shown that amphetamine increases the rate of metabolic conversion of intraventricularly injected [³H]NE to [³H]normetanephrine. This occurs because the drug blocks the uptake of NE from synaptic clefts where it is acted upon by COMT to form normetanephrine. Also, animals that are treated with drugs that block CA synthesis (e.g., AMPT or DDC) show a marked reduction of the behavioral reactions to amphetamine. Amphetamine effects are also attenuated when DA nerves are destroyed by administering 6–hydroxydopamine (6–OHDA). These experiments indicate that amphetamine causes the release of DA and NE from axon terminals (Stein and Wise, 1970; Moore and Kelly, 1978).

Amphetamine causes, in humans, a heightened alertness, euphoria, lowered fatigue, and decreased boredom. Its use permits sustained physical effort without rest and sleep. During World War II it was frequently given to soldiers who were required to make forced marches and to airmen who piloted aircraft for sustained periods without adequate rest. Amphetamine also depresses the appetite. Consequently it has been used as an anorectic to reduce body weight. When used over a prolonged period, tolerance develops, requiring increased intake to sustain the drug effects. This frequently leads to considerable weight loss, lack of sleep, and general deterioration of physical and mental condition. Continued use may ultimately lead to compulsive, agitated behavior, and symptoms may develop that appear almost identical to those of paranoid schizophrenia. This resemblance is so marked that many investigators have regarded the drug-induced toxic psychosis as virtually the same as some forms of schizophrenia. An understanding of this syndrome contributes to a better understanding of schizophrenia and its treatment (Chapter 13) (Snyder, 1974; Snyder et al., 1974; Angrist and Sudilovsky, 1978). The behavioral effects of amphetamine will be more fully described and discussed in a later section.

N-methamphetamine is related to amphetamine and seems to be somewhat more potent. However, it seems to have a different ratio of central to peripheral effects, that is, a small dose of *N*-methamphetamine has

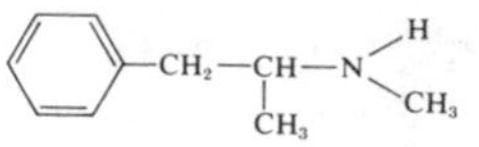

N-Methamphetamine

prominent central stimulating effects without the usually annoying peripheral effects of amphetamine such as hypertension, dilation of pupils, increased rate of respiration, dizziness, tremor, sweating, and nausea. But, the differences between this drug and amphetamine are of little consequence.

Tyramine also causes the release of endogenous amines. Tyrosine can be decarboxylated to form tyramine (Figure 14), but usually most of the tyramine is deaminated in the liver by MAO and ultimately excreted. The effect of tyramine in the CNS is not known. However, sizable amounts of tyramine, either from endogenous or exogenous sources, causes the release of NE and an increase in sympathetic activity. There is a second consequence of the presence of tyramine in the bloodstream. In the presence of MAO-inhibiting, antidepressant drugs, high levels of tyramine may not be deaminated, but rather tyramine may be β-hydroxylated to form octopamine,* which is considered to be an endogenous neurotransmitter in many species (Saavedra and Axelrod, 1976). (The chemical chain of events that mimics the purported normal synthesis is shown in Figure 22.) Octopamine is taken up in sympathetic nerve terminals, displacing NE. When these sympathetic nerves are stimulated, a substantial part of the released amines is octopamine, which mimics NE but is two orders of magnitude less effective than NE. Therefore, the release of octopamine results in a marked decrease of sympathetic tone. This explains the occasional observation of hypotensive effects found when MAO inhibitors are used.

Drugs That Block Catecholamine Reuptake

Reuptake has been found to be the principal mechanism responsible for the termination of NE and DA ef-

---

*p-Hydroxyphenylethanolamine. The name *octopamine* is derived from the fact that it was first found in the venom-producing salivary gland of the common octopus, *Octopus vulgaris* (Erspamer and Boretti, 1951).

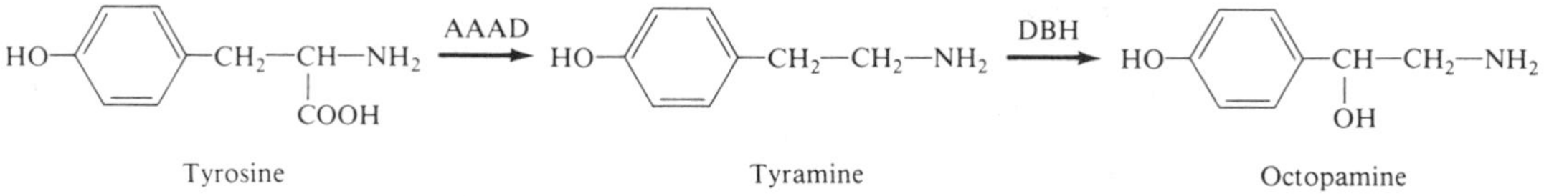

FIGURE 22   THE SYNTHESIS OF OCTOPAMINE.

fects at the synapse. Therefore, drugs that interfere with this reuptake process potentiate the activity at synapses by increasing the concentration of the transmitter at receptor sites: these are indirect catecholamine agonists. Some of the drugs in this category are important in the treatment of psychic depression, for example, the anticholinergic drug benztropine and the so-called tricyclic antidepressants imipramine (Tofranil), amitriptyline (Elavil), desipramine (desmethylimipramine; Norpramin).

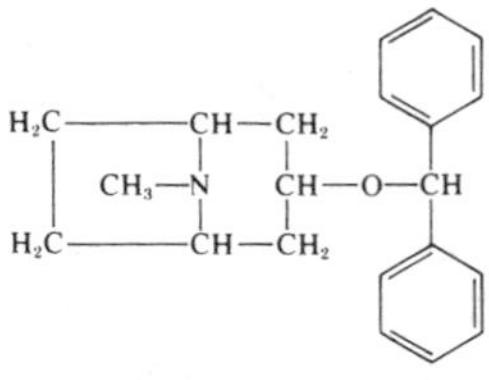

Benztropine

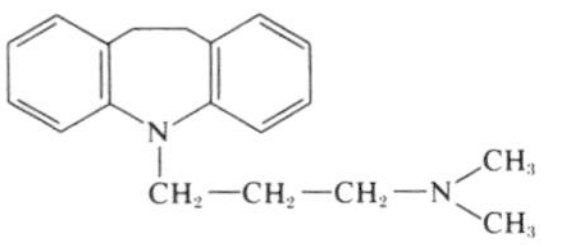

Imipramine

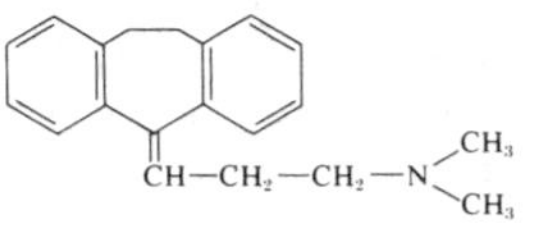

Amitriptyline

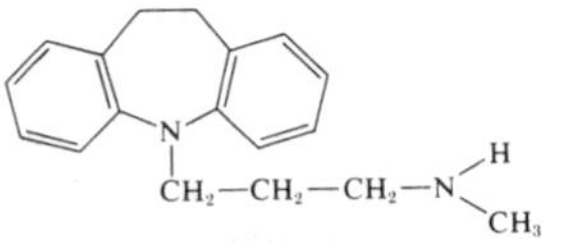

Desipramine

Amphetamine and cocaine also block CA reuptake. Cocaine has a long history of use not only as a central stimulant but also as a local anesthetic. Cocaine selectively blocks the initiation of nerve impulses in fibers that mediate pain, thus preventing pain impulses from reaching the brain. For centuries the natives of Bolivia

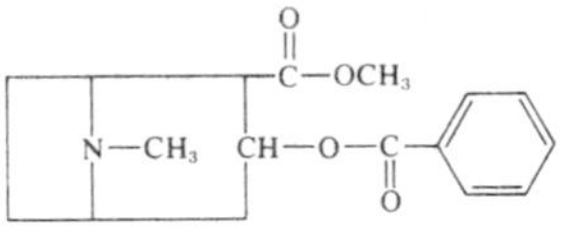

Cocaine

and Peru have chewed the leaves of the plant *Erythoxylon coca* (the source of cocaine) to overcome fatigue and increase endurance in the high altitudes in which they live. More recently the drug has been used to obtain an exhilarating effect that is compared, as one user described it, "to being Adam and having God blow life into your nostrils." It is still in use as a local anesthetic but is frequently replaced by the synthetic drug, procaine (Novocain). Although cocaine is a very potent

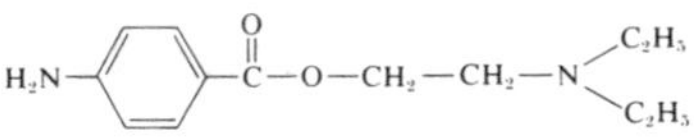

Procaine

stimulant it has no value as an antidepressive agent because of its short duration of action and its high toxicity, even in small doses. It also has a high potential for abuse and dependence because of the stimulation and the euphoria that it provides.

Another drug of recent interest is amantadine (Symmetrel). It was accidentally discovered that this drug, which is an antiviral agent for preventing influenza, reduces the symptoms of Parkinson's disease (Schwab et al., 1969). Experiments in cats showed that this drug, when placed in the cerebral ventricles, caused an increased concentration of dopamine in the CSF (Von Voigtlander and Moore, 1971). It is possible that amantadine either directly caused the release of dopamine from the caudate nucleus into the CSF or that it blocked the reuptake of this neurotransmitter, which then diffused into the CSF. In the latter case the drug would potentiate the action of dopamine and explain the amelioration of the parkinsonian symptoms.

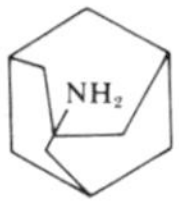

Amantadine

Drugs That Stimulate or Block Noradrenergic Receptors

Peripheral Effects

As mentioned earlier, there are in peripheral tissues two general types of noradrenergic receptors that are innervated by noradrenergic sympathetic nerves or by circulating epinephrine from the adrenal medulla. These receptors are designated as alpha (α) and beta (β), with subtypes α_1, α_2, β_1, and β_2. All four types are also found in the mammalian brain. The differences among them are defined by the differential effects of drugs that stimulate or block them. Thus, for example, epinephrine (EPI) is generally more potent for stimulating α-receptors, and isoproterenol, tazolol, and salbutamol are more potent for β-receptors. The receptor blockers phentolamine and phenoxybenzamine block α-receptors whereas propranolol, practolol, butoxamine, and IPS

Phentolamine   Phenoxybenzamine

339 have more specificity for blocking β-receptors. It should be emphasized that in many cases the differential drug effect is one of relative potency and not one of exclusive action on one receptor or the other. The receptors are designated as α or β only on this basis because no other set of characteristics applies exclusively to either of them (Lefkowitz, 1978).

The distribution of α- and β-receptors on the thoracic organs (heart, lungs, bronchi), the visceral organs (stomach, intestines, liver, pancreas, kidneys), and the pelvic organs (bladder, rectum, uterus, ejaculatory ducts, prostate) is very widespread, and each of the receptors can exert either excitatory or inhibitory effects, depending upon which organ is innervated. Recognizing that NE and EPI act on all of these receptors, investigators have discovered or formulated many drugs in attempts to exert specific effects on one type of receptor without affecting the others, for example, to exert antihypertensive effects without incurring sexual impotence (Tester-Dalderup, 1980). There are many useful sympathomimetic and sympatholytic drugs, but their application is usually limited by the wide range of autonomic side effects or central effects that can occur with the use of them. EPI is sometimes used as a drug to obtain a rapid stimulation of the cardiovascular system, but because it, as well as NE, causes such widespread autonomic effects and because it is so rapidly metabolized, it has few other medicinal uses. (Known side effects of catecholaminergic agents can be found in the Physician's Desk Reference.)

Most of the drugs that affect noradrenergic receptors are used to modulate peripheral sympathetic activity. For example, one other use for EPI is for the relief of congestion and spasm in the bronchi during asthma attacks by stimulating α-receptors that constrict blood vessels and reduce edema. EPI also stimulates β-receptors that inhibit bronchial muscles, thereby dilating the airways. Also, as is well known, EPI stimulates the heart by stimulating β-receptors, while at the same time raising blood pressure by affecting the vasocon-

strictor α-receptors. Because of this vasoconstricting action, EPI is also used in emergencies to stop bleeding in wounds.

Ephedrine also stimulates α- and β-receptors when used to relieve bronchial spasm and nasal congestion. Its advantages over EPI are that it can be administered orally, it has a longer duration of action, and it has a lower potency, making it somewhat safer.

Ephedrine   Phenylephrine (Neosynephrine)

Phenylephrine (Neosynephrine), which is chemically very similar to EPI, is used as a nasal spray to constrict the blood vessels and reduce congestion in inflamed and swollen nasal membranes resulting from colds and allergies. It is also used in eye drop solutions to stimulate sympathetic α-receptors of the iris to dilate the pupil during opthalmoscopic examinations of the interior of the eye and other ophthalmic procedures. Another drug, Long-lasting Neosynephrine, is the chemically distinct compond oxymetazoline (Afrin), a more potent α_2- than α_1-NE agonist, which has prolonged sympathomimetic effects when sprayed into the nostrils.

Oxymetazoline (Afrin)

Isoproterenol

Isoproterenol has strong effects on β-receptors that are inhibitory and that cause relaxation of the smooth muscles of the bronchi, blood vessels, and alimentary tract. It also effectively relieves the bronchial spasm of asthma when it is used (nearly always) as an aerosol-supplied inhalant.

Propranolol (Inderal) is a β-receptor blocker that is also used medicinally for a variety of cardiac conditions such as arrhythmias and tachycardias associated with pheochromocytoma. In addition, it has been

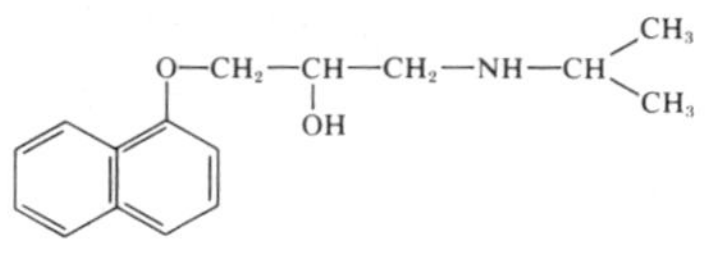

Propranolol

found to reduce the repetition of heart attacks (Kolata, 1981a). It is sometimes prescribed for patients who are subjected to acute periods of stress due to personal problems when the symptoms of the stress are sympathetic manifestations such as "fluttering" sensations in the chest (abnormal heart rhythms) and increased blood pressure. Frequently these symptoms are relieved by propranolol in appropriate doses without sedative side effects or the cultivation of dependence, both of which sometimes occur when other antianxiety drugs are used.

The discovery of the existence of β_1- and β_2-receptors and their distribution led to the development of drugs that were selective agonists and antagonists for each of these two subtypes. Thus, a β_1-agonist, tazolol, is used to stimulate heart rate, whereas a β_2-agonist, salbutamol, is used to induce bronchial relaxation in the treatment of asthma. It was hoped that this selective

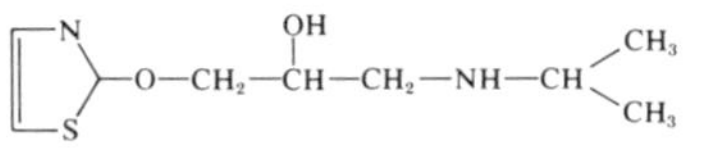

Tazolol

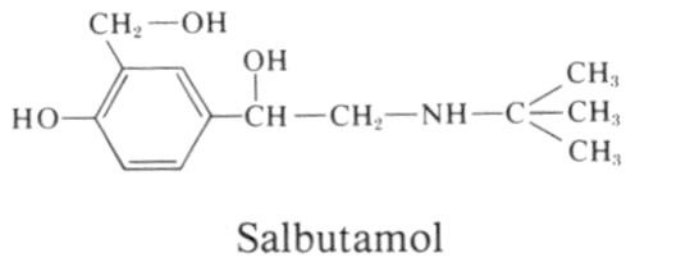

Salbutamol

potency would reduce the incidence of adverse side effects. This hope was borne out when it was found that salbutamol was an effective bronchodilator that caused only minimal cardiac stimulation.

Similarly, β-antagonists were developed. The β_1-antagonist practolol is useful in blocking the stimulating effects of the catecholamines in the treatment of cardiac arrhythmias and angina, whereas the β_2-antago-

Practolol

nist butoxamine has little effect on β_1-receptors, such as those mediating inhibition of the intestine and stimulation of the heart, but it does block vasodilation, uterine relaxation, and inhibition of the contraction of the guinea pig trachea. IPS 339 was found to be 100 times more potent in inhibiting the effect of CAs on the trachea than the effects of CAs on the heart of the guinea pig (reviewed by Minneman et al., 1981).

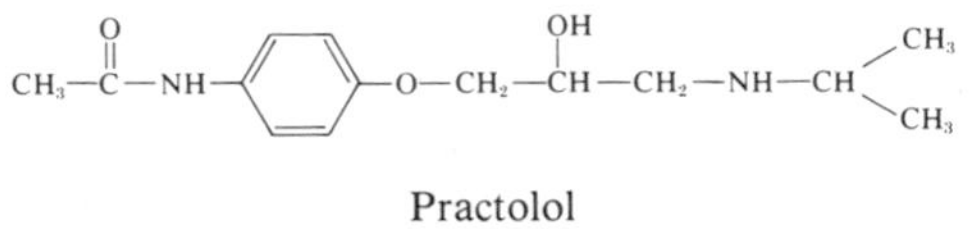

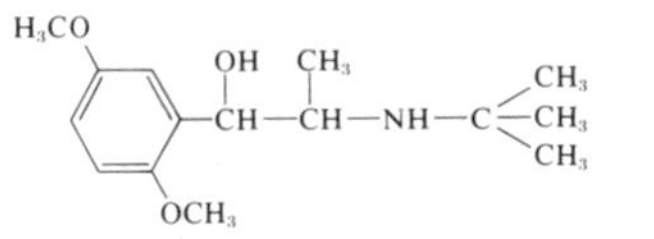

Butoxamine

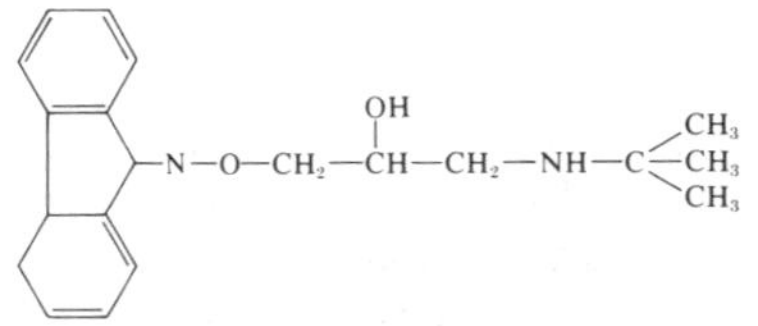

IPS 339

Central Nervous System Effects

NA receptors within the CNS appear to be similar to those in peripheral tissues as the drugs that are differentially potent for α- and β-receptors in the periphery have similar effects in the CNS. For example, the administration of noradrenergic drugs via cannulas implanted in the brains of animals elicit feeding in satiated rats or block feeding in hungry rats; these effects are reversed by appropriate antagonists (Leibowitz, 1974a). Some examples taken from experiments will make this argument clear.

When NE or EPI was injected into the hypothalmus of satiated rats, feeding behavior was elicited and the onset of feeding was inversely proportional to the dose (i.e., the higher the dose the sooner the rats began eating). However, as NE and EPI stimulate both α-and β-receptors, it was not known which receptor was responsible for the effect. A later test showed that the α-blocking drug phentolamine reliably reduced NE- and EPI-induced feeding, whereas the β-blocker propranolol did not. Also, the β-agonist isoproterenol strongly suppressed feeding by hungry rats, whereas prior injections of β-blockers eliminated the effect. Thus, stimulating α-receptors elicits feeding and blocking α-receptors reduces drug-induced feeding. Also, β-agonists suppress feeding, an effect that is reduced by β-blockers. Or, perhaps more simply, stimulating α-receptors induces feeding whereas stimulating β-receptors suppresses feeding (Leibowitz, 1971).

In other studies investigating the role of NE receptors on water intake, a specific site in the lateral hypothalamus was found that elicited drinking behavior when the site was stimulated by intracranial administration of the β-agonist isoproterenol. The effect was blocked by a β-antagonist but not by an α-antagonist. Thus, α- and β-receptors appear to play distinctive roles in drinking behavior as well as feeding behavior (Leibowitz, 1971). However, it is known that intravenous injection of isoproterenol releases renin from the kidney, which induces the formation of angiotensin I, which in turn is acted upon by another enzyme to form angiotensin II in the blood (see Chapter 11). Angiotensin II passes the blood brain barrier and induces drinking by stimulating the preoptic region of the hypothalamus. There is the possibility, therefore, that intracranial administration of isoproterenol in the rat could cause some leakage of the drug from the brain. The drug could then enter the general circulation and cause renin release from the kidney and thus induce drinking as a result of this peripheral effect rather than as a result of direct action of isoproterenol on β-receptors in the brain. This hypothesis is supported by the finding that surgical removal of the kidneys abolishes isoproterenol-induced drinking, regardless of the route of drug injection (Iversen and Iversen, 1981).

There are β-receptors in the pineal gland. Stimulating the nerves that originate in the superior cervical sympathetic ganglion and act upon the pineal gland leads to the production of melatonin, which among other things regulates sexual cycles (Axelrod, 1974b) (see Chapter 7). In support of the above, it was discovered that the stimulating effect of NE on melatonin synthesis was blocked by the β-antagonist propranolol, but not by an α-blocking agent.

Clonidine is an antihypertensive drug that reduces stimulation-produced release of NE from central and

Clonidine

peripheral noradrenergic neurons. Clonidine stimulates α₂-receptors (autoreceptors), which inhibit NE synthesizing activity. Intravenous and iontophoretic applications of clonidine had potent inhibitory effects upon the firing rates of single cells in the locus caeruleus (LC) of rats (A6 in Figure 4). Also, clonidine-sensitive receptors have been found on the cell bodies of NE cells that are in the LC and that are activated by axon collaterals of the LC neurons themselves, as well as by neurons from the EPI loci in the medulla oblongata (C1 and C2 in Figure 8).

Clonidine-induced inhibition of the LC neurons was also attained by iontophoretic applications of NE and EPI, but the effects of the α-agonist phenylephrine were weak. The α-antagonist piperoxane by itself enhanced the firing rate of LC neurons, and blocked the inhibitory effects of NE and EPI. However, the β-antagonist sotalol had no effect (Figure 23). These find-

Piperoxane

Sotalol

ings established the identity of the clonidine receptor as an α-receptor. Moreover, the sensitivity to various α-agonists of α-receptors in other parts of the body, and even those in distant centers receiving inputs from LC neurons, was in the order EPI ≥ NE > phenylephrine > α-methyl norepinephrine > clonidine ≫ isoproterenol = DA. However, the order of sensitivity by the receptors in LC was clonidine ≫ α-methyl norepinephrine ≥ NE = EPI ≫ phenylphrine. As mentioned earlier, the differences in drug sensitivity and in function of the LC receptors led to their designation as α₂-receptors as distinguished from the usual or α₁-receptors (Cedarbaum and Aghajanian, 1976; Aghajanian et al., 1977; Cedarbaum and Aghajanian, 1977). Clinically clonidine hydrochloride (Catapres) is used as an antihypertensive agent. Its mode of action appears to depend on its ability to stimulate the α₂-autoreceptors, thereby diminishing NE synthesis and/or NE release from sympathetic cardioaccelerator and vasoconstrictor neurons. However, because this

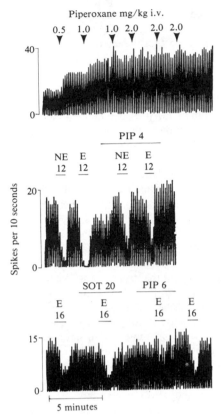

Piperoxane mg/kg i.v.

FIGURE 23   THE EFFECTS OF α- and β-NORADREN-ERGIC DRUGS ON SPONTANEOUS FIRING RATES in the locus caeruleus (LC). The vertical lines represent the integrated firing rates of a single cell during consecutive 10-second samples. The top trace shows the effects of intravenous piperoxane (PIP) on the firing rate of an LC cell. The numbers above the arrows indicate the doses in mg/kg given at intervals of about 2 minutes. The drug increases the firing rate. The middle trace shows the inhibitory effects of iontophoretically applied norepinephrine (NE) and epinephrine (E) on LC units. The bars above the trace indicate the time of drug injection. When PIP was also applied, the inhibition was attenuated. The bottom trace shows the failure of sotalol (SOT) to block the inhibitory effect of E during the second test, whereas PIP blocked the inhibitory effect of E in the third test. (From Cedarbaum and Aghajanian, 1976.)

drug also acts upon α_2-autoreceptors on the presynaptic terminals of sympathetic nerves, it can among other things diminish NE release from the nerves that innervate the vas deferens, the ejaculatory duct, the prostate, and erectile tissue, thereby making sexual inter-

course and ejaculation of seminal fluid difficult or impossible.

With respect to β-receptor-mediated drug effects in the CNS, the current status of research appears to be one of establishing more firmly the central distribution of the β subtypes and the development of drugs that can act differentially upon them. Behavioral studies must first wait for these developments.

Drugs That Inhibit Catecholamine Catabolism

It should be clear by now that there is no dearth of drugs that lead to noradrenergic stimulation. However, most substances that are responsible for these effects act by potentiating the effects of endogenous catecholamines. It has already been shown that this can be done by increasing the release of the transmitter or by blocking its reuptake. This section will deal with drugs that increase noradrenergic effects by interfering with the reactions that inactivate catecholaminergic transmitters.

It was mentioned earlier that catecholamine metabolism does not play a significant role in terminating the action of these transmitters. Nevertheless, there are some drugs having significant behavioral effects whose mode of action can be traced to interference with metabolic activities. The substances primarily responsible for catecholamine breakdown are monoamine oxidase (MAO) and catechol-O-methyltransferase (COMT). Consequently, drugs that block the activity of these two enzymes would presumably delay the degradation of the catecholamines and thereby potentiate their action.

Monamine Oxidase Inhibitors

MAO inhibitors were discovered among drugs that had been developed in the early 1950s for the treatment of tuberculosis. These drugs, of which isoniazid and iproniazid are examples, are rather specific in their toxic effects upon the tubercle bacillus, the mode of action not being completely known. It was soon discovered that iproniazid had a euphoric effect upon tuberculous patients, but it was not known whether

Isoniazid   Iproniazid (Marsilid)

this effect was a specific pharmacological attribute of the drug or simply due to the remission of the symptoms of tuberculosis (Bloch et al., 1954; Selikoff et al., 1952). This led to investigations on the use of isoniazid and iproniazid for depressed states. The results of clinical tests were found to be generally positive, and the drugs were adopted because they were preferable to the then-favored treatment of clinical depression by electroshock therapy. In early investigations it became apparent that iproniazid inhibited the enzyme MAO, an effect that lasted for days or weeks (Zeller et al., 1952; Pletscher, 1968) (Figure 19). Its mode of action was further demonstrated in rats by the finding that iproniazid, when used in conjunction with pretreatment by reserpine, caused excitement. This effect came about because reserpine presumably released NE from storage vesicles intraneuronally and the inhibition of MAO degradation of NE provided large amounts of NE in the synaptic cleft. MAO also controls NE levels by metabolizing excess DA before its incorporation into the vesicles, where it is subsequently acted on by DBH to form NE. In the presence of MAO inhibitors, higher levels of DA would also occur. However, there is no runaway buildup of CAs, probably because of end-product inhibition of the action of tyrosine hydroxylase.

Iproniazid has a hydrazine group (R_1—NH—NH—R_2) that caused toxic effects in the liver. Therefore, other hydrazines were developed that might be more potent and safer. Among these were isocarboxazide, nialamide, and phenelzine. Only phenelzine was found to be clinically useful, but it also had undesirable side effects. Nonhydrazine MAO inhibitors were also developed (e.g., pargyline and tranylcypromine), and

they seemed to help some depressed patients but not others—a characteristic that is typical of some of these drugs. The drug that is beneficial for each depressed patient must be sought by trial and error (Davis et al., 1968).

Animal studies have shown that MAO inhibitors increased brain levels of biogenic amines, decreased brain and urine levels of deaminated metabolites, and increased brain and urine levels of O-methylated metabolites. This finding suggested that MAO inhibitors increased synaptic release of CAs in central and peripheral sites (Pletscher, 1968). Also, terminally ill humans who died while being treated with MAO inhibitors showed upon autopsy that their brain biogenic amine levels peaked after about 2 weeks of drug treatment, a time that correlated well with the onset of the antidepressant action of the drugs (Berger, 1977). However, the supposed increased availability of synaptic CAs caused by the drugs cannot be the sole mechanism of action in the relief of depression. The sympathomimetic drug amphetamine also increased synaptic CAs. However, although it produced alertness and moderate elation in some patients for a few days, in other patients it produced anxiety, tension, and irritability. For the patients that were improved, the effect was soon followed by jitteryness, irritability, palpitations, postamphetamine fatigue, dejection, and in high doses, psychotic episodes. Thus, the mechanism of action of MAO inhibitors as antidepressants is not fully understood. The clinical use of these and the tricyclic antidepressants are discussed more fully in Chapter 11.

Different MAO isoenzymes have been discovered, and some of them respond specifically to different MAO inhibitors (see review by Musacchio, 1975). Two forms of MAO were designated as types A and B by Neff et al. (1974). Type A MAO acts upon the substrates DA, NE, tyramine, and serotonin. This MAO is inhibited by clorgyline. The substrates for type B

Isocarboxazide (Marplan)

Nialamide

Phenelzine (Nardil)

Clorgyline HCl

Pargyline (Benelin)

Tranylcypromine (Parnate)

Phenethylamine (PEA)

Deprenyl (E-250)

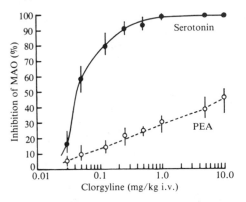

FIGURE 24 CLORGYLINE AND DEPRENYL BLOCK-ADE OF MAO ACTIVITY in the rat brain. Animals were sacrificed 2 hours after the drug injections and enzyme activity was assayed with serotonin or phenethylamine (PEA) as substrates. Serotonin is a substrate for type A MAO and is preferentially blocked by clorgyline, whereas PEA is a substrate for type B MAO and is preferentially blocked by deprenyl. (After Neff et al., 1974.)

MAO are dopamine, phenethylamine (PEA), and tyramine but not serotonin. Inhibitors of type B MAO are deprenyl and pargyline. At high doses, the specificity of these drugs decreases (Figure 24).

Catechol-O-Methyltransferase Inhibitors

Drugs that block the metabolic action of COMT are few in number and have no important therapeutic use. One of these is tropolone (Figure 25); another is pyrogallol, which is used in antimicrobial ointments. However, pyrogallol is highly toxic in the bloodstream and is only used experimentally in neurochemical research.

Tropolone   Pyrogallol

Drugs That Block or Stimulate Dopaminergic Activity

Because dopamine is a precursor for norepinephrine, drugs that interfere with the early stages of catecholamine synthesis such as the tyrosine hydroxylase and dopa decarboxylase inhibitors (α-methyl-p-tyrosine and carbidopa, respectively) will affect dopamine and NE to a similar extent. Also dopamine and NE are affected in similar ways by amphetamine, reserpine, and MAO inhibitors. The mechanisms of action of these drugs is similar for both transmitters so we shall proceed to describe drugs that have more specific effects upon dopamine synapses. (Figure 25.)

Dopaminergic Receptor Blockers

Of greatest interest and significance are those compounds that are classed as antipsychotic or neuroleptic drugs. Among these are the phenothiazines, for example, chlorpromazine, thioridazine, and promazine; the butyrophenones (phenylbutylpiperidines), of which haloperidol, fluoropipamide, and spiroperidol are the best examples; the diphenylbutylpiperidines, of which pimozide is a good example; and the dibenzodiazepines, which include clozapine, potentially a very important drug but not in wide use at the present time (Figure 26). It is well established that the one characteristic of the neuroleptic drugs that is most directly related to the potency of their antipsychotic effects is their ability to block DA receptors (even though most of them block NE receptors to some extent). More specifically, the antipsychotic potency correlates with the ability of these drugs to inhibit dopamine-sensitive adenylate cyclase (the enzyme that converts ATP to cAMP) in dopaminergically activated neurons. The implication is either that the inhibition of cAMP synthesis occurs because the dopamine receptor is blocked so that dopamine is ineffective as a synaptic transmitter in these systems, or that the receptor is stimulated but the activation of adenylate cyclase is blocked. At the present time it is not known which of these alternatives is correct.

Of related interest is the fact that phenothiazines

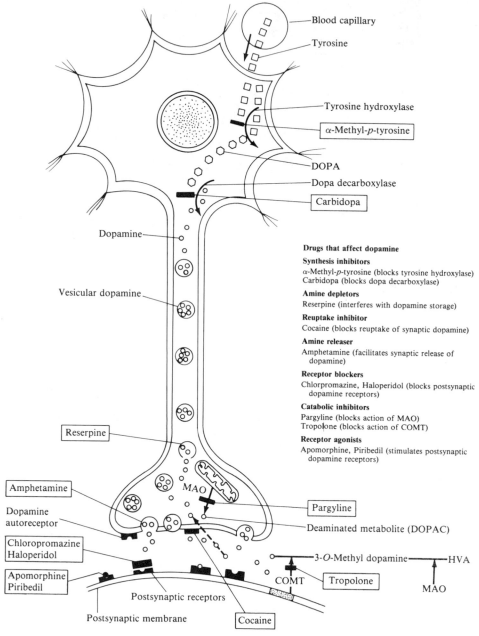

FIGURE 25   DOPAMINERGIC SYNAPSE indicating synthesis, catabolism, storage, release and the sites of action of the drugs listed on the right. (After Frohman, 1980.)

and butyrophenones, when used to treat schizophrenia, frequently produced parkinsonian symptoms such as tremors, reduction of voluntary movements, and spasticity. This is understandable as the antipsychotic drugs are effective because of their ability to block dopaminergic receptors, and parkinsonism has been traced to a deficiency of dopamine release in the caudate nucleus of the striatum (Hornykiewicz, 1966). Further-

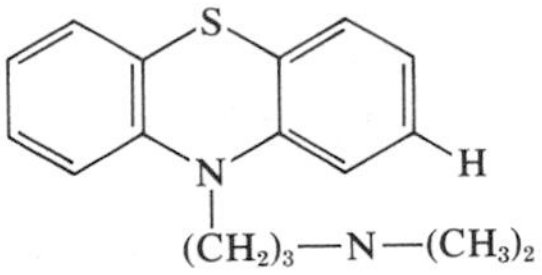

Chlorpromazine
(Thorazine)

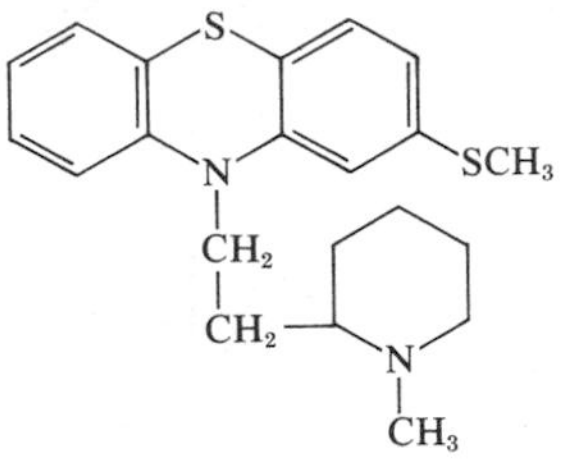

Thioridazine
(Melleril)

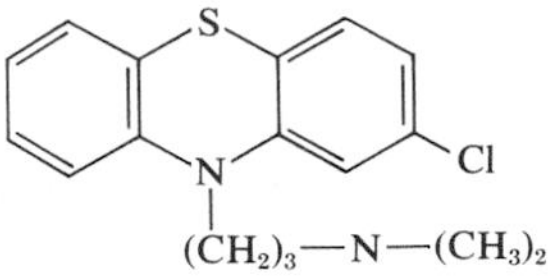

Promazine
(Prazine)

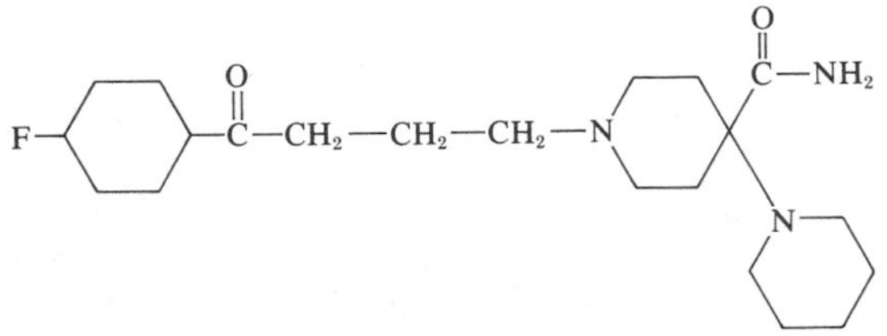

Floropipamide
(Pipamperone)

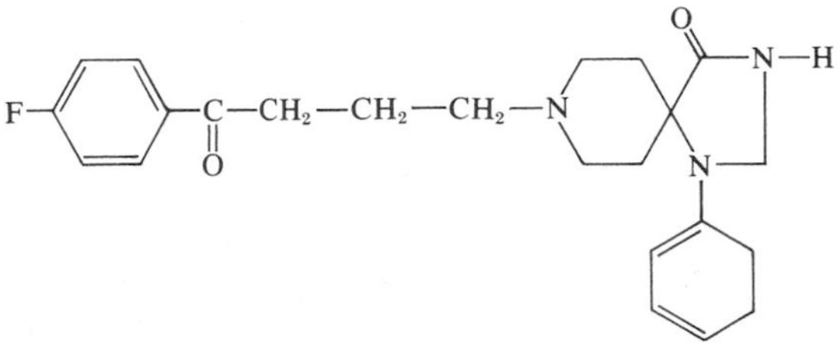

Spiroperidol

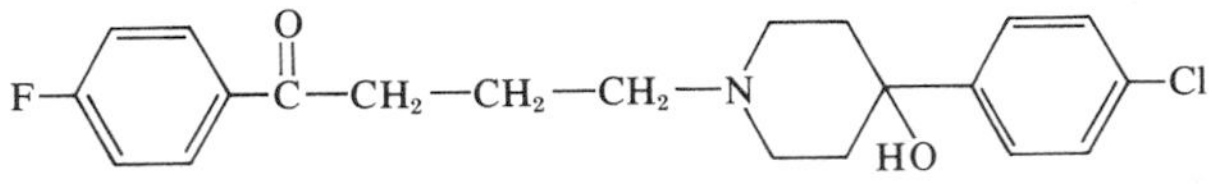

Haloperidol
(Haldol)

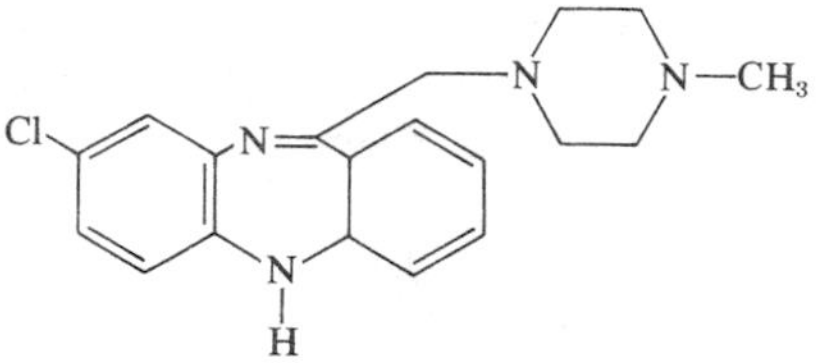

Clozapine

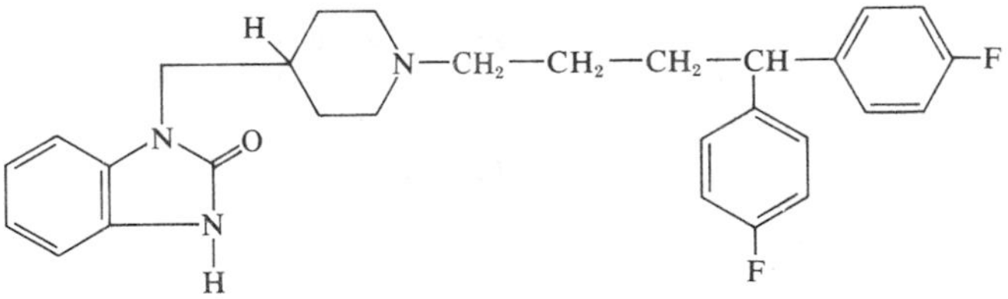

Pimozide

FIGURE 26   DRUGS THAT BLOCK DOPAMINE RE-
CEPTORS. These drugs are used principally for reducing the symptoms of schizophrenia.

more, there are cholinergic neurons in the striatum that are inhibited by dopamine. In the case of a dopamine deficiency, these cholinergic neurons become overactive and are presumed to be responsible for parkinsonism (Sethy et al., 1974). It had long been suspected that ACh was implicated in parkinsonism as the antimuscarinic drug atropine was sometimes effective in blocking the symptoms of the disease. Use of atropine gave way to use of other anticholinergic drugs such as benztropine mesylate (Cogentin) (which also blocks DA reuptake) and L-dopa when the overproduction of ACh was traced to a dopamine deficiency. Fortunately, new compounds have been produced (e.g., clozapine and thioridazine) that in addi-

Benztropine mesylate (Cogentin)

tion to blocking dopaminergic receptor sites also block muscarinic receptor sites in the brain. This development may soon lead to treatment for schizophrenia that can be undertaken with less risk of parkinsonian side effects. In summary, Parkinson's disease has been traced to a deficiency of dopamine in the striatum, and this condition can be corrected by supplying the precursor L-dopa to raise striatal dopamine levels. Schizophrenia, on the other hand, seems to be related to an abnormal sensitivity to or a surfeit of dopamine in the forebrain (Bird et al., 1979). This condition can be alleviated by administering a dopamine blocking drug. Unfortunately, drugs currently used do not specifically block only forebrain dopamine systems, hence they produce parkinsonian symptoms. But, fortunately, as parkinsonism is due to an overrelease of ACh, antipsychotic drugs that block both dopaminergic and cholinergic receptors may come to be the drugs of choice.

Dopamine Agonists

Amphetamine is active on dopaminergic systems as well as on noradrenergic systems. The action of amphetamine is presumed to involve leakage of dopamine from presynaptic terminals and blockade of the uptake process, the latter process being more pronounced than the former. The related drug methylphenidate (Ritalin) has similar effects. However, amphetamine seems to release newly synthesized DA, whereas methylphenidate seems to release vesicular (stored) DA. This hypothesis is based on the finding that drugs that interfere with DA storage (e.g., reserpine) block the action of methylphenidate (Chiueh and Moore, 1975). It was mentioned earlier that amphetamine and methylphenidate, after chronic use, may lead to schizophrenic-like psychotic episodes. When given to schizophrenics, the psychotic symptoms are exacer-

Methylphenidate (Ritalin)

bated even with low doses, and are so recognized by the patients themselves. Furthermore, as might be expected, the phenothiazines and other antipsychotic drugs are effective in reversing the psychotic episodes induced by these stimulants.

Strangely, it seems that d-amphetamine and methylphenidate inhibit firing of the DA cell groups A10 and A9. These effects may be due to the stimulation of the dendritic autoreceptors (described by Groves et al., 1975; Bunney and Aghajanian, 1975a; Costa and Trabucchi, 1975) or by a neuronal feedback pathway that runs from the corpus striatum to the substantia nigra and that regulates the activity of cells in A9 and A10 (Bunney and Aghajanian, 1978). Iontophoretic applications of NE and DA have similar effects on A10 cells, thus supporting the notion of negative feedback for these systems.

Apomorphine, a potent agonist, is a derivative of morphine that has long been used as an emetic (to induce vomiting). Its mode of action is to stimulate the chemical trigger zone (CTZ) in the medulla. However,

Apomorphine

like morphine, apomorphine is a CNS depressant. Therefore, if a suitable dose does not evoke emesis, successive doses are equally unsuccessful. Because rats are incapable of emesis, apomorphine can be used as a dopamine agonist for experimental purposes without concern for this side effect. Apomorphine-induced emesis in dogs frequently provides the standard in the assessment of the potency of antiemetic drugs such as chlorpromazine and other phenothiazines.

Because apomorphine is a potent dopamine agonist, it has been tried as an antiparkinsonian compound. It was found to be effective but caused abnormal formation of urea in the blood. Therefore, its use as an antiparkinsonian compound has been discontinued (Barbeau, 1978).

Applied iontophoretically upon DA cells, apomorphine inhibits their firing rate, as does d-amphetamine and methylphenidate. As might be expected, intravenous haloperidol and chlorpromazine (both potent dopamine receptor blockers) also block DA-induced inhibition of A10 cells. However, neither the α-antagonist piperoxane nor the β-antagonist sotalol showed any blocking activity. Thus the autoreceptors, at least in A10, are uniquely dopaminergic (Bunney and Aghajanian, 1978).

An interesting observation was reported on the effects of apomorphine on schizophrenic patients (Tamminga et al., 1978). The patients had prominent schizophrenic symptoms despite ongoing neuroleptic drug treatment. When they were given additional low doses of apomorphine (3 mg), they showed an immediate reduction of symptoms that lasted for about an hour. Some temporarily stopped hallucinating and others lost their delusions. The suggestion put forward by these investigators was that the presynaptic dopamine autoreceptor may have a higher affinity for apomorphine at low doses than the postsynaptic receptor, thus blocking DA synthesis and release.

Bromocriptine

Bromocriptine is an ergot derivative having DA agonist properties similar in many respects to those of apomorphine. Interest in this drug arose because of the possibility that it might be an effective antiparkinsonian agent. It is most effective against tremor, but only secondarily, at much higher doses, is it effective against akinesia (the inability to initiate a voluntary act or to stop one that is in progress). Although it does improve motor performance in parkinsonian patients, it does have side effects—nausea, vomiting, and abnormal involuntary movements. The use of this drug is still under experimental study (Barbeau, 1978).

Dopamine Release Blockers

Aside from depleting stores of DA, blocking its synthesis, or destroying its terminals, there is no specific drug that will block the release of DA. Destroying DA terminals with 6-hydroxydopamine (6-OHDA), will block the release of this transmitter, but this effect is irreversible.

Summary

A summary of dopaminergic drugs is presented in Table II. It should be appreciated that any compound that blocks the synthesizing enzymes tyrosine hydroxylase (e.g., α-methyl tyrosine) will block the synthesis of NE as well as of DA. Also, monoamine oxidase inhibitors will increase NE as well as DA levels in presynaptic terminals. Drugs that block dopamine-β-hydroxylase may block the conversion of DA to NE and thus increase the stores of DA. Chase et al. (1974) reported an attempt to raise endogenous striatal dopamine levels in parkinsonian patients by blocking dopamine-β-hydroxylase with fusaric acid. This treatment had no reliable effect on otherwise untreated patients. This result may be explained by an insufficient number of NE terminals in the striatum to provide the necessary increase of DA. We also mentioned earlier that compounds that cause vesicular release of neurotransmitters (e.g., reserpine) will in all probability be quite unselective, thereby causing the release of DA in addition to NE and serotonin. And last but not least, one should recognize that alterations in the physiology of any transmitter probably have indirect effects on other transmitters as well and that any drug effect is probably due to complex interactions among a number of neural mechanisms.

Part IV Behavioral Significance of Catecholamine Systems

Catecholamines and Reward

Studies of the functional significance of the catecholaminergic systems in the CNS and of their target centers indicate that catecholaminergic systems are the central adjunct to the peripheral noradrenergic sympathetic system. This means that the autonomic homeostatic mechanisms that control hunger and digestion, thirst and drinking, blood pressure and heart rate, respiration and body temperature, sexual expression and aggression all have their CNS noradrenergic and dopaminergic counterparts. It is believed that these central NA and DA systems respond to cues that

TABLE II   Drugs That Affect Dopamine Synapses

Drug	Mechanism of action	Major effects
ANTAGONISTS		
Chlorpromazine Fluphenazine Thioridazine Haloperidol Spiroperidol γ-Hydroxybutyrate	Receptor blockers	Tranquilizations, antipsychotic, and antinauseant
AGONISTS		
Apomorphine Piribedil Bromocriptine	Receptor stimulants	Antiparkinsonian and emetic
Amphetamine	Releases synaptic DA and blocks DA reuptake	Stimulant, anorexic
VESICLE DEPLETERS		
Reserpine Tetrabenazine	Block storage	Antihypertensive, tranquilization, and antipsychotic
REUPTAKE INHIBITORS		
Benztropine	Pump inhibitor	Antiparkinsonian
Amphetamine Cocaine Amantadine	Pump inhibitors	Stimulant, euphoriant
SYNTHESIS INHIBITORS		
α-Methyl-p-tyrosine	Tyrosine hydroxylase inhibition	Depressant
α-Methyldopa hydrazine (Carbidopa)	Dopa decarboxylase inhibition	
MAO INHIBITORS		
Iproniazid Pargyline Tranylcypromine	Broad spectrum MAO inhibition	Antidepressant
Clorgyline	Type A MAO inhibition	Experimental
Deprenyl	Type B MAO inhibition	
COMT INHIBITORS		
Tropolone Pyrogallol	COMT inhibition	Minimal effects
TOXIN		
6-Hydroxydopamine	Destroys DA cells	Experimental

emate from the external and internal environments and initiate and direct overt *behaviors* essential to self- and species preservation. We can develop this idea by considering the now familiar study by Olds and Milner (1954), who demonstrated that rats could be taught to lever-press to stimulate certain areas of their own brains. This phenomenon led to the conclusion that the stimulation had positive reinforcing effects.

Anatomical Considerations

Later studies showed that intracranial self-stimulation (ICS) rates seemed to be highest in those sites where CA neurons were most densely concentrated and that areas that were not CA innervated did not seem to support ICS. This was particularly true for the medial forebrain bundle (MFB). This fiber tract showed a high concentration of NE neurons and supported very high rates of ICS. Also, there was evidence that stimulating ICS loci caused a release of catecholamines and that damage to the CA systems or administration of drugs that blocked CA receptors or CA synthesis led to a proportional suppression of ICS. On the other hand, administration of drugs that enhanced transmission at CA synapses increased ICS rates (e.g., amphetamine, methamphetamine, phenethylamine, and monoamine oxidase inhibitors such as iproniazid, pargyline, and tranylcypromine). The MAO inhibitors probably had this effect by blocking the intraneuronal breakdown of CAs, thus raising the available supply of CAs for synaptic action (Stein, 1968; Stein and Wise, 1970, 1974).

Catecholaminergic brain areas and fiber systems that support ICS may play a crucial role in response acquisition and frequency. Indeed it has been proposed that the fibers that originate in the richly CA-staining locus caeruleus and that course rostrally in the dorsal noradrenergic bundle and MFB to the hypothalamus, limbic structures, and neocortex make up a "noradrenergic reward system" that serves in a significant way to increase response rates of behaviors having positively rewarding consequences (Stein et al., 1973; Wise et al., 1973). Somewhat later, other catecholamine systems were given a role in the "reward" process, namely, two dopaminergic fiber tracts—the mesolimbic and the nigrostriatal dopaminergic systems (German and Bowden, 1974).

Criticisms of the Catecholamine Reward Theory

Fibiger (1978) reviewed many of the studies that attempted to specify the nature of reinforcement mechanisms more precisely. The studies focused upon intracranial self-stimulation and its neural and biochemical substrates.

Neuroanatomy and ICS Rates. Causal implications could not be drawn from the correlational data of the presence of NA fiber systems at most electrode sites that support intercranial self-stimulation because NA systems are rather widespread in the brain. Even in the case of the MFB, there are other types of fibers in this fiber tract and in surrounding areas that could be responsible for high ICS from MFB electrodes.

Damage to NA Systems and Resultant ICS Rates. Experiments showed that intracisternal injections of 6-OHDA and other drugs that severely deplete brain NE had no effect on ICS rates; and lesions that destroyed the locus caeruleus and depleted cortical NE by 80 percent or more failed to attenuate ICS. Other lesions depleted brain NE by 97 percent without affecting amphetamine-facilitated ICS.

On the other hand, bilateral lesions of the locus caeruleus led to a decrease in cortical NE levels and a significant reduction in the rate of increase in running speed for food rewards during consecutive days of testing in an L-shaped runway with rats. It was suggested that the damage to this NE system impaired learning (Anlezark et al., 1973). Other investigators (Sessions et al., 1976) found that lesions of the locus caeruleus did not produce deficits in learning one-way active or passive shock avoidances, in acquisition or extinction of conditioned taste aversions, or in acquisition of lever-pressing responses for food reinforcements. However, they, like Anlezark et al., did find deficits in the increase of running speeds for food in L-shaped runways. These results failed to support a general learning role for the NE system arising from the locus caeruleus, though the deficits in the increase of running speeds could not be traced to any observed motor impairment during a battery of screening tests designed to identify such abnormalities. All of the treated animals eventually ran at normal speeds, although they required more training to do so.

Pharmacological Studies. Drugs that enhanced NE activity and ICS rates also enhanced dopamine activity, and drugs that blocked NE synthesis (e.g., α-methyl-p-tyrosine) and reduced ICS rates obviously blocked DA synthesis as well. This made it difficult to determine which transmitter, NE or DA, was involved in the effect. However, studies by Wise and Stein (1969) and Stein and Wise (1970) seemed to support a noradrenergic reward hypothesis. They blocked the conversion of DA to NE in rats by blocking the enzyme action of dopamine-β-hydroxylase with disulfiram and diethyldithiocarbamate (DDC) and with two newer, more specific compounds, U-14624 and fusaric acid (Stein, 1978). This treatment decreased ICS rates, and the effect could be reversed by subsequent intraventricular infusions of NE. However, Roll (1970) observed that disulfiram induced sedation and sleep during long pauses in bar-pressing and concluded that the lowered ICS rates could have been due to the nonspecific sedative effects of the drug, especially as the ICS current was at threshold intensities. She also observed that the sedated rats would bar-press for short times if they were dragged over and placed upon the bar. Rolls et al. (1974) obtained data that supported those of Roll. They found that disulfiram, as well as the α-nonadrenergic antagonist phentolamine, lowered arousal (as measured by locomotor activity and rearing) at doses that also lowered ICS of the lateral hypothalamus. Moreover, spiroperidol (a dopamine receptor blocker) suppressed arousal least and suppressed ICS the most (Figure 27).

Stein (1978) responded to these criticisms by pointing out that extinction of self-stimulation by turning off brain-stimulating currents also produces intermittent bar-pressing and sleep. This implies that the drowsiness reported by Roll was the consequence of the drug-induced loss of NE-mediated reinforcement and not the cause for it. In response to the conclusions of Rolls et al., Stein rightly pointed out that rearing and locomotion are probably not independent of reward effects. It is known that rats eagerly explore new environments and then go to sleep as the novelty wears off, that is, the reward value diminishes and extinction occurs. Thus, it could be argued that the disulfiram's depressant action on locomotion and rearing could have been due to an accelerated decline in the rewarding effects of novel stimulation and was a parallel effect and not a causal effect of the depression of the ICS rate. (For further discussion of these issues, see Stein, 1978.)

These experiments have raised some questions about the hypothesis that NA systems are essential for the maintenance of ICS, or for that matter whether NE plays a significant role in reinforcement at all. Moreover, the data seem to point to an essential role for dopamine. We will now consider some of Fibiger's arguments in support of that idea.

Dopaminergic Reward System

We have already pointed out that Rolls et al. (1974) found that spiroperidol suppressed ICS. Other neuroleptic drugs such as haloperidol, pimozide, and pipamperone also suppressed ICS when the ICS electrodes were in the lateral hypothalamus (Wauquier and Niemegeers, 1972). However, there was a question of whether the effects of the drugs were due to a reduction of the reinforcing value of the brain stimulation or to an impaired ability to perform the operant response. This latter consideration is significant. Dopamine is an important transmitter in the striatal system, which integrates motor behavior, and neuroleptic drugs (which block DA receptors) disrupt many types of learned responses, suggesting a common denominator, that is, a motor deficit.

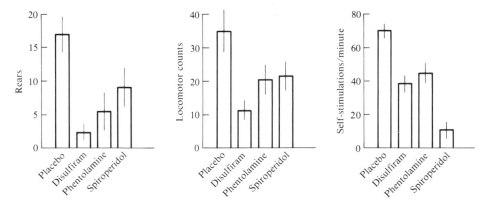

FIGURE 27   DISULFIRAM AND PHENTOLAMINE EFFECTS. Although disulfiram and phentolamine partially attenuated self-stimulation, they also produced sedation as shown by reductions in rearing and locomotor counts. In contrast, spiroperidol attenuated self-stimulation much more than arousal. Each column represents the mean ± SE. (From Rolls et al., 1974.)

Neuroleptic Drugs and Reinforcement Mechanisms

A number of strategies have been used to answer the "reinforcement versus performance" question. Spiroperidol depressed ICS responding but similarly depressed bar-pressing for food and water. The same doses had minor effects on eating and drinking in the home cage after 24 hours of food and water deprivation. This showed that hunger and thirst were not strongly affected by the drug. Spiroperidol depressed response rates equally well when the ICS electrodes were in nondopaminergic and dopaminergic areas. Some experiments reported that DA blocking drugs had a greater inhibitory effect on response rates for ICS than for food reward, but in these instances the baseline response rate for ICS was about six times higher than it was for food. We have already remarked that drug effects can be proportional to baseline rates so that these differences in drug effects may not have meant very much. Fibiger et al. (1976) attempted to clarify this situation by testing the effects of haloperidol on equal response rates on a VI-60 second schedule for ICS or food. In this experiment, the drug-induced depressions of response rates for the two reinforcers were the same. These studies suggested that the drug interfered with mechanisms involved with the initiation and maintenance of operant behavior rather than with the reward process.

Wise (1978) examined the mechanism of action of dopamine antagonists on ICS. Although it was clear that these drugs decreased ICS rates, he also raised the question as to whether this effect was due to a specific effect on catecholamine reward systems or whether the effect was due to a nonspecific performance deficit caused by the commonly observed sedative effects of these drugs. Relevant to a solution of this problem was the finding that pimozide at a dose that depressed ICS rates actually increased lever-pressing rates in rats that were self-injecting the psychomotor stimulants amphetamine and cocaine. At higher doses of pimozide, there was an early period of accelerated responding for self-injection followed by cessation of lever-pressing. These findings are understandable if one first appreciates what undrugged rats do during self-injection of stimulants. These animals wait several minutes between responses, suggesting that each self-injection is temporarily satiating. When the animal is treated with pimozide, the "reward" value of the stimulant is presumably reduced, causing the animals to press at a

higher rate to make up the deficit. At higher pimozide doses, the rewarding effect of the psychostimulants is completely blocked; thus, extinction of lever-pressing occurs. However, self-stimulation is not satiating. If brain-stimulating current is lowered, reduced reward immediately leads to reduced response rates. Increased pimozide doses (0.125 to 0.5 mg/kg) lead to lowered self-stimulation rates in the same manner as that caused by graded reduction of stimulation current intensity. Furthermore, rats with ICS experience, when tested without brain-stimulating current, will initially lever-press at normal rates before extinction. Likewise animals pretreated with an extinction-producing dose of pimozide will show a similar pattern, presumably because brain-stimulating current, although available, has no rewarding effect.

These studies show that in all cases dopamine receptor blockers caused a deterioration of lever-pressing performance; after high doses of pimozide, the decline in performance was typical of situations wherein rewards are completely withheld. With low doses, the increase in performance rates resembled the activity seen with reward reduction. These findings thus support the contention that neuroleptic drugs do not disrupt lever pressing per se. Rather, by blocking the dopaminergic component of the reward system, they can either increase or decrease response rates according to the rewarding and satiating features of the incentives.

Lesion Studies of Dopaminergic Systems

In examining the effects of lesions in DA systems upon response rates for ICS, the question of the reward versus the performance aspects of the response again appears. Although it has been shown that intraventricular injections of 6-OHDA produced extensive lesions of central DA neurons and long-term depression of ICS, the effect could be due to lesion-induced motor impairments or changes in the reward value of the brain stimulation. Phillips et al. (1976) attempted to answer the question by implanting an electrode unilaterally in the striatum of rats and establishing baseline ICS rates. After baseline establishment, 6-OHDA-induced lesions were made in the ipsilateral or contralateral substantia nigra (zone compacta), which contains the cell bodies of the DA fiber terminals in the striatum. Total brain DA dropped by 95 percent. The ipsilateral 6-OHDA lesions caused a 90 percent drop in ICS, whereas contralateral lesions caused a drop followed by recovery to 72 percent of control by the twenty-eighth postoperative day. These results were interpreted to mean that the ipsilateral lesion caused a motor deficit that was added to the loss of brain stimulation reward due to the drop in brain DA; the contralateral lesion affected the response by producing only a temporary motor deficit plus a longer-lasting loss of reward value for ICS.

In a similar experiment by Clavier and Fibiger (1977), the ICS electrodes were placed in the substantia nigra (SN) and ipsilateral or contralateral lesions were made (with 6-OHDA) in the fibers leading from the SN to the striatum. Ipsilateral lesions caused a large but temporary drop in ICS rates (the ICS rate returned to normal 8–10 days postoperatively). The same result was obtained by contralateral lesions. It was concluded (1) that unilateral lesions caused transient motor deficits and (2) as shown by the ipsilateral lesion, that this pathway from SN to the striatum was not the exclusive nor essential neuronal pathway responsible for the reinforcing properties of nigral ICS. Thus, it is probable that systems other than DA systems can support responses for brain self-stimulation.

Summary

This discussion has considered the role of the catecholaminergic systems in ensuring the acquisition and repetition of behavior having rewarding consequences. Intracranial self-stimulation (ICS) was assumed to represent the "purest" example of a stimulus–reinforcement system, and the system's anatomical and neurochemical substrates were examined. The evidence to date suggests that data from ICS studies can be easily reconciled with data from other stimulus–response systems. Therefore, ICS continues to serve as an acceptable model to study reinforcement mechanisms. At the present time it appears that NA systems are at best only correlationally related to ICS. A better case can be made for a significant role for DA systems in ICS phenomena. However, disruption of DA systems by surgical lesions or pharmacological methods has multiple effects. Isolating the "reward" effects from motor deficits and changes in subtle response-initiating mechanisms requires highly sophisticated experimental strategies and cautious interpretations. Finally, there is some evidence that systems other than CA systems can be functionally related to ICS phenomena, a situation that requires further study.

Differential Drug Effects on Dopaminergic Systems

Effects of Amphetamine

A common feature of behavior following low doses of amphetamine in rats (0.25–1.0 mg/kg) is general activation consisting of sniffing, locomotion, and rearing. Gradually increasing the dose in the 1–10 mg/kg range leads to a decrease in locomotion and rearing so that only sniffing remains. At 10 mg/kg, the sniffing response becomes maximally stereotyped and is accompanied by licking and biting that is typically performed in a small confined area at the bottom of the cage. After a single large dose given subcutaneously, the animal's behavior goes through the same stages that are followed by increasing amphetamine doses.

These same effects are seen after amphetamine administration to many other animal species. Stereotypy may take many forms and depends upon the animal species, the dose of amphetamine, time after injection, environmental conditions, and previous experiences. For example in mouse, rat, and guinea pig, there is sniffing, licking, and biting; in cats, looking from side to side, sniffing, and grooming activities; in dogs, circling and running to and fro on a fixed route; in monkeys, grooming, staring, seizing bars, and repertoires of body and limb movements, chewing, protrusions of the tongue, and jerking of the neck and shoulders. In humans, amphetamine elicits stereotypies of bathing, house cleaning, mechanical work on machinery (cars), continuous sorting of the contents of one's purse, combing hair, persistent repetitions of words or sentences, walking the street; in some cases there is compulsive examinations of the skin and attempts to dig out imagined encysted parasites (Randrup et al., 1975).

Mediation of Amphetamine Effects by Dopaminergic Systems

There is abundant evidence that dopamine alone is responsible for the locomotor effects and the stereotypy induced by amphetamine. First, α-methyl-p-tyrosine (which blocks DA and NE synthesis) reduced the locomotor effects of amphetamine; but U-14624 (a dopamine-β-hydroxylase inhibitor that blocks the synthesis of NE from DA) failed to block the amphetamine effect. Thus, DA is necessary for the effect but NE is not (Weissman et al., 1966; Hanson, 1967; Hollister et al., 1974; Breese and Cooper, 1975). Furthermore, the nucleus accumbens, which has a dense noradrenergic innervation in addition to many dopaminergic nerve endings, might be mediating the amphetamine effects through its NA input. However, neither the α-NA receptor blocker phentolamine nor the β-NA receptor blocker propranolol, when injected into the nucleus accumbens, blocked amphetamine-induced locomotion.

Other studies have shown that neither α- nor β-adrenergic receptor blockers alter the stereotypic behaviors in animals or the euphoria in man induced by amphetamine. High doses of noradrenergic receptor blocking drugs reduced d-amphetamine-induced exploratory behavior in rats but only at doses that caused severely depressed activity in control animals. Furthermore, when DA was injected directly into the nucleus accumbens of rats that had been pretreated with an MAO inhibitor, there was an enhancement of locomotor activity. This effect was diminished by the DA receptor blocker haloperidol but not by phentolamine. Also, injection of haloperidol into the nucleus accumbens, but not in the striatum, blocked the locomotor effect of amphetamine. But, again, this blocking effect did not occur with injections of phentolamine or propranolol. Thus, amphetamine-induced locomotor activity is largely mediated by a DA system, whereas the role of NA systems seems obscure (Moore, 1978).

The overall conclusions from these studies are that dopaminergic neurons seem to be more sensitive to the uptake-blocking and DA-release effects of amphetamine than NA neurons and that the behavioral effects of amphetamine-type drugs are largely due to the activation of DA systems (Randrup et al., 1975). The consequences of these studies was that more attention has been directed to the role of different structures of the DA system to differentiate the behavioral effects of catecholamine agonists.

Effects of Agonist Drugs on the Mesolimbocortical and the Nigrostriatal Dopaminergic Systems

The two major dopaminergic pathways to the forebrain are the mesolimbocortical (MLC) and the nigrostriatal systems (Figures 6 and 7). These two systems seem to be the focal points for amphetamine-induced locomotor and stereotyped behaviors. There is considerable evidence that amphetamine-induced locomotor activity is mediated by the MLC DA neurons whereas stereotypic behavior is related to the activity of the nigrostriatal neurons. The evidence for this may be summarized as follows.

1. Microinjections of DA, d-amphetamine, and other DA agonists directly into the nucleus accumbens (of the MLC system) increased locomotor activity, whereas similar injections into the caudate nucleus (of the nigrostriatal system) did not have this effect.
2. DA antagonists (e.g., haloperidol) blocked the locomotor effects of d-amphetamine injected into the nucleus accumbens, but noradrenergic receptor blockers (e.g., phentolamine and propranolol) did not. Also, injections of DA antagonists directly into the nucleus accumbens blocked the locomotor effects of systemic injections of amphetamine, but injections of DA antagonists into the caudate nucleus did not.
3. Injections of haloperidol into the caudate nucleus blocked amphetamine-induced behavior stereotypies.
4. Destruction of MLC neurons with 6-OHDA injected into the nucleus accumbens blocked the locomotor effects of d-amphetamine but not the drug-induced stereotypic behavior. The opposite effects occurred when 6-OHDA was injected into the striatum.
5. In animals with 6-OHDA lesions in the nucleus accumbens or the striatum, apomorphine (a direct DA agonist acting on DA receptors) had an enhancing effect on locomotion and stereotypic behavior, probably as a result of the development of receptor supersensitivity in these two regions (Moore and Kelly, 1978; Moore, 1978).

Summary

Amphetamine and related drugs such as N-methamphetamine and methylphenidate block reuptake and enhance the release of DA and to some extent NE. The NE effects are particularly manifest in the peripheral autonomic nervous system, and centrally NE appears to play a significant role in intracranial self-stimulation. With respect to the frequently demonstrated locomotor and stereotypic behavior elicited by amphetamine, the evidence favors the view that DA activity is enhanced in the MLC and the nigrostriatal systems, respectively, for these two phenomena. The evidence consists of demonstrations that amphetamine-induced locomotor and stereotypic behavior was abolished by inhibiting DA synthesis but not by inhibiting NE synthesis. Also, amphetamine effects were blocked by DA receptor blockers, but not by NA receptor blockers; and the selective destruction of MLC or nigrostriatal neurons with 6-OHDA interfered with amphetamine-induced locomotor and stereotypic behavior, respectively.

Amphetamine effects are suppressed by AMPT, which blocks DA synthesis. This suggests that newly synthesized pools of DA are released and confined in the synaptic space by reuptake blockade. The rapid availability of this source of DA could account for the central sensitivity of DA systems to amphetamine. In the periphery, the sympathomimetic effects of amphetamine depend upon NE release. Reserpine blocks the peripheral but not the central effects of amphetamine. Reserpine depletes the NE storage vesicles and blocks the transport of DA into the storage vesicles (where it is acted upon by DBH to form NE). In the absence of any significant DA innervation in the periphery (except for SIF cell activity), amphetamine effects in the periphery depend upon NE release (Moore, 1978).

Catecholamines and Homeostasis

A further appreciation of the role of CA systems can be found amidst the prodigious efforts to understand motivational systems as they pertain to feeding. Long before it was known that there were important CA systems coursing through the brain stem and forebrain or how to detect them, a number of animal studies appeared that suggested feeding behavior could be manipulated by selective lesions in the diencephalon. The same was true for drinking behavior, temperature regulation, aggression, and other behaviors relating to homeostasis. This was not surprising because there already was an abundance of clinical evidence showing that brain stem lesions from invasions of neoplasms, stroke, and degenerative diseases produced the same effects. The literature covering this subject is so extensive that the mere citation of representative references would take many pages. Consequently, as this discussion develops we will cite only a few recent reviews in the text and more in the suggested reading list at the end of this chapter. These can serve as a beginning source for readers who wish to pursue these matters in greater depth and detail.

Effects of Lesions in Catecholaminergic Systems on Ingestive Behavior

Lesions that disrupted feeding behavior in many instances were found to be accompanied by widespread depletion of brain norepinephrine and dopamine (Ungerstedt, 1974a). Earlier conceptions of neural mechanisms of feeding proposed that there were hunger centers and satiety centers that were triggered by nutritional needs or the lack thereof, possibly via hormonal vectors. It later developed that the lesions in the ventromedial hypothalamic nucleus, which were presumably responsible for hyperphagia, and in the lateral hypothalamic nucleus, which were responsible for aphagia (loss of appetite), were not critical for those particular nuclei. Rather, lesion effects were better understood in terms of disrupted catecholaminergic pathways that coursed in the vicinity of the treated sites. Ahlskog and Hoebel (1973) claimed that lesions in the ventromedial nucleus caused hyperphagia by interrupting the ascending ventral noradrenergic bundle, and Gold (1967) and Ungerstedt (1974b) presented evidence suggesting that lateral hypothalamic lesions produced aphagia by interrupting the ascending dopaminergic nigrostriatal bundle. This latter finding has been confirmed repeatedly (Stricker and Zigmond, 1974), although there is a strong possibility that the nigrostriatal bundle is involved with the motor coordination associated with eating rather than with appetite regulation. Leibowitz (1971, 1974b) showed that discrete applications of CA agonists and antagonists in the paraventricular nucleus of the hypothalamus, which has an extensive noradrenergic input, elicits vigorous eating and drinking. It should not be concluded from the foregoing that the hypothalamus and the catecholaminergic bundles associated with it serve as hunger and satiety centers controlling food intake. Evidence now suggests that nutritional needs are signaled to the brain from the liver, and as we shall see these brain centers probably serve to give direction and vigor to eating behavior (Friedman and Stricker, 1976).

Zigmond and Stricker (1974) and Stricker and Zigmond (1974) have reviewed a number of their own studies and those of others detailing the effects of damage to dopaminergic systems on feeding and other homeostatic functions. They were able to deplete selectively dopamine or norepinephrine from the brain by intraventricular injections of 6-hydroxydopamine (6-OHDA) alone and in combination with other drugs.

This drug is taken up by CA nerve terminals and destroys them, thereby causing substantial depletions of catecholamines. Given by itself, 6-OHDA mainly destroys NE terminals, but pretreatment with the MAO inhibitor pargyline causes destruction of both NE and DA terminals. By combining administration of 6-OHDA with systematic pargyline and desmethylimipramine (DMI), which blocks the uptake pump of NE neurons, a selective depletion of dopamine was obtained.

The general appearance of rats treated with 6-OHDA alone was largely indistinguishable from control rats given the vehicle solution. The DA-depleted animals did not eat when challenged by high doses of 2-deoxy-*D*-glucose (2-DG) (a drug that produces a functional hypoglycemia), although they did show the usual compensatory autonomic responses such as increased glycogenolysis in response to hypersecretion of epinephrine from the adrenal glands. However, with gradually increased doses of hypoglycemic drugs over a 2–3 week period, the DA-depleted rats did overeat. Similar effects were obtained by bilateral lesions of the nigrostriatal dopamine bundle.

Rats were shaved and subjected to acute cold stress (5 °C). Normal rats were able to maintain their body temperature and significantly increased their food intake. However, shaved rats with lesions of the lateral hypothalamus showed appropriate thermoregulation but did not increase their food intake during the first 48-hour period of exposure. In another experiment, rats were treated with subcutaneous polyethylene glycol (which causes a loss of plasma fluid). Normals showed an immediate thirst with lowered urine volume. 6-OHDA-treated rats showed lowered urine volume but no increase in fluid intake (Stricker et al., 1975).

These results revealed that 6-OHDA rats failed to behave normally during severe homeostatic imbalances even though physiological responses seemed to be intact. Rats with small lateral hypothalamic lesions showed similar deficits, suggesting that brain CA depletion impairs the expression of motivated ingestive behaviors. In a sense these observations are similar to those obtained with animals that are deprived of adrenergic fibers of the sympathetic nervous system or undergo the removal of the adrenal medulla. In a benign environment these animals appear quite normal, but when these sympathectomized animals are stressed by hemorrhage, hypoglycemia, or cold, they

often die. On a different scale, these effects are similar to the action of transplanted hearts whose sympathetic and parasympathetic input unfortunately must be severed. Transplanted hearts beat quite normally, but they do not respond to stress or increased demand by increasing heart rate.

When rats were treated with 6-OHDA, pargyline, and DMI (resulting in more specific and complete DA depletion), the animals were hypokinetic and ataxic, displayed rigidity in the hind limbs, and failed to respond to sensory stimuli. Most important, these animals were aphagic and adipsic and had to be intubated with food and water to survive. This syndrome was also similar to that produced by lateral hypothalamic and nigrostriatal lesions. In addition, both animals with electrolytic lesions and animals with 6-OHDA lesions could ultimately be induced to eat by first offering them highly palatable foods and fluids and gradually switching them over to lab chow and water. This is an illustration of the well-known fact that the mere taste of food can serve as a powerful stimulus to eating. Nevertheless, these animals did not show increased ingestive behaviors when challenged by acute glucoprivation, dehydration, and cold stress.

Lesions in Dopaminergic Systems and Parkinsonism

As previously noted, parkinsonism is related to the destruction of the dopaminergic nigrostriatal fibers emanating from the zona compacta of the substantia nigra with a consequent loss of DA in the caudate nucleus and putamen. How then can L-dopa compensate for the loss of nigrostriatal fibers when active DA terminals are needed to convert L-dopa into transmitter DA? Hornykiewicz (1974) explains this in part by pointing to the high rate of activity of the remaining nigrostriatal fibers in parkinsonian patients, as judged by the ratio of DA to its metabolite HVA in the striatum. This finding is supported by studies with rats, which showed that partial destruction of the nigrostriatal DA pathway increased the turnover of labeled DA (formed from [³H]tyrosine) in the remaining DA neurons. It can be concluded (1) that compensatory mechanisms have already begun in response to damage to DA neurons as judged by the fact that even an extensive DA deficiency is correlated with only mild symptomatology, and (2) that parkinsonism represents a late decompensated stage due to progressive deterioration of DA neurons and a 70 to 90 percent decrease in dopamine levels. Thus, more severe symptoms do not appear until the damage is nearly total. (3) The efficacy of L-dopa rests on its ability to serve as a substrate for the increased synthesis rate and release of DA and the availability of this DA to the striatal postsynaptic receptors. Thus, L-dopa is able to revert the decompensated stage of the DA deficiency to a state of functional recompensation.

The Neurochemistry of Recovery of Function

Earlier sections of this chapter have mentioned that there are a number of mechanisms that are called into play when there is a drop in the effective concentrations of synaptic neurotransmitters. When receptors are blocked, there is an increase in transmitter synthesis and release. This in turn is responsible for the induction of increased synthesizing enzyme production. Furthermore, when transmitters are depleted by disrupting presynaptic fibers, by using synthesis blockers such as α-methyl-p-tyrosine, or by reserpine (which interferes with vesicular storage) supersensitivity devel-

ops in receptor membranes and is correlated with increased numbers of receptor molecules.

An explanatory model for partial recovery of ingestive behavior following subtotal nigrostriatal lesions is shown in Figure 28. There is ample evidence to support the hypothesis that recovery of function is the result of compensatory mechanisms that develop within the synaptic area. First, there is an increase in CA synthesis rate and turnover in fibers that were spared from the disruptive lesion. Second, there is a decrease in uptake in CA fibers that is probably due to a decrease in affinity for uptake as well as to the loss of uptake sites. The decrease in uptake has the probable consequence of increasing the duration of synaptic transmitter action. Third, the sensitivity of postsynaptic membranes of treated rats is increased. This idea is based on the finding that L-dopa increases the motor activity of 6-OHDA-trated rats at an L-dopa dose that is ineffective in nontreated controls. Also, there is increased binding of haloperidol (a dopamine receptor blocker) to striatal dopamine receptors after 6-OHDA-induced

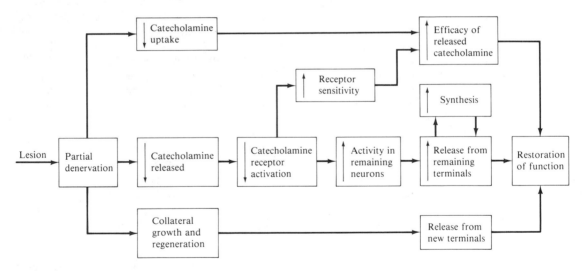

FIGURE 28   RECOVERY OF FUNCTION FOLLOWING NEURAL DAMAGE. Immediately following administration of the lesion, a reduced release of CAs occurs because of the reduced number of CA neurons that remain. Though the loss of some neurons also reduces the number of uptake sites and increases the efficacy of the released amines, there will be still a net loss of receptor stimulation. This has the effect of reflexly inducing an increased release of CAs from the residual neurons. This, in turn, induces more CA synthesis through the induction of tyrosine hydroxylase to sustain the increase of CA turnover. At the same time, an increased sensitivity of postsynaptic receptors further increases the effectiveness of the released CAs and promotes the recovery of function. Collateral growth from intact axons and regeneration from damaged fibers may also contribute to recovery of function, although the nature of these processes is unknown. (From Zigmond and Stricker, 1974.)

lesions of the nigrostriatal dopamine bundle (Creese et al., 1977). Further support for these conjectures comes from the fact that rats with greater than 98 percent depletion of striatal dopamine never seem to recover ingestive functions, even after extensive efforts to wean them from tube feeding, whereas rats with 90 to 98 percent depletion show gradual recovery from aphagia and adipsia. Thus, there seems to be a minimum number of intact terminals for effective compensation. What is surprising is the paucity of the required number of terminals, indicating the extraordinary range of tissue damage that can be overcome.

Another supporting observation is that recovery of function requires, as expected, some time for its development. That is, shortly after the administration of nigrostriatal lesions, aphagia and adipsia are very persistent, probably because the compensatory physiological changes have not had a chance to develop. There is even some evidence that some compensation can occur in quite usual ways. Powley and Keesey (1970) found that if rats were subjected to food deprivation just prior to receiving small lateral hypothalamic lesions, they were able to avoid the brief postoperative aphagia and adipsia. This suggests that the induced hunger was sufficient to initiate postsurgical eating.

The foregoing material is gratifying because we see an example of the confluence of neurochemical, neuroanatomical, and behavioral data that give substantial insights into the role of catecholaminergic systems as they pertain to exceedingly complex interactions between physiological and behavioral factors of homeostasis. Perhaps there is significance in the fact that the noradrenergic branch of the autonomic nervous system (sympathetic) plays a major role in visceral function, whereas the noradrenergic and dopaminergic systems play a complementary role in the diencephalon. Certainly, gaps remain in our knowledge, but these observations and speculations can inspire high levels of confidence that more and more of the story about the brain and behavior will be forthcoming.

Recommended Readings

Angrist, B. and Sudilovsky, A. (1978). Central nervous system stimulants: historical aspects and clinical effects. In *Handbook of Psychopharmacology, Vol. 11* (L.L. Iversen, S.D. Iversen and S.H. Snyder, Eds.), pp. 99–165, Plenum Press, New York.

Antelman, S.M. and Caggiula, A.R. (1977). Norepinephrine-dopamine interactions and behavior. *Science*, 195, 646–653. The presentation of a new hypothesis concerning stress-related interactions between brain norepinephrine and dopamaine.

Biel, J. H. and Bopp, B.A. (1978). Amphetamine: structure-activity relationships. In *Handbook of Psychopharmacology, Vol. 11* (L.L. Iversen, S.D. Iversen and S.H. Snyder, Eds.), pp. 1–39. Plenum Press, New York. Excellent coverage and extensive reference lists on the development, biochemistry, physiology, behavioral effects and clinical significance of amphetamine-like drugs.

Fuxe, K., Hökfelt, T., Agnati, L.F., Johannson, O., Goldstein, M., Perez de la Mora, M., Possani, L., Tapia, R., Teran, L., and Palacios, R. (1978). Mapping out central catecholamine neurons: immunohistochemical studies on catecholamine-synthesizing enzymes. In *Psychopharmacology: A Generation of Progress* (M.A. Lipton, A. DeMascio and K.F. Killam, Eds.), pp. 67–94. Raven Press, New York. A review of the central distribution of catecholamine systems.

Guroff, G. (1975). Some aspects of aromatic amino acid metabolism in the brain. In *The Nervous System, Vol. 1, The Basic Neurosciences* (D.B. Tower, Ed. in chief), pp. 553–564. Raven Press, New York. A clear account of the structure and action of the pteridines.

Jacobowitz, D.M. (1978). Monoaminergic pathways in the central nervous system. In *Psychopharmacology, A Generation of Progress* (M.A. Lipton, A. De Mascio and K.F. Killam, Eds.), pp. 119–129. Raven Press, New York. A good review of monoaminergic pathways.

Lindvall, O. and Björklund, A. (1978). Organization of catecholamine neurons in the rat central nervous system. In *Handbook of Psychopharmacology, Vol. 9, Chemical Pathways in the Brain* (L.L. Iversen, S.D. Iversen and S.H. Snyder, Eds.), pp. 139–222. Plenum Press, New York. A detailed treatise on the catecholamine systems in the rat brain.

McGeer, P.L., Eccles, J.C. and McGeer, E.G. (1978). *Molecular Neurobiology of the Mammalian Brain.* Plenum Press, New York. An outstanding review of the anatomy, physiology, neurochemistry and function of the nervous system.

Moore, K.E. (1978). Amphetamines: biochemical and behavioral actions in animals. In *Handbook of Psychopharmacology, Vol. 11, Stimulants* (L.L. Iversen, S.D. Iversen and S.H. Snyder, Eds.), pp. 41–98. Plenum Press, New York. A review of animal studies on the action of amphetamines.

Musacchio, J.M. (1975). Enzymes involved in the biosynthesis and degradation of catecholamines. In *Handbook of Psychopharmacology, Vol. 3, Biochemistry of Biogenic Amines* (L.L. Iversen, S.D. Iversen and S.H. Snyder, Eds.), pp. 1–35. Plenum Press, New York. A review of MAO inhibitors.

Sedvall, G. (1975). Receptor feedback and dopamine turnover in CNS. In *Handbook of Psychopharmacology, Vol. 6, Biogenic Amine Receptors* (L.L. Iversen, S.D. Iversen and S.H. Snyder, Eds.), pp. 127–177. Plenum Press, New York. A thorough review of dopamine synthesis control.

CHAPTER EIGHT

Serotonin

Part I Physiology and Neuropharmacology of Serotonergic Systems

Rapport et al. had been searching for the vasoconstrictor component in the serum of clotted blood that might be a possible cause of cardiovascular hypertension. They finally isolated this substance and named it serotonin, to suggest its origin from blood *serum* that has *tonic* effects upon the cardiovascular muscles (1948). In 1951 Erspamer and Boretti isolated a substance from the mucous membranes of the gastrointestinal tract that caused contractions of smooth muscles. It was later established that serotonin and Erspamer's substance, enteramine, were one and the same.

Further extensive investigation demonstrated that this substance was found in the blood and intestinal tract of virtually every animal species, as well as in such diverse places as the venom of certain amphibians, wasps, and scorpions; the salivary glands of the octopus; and the nematocysts of the sea anemone. Serotonin was also found in many plants and fruits. Interestingly, it is abundant in pineapples and in the pulp of bananas (at the relatively high concentration of 28 μg/gm).

Studies with humans, dogs, and rats showed that the substance is widely distributed in the animal body (Twarog and Page, 1953). It is found not only in blood serum and the digestive tract, but also in the spleen, liver, lungs, and skin; and it was these authors who first reported its consistent presence in nervous tissue. It is now estimated that in humans 90 percent of the body's serotonin occurs in the mucous membrane of the digestive tract, 8 to 10 percent in the blood

platelets, and 1 to 2 percent in the central nervous system. Within the brain, the highest concentration occurs within the pineal gland (Snyder, 1972).

Shortly after Rapport's discovery, the chemical identity of serotonin was elucidated; and this was quickly followed by its synthesis. Serotonin was identified as an indolealkylamine: 5-hydroxytryptamine (5-HT) or more specifically, 3-(2-aminoethyl)indol-5-ol.

The chemical formula of 5-HT revealed a close relationship to the dietary amino acid tryptophan (α-aminoindole-3-prop from which ionic acid) 5-HT is synthesized. Similarly its degradation was found to be primarily a process of deamination. A number of drugs were found that affected serotonin's synthesis and metabolism, and serotonin was found to play a role in a number of diseases. It was suspected that serotonin might play a significant role in mental illness, but many suggestive leads have turned out to be unproductive.

An early review reported that there was no conclusive evidence for any specific physiological role for serotonin in an organ system but that it was probably a chemical mediator of some sort (Maupin, 1961). Two decades later, a prodigious amount of research on this substance has clearly defined a role for serotonin as a neural transmitter subserving a number of important physiological and psychological functions.

A variety of methods, both chemical and biological, were developed for the identification of 5-HT. The chemical methods included chromatographic and fluorimetric techniques. The biological techniques measured the effects of various concentrations of 5-HT on contractions of annular sections of sheep carotid artery and on contractions of rat uterus. One of the most sensitive techniques was developed in 1943 by Welsh, who found that concentrations as low as 0.00018 μg/ml induced measurable contractions in the heart of the large mollusc *Venus mercenaria* (Welsh, 1954).

The histochemical fluorescence technique (Hillarp et al., 1966) enabled accurate CNS localization of 5-HT neurons. The technique involves an interaction of serotonin with formaldehyde in the presence of protein to yield fluorescent 3,4-dihydro-β-carboline. The fluorescence emission peak differs from that of the blue-green emissions of catecholamines and is seen as yellow, with a maximum emission peak at 525 nm.

3,4-Dihydro-β-carboline   5,6-Dihydroxytryptamine

Another technique for studying the distribution of serotonergic fibers involved the use of the neurotoxin 5,6-dihydroxytryptamine (5,6-DHT), modeled after the catecholamine neurotoxin 6-hydroxydopamine (6-OHDA) (Björklund et al., 1974). Incubation of brain tissue with radioactive 5,6-DHT showed that the neurotoxin was readily taken up by the serotonergic neurons. Although 5,6-DHT is also taken up by NE and DA neurons, the affinity for 5-HT neurons is about seven times higher than that for the CA neurons. 5,6-DHT also gives rise to a yellow to yellow-green fluorescence after formaldehyde treatment and thus can be visualized fluorimetrically. 5,6-DHT causes a degeneration of unmyelinated axons and nerve terminals, signs of which appear as early as 2 hours after drug injection, although adjacent nonserotonergic neurons are generally unaffected.

It is of related interest to note that 5,6-DHT causes a selective decrease of brain 5-HT. However, in some parts of the brain, there is some recovery of 5-HT levels. Björklund et al. (1974) injected 5,6-DHT into the ventricles of rats and examined whole brains after various intervals (3 hours to 6 months). They found, for example, that there was a 90 percent depletion of brain 5-HT after 1 day and the effect was the same 6 months later. On the other hand, in the hypothalamus,

after 1 day the depletion was 60 percent, but after 6 months there was a 30 percent increase over the normal level. There also was evidence that the damaged axons sprouted new extensions. This was a finding of considerable interest because regrowth of damaged axons within the CNS indicates a kind of repair that is generally thought not to be possible in higher organisms.

Distribution of Serotonergic Neurons in the Central Nervous System

For the most part the cell bodies of 5-HT neurons are localized in nuclei of the raphe and reticular region of the lower brain stem. Dahlström and Fuxe (1964) described nine 5-HT-containing nuclei, labeled B1 to B9 (Figure 1). It is estimated that the nuclei contain an average of a few thousand cells each. Other authors have given anatomical names to some of these nuclei and these are given in parentheses (Chan-Palay, 1977). The caudal group, consisting of B1 (raphe pallidus), B2 (raphe obscurus), and B3 (raphe magnus) is located in the ventromedial area of the medulla-pons. These cells give rise to axons that descend in the spinal cord and terminate in the cervical and lumbar enlargements and the sacral segments (Jacobowitz, 1978). The 5-HT terminals of these axons are found in the dorsal, intermediate (sympathetic), and ventral horns of the spinal cord.

The axons of the pontine and mesencephalic raphe nuclei (B4–B9) make up the ascending 5-HT pathways (Figure 1B). Neurons from B7 (raphe dorsalis) and B8 (raphe medianus) account for about 80 percent of the forebrain serotonin terminals, and therefore can be considered as the major source of the ascending pathways (Azmitia, 1978). In the rat, the principal ascending 5-HT pathways consist of medial and lateral bundles along the ventral aspect of the medial forebrain bundle (MFB) (Dahlström and Fuxe, 1965; and Fuxe and Jönsson, 1974). The medial (subcortical) pathway emanates from the mesencephalic raphe nuclei B7 and B8, and from those of the pons, B5 (raphe pontis) and B6 (not otherwise named). This pathway innervates the limbic structures, especially by fibers from raphe medianus (Cooper et al., 1978), the hypothalamus and the preoptic area. The lateral (cortical) pathway also emanates from the mesencephalic group B7, B8, and B9 (nucleus centralis superior), and innervates the cingulate cortex. A third minor pathway, the far lateral 5-HT pathway, similarly originates from B7–B9, and primarily innervates the extrapyramidal motor pathways whose origins are in the caudate nucleus. The

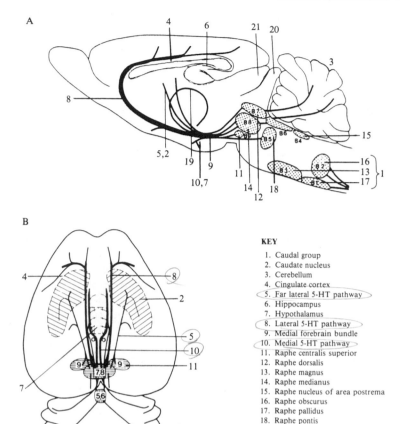

KEY

1. Caudal group
2. Caudate nucleus
3. Cerebellum
4. Cingulate cortex
5. Far lateral 5-HT pathway
6. Hippocampus
7. Hypothalamus
8. Lateral 5-HT pathway
9. Medial forebrain bundle
10. Medial 5-HT pathway
11. Raphe centralis superior
12. Raphe dorsalis
13. Raphe magnus
14. Raphe medianus
15. Raphe nucleus of area postrema
16. Raphe obscurus
17. Raphe pallidus
18. Raphe pontis
19. Stria terminalis
20. Inferior colliculus
21. Superior colliculus

FIGURE 1 SEROTONERGIC NUCLEI AND PATH-WAYS in the rat brain. (A) Medial view showing ascending and descending fiber systems emerging from the serotonergic nuclei of the brain stem. Most of the cell groups, except B3, B6, and B9, lie alongside the midline (the raphe). The exceptional ones lie more laterally in the reticular formation. Nuclei B1, B2, and B3, the caudal group, give rise to descending pathways; the rest to ascending pathways. (B) Horizontal view showing the medial ascending 5-HT pathway from B5-B8 that innervates limbic structures, the hypothalamus, and the preoptic area. The lateral pathway from B7-B9 innervates the cingulate cortex. The far lateral pathway innervates the caudate nucleus, which is part of the striatum and gives rise to extrapyramidal motor systems. Cerebellar connections arise from B7 and B8, and possibly from B5 and B6. (After Fuxe and Jonsson, 1974.)

cerebellum is also innervated by 5-HT neurons, those that emerge from B7, B8, and possibly from B5 and B6. Fibers from B4 (nucleus of the area postrema) also contribute to the medial forebrain bundle (Fuxe and Jonsson, 1974). The ascending pathways were first found to project to the suprachiasmatic nucleus of the hypothalamus, the globus pallidus, certain amygdaloid nuclei, and the ventral part of the lateral geniculate nucleus. However, because the 5-HT content of some ascending fibers was very small, special procedures were necessary to make them visible by histochemical treatment. The special process involved the use of MAO inhibitors and precursor loading to selectively increase the brain levels of 5-HT. In this way, very fine 5-HT neurons were traced to the septal area, the superior colliculi, the hippocampus and into the neo- and mesocortex.

Other techniques were used to localize 5-HT

pathways, and the overall results were quite consistent with one another. For example, Pierce et al. (1976) injected radioactive proline (an amino acid) into the dorsal raphe nucleus in cats. This was rapidly taken up by the serotonergic cells and distributed to the end terminals. Using autoradiographic techniques, she traced serotonergic fibers in the medial forebrain bundle, the diagonal band of Broca, stria medullaris, stria terminalis, cingulate bundle, fornix, and the fasciculus retroflexus. Other fibers, few in number, were dispersed within the periaquaductal gray, the medial longitudinal fasciculus, and the tegmentum. Descending fibers were traced to the medulla. The terminals were localized in the rostral terminal sites described by other authors, but probably because of the restricted injection area in her study, Pierce and her co-workers found only a very light projection to the ventral lateral geniculate and no projection to the caudate nucleus.

A detailed study by Geyer and his associates (1976a) described the extent of selective lesions among the raphe nuclei of rats and related them to changes in 5-HT synthesizing enzymes in 5-HT axon terminals in the forebrain. For example, lesions in the dorsal raphe (B7) led to decreased enzyme activity in the striatum, thalamus, cortex, and hypothalamus; whereas lesions in the median raphe (B8) caused enzyme decrement in septal nuclei, hippocampus, cortex, and hypothalamus. In this way they established two distinct, though possibly overlapping, serotonergic systems innervating the forebrain.

In a companion study, Geyer et al. (1976b) compared the extent of raphe lesions to behavioral changes in rats. The general findings were that raphe lesions induce hyperactivity and hyperresponsivity. They concluded that a pathway originating in the median raphe (B8) exerts some of the inhibition necessary to control behavioral responsivity. This result supported the findings of Jacobs et al. (1974), who made selective lesions either in the median or dorsal nuclei of the raphe and found that lesions in the median raphe significantly increased locomotor activity in rats, which is presumed to be a disinhibitory effect. This effect was correlated with a selective depletion of hippocampal serotonin (82 percent depletion after a median raphe lesion, versus a 10 percent depletion following a dorsal raphe lesion).

The role of the serotonergic system would be better understood knowing the afferent inputs to the raphe nuclei. Whereas histochemical studies revealed that catecholamine neurons innervate the raphe, it was not clear what the origins of those fibers were. However, using horseradish peroxidase (HPR) researchers have been able to clarify this issue. HPR is injected into the raphe nuclei where it is taken up by axon terminals innervating these cells and carried by retrograde axoplasmic flow back to the perikarya of those axons (which can be identified by suitable staining techniques). Aghajanian and Wang (1977) using this technique found afferent fibers that originated in the prefrontal cortex, the spinal cord, cerebellum, the rostral basal forebrain, the preoptic and lateral region of the hypothalamus, the medial forebrain bundle, the brainstem reticular formation, the nucleus solitarius, and perhaps most strikingly in terms of selectivity and density, the lateral habenula. This latter pathway is considered to serve a pivotal role in funneling information from the limbic forebrain to the limbic midbrain area. Azmitia (1978) has summarized similar findings from other investigators and these are illustrated in Figure 2.

In summary, whereas serotonergic neurons comprise less than .01 percent of neurons in the brain (which is comparable to the concentration of noradrenergic neurons in the CNS) serotonergic axons ramify widely throughout the brain with many forebrain structures projecting back to the raphe via similar routes. Other brain structures feed back to the raphe by intermediary structures such as the habenula which receives hippocampal and amygdaloid inputs. Axons from the habenula seem to terminate in areas immediately surrounding the clusters of the raphe cells, suggesting that habenula-induced effects are mediated through raphe interneurons (Aghajanian and Wang, 1978). There are also serotonergic influences (mostly inhibitory) on neuroendocrine systems by virtue of pathways from the medial and dorsal raphe nuclei to hypothalamic nuclei and the median eminence where hormone releasing factors are secreted and concentrated in response to stress and other events calling for homeostatic modulation. The raphe cells also maintain contacts with nonneuronal elements such as glial cells, blood vessels, the subarachnoid space and even the ventricular fluid (Azmitia, 1978).

Neurophysiology of Serotonin Systems

The serotonergic neurons of the raphe in the rat brain are characterized by a regular and slow spontaneous firing rate of about 0.5–2.5 spikes/sec. This autoactivity is very constant among the various nuclei; it has been found in the brain of three-day-old rat pups

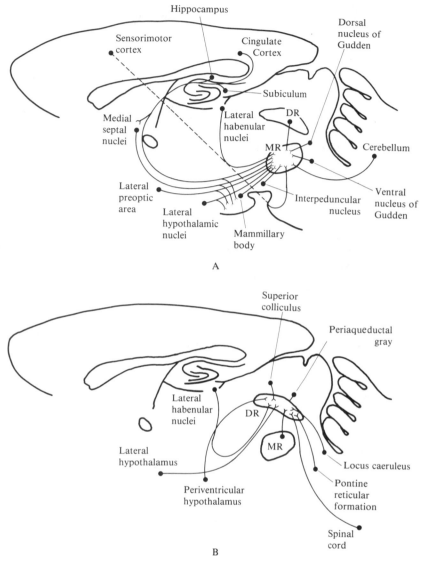

FIGURE 2   AFFERENT PATHWAYS TO THE RAPHE
NUCLEI. (A) Afferent pathways to the median raphe nu-
cleus (MR). (B) Afferents to the dorsal raphe nucleus (DR).
(After Azmitia, 1978.)

and can even be observed in serotonergic tissue *in
vitro*. In the unanesthesized cat, the firing rate ranged
from 0.5–5.0 spikes/sec in the awake state. Microiontophoretic applications of 5-HT have inhibitory effects
upon raphe neurons as does raising brain levels of
5-HT by supplying its precursor 5-hydroxytryptophan
(5-HTP). This indicates that the pacemaker-like con-

stancy of the raphe cell activity can be maintained by
axon collaterals and autoreceptors mediating 5-HT effects upon themselves. Any increase in firing rate
would cause an increase in collateral inhibition which
would tend to dampen the increase, whereas any decrease in firing rate would diminish collateral inhibition and thereby oppose a further decrease in firing

rate. Also, the fact that there are reciprocal connections among the raphe nuclei suggests a mutual inhibition among them (Aghajanian and Wang, 1977).

The constancy of the firing rates is resistant to any but extreme external stimuli. However, chronic single cell recordings indicate that the firing is all but eliminated during REM or dream sleep, or when the pontine reticular formation is stimulated, an area that projects an inhibitory pathway to the dorsal and median raphe nuclei. The cells in the pontine reticular formation selectively increase their firing rate just prior to the onset of REM sleep and maintain their high activity during the entire REM sleep episode (Aghajanian and Wang, 1978).

The axons that emerge from the raphe are fine (0.15–1.5 μm in diameter) and unmyelinated and have a slow conduction velocity (about 0.5–1.5 m/sec), and firing rates of from 0.1 to 5.0 spikes/sec. Labeled 5-HT axons in the frontal parietal cortex of the rat contained dense core vesicles and had varicosities (0.7 μm in diameter) about every 1 to 3 μm, but it was estimated that only about 5 percent of them made synaptic contacts. The 5-HT axon terminals in many instances similarly showed few postsynaptic specializations suggesting that serotonergic neurons can invade a neuropil more extensively by not being encumbered by rigid synaptic connections. This arrangement further suggests that these neurons are involved in a neuromodulator capacity, biasing the neuronal activity of a region rather than supplying precise information from one part of the brain to another. The postsynaptic effect of serotonergic terminals is usually a short latency (5–15 msec) long-lasting inhibition of from 50–400 msec, which compensates for the slow firing rate, and is compatible with a neuromodulator role for this system. It has also been established that there is a substantial network of interconnections among serotonergic, NE, and DA systems which provides a mechanism for coordinating these systems (Azmitia, 1978).

Part II Serotonin Neurochemistry

Serotonin Synthesis

Tryptophan Uptake and Hydroxylation

Figure 3 shows the steps of serotonin synthesis and degradation. The primary precursor is tryptophan, which is one of the least plentiful among the dietary amino acids. It is an "essential" amino acid, meaning that (unlike tyrosine) it cannot be synthesized in mammalian cells. Consequently, diets low in tryptophan can have profound effects on neural levels of 5-HT. Eating foods rich in 5-HT has no appreciable effect on brain levels of the amine as 5-HT does not pass the blood brain barrier. There is evidence that there are cyclic fluctuations of plasma tryptophan levels, as well as of other amino acids, during each 24-hour day. This also influences brain levels of 5-HT (Fernstrom and Wurtman, 1974). It should be noted that the conversion of tryptophan to 5-HT is a minor metabolic pathway for tryptophan and represents only 1 percent of tryptophan turnover.

Tryptophan is taken up from blood plasma by cells in the brain primarily by an active, high-affinity transport process, although Hamon et al. (1974) report that in synaptosomes there is a low-affinity process as well. These investigators have also shown a high- and low-affinity transport of tryptophan in glial cell preparations. Glial and synaptosomal uptake may buffer the overall availability of tryptophan for neurons by absorbing excess tryptophan and releasing it when it is needed.

Within neurons, tryptophan is hydroxylated in the 5-position to form 5-hydroxytryptophan (5-HTP). This synthetic step requires the enzyme tryptophan hydroxylase, a pteridine cofactor (which is probably tetrahydrobiopterin), and oxygen. The marked sensitivity of the synthetic process to oxygen is shown by the fact that breathing pure oxygen elevates brain concentrations of 5-HT several fold in rats.

Tryptophan hydroxylase is synthesized in neuronal cell bodies and undergoes axonal transport to the nerve terminals, where 5-HT synthesis occurs (Meek and Neff, 1972). Attempts to purify and identify tryptophan hydroxylase by subcellular fractionation of pig brain stem revealed a particulate fraction that accounted for about 65 percent of the enzyme activity and a soluble fraction that accounted for 25 percent (Moussa et al., 1974). The particulate fraction is assumed to be associated with serotonergic synapses,

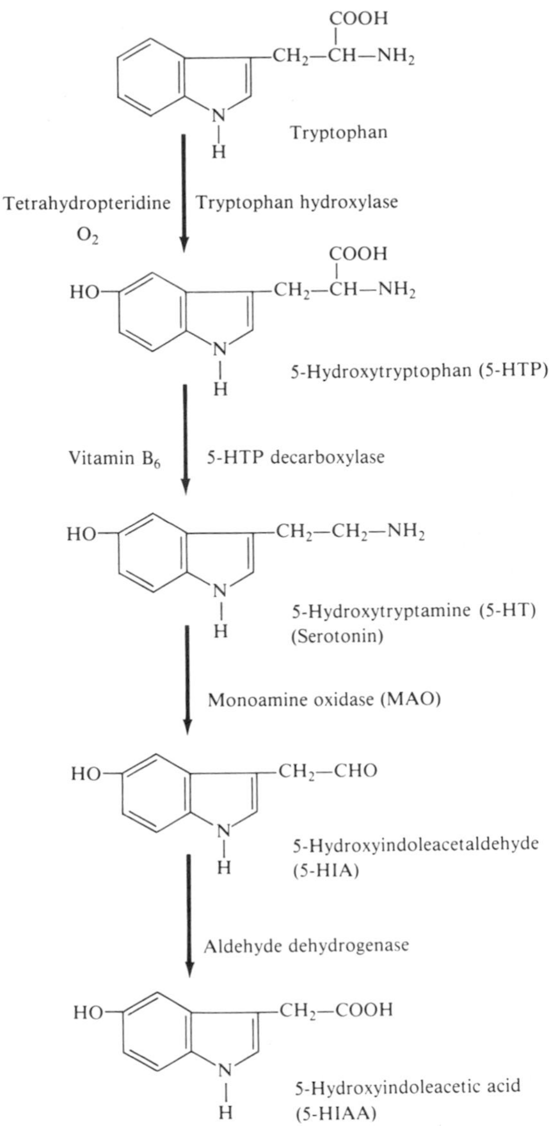

FIGURE 3 SYNTHESIS AND CATABOLISM OF SERO-
TONIN. The enzymes involved in the reactions are on the
right of the arrows, the cofactors are on the left.

whereas the soluble fraction is more likely linked to the
perikaryal cytoplasm (Cooper et al., 1978). As expected, the highest enzyme activity was found in beef
and rat pineal gland and in rat and rabbit brain stem.

The chemical p-chlorophenylalanine (PCPA) has a
high, irreversible affinity for tryptophan hydroxylase

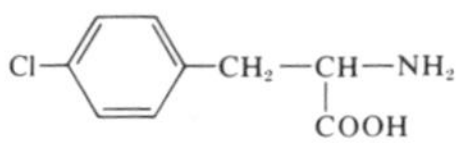

p-Chlorophenylalanine

and thereby blocks the synthesis of 5-HTP and 5-HT.
A single intraperitoneal injection of 300 mg/kg of
PCPA in a rat lowers cerebral serotonin to less than 20
percent within 3 days, and the level does not return to
normal for up to 2 weeks—the time it takes to synthesize new stores of tryptophan hydroxylase (Koe and
Weissman, 1966). This and other experiments showed
that brain 5-HT levels paralleled the activity of tryptophan hydroxylase when it was deactivated by PCPA,
suggesting that tryptophan hydroxylase was the rate-
limiting factor in 5-HT synthesis. However, other
studies have shown that tryptophan hydroxylase has a
Michaelis constant (K_m) for its substrate that is much
higher than the total concentration of tryptophan in
the mammalian brain (Lovenberg et al., 1968).
Therefore, the enzyme is probably unsaturated, or in
other words, there is more than enough enzyme present to catalyze all the tryptophan that is available at a
given time. This view agrees with the previously mentioned statement that a low plasma level of tryptophan
caused by dietary deficiencies or cyclic variations
lowers CNS levels of 5-HT (Fernstrom and Wurtman,
1974). Furthermore, a study by Goodwin and Post
(1974) showed that the accumulation of the 5-HT
metabolite, 5-hydroxyindoleacetic acid (5-HIAA), in
the cerebrospinal fluid of humans was raised by exogenous administration of tryptophan and lowered by
PCPA (Figure 4). If we assume that the rate of accumulation of 5-HIAA is an index of 5-HT synthesis
and metabolism, then these data support the idea that
within certain limits the plasma tryptophan level is also
a rate-limiting factor in 5-HT synthesis.

5-Hydroxytryptophan Decarboxylation

In the next stage of 5-HT synthesis, 5-HTP
undergoes decarboxylation to form 5-HT. (That is, a
hydrogen atom is substituted for the carboxyl group
that is removed from the α-carbon on the side chain.
The α-carbon is the first one to the left of the amine
group.) This reaction involves the enzyme 5-HTP decarboxylase (5-HTP-D) and pyridoxal phosphate (vitamin B_6). The decarboxylase in this reaction was
formerly presumed to be identical to DOPA decarboxylase (DOPA-D). 5-HTP-D and DOPA-D both have

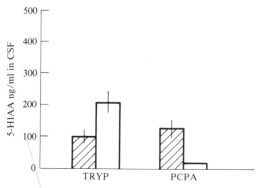

FIGURE 4 TRYPTOPHAN AND PCPA EFFECTS ON CEREBROSPINAL 5-HIAA. Tryptophan (TRYP) increases and PCPA diminishes the accumulation of the metabolite 5-HIAA. The patients were pretreated with probenecid to prevent the transport of 5-HIAA from the CSF. Open bar is the drug period; shaded bar is the control period. (After Goodwin and Post, 1974.)

a very high K_m. Thus, there is always a surplus of decarboxylating enzymes so that all available substrate (DOPA or 5-HTP) is easily converted to dopamine or serotonin, respectively. The surplus of decarboxylating enzymes accounts for the fact that only small amounts of DOPA and 5-HTP can be recovered from blood or brain plasma.

However studies have shown that there are significant differences between the two enzymes. First, decarboxylation activity in brain homogenates for DOPA-D and 5-HTP-D differed with respect to optimal pH, temperature, and level of available substrate (reviewed by Cooper et al., 1978). Furthermore, Sims (1974) reported that the decarboxylase activities are different in homogenate subfractions. He showed that 5-HTP-D activity was almost four times greater than DOPA-D activity in synaptosomal and mitochondrial subfractions. Additional evidence for differences between DOPA-D and 5-HTP-D was found in the experiment by Sims and Bloom (1973). They gave rats intracisternal injections of 6-hydroxydopamine, which is selectively absorbed into adrenergic nerve terminals and destroys them. After drug treatment, the same tissue sample showed that a marked fall in DOPA levels was paralleled by a marked decline in DOPA-D activity (⅓ to ½ of control). However, there was no decrease in 5-HTP-D activity. Also, there was a surprising selective increase in 5-HTP-D activity in hypo-

thalamus, cerebellum, and the medulla-pons areas of the brain. These findings point to highly specific decarboxylating enzymes for NE and 5-HT synthesis (Green and Grahame-Smith, 1975). On the other hand, antibodies to hog kidney DOPA-D will react equally well with DOPA-D and 5-HTP-D, implying that the two enzymes are immunologically very similar (McGeer et al., 1978).

Serotonin Synthesis Regulation

We have described the role of tryptophan hydroxylase and its precursor, tryptophan, in 5-HT synthesis. In this section we will examine arguments about other mechanisms that control 5-HT synthesis. For catecholamine and acetylcholine synthesis, we saw that increases in synthesis rate were proportional to the activity and demands of the respective system, and that decreases in synthesis occurred by means of end-product inhibition. The evidence to support these conclusions came from studies of peripheral neurons that were clearly adrenergic or cholinergic, and the assumption was made that similar events occur for these transmitters centrally. However, as there seem to be no purely serotonergic neural systems in the periphery, control mechanisms for 5-HT synthesis are more hypothetical.

There is some evidence that increased demand results in an increased 5-HT turnover,* and thus, presumably, there is increased synthesis. For example, subjecting rats to foot shock stimulated central 5-HT turnover (Thierry et al., 1968) and increased synthesis occurred in heat-stressed mice (Hamon et al., 1974). Also, deprivation of paradoxical sleep increased 5-HT synthesis (Hery et al., 1970). Carlsson (1974) reported that after acute spinal transection (which severed descending serotonergic axons) there was a 50 percent decrease of 5-HTP formation in the spinal cord of rats. This effect occurred before there could be a loss of enzyme molecules and was attributed to a change in activity of tryptophan hydroxylase resulting from the absence of nerve impulses.

Feedback inhibition has been investigated by Macon et al. (1971), who measured the rate of conversion of intracisternal radioactive tryptophan ([3H]-TRP) to [3H]-5-HTP in rats previously treated with MAO inhibitors pheniprazine or pargyline. At first there was a

*Turnover rates reflect the rate of incorporation of a labeled precursor such as [3H]tryptophan into an end product such as [3H]5-HT, or [3H]5-HT into [3H]5-HIAA.

Pheniprazine

significant rise in brain levels of nonradioactive 5-HT, to two- and threefold higher than normal. However, after the initial increase in [³H]-5-HT, there was a 40 percent decline. These results were interpreted to mean that the high rise of nonradioactive 5-HT caused by the MAO inhibitors eventually blocked synthesis of [³H]-5-HT from [³H]-tryptophan. This would be consistent with the end-product inhibition of 5-HT synthesis.

Despite the foregoing evidence, Cooper et al. (1978) reported that MAO inhibitors caused a two- to three-fold increase in brain accumulation of 5-HT and that the blockade of efflux from the brain of the 5-HT metabolite 5-HIAA by the drug probenecid also caused a linear rise in 5-HIAA levels for prolonged periods. This suggests that the initial synthesis step is not significantly affected by any of the naturally occurring end products and that feedback inhibition is at best trivial.

Carlsson (1974) reported that after administration of the MAO inhibitor pargyline there was a 60 percent increase in mouse brain 5-HT, and this in turn caused a significant drop of 5-HTP synthesis. The 5-HTP was measurable because a 5-HTP decarboxylase inhibitor was simultaneously administered. This finding indicated the existence of some feedback control.

Another study showing feedback inhibition utilized chlorimipramine, a drug that blocks reuptake of 5-HT. The drug raised the concentration of synaptic 5-HT and retarded 5-HTP synthesis in the central nervous system in rats. Carlsson also found that the depletion of 5-HT with reserpine *increased* 5-HTP formation in rat brain but not in mouse brain. All of these studies support the idea that tryptophan hydroxylase activity can be modulated to some extent by nerve impulses and by intra- and extraneuronal concentrations of 5-HT.

Carlsson suggested a mechanism of synthesis regulation whereby nerve impulses deplete a strategic intraneuronal pool of 5-HT that controls tryptophan hydroxylase activity. He favored the view that 5-HT alters the conformation of the enzyme molecule and thereby renders it less active. He also cited the study by Aghajanian and Haigler (1974), who showed that 5-HT neurons can be inhibited by local applications of 5-HT. Thus, feedback control could be mediated in-

directly by altering nerve impulse frequency. Macon et al. (1971) proposed that feedback inhibition is due to the blockade of tryptophan transport into the cells. Clearly, the issue of synthesis regulation and its mode of action does not seem to be settled and more work is needed (Glowinski et al., 1973; Green and Grahame-Smith, 1975).

Serotonergic Receptors

Little is known about the precise chemical structure of neurotransmitter receptors. However, information is available with respect to the locus of serotonergic receptors and their interactions with certain drugs (Garattini and Valzelli, 1965). Gaddum (1958) identified two types of 5-HT receptors, M and D, in peripheral sites. The M-receptor is blocked by morphine and atropine, and the D-receptor is blocked by phenoxybenzamine, LSD, methysergide, and cyproheptadine. The differential drug effects makes it possible to delineate the receptor site in different organs and species. For example, rat uterus is similar to rat stomach and rat colon. All contain D-receptors because they are all insensitive to the inhibitory action of morphine.

The M-receptors are presumably in neural tissue (sympathetic ganglia or postganglionic fibers to guinea pig intestines); the D-receptors are located in smooth muscle fibers. To distinguish these receptors from cholinergic receptors, tests were performed with cholinergic blocking agents. M-receptors were blocked by neither hexamethonium nor large doses of nicotine, thus arguing for their specificity for 5-HT. Both receptor types were found in the guinea pig ileum* as either morphine or phenoxybenzamine alone only partially antagonized effects of 5-HT, even when drug concentration was high.

In other attempts to identify the serotonergic receptor, Fiszer and DeRobertis (1969) did *in vitro* binding experiments on subcellular fractions of cat brain. They observed that the highest affinity for [¹⁴C]-5-HT occurred in nerve-ending membranes isolated from the hypothalamus, basal ganglia, and gray areas of the midbrain. All of this correlated well with histochemical studies showing the locus of 5-HT terminals.

*In the intestines, 5-HT is probably not of neural origin. Rather, it is found in the enterochromaffin cells of the mucosa. In response to internal pressure, 5-HT is released into the gut lumen, where it then stimulates receptors and causes smooth muscle contraction.

Their chemical analysis suggested that the receptor was a PROTEOLIPID (a macromolecule containing protein and lipid components). What was not clear, however, was whether these receptor sites were on pre- or post-synaptic membranes.

Affinity chromatography is another technique used to identify receptor structure. A tissue suspected of having 5-HT receptors is prepared and incubated in a solution containing 5-HT, some of which binds to the receptors. After the incubation period, the 5-HT–receptor mixture is washed with a solution containing a drug that is known to have either a stimulating or a blocking effect on 5-HT receptors. It is assumed that the drug will bind to the receptor and displace the 5-HT. Then the receptor will be carried out of the tissue mixture, where the drug–receptor combination can be analyzed. Shih and her co-workers (1974) obtained tissue samples from the hypothalamus and spinal cord of rats, and washed them with solutions of LSD and chlorimipramine (CIP), two drugs that have different effects on 5-HT systems. Two different proteins were obtained by this method—each bound to a single drug. Because LSD seems to act upon cells as a transmitter and because CIP blocks reuptake of 5-HT, the evidence suggested that LSD was bound to post-synaptic receptors and CIP was bound to presynaptic receptors. However, these data alone do not validate this idea.

Shih et al. repeated the preceding procedures after pretreatment of the rats with intraventricular injections of 6-hydroxydopamine (a drug that destroys noradren-ergic nerve terminals). The results were the same, indi-cating that the serotonin-binding proteins were not lo-cated in the membranes of noradrenergic cells.

Serotonergic Autoreceptors

An early study by Chase et al. (1967) showed that LSD blocked the release of 5-HT from rat brain slices containing 5-HT terminals. In their experiment, brain slices were taken from rats that received intracisternal injections of radioactive 5-HT, or rat brain slices were incubated in vitro with the labeled amine. In both cases, when the brain slices were electrically stim-ulated, there was a release of the labeled exogenous 5-HT that had previously been taken up by the seroto-nergic cells. The amount of release was correlated with the endogenous 5-HT content of the tissue studied. However, when the tissue was treated with LSD, the re-lease of 5-HT was reduced by about 63 percent. This could mean that LSD affected autoreceptors that were on 5-HT terminals and that blocked the release of 5-HT.

Later experiments have shown that 5-HT does in-hibit raphe neurons, which suggests that 5-HT auto-receptors may occupy sites on the soma of 5-HT neurons and that 5-HT neuron terminals and 5-HT autoreceptors could be responsible for feedback ef-fects (Aghajanian and Haigler, 1974). For example, if large amounts of 5-HT were released into the synaptic cleft, receptors on the presynaptic terminals could act to prevent further release. Or receptors on the soma could respond to serotonergic inhibition via recurrent collaterals or by other serotonergic cells in the raphe region. Strong evidence in support of this view comes from the observations that MAO inhibitors, which block 5-HT catabolism; L-tryptophan, which stimulates 5-HT synthesis; and drugs that block 5-HT reuptake all depress the firing rates of raphe neurons (Aghaja-nian et al., 1970). The common mechanism resulting in the depressed firing rate is an increase in the availabil-ity of 5-HT, which can act upon local autoreceptors (Aghajanian et al. 1975). It also turns out that these autoreceptors are more sensitive to LSD than to 5-HT. Thus it appears that drugs that have a direct action on 5-HT autoreceptors and those that increase 5-HT availability induce an inhibition of 5-HT neuronal fir-ing (Figure 5) (Aghajanian and Wang, 1978).

Termination of 5-HT Action in the Synaptic Cleft: The Reuptake Process

Termination of the effects of 5-HT in synaptic func-tion occurs in two ways, by an uptake process, which recycles the transmitter for continued use, and by degradation (catabolism) of the transmitter. Although the details of 5-HT catabolism have been clearly established, the process probably plays a minor role in terminating the action of 5-HT at the synaptic junc-tion. The most likely terminating process is the reup-take of 5-HT by the presynaptic terminal (Kuhar et al., 1974). Small amounts of 5-HT injected into the cere-brospinal fluid rapidly accumulate in neurons con-taining 5-HT, and labeled 5-HT is rapidly taken up by brain tissue containing 5-HT synaptosomes. A high-affinity uptake of $[^3H]$-5-HT by synaptosomes in rat brain homogenates was blocked when the homoge-nates were prepared from rats that had lesions of the raphe nuclei that caused the loss of the end terminals. It is true that under the experimental conditions described above 5-HT is also taken up by catechola-

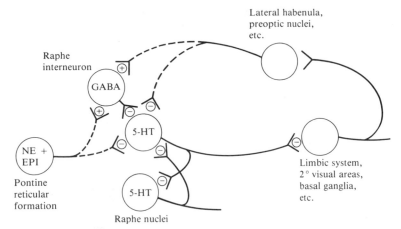

FIGURE 5 ANATOMICAL CONNECTIONS OF THE RAPHE NUCLEI. Inhibitory synapses are indicated by circled minus signs, excitatory synapses by plus signs. Dashed lines indicate uncertain connections. Reciprocal connections are proposed between the raphe and limbic systems and secondary visual areas. The feedback connections pass through the lateral habenula and preoptic nuclei. These connections project directly or via GABAergic inhibitory interneurons upon the 5-HT neurons. Direct 5-HT to 5-HT inhibitory collaterals are shown. A direct and indirect inhibitory pathway from the reticular formation is also shown. This innervation may be both adrenergic and noradrenergic (Fuxe et al., 1978). (From Aghajanian and Wang, 1978.)

minergic end terminals. But under normal conditions the concentration of 5-HT is probably too low for this to occur.

A number of drugs have been found that block the 5-HT reuptake process, and these potentiate the action of 5-HT systems. This would not be as likely if the reuptake system played a secondary role to 5-HT catabolism.

Serotonin Catabolism. The first step in serotonin catabolism involves oxidative deamination by monoamine oxidase. MAO is quite abundant intra-and extraneuronally and is located on mitochondrial outer membranes. Type A MAO is the most potent isoenzyme for 5-HT deamination. In the oxidative deamination process, the terminal carbon loses the amine group and becomes doubly bonded to oxygen (oxidized) to form an aldehyde. The resulting product is 5-hydroxyindoleacetaldehyde (5-HIA) (Figure 2). In the next step 5-HIA is further oxidized by aldehyde dehydrogenase to form 5-hydroxyindoleacetic acid (5-HIAA). 5-HIAA enters the cerebrospinal fluid and the bloodstream and is eventually excreted.

We cannot assume that urine levels of 5-HIAA indicate levels of 5-HT activity in the brain, as urine levels of 5-HIAA also reflect the rate of 5-HT metabolism in the gut and elsewhere. A better indication of 5-HT activity in the brain is the level of 5-HIAA in the cerebrospinal fluid and brain after the animal has been pretreated with probenecid, a drug that blocks acid transport from the brain.

$$CH_3-CH_2-CH_2 \diagdown N-SO_2- \diagdown -COOH$$
$$CH_3-CH_2-CH_2 \diagup$$

Probenecid

The Pineal Story

Technically speaking, the pineal gland is outside the CNS and its physiology ought to be minimized in this discussion. However, in response to neural stimulation, indoleamines that play a significant role in brain function are synthesized in this structure.

Circadian Rhythm of Serotonin Levels

The pineal gland has the greatest concentration of 5-HT per gram of tissue—more than 200 times greater than in the brain of the rat—of any tissue in the body. Pineal serotonin undergoes circadian (daily) fluctuations. Under normal lighting conditions, the 5-HT level at noon is 10 times the level found at midnight, and 5-HT levels will double in 14 minutes in rats after first exposure to light (Green and Grahame-Smith, 1975). This circadian variation continues in rats kept in continuous darkness and in blinded animals kept in continuous light, but the cyclicity is abolished in sighted animals kept in continuous light. Reversal of the lighting schedule—lights on at night, off during the day—changed the 5-HT rhythm by 180° within 6 days. Thus, the daily rhythm is endogenous but is synchronized (entrained) by environmental light.

The pineal gland is innervated by postganglionic noradrenergic axons from the superior cervical sympathetic ganglia (see Figure 1 in Chapter 6). Denervation of the pineal gland, achieved by sectioning the pre- or postganglionic fibers, suppressed the pineal rhythm. Thus, there is a "clock" in the brain that generates the circadian rhythm via these nerve fibers.

Some serotonin in the pineal gland is metabolized to 5-HIAA in the usual way, and some leaves the pineal cells and is stored along with NE in the presynaptic noradrenergic terminals. But a significant portion of pineal 5-HT undergoes a unique transformation. Within the pineal cells is the enzyme N-acetyltransferase (NAT). The concentration of this enzyme is 180° out of phase with that of 5-HT, that is, in darkness there is as much as a 15- to 70-fold increase in NAT activity. The dark activity, in turn, is reduced by half 3 minutes after exposure to light (Green and Grahame-Smith, 1975). NAT is the first enzyme in the metabolic pathway for conversion of 5-HT to melatonin. Melatonin has widespread effects and may account for the diurnal loss of pineal 5-HT. What is most important here is that the NAT rhythm is also circadian; it also persists in sighted animals kept in constant darkness and in blinded rats kept in constant light. Moreover, it seems that the NAT rhythm is the key to the rhythmicity of all the other substrates and end products involved in the conversion of 5-HT to melatonin.

The mechanism by which light entrains the NAT rhythm was investigated by Moore (1974). Moore and his co-workers injected directly into the eyes of rats radioactive amino acids (proline and leucine), which were taken up and incorporated into the proteins of the optic tract. The radiolabeled proteins were carried to the nerve terminals by axoplasmic flow and were detected autoradiographically in the terminals ending in all known nuclei of the optic system. In addition, however, labeled protein was found in the suprachiasmatic nucleus (SCN) of the hypothalamus, a nucleus that directly overlies the optic chiasma. No other hypothalamic area was significantly labeled. The presence of this retinohypothalamic pathway has since been confirmed using electron microscopy, and it has been demonstrated in a number of mammalian species.

Other experiments showed that bilateral electrolytic lesions of the SCN abolished the pineal NAT rhythm (Moore and Klein, 1974). Although knife cuts rostral to the SCN had no effect, caudal knife cuts also abolished the NAT rhythm (Moore and Eichler, 1972). It is important to note that the SCN does not drive pineal indole metabolism exclusively; SCN lesions also interfere with circadian rhythms of water intake, running wheel activity, adrenal corticosterone output, and other hormonally determined functions. It was also determined that the neural input to the pineal acts upon the noradrenergic β-receptors on the pineal cells, is increased at night, and leads to the production of cAMP, which apparently increases protein synthesis related to NAT activity.

In summary, environmental darkness leads to a neural input to the suprachiasmatic nucleus via the retinohypothalamic tract (Figure 6). The SCN seems to be a focal point for a "brain clock" governing rhythmicity for a number of physiological functions. The efferents from SCN proceed caudally (by unknown fiber systems) to the intermediolateral cell column in the lateral (sympathetic) horn of the thoracic spinal cord, which gives rise to preganglionic fibers leading to the superior cervical ganglion of the sympathetic chain. At night, sympathetic postganglionic fibers release norepinephrine, which activates cAMP production in pineal cells. The cAMP increases NAT activity (by a process probably involving protein synthesis), and NAT initiates conversion of 5-HT to melatonin. Environmental light inhibits these processes and darkness stimulates them.

Conversion of Serotonin to Melatonin

Activation of N-acetyltransferase leads to the acetylation of serotonin to N-acetylserotonin with acetyl CoA supplying the acetyl radical for this step (Figure 7). N-acetylserotonin is then methylated by the action of hydroxyindole-O-methyltransferase (HIOMT), with S-adenosylmethionine (SAM) serving as the methyl donor. HIOMT is found predominantly in the pineal glands of mammals and birds, but it is also found in the retina of the rat and in the eye and brain as well as the pineal gland in reptiles, amphibians, and fishes.

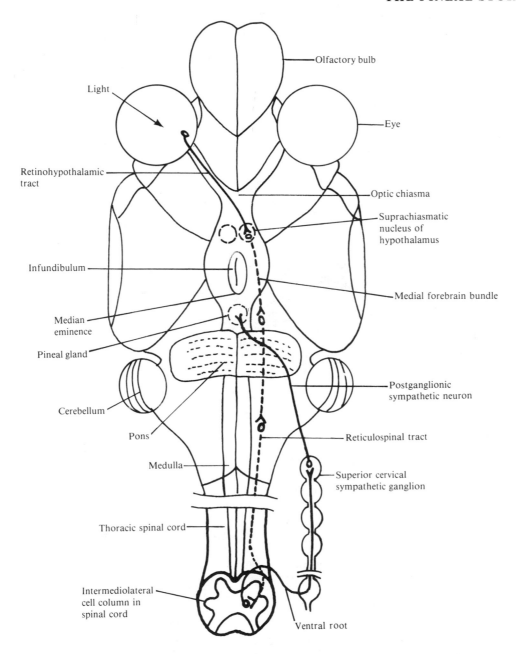

FIGURE 6. RETINAL-PINEAL PATHWAY. This ventral view of rat brain shows that photic input to the eyes leads to nerve impulses that traverse the axons of the retinal ganglion cells. The axons make up the inferior accessory optic tract and the retinohypothalamic tract which converge upon the suprachiasmatic nuclei. From these nuclei stimulation passes through the hypothalamus and the brain stem presumably via the medial forebrain bundle and a reticulospinal tract to the intermediolateral cell column whose neurons provide preganglionic fibers to the superior cervical sympathetic ganglia. Postganglionic noradrenergic fibers then proceed to the pineal gland. (After Wurtman, 1980.)

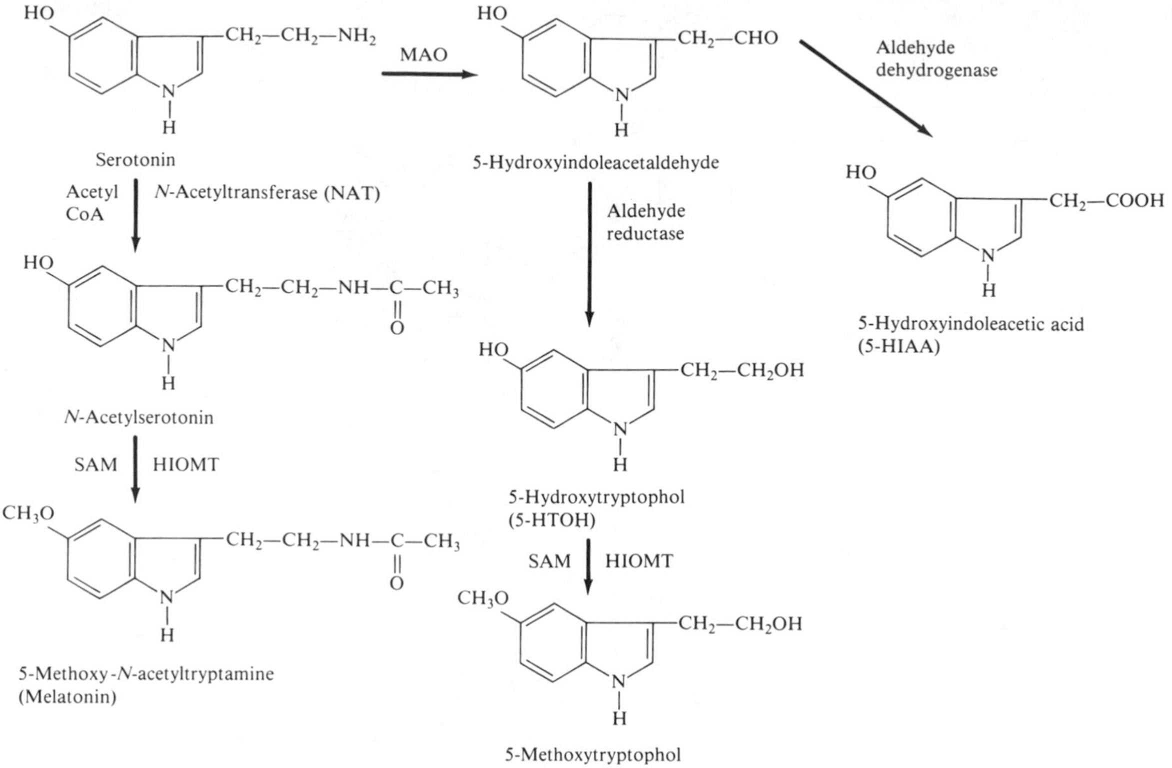

FIGURE 7 SEROTONIN CATABOLISM IN THE PINEAL GLAND. HIOMT, hydroxyindole-O-methyltransferase; SAM, S-adenosylmethionine; MAO, monoamine oxidase.

The methylated end product is 5-methoxy-N-acetyl tryptamine, or melatonin.

An alternative metabolic route is available for pineal 5-HT. After deamination of 5-HT by MAO to form 5-hydroxyindoleacetaldehyde (5-HIA), aldehyde reductase reduces 5-HIA to 5-hydroxytryptophol. This product, in the presence of SAM and HIOMT, is converted to 5-methoxytryptophol. The latter compound is, like melatonin, biologically active, but it is not nearly as potent as melatonin.

Effects of Melatonin

Melatonin has a wide range of effects, some of which are listed below. (1) Melatonin causes contraction of MELANOPHORES in frog and fish skin, resulting in a rapid blanching of the skin that presumably results in protective camouflage. (2) When melatonin is injected into birds, it causes a decrease in the weight of ovaries, testes, and oviducts. (3) Melatonin delays the

vaginal opening and reduces ovary weight in young rats. (4) Blinding male hamsters lowers the weight of the testes. However, when nerves to the pineal are cut or when the pineal is removed, the loss in testes weight is prevented. (5) During proestrus (before estrus), melatonin inhibits ovulation (Axelrod, 1974b).

It seems that melatonin is involved in fear-induced protective responses and has inhibitory effects on the gonads. But just how these effects fit into the various patterns of reproductive behavior is difficult to ascertain. Considering the fact that some animals are diurnal whereas some are nocturnal, and some females ovulate but once a year whereas others ovulate as often as every 4 days, it is hard to adapt diurnal fluctuations of melatonin synthesis to all these events in meaningful ways. For example, Reiter (1976) attempted to fit melatonin physiology to the reproductive pattern of the golden hamster. This species is monoestrus: it breeds only once a year, in the summer months.

Melatonin levels would serve as an index to the length of the day, thereby providing the species with an internal calendar. During the summer months the days are long, melatonin synthesis is inhibited, the gonads are matured, and reproduction occurs at a time of year favoring offspring survival during the summer and fall. During the winter months the species is sexually inactive, and the genitalia involute, a process that is prevented by pinealectomy (Reiter, 1976).

However, another monoestrus species, sheep, have a period of sexual activity in the fall, which makes sense because the sheep has a longer gestation period and produces offspring in the spring. However, in this case, the sexual activity of the sheep occurs when the days are getting shorter and melatonin synthesis is increasing with subsequent inhibition of gonadal function. Other factors must certainly be operating here—factors that would seem to defeat the function of the pineal gland. These examples illustrate the complexity of any potential model of pineal function.

Part III   Serotonergic Drugs

A wide variety of drugs have been found that effect serotonergic mechanisms. Some of the drugs have been designed for that purpose; other drugs have serotonergic effects that are incidental to effects on other transmitters; and some serotonergic effects were discovered long after a drug substance had been used and found to have pronounced behavioral effects. (LSD is a good example of this latter situation.) Figure 8 shows a serotonergic neuron and the sites of action of the drugs discussed in this section. Table I also summarizes information on serotonergic drugs.

Inhibitors of Serotonin Synthesis

The synthesis of 5-HT is a two-step process involving hydroxylation of tryptophan to form 5-hydroxytryptophan, followed by decarboxylation to form 5-HT. It has already been mentioned that p-chlorophenylalanine reduces brain levels of 5-HT by blocking tryptophan hydroxylase. This and related investigations pointed to the hydroxylating process as the rate-limiting step in 5-HT synthesis.

Koe and Weissman (1966) were the first to report the effect of PCPA on 5-HT synthesis. They found that PCPA significantly depleted 5-HT stores and 5-HIAA in the brain and in peripheral tissue and blood. They also reported that PCPA blocked the increase in brain 5-HT induced by pargyline (a MAO inhibitor) and by tryptophan loading. However, PCPA did not block uptake of tryptophan, suggesting that PCPA acted on the hydroxylating enzyme itself.

PCPA acts in two ways. At first there is an inhibition of tryptophan hydroxylase that disappears within a few hours as brain levels of PCPA fall. An irreversible inhibition, however, persists for several days (Jequier et al., 1967; Sanders-Bush et al., 1974). Later studies claimed that the irreversible inhibition occurred because PCPA (an amino acid analog) was incorporated into the enzyme protein, thereby inhibiting enzyme activity. But other experiments revealed that PCPA was just as effective below a spinal transection, indicating that PCPA could inactivate already existing enzyme. Because PCPA treatment (300 mg/kg in a rat) can depress brain 5-HT levels for as long as 2 weeks, synthesis of new stores of tryptophan hydroxylase seem to be necessary for the return of normal rates of 5-HT synthesis. Perhaps all that can be confidently stated at this point is that PCPA competes with substrate tryptophan for the enzyme tryptophan hydroxylase.

Another synthesis inhibitor is α-n-propyldopacetamide (H22/54). This substance also blocks the hydroxylation of tryptophan but not nearly as effectively as PCPA. Moreover H22/54 also depletes catecholamine levels. Its mode of action is said to involve competition with tryptophan hydroxylase for the pteridine cofactor.

α-n-Propyldopacetamide

Two other substances have been found to block 5-HT synthesis. 6-Fluorotryptophan has effects similar to those of PCPA, except that the effects are more transient and the side effects are different. p-Chloroamphetamine (PCA) (as well as its congener p-chloromethamphetamine) is a more widely studied drug, but its mode of action is complex (Sanders-Bush et al., 1974). Evidence indicates that PCA inhibits

TABLE I   Drugs That Affect Serotonergic Synapses

Drug	Mechanism of action	Major effects
5,6-Dihydroxytryptamine	Serotonergic neurotoxin	Destroys 5-HT cells
p-Chloroamphetamine (PCA)	Releases 5-HT, then destroys neuron	5-HT agonist and neurotoxin
Fenfluramine	Releases 5-HT	Anorectic
p-Chlorophenylalanine α-n-Propyldopacetamide 6-Flurotryptophan	Inhibit tryptophan hydroxylase	Block 5-HT synthesis
α-Methyldopa α-Methyl 5-HTP	Block 5-HTP decarboxylase	Block 5-HT synthesis
Clorgyline Iproniazid Tranylcypromine	Type A MAO inhibitor Broad spectrum MAO inhibitors	5-HT potentiation Antidepressants
Chlorimipramine Nortryptiline Fluoxetine	Block 5-HT reuptake	Antidepressant Antidepressant 5-HT agonist
Reserpine Tetrabenazine	Release vesicular monoamines	Hypotensives
LSD-25 Bufotenine Psilocin Dimethyltryptamine (DMT) Isoergine (lysergic acid amide) Mescaline	Interact with 5-HT receptors Interaction unknown	Phantasticants
2-Bromo-LSD Methysergide Cinanserin	Peripheral 5-HT receptor blocker 5-HT receptor blockers	5-HT antagonist
Cyproheptadine Metergoline Methiothepin	5-HT receptor blockers at excitatory synapses but enhance 5-HT inhibitory action	Experimental
α-Methyltryptamine	Stimulates 5-HT receptors	5-HT agonist
Chlordiazepoxide Diazepam Oxazepam	Block 5-HT turnover	Anxiolytics

tryptophan hydroxylase and that it does so even longer than PCPA. The result, as expected, is reduced brain 5-HT and 5-HIAA and lower brain turnover of 5-HT, which may only begin to recover after 4 months. PCA also inhibits the reuptake of 5-HT by presynaptic nerve terminals and increases the release of 5-HT from these terminals, but PCA does not inhibit 5-HT synthesis in peripheral tissue. Fuller and Molloy (1974) also found that PCA inhibits MAO in both *in vitro* and *in vivo* preparations when 5-HT is the substrate. They also proposed that the long duration of PCA effects are due to the drug's high affinity for the 5-HT uptake pump on synaptic terminals. Thus, PCA might be recycled over and over again. This proposal is supported by experimental results that showed that if after PCA administration continued reentry of PCA into the

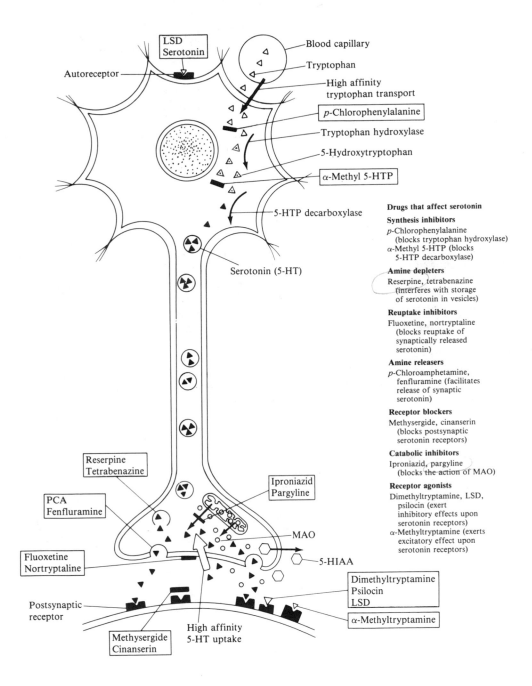

FIGURE 8 SEROTONERGIC NEURON. Synthesis of serotonin is shown in the perikaryon along with the sites of action of drugs that can block the synthesizing steps.

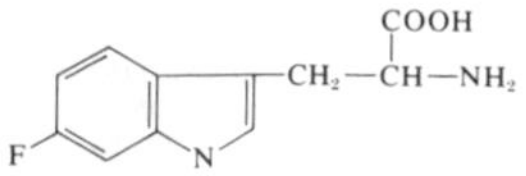

6-Fluorotryptophan

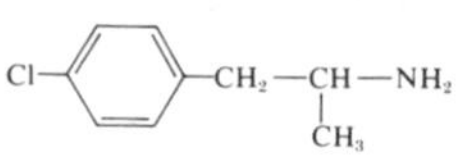

p-Chloroamphetamine

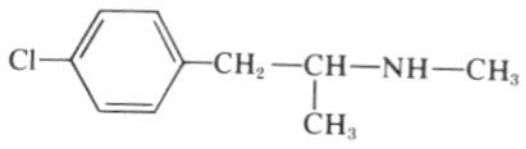

p-Chloromethamphetamine

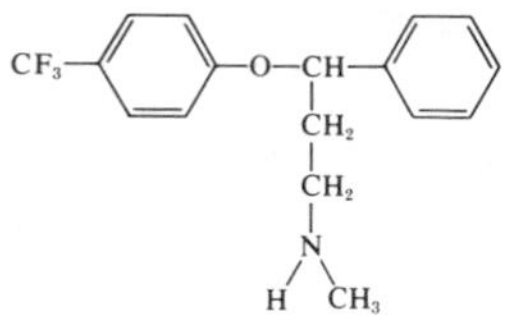

Fluoxetine

nerve terminal is blocked by the reuptake inhibitor chlorimipramine, brain levels of 5-HT are quickly restored to normal (Meek et al., 1971).

Further studies showed that there are reversible and irreversible phases of serotonin depletion by PCA. Fuller et al. (1975a, 1975b) used a 5-HT reuptake blocker fluoxetine that had a marked specificity for 5-HT neurons over catecholamine neurons (Wong et al., 1974). They found that pretreating rats with fluoxetine (FXT) completely blocked the 5-HT depletion by PCA. Furthermore, they found that treating rats with FXT as much as 4 hours after PCA treatment, when tryptophan hydroxylase (TPH) and 5-HT levels were already lowered, completely reversed the depletion of both the enzyme and the transmitter, as indicated by measurements of TPH and 5-HT at later intervals. When FXT was administered 8 to 16 hours after PCA, later measures (40 hours after PCA) showed less reversal than when FXT was given earlier. Finally, when FXT was given between 32 and 48 hours after PCA, there was no reversal of PCA-induced 5-HT depletion at all. Measures of 5-HT and 5-HIAA made a week after giving FXT still showed no reversal, and giving FXT 10 weeks after PCA did not significantly alter the depression of 5-HT and 5-HIAA.

These results led to the conclusion that 5-HT depletion by PCA is not irreversible initially but becomes so within 24 to 48 hours. That inhibiting uptake not only prevents but also reverses the action of PCA suggests that the entry of PCA into the axon terminal is necessary for 5-HT depletion and that continual reuptake of PCA is necessary for the depletion to be maintained. It is not clear how continual reuptake of PCA causes all but permanent damage to 5-HT neurons—in the sense that they are no longer able to syn-

thesize 5-HT. It appears that tryptophan hydroxylase activity fails because of the prolonged presence of either PCA or some neurotoxic metabolite that is reactive to nucleic acids and proteins. More work is necessary to resolve these issues.

Finally, while examining the effect of PCA on single neurons in the raphe, Sheard (1974) found that an intravenous injection of PCA led within 30–45 seconds to a marked depression in firing rate. However, this is now thought to have been due to an initial increase in 5-HT at the presynaptic autoreceptors, causing direct inhibitory effects on raphe neurons.

Inhibition of 5-Hydroxytryptophan Decarboxylating Enzymes

Theoretically, serotonin synthesis can be blocked by interfering with the decarboxylating enzyme 5-HTP decarboxylase. However, it is questionable whether this can be done effectively because the decarboxylating enzyme is so plentiful. In an earlier section we discussed the question whether 5-HTP decarboxylase is distinct from DOPA decarboxylase. Now it should be asked whether one decarboxylating enzyme can be blocked without affecting the other. Whereas DOPA decarboxylase is effectively inhibited by MK 485, α-methyldopa hydrazine (Carbidopa), effective 5-HTP decarboxylase inhibitors are α-methyldopa (Aldomet) and α-methyl 5-HTP. The inhibition by these sub-

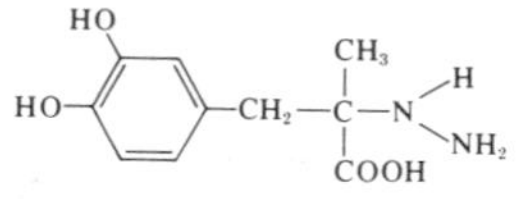

α-Methyldopa hydrazine (Carbidopa)

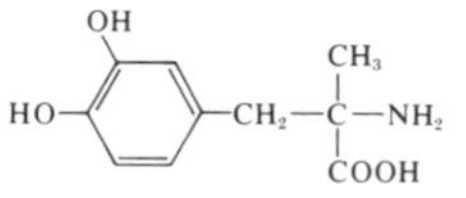

α-Methyldopa (Aldomet)

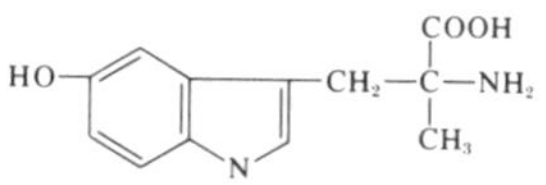

α-Methyl 5-HTP

stances can be reversed by adding more of the coenzyme pyridoxal 5–phosphate (vitamin B_6) suggesting that the effect of the inhibiting drugs is by preempting the coenzyme. Brain 5-HTP decarboxylase in rats can be rapidly inhibited by α-methyldopa, with normal enzyme activity returning in about 1 day. However, high single doses or repeated injections will not decrease brain 5-HT levels by more than 50 percent. Also, phenylalanine hydroxylase, tyrosine hydroxylase, and tryptophan hydroxylase are inhibited by α-methyldopa thereby limiting its value as a research tool (Green and Grahame-Smith, 1975).

Drugs that Block Serotonin Catabolism

The first step in serotonin catabolism is oxidative deamination by monoamine oxidase. Therefore, inhibition of deamination would be expected to block 5-HT degradation. However, as mentioned earlier, other monoamines are effected by MAO inhibitors. The termination of synaptic action occurs primarily by transmitter reuptake, but 5-HT catabolism by MAO still is significant—probably not in terminating the synaptic action of 5-HT but in modulating the intraneuronal 5-HT concentration. Green and Graham-Smith (1975) proposed that there are two pools or compartments of 5-HT in nerve endings. One pool provides the immediate source of functionally active 5-HT, and the other is the vesicular pool that provides a reserve source of the transmitter. The functionally active pool is controlled by the rate of synthesis, the rate of vesicular binding, and the rate of intraneuronal MAO activity. When an excess amount of tryptophan (the 5-HT precursor) is given to rats, there are no gross behavioral changes. However, if it is given to rats pretreated with a MAO inhibitor, gross behavioral changes occur. With tryptophan alone, 5-HT is synthesized and metabolized to 5-HIAA. However, after administration of an MAO inhibitor, 5-HT is synthesized but not metabolized, resulting in saturation of storage (vesicular) sites and "spill over" into the functional pool, thereby leading to excess 5-HT activity.

One consequence of MAO inhibitor treatment is a depression of the firing rate of serotonergic neurons of the raphe. It is believed that the depression is indirectly triggered by a rapid accumulation of brain 5-HT. This hypothesis is borne out by the fact that PCPA (which inhibits 5-HT synthesis) blocked the MAO inhibitor-induced inhibition of the raphe neurons. Thus, MAO inhibitor-induced inhibition of raphe neurons is secondary to the accumulation of 5-HT, which probably acts upon the inhibitory receptors of the raphe neurons (Aghajanian et al., 1970, 1975). As discussed in an earlier chapter, it is likely that serotonin deamination takes place with type A MAO, whose most active inhibitor is clorgyline. At high doses, however, other MAO inhibitors can be nearly as effective. Other MAO inhibitors are described in Chapter 7.

Aldehyde Oxidation versus Reduction

Another step in 5-HT degradation occurs via the activity of aldehyde dehydrogenase, which oxidizes 5-hydroxyindoleacetaldehyde (5-HIA) to form 5-hydroxyindoleacetic acid. Thus far it has not been reliably demonstrated that aldehyde dehydrogenase can be inhibited.

5-HIA also can be reduced by aldehyde reductase to form the alcohol 5-hydroxytryptophol (5-HTOH) (Figure 7). Both 5-HIAA and 5-HTOH are formed in the liver, but there is little evidence that 5-HTOH is formed in the brain. Some work was done to explore the possibility that ethanol in the brain shifts the metabolism of 5-HIA to 5-HTOH instead of 5-HIAA, but the experimental results were essentially negative. Nevertheless, 5-HTOH and a few of its congeners (tryptophol and 5-methoxytryptophol) do seem to be physiologically active: they induce sleep in mice and decrease body temperature. However, there is nothing to suggest that these indoles play a significant role in brain function (Green and Grahame-Smith, 1975). Consequently, there is little interest in finding or fabricating drugs to block the conversion of 5-HIA to 5-HIAA.

d-Lysergic Acid Diethylamide (LSD-25)

LSD-25 or just LSD was first synthesized in 1938 by the Swiss chemist Albert Hofmann* (1970). It contains lysergic acid and diethylamide. Lysergic acid is an alkaloid obtained from ergot (Claviceps purpurea), a parasitic fungus found on rye and wheat; diethylamide is a synthetic compound. Hofmann and his associates were studying ergot compounds, which are vasoconstrictors and are useful in controlling migraine headaches and postpartum hemorrhage. LSD was not noteworthy in early experimental tests with animals, and the compound was shelved. Five years later, while searching for an ANALEPTIC drug (respiratory stimulant), Hofmann compared LSD effects with those of nikethamide (another diethylamide com-

*It was the twenty-fifth compound synthesized in the series of experiments; hence, LSD-25.

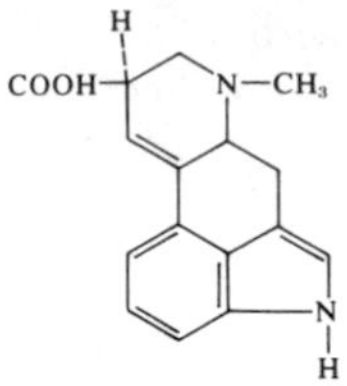

Lysergic acid

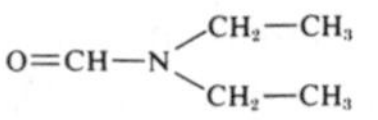

Diethylamide

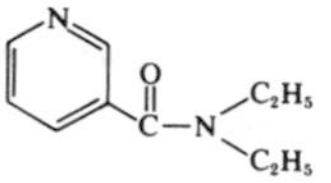

Nikethamide

pound having central stimulatory effects). During these investigations, Hofmann accidentally ingested a small amount of LSD and experienced a very unusual reaction. He reported vertigo and restlessness, optical distortions, a dreamlike state, feelings similar to drunkenness, and exaggerated imagination.

Subsequently he investigated his suspicion that he had ingested some LSD and intentionally ingested 0.25 mg orally, a dose based on doses of other ergot alkaloids. However, this dose was 5 to 10 times larger than the dose that was later found to be adequate for the reaction. This time Hofmann's reactions were quite spectacular. The first printed account of these phenomena appeared when Stoll (1947) reported the results of studies done on human subjects at a psychiatric clinic at Zurich, a report that confirmed Hofmann's original findings. These effects provided the impetus for further pharmacological studies of LSD because the subjective effects seemed in many ways to be similar to some schizophrenic symptoms. It was thought, therefore, that LSD might be the means of experimentally inducing schizo-

phrenia, thereby aiding research and perhaps leading to the cure and prevention of schizophrenia.

During this same period serotonin was also being studied, and it was soon noted that LSD and serotonin were related chemically—at least they both contained the indole nucleus (Figure 9). The early studies also suggested that LSD blocked the effects of serotonergic systems, for example, it blocked the stimulating effect of 5-HT on smooth muscle of the intestine and the rat uterus. These facts and the fact that 5-HT was found in the brain (a decade before the confirmation of the histochemical fluorescence studies of Dahlström and Fuxe, 1965) made it seem quite probable that schizophrenia, serotonin, and LSD were related in significant ways.

A related compound, 2-bromo-LSD (BOL), was found to be a 5-HT antagonist in peripheral structures, but it produced none of the subjective experiences of LSD even though it freely passed the blood brain barrier. This created some doubt about the assertion that LSD blocked 5-HT systems in the brain, but it did not rule out the possibility that central receptors reacted differently to BOL.

Tissue Binding of LSD. In extensive studies conducted to examine the binding properties of LSD and related compounds, Bennett and Snyder (1975) found that LSD binding sites in rat brain had a high degree of structural specificity. *d*-LSD had a high affinity for binding sites whereas psychotropically inactive *l*-LSD had a binding potency 1000 times weaker. The configurational changes in the LSD molecule that reduced

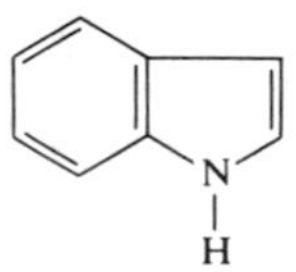

Indole nucleus

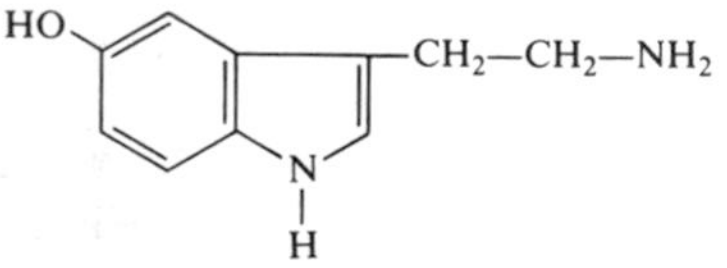

Serotonin

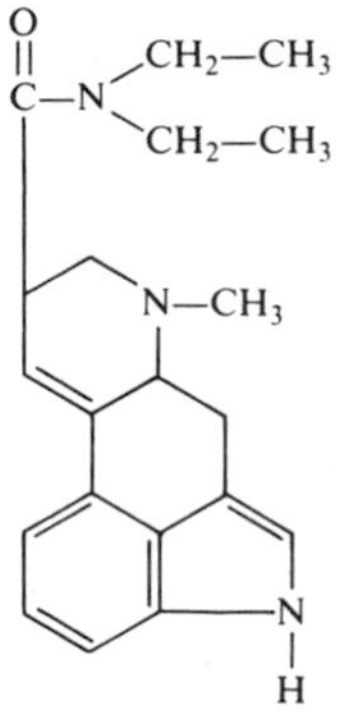

LSD-25

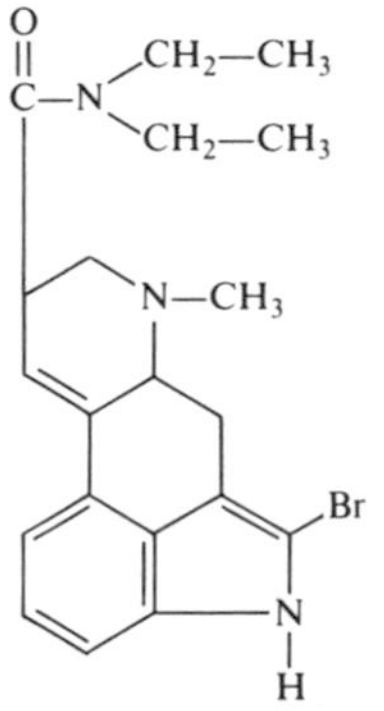

2-Bromo-LSD (BOL)

FIGURE 9   SEROTONIN AND INDOLE COMPOUNDS.

psychotropic potency also diminished binding potency. The one exception to this rule was 2-bromo-LSD, which equaled *d*-LSD in binding affinity although it was psychotropically inactive. A wide range of tryptamine compounds, serotonin antagonists, and other psychotropic alkylindoleamines were tested for their ability to displace LSD from cortical binding sites. In general, psychotropic potency correlated positively with potency for replacing LSD at binding sites. Furthermore, they found that tissue samples from various monkey brain areas that showed high degrees of LSD binding showed high levels of 5-HT uptake as well. Highest binding occurred in cerebral cortical regions; lowest binding occurred in white matter and cerebellum; and diencephalic areas showed intermediate binding.

Perhaps most noteworthy was their finding that destruction of the nuclei of the midbrain raphe did not change the affinity or maximum number of detectable *in vitro* LSD binding sites in brain tissue. This imples that LSD binds to postsynaptic serotonin receptors. However, this did not rule out the possibility that LSD could bind to receptors located on the soma and dendrites of 5-HT cells of the raphe nuclei.

Physiological Effects of LSD. LSD is usually ingested orally and is rapidly absorbed. The potency of LSD is so high that the substance is diluted many times in order to measure doses more conveniently. Oral ingestion of 100 μg is usually sufficient for a significant effect in man, and as little as 0.3 μg/kg is subjectively detectable. LSD is rapidly distributed to all parts of the body including the brain, but surprisingly, only a small part of the dose (about 1 percent) is found in the brain; the biggest concentration is found in the liver, where it is degraded before being excreted. Tolerance to LSD occurs rapidly so that after three or four daily doses the usual doses become quite ineffective. There is a cross tolerance to psilocin* and mescaline, suggesting that all of these substances have a common mode of action. LSD is degraded rather rapidly in man; the plasma half-life is about 175 minutes.

Physiologically LSD has sympathomimetic effects, which probably come about by upsetting the balance between cholinergic and catecholaminergic systems. It induces tachycardia, increased blood pressure, dilated pupils, piloerection, increased body temperature, sweating and chills, increased blood glucose levels, and

*The active ingredient of psilocybin.

sometimes headache, nausea, and vomiting. However, these effects seldom interfere with the perceptual effects described by Hofmann.

Biochemical Effects of LSD. The effects of LSD on serotonergic neurons have been investigated in many ways, and the methods and results of these experiments have been reviewed by Aghajanian et al. (1974, 1975). Aghajanian and his co-workers showed that electrical stimulation of the midbrain raphe in rats led to a reduction of forebrain 5-HT levels and an increase in brain 5-HIAA. After the introduction of unilateral lesions of the medial forebrain bundle, the usual changes in brain 5-HT concentration after electrical stimulation were prevented on the side with the lesion but not on the control side (Aghajanian et al., 1967). This and similar experiments revealed the presence of a neuronal system appropriate for investigations of serotonergic drugs free of the complications that arise because of the special characteristics of peripheral serotonergic systems.

Other studies showed that systemic administration of LSD produced a slight increase in brain 5-HT, a decrease in brain 5-HIAA, and a decrease in brain 5-HT synthesis. These findings led to the conclusion that LSD slows the turnover of 5-HT. Because electrical stimulation of the raphe had the opposite effects, it was proposed that LSD might be suppressing the firing of 5-HT neurons in the raphe. Also, when 5-HT synthesis was inhibited, LSD reduced the rate of 5-HT depletion that normally occurred. This also supported the idea that LSD slows the action of 5-HT neurons. However, an alternate interpretation was proposed, namely, that LSD stimulated postsynaptic 5-HT receptors, which, by way of a negative feedback system, caused an inhibition of the presynaptic neurons.

Single Cell Studies. To resolve the differences in the interpretation of the data, studies were done on the effects of LSD on single serotonergic neurons (Aghajanian and Haigler, 1974). This was feasible because the histochemical mapping by Dahlström and Fuxe (1965) made accurate placement of microelectrodes possible. Experiments showed that small intravenous doses of LSD (10–20 μg/kg) produced brief, but total, inhibition of firing of 5-HT neurons of the dorsal and median raphe nuclei (Figure 10A). However, larger doses (more than 100 μg/kg) that increased the duration of inhibition were required to alter the brain levels

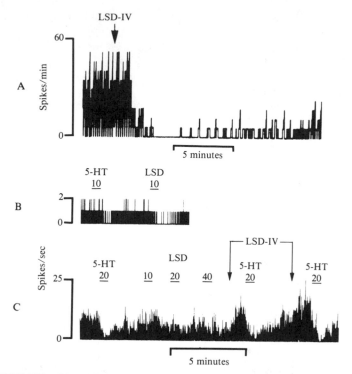

FIGURE 10 LSD EFFECTS ON DORSAL RAPHE NEURONS. (A) The baseline rate of a raphe cell from a rat midbrain; a rate of about 1 spike/sec. LSD bitartrate (20 μg/kg) was slowly intravenously administered where indicated by the arrow. An almost total inhibition of the firing for about 2 minutes was followed by a gradual recovery. Each deflection is the integrated firing rate during a 10-second sample period. (B) The effect of 5-HT and LSD on a dorsal raphe neuron during iontophoretic administration. The numbers above the bars give the ejection current in nA. Recovery from 5-HT is more rapid than from LSD. (C) The effect of 5-HT and LSD on a cell in the ventral lateral geniculate nucleus (VLG). This cell is also inhibited by iontophoretic 5-HT but is relatively insensitive to LSD. When LSD was administered as an intravenous dose (10 μg/kg), there was an acceleration of firing in this cell, but the inhibition by iontophoretic 5-HT during the infusion was not blocked. The baseline firing of this neuron was a response to a steady light. Each deflection in this trace is the integrated firing rate during a 1-second sample time. (From Aghajanian and Haigler, 1974.)

of 5-HT and 5-HIAA. It was also found that BOL (the nonpsychotropic analog of LSD) had less than 1 percent of the activity of LSD on raphe neurons. These findings supported the hypothesis that LSD led to decreased 5-HT turnover by reducing impulse traffic in 5-HT neurons. However, these findings did not resolve the issue of whether the effect of LSD was direct or indirect (i.e., by way of a compensatory feedback mechanism). To answer this question, the effects of LSD applied directly to serotonergic neurons needed to be known.

Consequently, another series of studies used micro-iontophoretic techniques to examine the effects of LSD that was directly applied to raphe neurons. These studies used multibarreled micropipettes that allowed controlled ejection of a drug upon neurons while simultaneously recording neural activity. Accordingly, raphe neurons were found to be extremely sensitive to LSD ions, and their firing rate was clearly inhibited in anesthetized and unanesthetized rats. It was also found that 5-HT itself inhibited raphe neurons, but LSD was much more potent in this respect (Figure 10B). When LSD and 5-HT were combined, the effect was additive, and there was no evidence that LSD blocked the action of 5-HT or vice versa. Therefore, the evidence supported the view that LSD had direct effects on raphe neurons, but it still did not rule out the possibility that feedback effects could occur. This could be ascertained by investigating the effects of LSD on 5-HT target neurons (i.e., cells with a probable 5-HT input).

Again, with the aid of histochemical fluorescence techniques, it was possible to localize accurately terminals of raphe neurons in forebrain areas such as the ventral lateral geniculate nuclei, the basolateral and cortical amygdala, and optic tectum. Assuming that the cell bodies juxtaposed to the 5-HT terminals had a serotonergic input, microiontophoretic studies tested the sensitivity of these postsynaptic elements to 5-HT and to LSD. The postsynaptic cells were inhibited by 5-HT but were quite insensitive to LSD at ejection currents that were highly effective on raphe neurons (Figure 10C). However, the postsynaptic cells could be inhibited by very high concentrations of LSD. When LSD (10 μg/kg) was administered intravenously, the postsynaptic neurons appeared to be stimulated, but the LSD did not block the inhibitory effects of 5-HT applied iontophoretically (Figure 10C, end of trace). Thus, high iontophoretic doses did inhibit the postsynaptic neurons, but intravenous doses appeared to stimulate them.

The next question was which receptors were the more important as the locus of action of LSD: the receptor on the raphe cell bodies or those on the postsynaptic target cells? Logically the question was considered as follows. Given that low doses of LSD inhibit raphe neurons and that raphe neurons exert an inhibitory effect on postsynaptic cells, one would expect LSD-induced inhibition of raphe neurons would result in a disinhibition of the target cells, causing an acceleration of their firing rates. As mentioned previously, experiments show just that: intravenous administration at a dose sufficient to inhibit raphe neurons caused an acceleration of firing in postsynaptic cells.

The assumption of LSD action on raphe neurons is also supported by the fact that when the brain stem was transected above the midbrain, thereby separating it from the forebrain, LSD still inhibited the firing rate of the dorsal raphe neurons. This procedure eliminated the possibility that the depressant effect of LSD on raphe neurons resulted from negative feedback, due to postsynaptic excitation from the forebrain.

Many of the postsynaptic neurons are in structures of the visual system, such as the lateral geniculate

nucleus and the optic tectum, and limbic structures. Excitation of these areas as a result of their release from inhibitory influences may account for the distortions of visual perceptions that are characteristic of LSD effects.

Parenthetically, it was found that BOL, even at iontophoretic ejection currents ten times greater than that for LSD, had no effect on raphe neurons, nor did BOL block the effects of 5-HT. This evidence showed that LSD and BOL act differently from one another on central 5-HT receptors. Moreover, LSD mimics the inhibitory action of 5-HT at central receptors, whereas it and BOL both block the action of 5-HT on peripheral receptors.

There is some evidence that 5-HT has excitatory effects on some neurons in the cerebral cortex and brain stem and that these effects are blocked by LSD. Aghajanian and Haigler (1974) corroborated these findings in experiments showing that microiontophoresis of 5-HT in rat midbrain reticular formation caused some cell excitation and that these effects were also blocked by LSD. However, it was not certain that the excited cells normally receive a serotonergic input, so there is a question as to whether or not these data are relevant to 5-HT systems.

Raphe Neural Unit Activity and the Behavioral Effects of LSD. The evidence thus far suggests that the dramatic physiological and perceptual effects of LSD are mediated by the depression of the discharge rates of 5-HT neurons in the raphe nuclei. However, the electrophysiological data has been obtained from anesthetized or immobilized animals, while the behavioral data is taken from freely moving animals or obtained from human reports after drug ingestion. To obtain correlative data, Trulson and Jacobs (1979) utilized the technique of measuring the activity of single neurons in the dorsal raphe nucleus of freely moving cats along with measures of the electroencephalogram, the electrooculogram (eye movements), and the neck electromyogram (neck movements) (Jacobs, 1973). They found that LSD (50 μg/kg, i.p.) administration caused limb flicking, abortive grooming, head shaking, staring, and investigatory behavior. Raphe unit activity was significantly decreased (48 percent), with the maximal decrease occurring 1 hour after drug administration, and the peak level of behavioral effects occurring at about the same time. Unit activity remained depressed for about 3 hours after the injection, but some of the behavioral effects, especially limb flicking, were significantly higher than baseline for as long as 8 hours. Twenty-four hours after the first injection, a second injection (50 μg/kg) was given. This dose was virtually without behavioral effects, but there was an even greater suppression of raphe unit activity (62.4 percent). There were no changes in the discharge rate that were correlated with the limb flicks, but some neural units were completely surpressed during staring and increased during digging or grooming (normal) behavior. A lower dose (10 μg/kg) produced a smaller decrement of discharge from raphe units (18 percent) that lasted for about 2 hours, but limb flicks lasted about 4 hours. Neither saline nor BOL had any effect on raphe unit activity or behavior; nor did LSD effect nonserotonergic cells outside the raphe nucleus.

Thus, (1) there was an LSD dose-related change in the depression of raphe unit activity and the elicitation of behavioral effects characteristic of LSD and related drugs. (The smaller dose led to less raphe unit depression and a shorter duration of the behavioral effects.) (2) The LSD-induced behavioral changes persisted much longer than the depression of raphe unit activity. (3) The tolerance to the drug, shown by the absence of behavioral effects after a second dose, was accompanied by an even greater depression of the raphe units.

At first glance, these results showing the dissociation between raphe unit activity and LSD-induced behavior suggested that there was no causal connection between these two phenomena. However, it was argued, first, that the decrease in unit activity that accompanied a significant behavioral effect after the lower dose could mean that small changes in unit activity are sufficient for the behavioral effect. Second, the fact that the behavioral effect outlasted changes in the raphe units could mean that serotonin release could still be depressed even after unit activity was restored to baseline levels or that the neurons receiving input from the raphe units had become less responsive to those inputs. Third, after the second dose, although unit depression continued, the tolerance for the behavioral effect could mean that the repeated depression of the raphe units was offset by a compensatory change in the raphe target neurons.

These results did not invalidate the serotonergic basis of LSD effects proposed by Aghajanian and Haigler (1974). Rather, they only pointed to the possibly greater importance of the LSD effects on the raphe target neurons and to the lesser importance of the depression of raphe unit activity.

Other "Hallucinogenic" Drugs (Phantasticants)

A number of other compounds that elicit similar physiological and behavioral effects are chemically related to LSD. A few of these compounds are shown in Figure 11, illustrating the relationship of these drugs to serotonin. As previously mentioned, acute tolerance to LSD occurs after a few doses in animals and man, with cross tolerance extending to chemically related compounds such as BOL and psilocybin (Isbell et al., 1959, 1961) but not with d-amphetamine (Isbell et al., 1962). There are other hallucinogens such as mescaline that have effects similar to those of LSD, but they are chemically similar to catecholamines such as dopamine. The major difference between mescaline and LSD is that the hallucinogenic effect from 5 mg/kg of mescaline is equivalent to that from a dose of 1.5 μg/kg of LSD. Interestingly, there is also a cross tolerance between LSD and mescaline (Appel, 1968). Other hallucinogens such as atropine, scopolamine, and ditran are anticholinergics. Ditran is a combination of two isomers of 3-N-substituted piperidyl benzilates. There is no cross tolerance between these anticholinergics and LSD, mescaline, or psilocybin (Cohen, 1970). The active ingredient of marijuana, Δ^9-tetrahydrocannabinol, in high doses can produce some LSD-like effects.

It is a misnomer to label these drugs as hallucinogens as their effects are not truly hallucinogenic. Genuine hallucinations are characterized as perceptions that are usually auditory and threatening and the subjects tend to think of the voices as real. The perceptual effects of LSD and related substances are more likely to be visual and interesting, with the subjects being aware that they are experiencing these strange perceptions—as though they were watching a private television show. Referring to these compounds as psychotogenic or psychotomimetic, implying that the induced effects are similar to psychotic states, is also misleading as resemblance to psychotic states is only superficial; and well-trained observers can easily discriminate between drug-induced effects and schizophrenia (Hollister, 1978). (This is not true of the psychotic states induced by amphetamine and some of its derivatives.) A number of these substances, as well as others of different chemical structure, are being classified as phan-

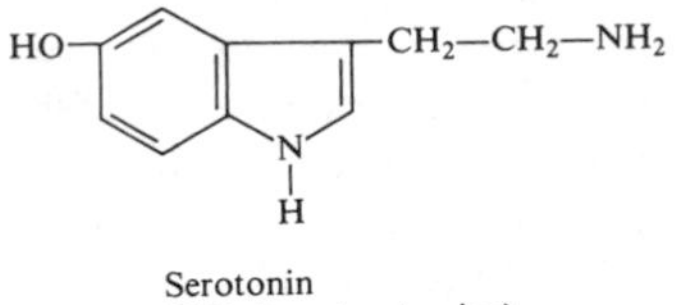

Serotonin
(5-Hydroxytryptamine)

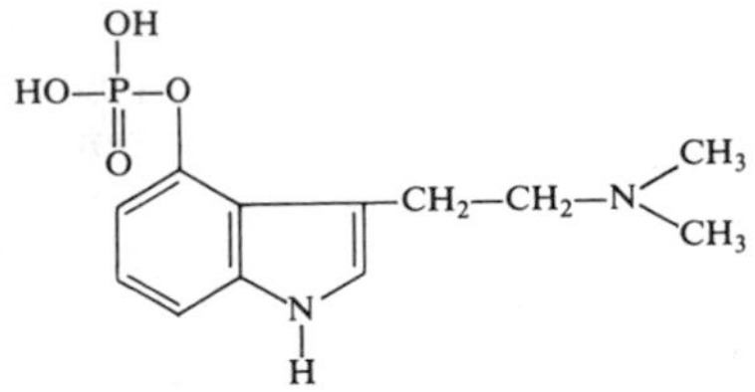

Psilocybin
(*N,N*-Dimethyl-4-phosphoryltryptamine)

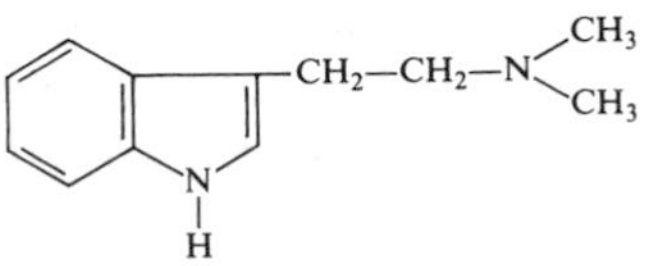

DMT
(*N,N*-Dimethyltryptamine)

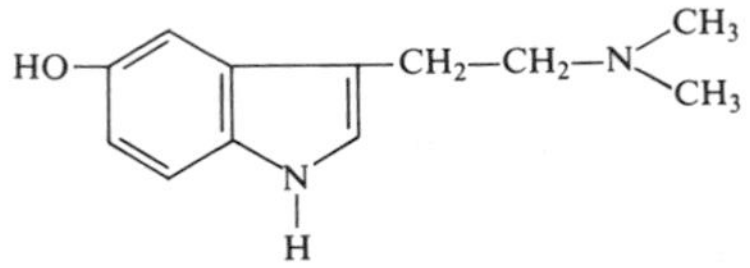

Bufotenine
(*N,N*-Dimethyl-5-hydroxytryptamine)

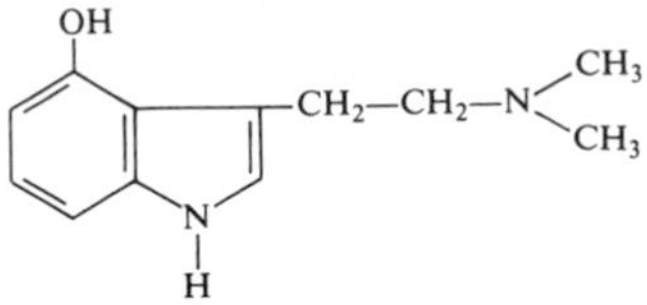

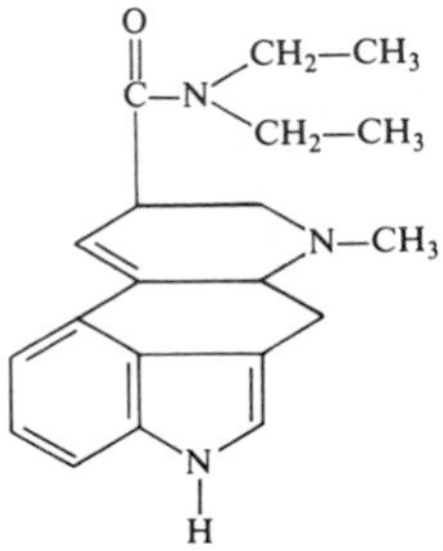

LSD
(Lysergic acid diethylamide)

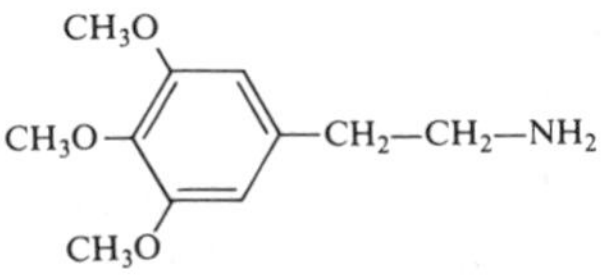

Psilocin
(*N,N*-Dimethy-4-hydroxytryptamine)

Mescaline
(3,4,5-Trimethoxyphenethylamine)

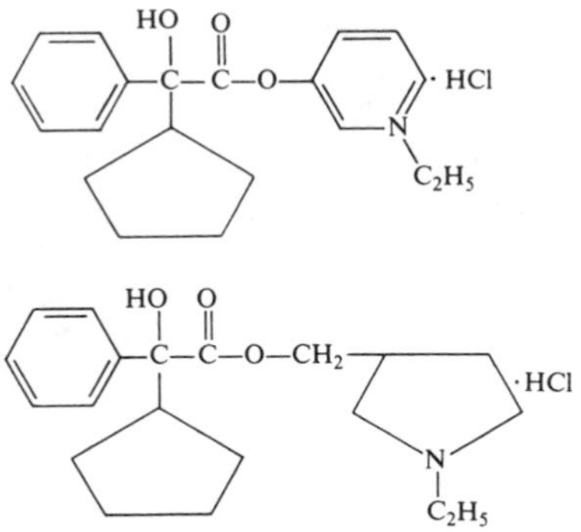

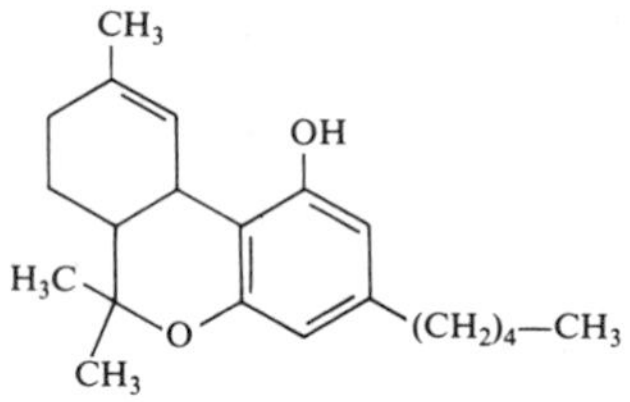

Marijuana
(△τ—Tetrahydrocannabinol)

Ditran

FIGURE 11 PHANTASTICANTS AND MONOAMINE TRANSMITTERS. There is a chemical resemblance between serotonin and the indole phantasticants. Mescaline (which resembles dopamine) is *not* an indoleamine, yet its pharmacological effects are similar to those of LSD and there is a cross tolerance between them. Ditran and marijuana have similar effects to those of LSD but are not related to serotonin.

tasticants to denote the type of experiences (phantasmagoria) associated with their use (Shulgin, 1978).

As mentioned earlier, LSD is derived from the ergot fungus. The other indoleamines are also of plant origin. Psilocybin is obtained from the mushroom *Psilocybe mexicana*. These mushrooms have been used for centuries by the native inhabitants of Central America in their religious ceremonies. Dimethyltryptamine (DMT) is derived from *Mimosa hostilis* and is an ingredient of Cohoba snuff, which is used by South American and Caribbean Indians. This compound becomes inactive when taken orally, hence it must be taken as snuff or injected. Bufotenine is believed to exist in small amounts in the mushroom *Amanita muscaria* and is also found in the skin and the poison glands of some toads. There is some evidence that bufotenine is found in the urine of schizophrenic patients, but other investigators report less in schizophrenics than in normals (Gillin et al., 1978). Behaviorally and physiologically, the effects of these substances are quite similar, except that the potency of LSD far exceeds that of DMT (by 250-fold) and of psilocin (by 100-fold).

Isoergine (Lysergic Acid Amide)

An interesting account of the possible role of another hallucinogen in an important historical event has been told by Caporael (1976). This author sought to find a rational basis for the accusations that were made and acted upon during the Salem witchcraft crisis of 1692. She examined numerous historical narratives and documents that might explain the strange events of that time. For the most part, the episode at Salem started in December 1691 with an affliction of "distempers" suffered by eight girls of Salem. The distempers were characterized by disorderly speech, odd postures and gestures, and convulsive fits. Because there was no logical explanation of these phenomena, the New England Puritans looked upon them as the work of Satan, brought about by the practice of witchcraft by some women of ill repute as well as by some respected members of the community. By the end of September 1692, 19 men and women were sent to the gallows, one man was pressed to death (a procedure designed to force him to enter a plea to the court so that he could be tried), and two of the accused died in prison.

During the trials, the girls described the activities of invisible specters and "agents of the devil in animal form"; they often had violent fits that were attributed to torture by apparitions; they complained of being choked, pinched, pricked with pins, and bitten by the accused. One man volunteered that he also had been choked and strangled by an apparition of a witch sitting on his chest, and that a black thing came through the window and stood before his face; "the body of it looked like a monkey, only the feet were like cock's feet, with claws, and the face somewhat more like a man's than a monkey. . . ."

After discounting fraud and hysteria, Caporael proposed that there were physiological bases for these behaviors stemming from ergot contamination of the food grains used in the area. Ergot is a parasitic fungus that grows on cereal grains. It contains a number of potent pharmacological agents, one of the most potent being isoergine (lysergic acid amide), an alkaloid having 10 percent of the potency of LSD-25. From written

Lysergic acid amide

records it was established that weather conditions were favorable in the 1691 growing season for an ergot infestation (i.e., a warm, rainy spring and summer), and that other factors favored the ingestion of contaminated cereal products by the residents of the town. It was the practice to harvest grain in August and store it in barns until cold weather, when it was threshed, usually in November, and then used as food. Until the midnineteenth century, ergot was not known to be a parasitic fungus; rather the ergot infected grain was regarded as sunbaked kernels.

The children's symptoms appeared in December of that year. It is to be noted that these events were sharply localized in the village of Salem, and there was no support from neighboring areas for what had transpired. It is not known how far the ergot-infected grain was distributed. In Salem most of the food was grown locally, and it was there that the accusations, convictions, and executions occurred.

In the summer of 1692 there was a drought that did not favor another ergot infestation. In late 1692 the accusations and trials ceased as suddenly as they had begun. In the following years nearly all who were responsible for the accusations and sentences publicly admitted to errors in judgment. Thus it was proposed that ergotism and the ingestion of isoergine, coupled with the ignorance and superstitions of the times were responsible for the Salem affair.

However, Spanos and Gottlieb (1976) took exception to Caporeal's conclusions after careful examination of early descriptions of ergotism and records of Salem witchcraft. They failed to find support for Caporeal's assertion that the accusers had symptoms of ergotism, and suggested that the behavior strongly favored an hypothesis that the accusers had faked the symptoms of "demonic possession" as the stereotypes of this affliction became known to them. The authors contended that the hypothesis is supported by many instances of sixteenth century demoniacs who displayed all the symptoms of the Salem girls who later confessed that they had faked their displays and confirmed their confessions by publicly enacting their supposedly involuntary symptoms. This method of analysis does not supply proof that the Salem girls were totally guilty of conscious faking, but it does suggest that this behavior could be accounted for without recourse to explanations based on an unusual disease.

Therapeutic Use of Hallucinogens

LSD and related compounds were tested in efforts to find ways to treat mental illness. They were used to treat psychoneuroses, schizophrenia reactions, depressions and alcoholism. The drugs were presumed to be able to facilitate insight on the part of the patient about the repressed memories that were the root causes of the present illness. However, these investigations did not yield much in the way of new-found approaches to these difficulties. First of all the studies frequently included poorly defined patient samples, vague goals of treatment, lack of control groups, and unorthodox investigators. Most of the claims that these drugs were beneficial could not be substantiated by replicated studies, and many favorable outcomes were deemed to be no better than placebo effects. In an evaluation of a study claiming success in treating depression with a single dose of ditran (an anticholinergic drug having severe autonomic side effects), it was proposed that the reported beneficial response might just as well have been based on the patient's fear that he might receive a second dose (Hollister, 1978).

LSD and other phantasticants were embraced in the 1960s by hundreds of thousands of American and European youths, who used these substances for an occasional thrill experience or because they thought the drugs were "consciousness expanders" and would open up their minds and provide insight into religious, sensual, esthetic, artistic, and creative endeavors of all sorts, as well as provide a profound understanding of one's place in society and the world. Because the drugs can only act upon the nervous system, whose mental content for all intents and purposes is derived from individual experiences, there are as many drug-induced experiences as there are drug takers. Thus, those seeking religious insights will see a diety in altered perceptions, the writer will see his experiences and hopes rearranged, the artist will see new geometric and color arrangements, and the disenchanted, the alienated, and the lonely will experience what they think is love, gentleness, innocence, and freedom. As Theodore Roszak (1969) wrote decrying the commitment to drug use by the youth of the counter culture (those expressing opposition to the then alleged "materialistic" society).

> Perhaps the drug experience bears significant fruit when rooted in the soil of a mature and cultivated mind. But the experience has, all of a sudden, been laid hold of by a generation of youngsters who are pathetically a-cultural and who often bring nothing to the experience but a vacuous yearning. They have, in adolescent rebellion, thrown off the corrupted culture of their elders and, along with that soiled bath water, the very body of the Western heritage—at best, in favor of exotic traditions they only marginally understand; at worst, in favor of an introspective chaos in which the seventeen or eighteen years of their unformed lives float like atoms in a void.

Not surprisingly, the anticipated promise of the phantasticant drugs could not be fulfilled; and because unique experiences are no longer unique when frequently repeated, the use of these substances markedly declined within a relatively short time (McGlothlin and Arnold, 1971). It obviously did not end, because new thrill-seekers can always be found. However, aside from the scientific interest in the physiological antecedents of the most unusual effects of these drugs, their serious use for restructuring the sick or dissatisfied personality is about over for now.

Summary

LSD and related indoleamines have significant effects upon the serotonergic cells of the raphe, and it is quite clear that the effect is an inhibition of the firing rate of these neurons. Normally these neurons exert a tonic inhibition on most of their target cells in the diencephalon and forebrain (Figure 12). The target cells of the raphe neurons seem to be quite insensitive to LSD, but at high doses LSD (like 5-HT) inhibited most of those target neurons as well. In cases where LSD seemed to block excitatory effects of 5-HT, it is possible that the excited cells were not normally excited by 5-HT inputs to begin with. In any case, the raphe cells do seem to be most sensitive to LSD and are probably the cells where LSD initiates the neural changes responsible for LSD effects. However, because LSD-induced cellular responses do not correlate in some respects with the behavioral effects and because LSD binding sites were found in various areas of the forebrain, the neural antecedents of LSD effects remain unclear (Watson, 1977).

Although LSD and related indoleamines have been, and remain, valuable tools for studying brain function, much behavioral research that is described in this volume is difficult to interpret because of the wide gamut of physiological effects that are characteristic of these drugs. The therapeutic and recreational use of the indoleamines was briefly mentioned, as well as their use in attempts to expand awareness or consciousness for the purpose of self-realization. It is our belief that there is meager evidence for sustained benefit. For contrary views, see Aronson and Osmund (1970) and Wells (1973).

Serotonin Antagonists

We have already mentioned that LSD and BOL inhibit the smooth muscle contraction that is mediated by 5-HT. It has also been well established that instead of blocking 5-HT effects in the CNS, LSD mimics the action of 5-HT and inhibits the neurons of the raphe and other neurons having serotonergic receptors. Whether or not LSD blocks the excitatory effects of 5-HT is not clear. Studies by Aghajanian et al. (1975, 1978) attempted to determine whether intravenous or microiontophoretic application of drugs that block peripheral 5-HT receptors would have similar effects on 5-HT receptors in the CNS. Using recording microelectrodes, cells were found in the reticular formation that were either stimulated or inhibited by 5-HT. The microiontophoretic application of the peripheral receptor blocking drugs, METHYSERGIDE (lysergic acid butanolamide, a congener of LSD) and LSD, blocked

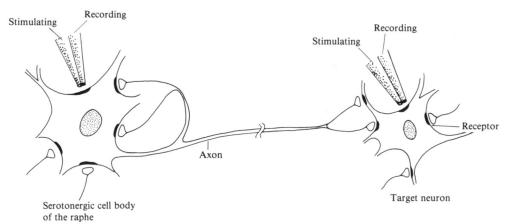

FIGURE 12 STIMULATION AND RECORDING FROM 5-HT and TARGET CELLS. The serotonergic cell on the left represents a cell in a nucleus of the raphe. It has two types of receptors: one type is more sensitive to 5-HT, the other to LSD. Both receptors exert inhibitory influences on the cell, and the effects are additive. These neurons may also inhibit themselves by releasing 5-HT via short recurrent collaterals ending on their own soma or dendrites. The target neuron on the right, found in areas such as the cortex,

amygdala, and lateral geniculate, is also inhibited by 5-HT and LSD. However, target neurons are more sensitive to 5-HT than LSD. LSD appears to have greater inhibitory effects on raphe cells, thereby disinhibiting target cells and causing them to increase their firing rate. Multi-barreled micropipettes on these cells permit simultaneous stimulation by drugs and recording of the resulting action potential firing rates.

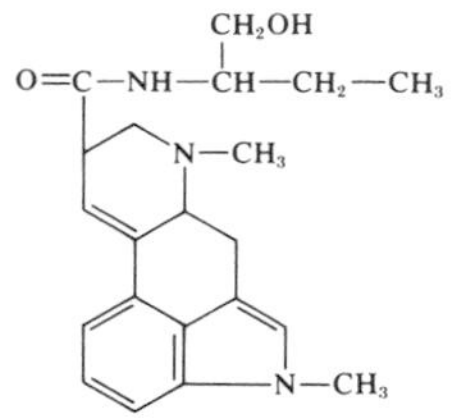

Lysergic acid butanolamide (Methysergide)

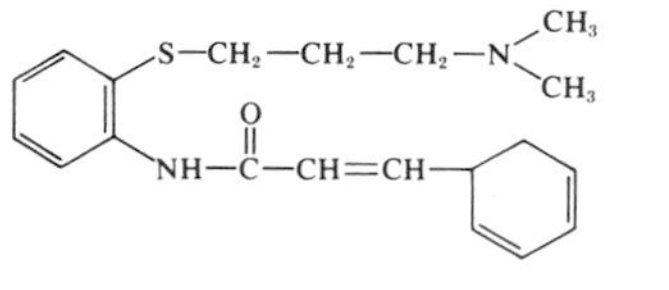

Cinanserin

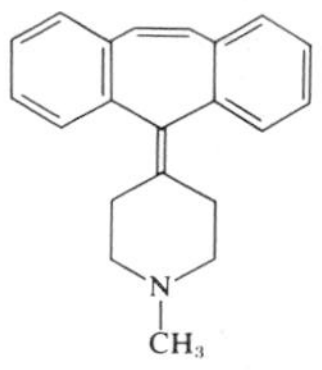

Cyproheptadine

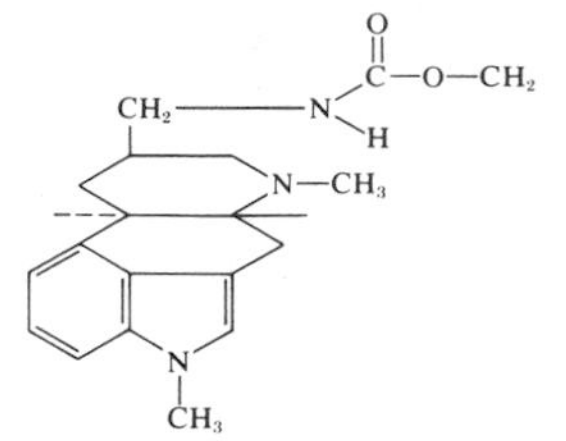

Metergoline

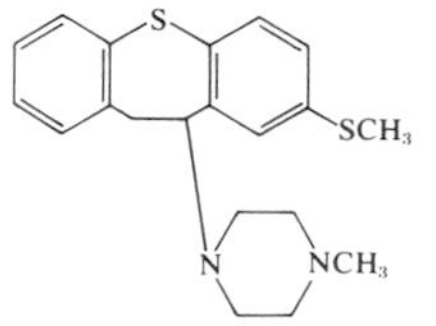

Methiothepin

the excitatory but not the inhibitory effects, and these two drugs plus another 5-HT receptor blocker, cinanserin, had the same effect in the cortex. These results suggested (1) that perhaps the two different receptors (the M and the D types) also exist within the CNS, (2) that one is responsible for excitatory effects and can be blocked by the antagonist drugs, and (3) that the other is responsible for inhibition and is not effected by the drugs. However, the excitatory effects of 5-HT can also be explained as pH artifacts of the procedures. Also, 5-HT induced inhibition was not blocked by the drugs. Therefore, it is possible that the drugs are not effective 5-HT antagonists within the CNS.

In some studies, methysergide did not block the inhibitory effects of 5-HT in the lateral geniculate in the cat—an area that has a high density of 5-HT terminals and that shows only inhibitory responses to 5-HT. In other studies, five different 5-HT antagonists (cinanserin, cyproheptadine, methysergide, metergoline, and methiothepin) given intravenously failed to block inhibitory effects of microiontophoretic ejection of 5-HT in the amygdala and lateral geniculate (also areas of high 5-HT terminal density), even when the doses of the drugs were high enough to depress spontaneous firing by themselves. As a matter of fact, when the drug doses were high, they potentiated the 5-HT-induced inhibition. Even when the antagonistic drugs and 5-HT were both applied microiontophoretically, the results were the same—no blockade of 5-HT depression and potentiated depression at higher drug doses (see Aghajanian et al., 1975).

The net results of these studies is that in the areas

tested these 5-HT antagonists did not block, but rather enhanced, the depressant effects of 5-HT; and in cases where excitatory effects of 5-HT were blocked, the possibility existed that cells not usually subject to 5-HT inputs were involved. The results also showed that at least some serotonergic receptors in the CNS have pharmacological properties that are different from the ones in smooth muscle. However, it is also possible that antagonistic drugs may have different effects in other parts of the CNS. This latter point deserves some emphasis because these drugs have important behavioral effects—effects that cannot easily be ascribed to peripheral drug action.

Physiological Effects of Serotonin Antagonists. Bennett and Snyder (1975) found that methysergide, cyprohetadine, and methiothepin are all fairly potent in their ability to displace LSD binding on rat brain membranes. This, of course, suggests that the drugs occupy the 5-HT receptor sites in place of LSD. Jacoby et al. (1975) investigated the mechanism by which methiothepin elevates brain levels of tryptophan and serotonin. They concluded that blockade of pre-or postsynaptic receptors could cause a compensatory increase of 5-HT synthesis. However, they also found evidence that methiothepin acting upon the pancreas elevated insulin levels, which raised brain tryptophan levels, which may have contributed to increased 5-HT synthesis. Furthermore, they found in cord-transected rats that tryptophan caused accelerated 5-HT synthesis both rostrally and caudally to the transection. However, in methiothepin-treated animals, the effect was absent in the caudal portion of the cord. Accordingly, the increase in amine synthesis in this case seemed to be secondary to impulse flow. The above results notwithstanding, Tebecis (1972) found that methiothepin alone among other 5-HT antagonists was able to block the effects of central 5-HT receptor stimulation that led to depression of PGO spikes, induction of sleep in immature chicks, and induced extensor reflexes in hindlimbs of spinal-transected animals. On the other hand, Monachon et al. (1972) found that methiothepin only partially blocked the 5-HT-induced hyperreflexia in spinal animals, and then only at high doses. Thus, the case for methiothepin as a CNS serotonin blocker is somewhat questionable.

Fenfluramine (Pondimin), a 5-HT agonist, has been widely used as an ANORECTIC (appetite suppressing) DRUG to aid in the control of obesity. However, its use

Fenfluramine

has declined because physicians have become increasingly reluctant to promote weight control by biochemical means; and there are reports that the drug causes cell damage in the raphe (Harvey and McMaster, 1977). Of interest here are the facts that 5-HT is involved in the anorectic action of fenfluramine (FEN) and that these effects could be blocked by 5-HT antagonists. The mechanisms of action of FEN were found to involve reduction of brain levels of 5-HT and increase of 5-HT turnover rate. At the synapse FEN increases 5-HT release from presynaptic terminals (Southgate et al., 1971; Jespersen and Sheel-Krüger, 1973), inhibits 5-HT reuptake (Belin, et al., 1976), and stimulates postsynaptic receptors (Funderburk et al., 1971). Also, FEN causes effects similar to those caused by raising brain levels of 5-HT in dogs by injecting 5-HTP. The fenfluramine effects were sedation, dilated pupils, apparent blindness, whining during petting, diarrhea, hypothermia, and unwillingness to keep still during measurement of rectal temperature. All of these FEN-and 5-HTP-induced effects were more or less reduced with methysergide (Jespersen and Scheel-Krüger, 1970).

Jespersen and Scheel-Krüger (1973) found that metergoline effectively blocked the anorectic effect of FEN, but methysergide failed to do so in rats and mice. However, in other studies, methysergide in high doses did block 5-HTP- and FEN-induced behavior in mice, even when the animals were also pretreated with a MAO inhibitor (Southgate et al., 1971). The lack of potency of methysergide may also be species related, because as noted earlier, it effectively reversed 5-HT and FEN effects in dogs (Jespersen and Scheel-Krüger, 1970).

The benzodiazepines constitute a group of ANXIO-LYTIC (antianxiety) drugs whose mode of action is related to the blockade of 5-HT in the CNS (Chase et al., 1970; Lidbrink et al., 1973; Stein et al., 1973). Geller and Seifter (1960) trained rats to lever-press for food reward, which on occasion was accompanied by foot shock, a condition that suppressed lever-pressing rates. Using this technique, Geller and Seifter evaluated the benzodiazepines (Librium, Valium, and Serax) in terms of each drug's ability to increase the response rates of the punished behavior. The benzodiazepines were quite effective in increasing the response rates—an effect that was considered to be due to the anxiolytic property of the drugs. These behavioral results have been repeated in many experiments, using different animal subjects and related experimental procedures. The role of 5-HT was further implicated as the same behavioral effects occurred when 5-HT levels were reduced with PCPA; and the PCPA effect was reversed by intraperitoneal injections of 5-HTP (the precursor of 5-HT). Furthermore, the 5-HT receptor agonist α-methyltryptamine strongly suppressed punished and nonpunished behavior alike (Graeff and Schoenfeld, 1970), and these same authors found that methysergide (a 5-HT receptor blocker) and BOL increased the rate of punished behavior. The same effect was found using the 5-HT receptor blocker cinanserin (Geller et al., 1974).

α-Methyltryptamine

Conclusions. The foregoing evidence would seem to show that 5-HT antagonists, which were mostly identified by their peripheral 5-HT blocking characteristics, exert, at least to some extent, 5-HT blocking effects in the CNS. However, this conclusion has to be accepted with some caution. The fact that 5-HT antagonists displaced LSD from binding sites in rat brains does not necessarily mean that the antagonists were occupying 5-HT sites, for it is possible that LSD occupies receptor sites of its own. With respect to the blockade of fenfluramine-induced effects, especially anorexia, it should be recalled that 90 percent or more of the body 5-HT is found in the smooth muscle of the GI tract, and 5-HT blocking drugs have strong effects on these stores of 5-HT. Also, there are 5-HT-mediated afferent nerves in the vagus nerve that may be the ones carrying "satiety signals" to the brain stem as the satiating effects of glucose infusion into the duodenum is blocked by vagotomy (Blundell, 1977).

The mimicking effects by methysergide and cinanserin of the anxiolytic drugs that block 5-HT release show most convincingly that central 5-HT receptors are involved in the methysergide effect. The blockade of 5-HT release by the benzodiazepines is an indirect effect (i.e., the benzodiazepines potentiate GABA inhibitory effects on 5-HT neurons—effects that only occur centrally as there are virtually no benzodiazepine binding sites outside of the CNS). Thus, suppression of central 5-HT systems can account for the anxiolytic effects of the benzodiazepines. If methysergide and cinanserin block central 5-HT receptors, the effects should be the same—as the evidence shows. If a 5-HT-blocking drug acting in the periphery had sympatholytic properties, it could account for its anxiolytic effects. Peripheral sympatholytic drugs do have anxiolytic effects, and propranolol (Inderal) (a β-noradrenergic blocker) is sometimes used in this capacity. However, there is no evidence that 5-HT receptor blockers share these properties. However, the fact that BOL also mimics the effect of the benzodiazepines does impose some constraints upon these interpretations as the central effects of BOL are unclear. In conclusion, more evidence will be required to firmly establish whether central effects are possible with 5-HT blocking drugs.

Part IV   Serotonin and Behavior

In the foregoing sections of this chapter there have been many examples of behavioral effects that occur when serotonergic systems have been manipulated. At this point it might be useful to describe in a more general way the changes that take place in broader behavioral categories that seem to be particularly dependent on serotonergic systems. It is implicit in this discussion that collateral changes in serotonergic systems and in behavior are insufficient to prove that there is a causal connection between the two phenomena. Rather the causal connection is established when the rise and fall of serotonergic activity is responsible for behavioral changes that are not readily duplicated by changes in other transmitter systems or by nonserotonergic drugs.

Ergotropic versus Trophotropic Systems

Serotonergic systems may have a well-defined role as a counterbalance to the activities of the catecholaminergic systems. This idea was put forward by Hess (1954), who proposed that an animal's reactions to environmental stimuli are affected by subcortical neural systems that coordinate autonomic, somatic, and psychic functions. The limbic system and the reticular activating system are examples of the subcortical neural systems structures. Within subcortical neural regions, there are two functionally antagonistic systems, which Hess termed the ergotropic system and the trophotropic system. The ergotropic system mobilizes functions that prepare the animal for arousal, excitement, increased muscle tone, and sympathetic nervous activity, whereas the trophotropic system is associated with decreased responsiveness, decreased muscle tone, and increased activity of the parasympathetic system. When efforts were made to correlate these behavioral attributes with the activity of drugs, it seemed that increasing noradrenergic functions were characteristic of the ergotropic system, whereas serotonin played a significant role in the trophotropic system (Brodie and Shore, 1957). It was even shown that the diurnal (24-hour) variations of tryptophan transport and 5-HT synthesis in hypothalamic tissue was the opposite of that for tyrosine and NE synthesis. In rats subjected to alternate 12-hr periods of light and dark, the high point of tryptophan transport was at 15:00 hours (light) and the low point at 21:00 hours (dark); the opposite was the case for tyrosine transport. To investigate the relationship between the diurnal variations in amine transport and states of arousal, rats received

6-OHDA into the cerebrospinal fluid and were sacrificed 3 weeks later. The drug injection led to degeneration of catecholamine neurons and a significant reduction of 5-HT synthesis and metabolism at 15:00 hours and the reverse at 21:00 hours compared to controls. Thus, the degeneration of CA neurons reversed the normal diurnal cycle of 5-HT synthesis, suggesting that the daily serotonin cycle is under the control of central catecholamine neurons (Héry et al., 1974).

Later, there were additional refinements of the ergotropic–trophotropic principle that suggested that rewards that followed responses and acted as positive reinforcers activated ergotropic CA systems, whereas the absence of reward or the consequence of punishment activated behavioral suppressant, trophotropic, serotonergic systems. The behavior-facilitating effects of CA systems and the behavior-suppressant effects of serotonergic systems is strikingly demonstrated in yet another experiment with intracranial self-stimulation as the behavioral end point. After rats had been trained to lever-press to deliver electrical brain stimulation to the hypothalamus, they were tested after intraventricular administration of L-norepinephrine HCl or serotonin HCl (Stein and Wise, 1974). Between 8 and 16 minutes after injection of NE there was a marked dose-dependent increase of lever-pressing followed by a gradual decline toward the baseline rate. In contrast, after 5-HT administration there was a decline in lever-pressing followed by a return to the baseline rate (Figure 13). Thus, following NE treatment, electrical brain stimulation seemed to be more reinforcing; however, after 5-HT treatment, the stimulation was either less reinforcing or even aversive.

Catecholamine and Serotonin Synergism

Although there are many examples of the counterbalancing relationship between adrenergic and serotonergic systems, it should be emphasized that this is probably not the exclusive relationship between these two systems. Most adrenergic and cholinergic systems within the autonomic nervous system are antagonistic, but in some ways they are synergistic. For example, excitatory fibers to the adrenal gland are cholinergic, but the secretion of the adrenal gland is epinephrine, which can also have excitatory effects. Within the central nervous system, similar synergistic relationships appear with respect to adrenergic and serotonergic systems. Jacobs (1974) observed that rats that were pretreated with the MAO inhibitor pargyline and then given

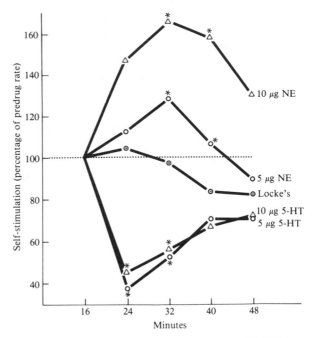

FIGURE 13 NE AND 5-HT EFFECTS ON HYPOTHALAMIC SELF-STIMULATION TESTS. Rats were trained to lever-press for hypothalamic self-stimulation. Sixteen minutes after the start of each test the rats were given an intraventricular injection of either L-NE•HCl or 5-HT•HCl in the doses shown. The data are expressed as a percentage of the self-stimulation rate in the second 8-minute test period (8 to 16 minutes after the start of the test). The data points were obtained by averaging the percentage scores of 11 rats. Starred points differ significantly (0.05 level or beyond) from Locke's solution (control) at the same time point. (From Stein and Wise, 1974.)

either L-tryptophan or L-dopa showed strikingly similar behavior syndromes. For examples, when pargyline (50 mg/kg, i.p.) and L-tryptophan (50 mg/kg, i.p.) were administered to rats, within 40 to 60 minutes the animals showed hyperactivity, hyperreactivity, salivation, head weaving, reciprocal treading with forepaws, tremor, and abduction of the hindlimbs. When L-dopa (100 mg/kg, i.p.) was substituted for L-tryptophan, many of the same changes occurred within 20–25 minutes, particularly tremor, head weaving, and the reciprocal treading of the forepaws. There was also hyperactivity, hyperreactivity, and salivation. However, with L-dopa, there was less rigidity and hindlimb abduction, but in addition, there was piloerection, exophthalmos (protruding eyes), and opisthotonus (arching of the back). In contrast, neither pargyline, L-tryptophan, nor L-dopa given alone produced any of these signs.

Jacobs was interested in whether or not a single neurochemical substrate was responsible for the symptoms that were induced by these two neurotransmitter precursors when potentiated by pargyline. Consequently, he selectively blocked the synthesis of serotonin or norepinephrine and observed the effect of later administration of pargyline and the precursors. That is, he blocked 5-HT synthesis with PCPA and tested animals with pargyline and L-tryptophan or L-dopa; or catecholamine synthesis was blocked with α-methyl-p-tyrosine (AMPT) and tested with pargyline combined with each of the two precursors. The results showed that prior blocking of CA synthesis with AMPT had little effect on the syndromes caused by pargyline and the two precursors. However, blocking 5-HT with PCPA abolished the pargyline + L-tryptophan syndrome, making the animals appear as untreated normals. When pargyline + L-dopa was given to the PCPA-treated animals, the rigidity, lateral head weaving, forepaw treading, and tremor were totally abolished, but the responses that would be expected of an animal with heightened CA activity (hyperactivity, hyperreactivity, salivation, philoerection, opisthotonus, exophthalmos, rearing, and jumping) were present.

Additional tests showed that animals that were pretreated with pimozide (a dopamine receptor blocker) showed the same effects from pargyline and the two precursors. However, when the rats were first treated with cinanserin (a 5-HT receptor blocker), the syndromes from pargyline and the two precursors were almost totally blocked, with occasional head weaving and forepaw treading occurring with each precursor. This evidence quite clearly indicated that heightened serotonergic activity was responsible for the syndrome whether it was induced by L-dopa or L-tryptophan. When the symptoms were induced by L-tryptophan, a higher synthesis and discharge rate of 5-HT, which is further potentiated by pargyline, would be the likeliest explanation. In the case of L-dopa, the syndrome is an indirect effect. It is known that L-dopa can be taken up by serotonergic axon terminals, thereby displacing and releasing 5-HT. When this synaptic release of 5-HT is potentiated by pargyline, the behavioral manifestations are almost the same.

There is a question here as to whether Jacob's experiment represents a natural *in vivo* effect or one that is dependent upon artificially high levels of transmitter precursors and potentiated transmitter action. This question cannot be answered by the results of this experiment, except that the results do indicate the possibility that dopaminergic and serotoninergic systems can act synergistically.

Serotonin and Sensitivity to Pain

A number of experimenters have investigated the role of serotonin in the perception of pain (for a review, see Seiden and Dykstra, 1977). Lesions in the medial forebrain bundle led to decreased brain serotonin and increased sensitivity to electric shock in rats. Increased sensitivity developed over the corresponding period necessary for nerve degeneration, and administration of the serotonin precursor L-5-HTP reversed the 5-HT depletion in the brain and decreased pain sensitivity; the correlation of brain 5-HT levels and pain threshold was 0.80. Administering D-5-HTP (which is not metabolized to 5-HT) or L-dopa had no effect. When lesions were made in septal areas, dorsal medial tegmentum, and the medial raphe nucleus, there were brain 5-HT depletions that were also accompanied by increased sensitivity to pain (Lints and Harvey, 1969). In other studies lesions that depleted brain serotonin were not accompanied by significant increases in pain sensitivity, but these paradoxical effects were believed to be due to lesion damage that encroached upon the central gray areas of the midbrain, an area that is traversed by pathways that mediate responses to painful stimuli (Harvey et al., 1974).

Morphine-induced analgesia was studied to determine whether there was a link with 5-HT levels. Tenen (1968) found that depleting 5-HT with PCPA blocked the analgesic effect of morphine, and another study (Samanin et al., 1970) showed that raphe lesions had the same effect. However, the results of neither study could be confirmed by other investigators. Also, there were disagreements as to whether chronic or acute morphine administration altered brain levels of 5-HT and whether the rates of 5-HT turnover were different in morphine-tolerant and non-tolerant animals.

The 5-HT pain sensitivity phenomenon is related to the observation that decreased levels of brain 5-HT lead to more rapid acquisition of conditioned avoidance responses (CARs) to aversive stimuli (e.g., learning to jump to a platform to avoid foot shocks) (Tenen, 1967). Rats treated with PCPA acquired an avoidance response in an average of 4.5 trials, the no-drug controls needed 23 trials; and the effect of PCPA was antagonized by 5-HTP. Because this result could have been due to increased sensitivity to shock, a second test was done in which the shock was increased for both groups, with the result that both groups acquired the avoidance response in less than five trials. Thus, the increase in shock intensity apparently led to more rapid acquisition of avoidance responding, and PCPA-induced 5-HT depletion presumably increased shock sensitivity with the same result.

Whereas PCPA did not facilitate learning in a T-maze, it did facilitate acquisition of one-way and two-way responding to avoid foot shocks. Conversely, potentiating 5-HT activity by blocking 5-HT reuptake with fluoxetine or increasing 5-HT turnover with fenfluramine hindered acquisition of CARs in a two-way shuttle box (Figure 14). Moreoever, these same effects were found in the shuttle box when the grid shock was intensified, i.e., higher levels of foot shock hindered CAR acquisition (McElroy et al., 1982). On the other hand, blocking 5-HT turnover with chlor-

diazepoxide (presumably by reducing 5-HT synaptic activity) facilitated CAR acquisition (Quenzer and Feldman, 1976) (Figure 15).

However, Tenen argued that because increased grid shock increased CAR acquisition, the effect of PCPA was to increase pain sensitivity, whereas other studies showed that raising grid shock impeded CAR acquisition. This contradiction might be explained by differences in the effectiveness of the grid shocks in these two different experiments. When grid shock is used as punishment in CAR paradigms, it is generally found that low shock levels may not sufficiently motivate shock avoidance, whereas moderate levels may do so, and high shock levels cause panic and "freezing" with poor CAR acquisition. It is the effects of moderate and high levels of shock that are most effectively blocked by antiserotonergic agents such as PCPA and chlordiazepoxide presumably by blocking fear and panic (see Chapter 11). When shock levels are low or moderate, drugs like fluoxetine and fenfluramine, which increase 5-HT effects, exacerbate fear and panic and hinder CAR acquisition. Thus, paradigms that ex-

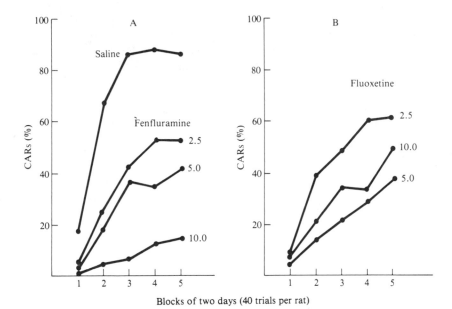

FIGURE 14 SEROTONIN AGONISTS INHIBIT ACQUISITION OF CARs. (A) Comparisons among the effects of saline and three doses of fenfluramine given i.p. one hour before ten daily avoidance tests (20 trials each) in a two-way shuttle box. Each data point represents the mean percentage of avoidances during two daily tests of 20 trials each (40 trials) for six rats. The numbers at the end of the curves represent the drug doses (mg/kg). (B) The effects of fluoxetine injections (McElroy, Dupont and Feldman, 1982).

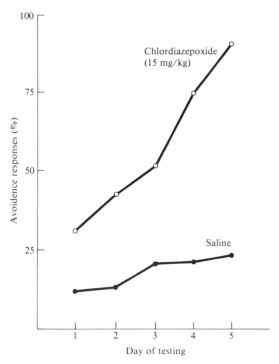

FIGURE 15 CHLORDIAZEPOXIDE FACILITATES
ACQUISITION OF CARs. Five rats were treated with saline
or chlordiazepoxide (15 mg/kg, i.p.) half an hour before 20
daily avoidance trials in a two-way shuttle box for 5 days.
(From Quenzer and Feldman, 1976).

amine the effects of 5-HT on the perception of pain
must consider the possibility that lowering 5-HT activity may disinhibit behavior that is suppressed by
punishment despite increases in pain sensitivity.

Serotonin is related to pain in a more direct way by
being associated with substance P, a putative neurotransmitter that mediates the perception of pain (see
Chapter 10), and enkephalins which are endogenous
opiate-like substances that produce analgesia (see
Chapter 13). All three of these substances are found in
neurons closely juxtaposed in the amygdala, periaquaductal gray, the raphe nuclei, and the substantia
nigra—all areas that are associated with the perception
and reaction to pain. Also, stimulation of the nucleus
raphe magnus (B3) activates a serotonergic descending
pathway to the spinal cord which elicits analgesia. Furthermore, certain raphe nuclei contain substance P
and serotonin which may interact in pain phenomena
(Snyder, 1980b). This finding is another piece of

evidence showing that a single neuron may contain
more than one neurotransmitter.

Serotonin and Sleep

A Brief History of Sleep Physiology

One of the most interesting aspects of our daily
existence is the phenomenon of sleep. Consequently
there is a long history of speculations attempting to explain this state. Discussions of sleep have been found
in the writings of antiquity but the earliest experiment
cited by Howell (1942) was one by Kohlschutter who in
1863 reported a study wherein a weight, fastened at the
end of a pendulum, was dropped from different
heights onto a "sounding plate" to make a noise to
waken a sleeping subject. The data were expressed as
the height that the pendulum was lifted as a function
of the duration of sleep. The sound tests occurred at
half hour intervals. The results showed that the loudest
noise necessary to wake the subject was needed about 1
hour after falling asleep after which there was a rapid
decline so that little noise was needed after 2 or 2½
hours. Similar experiments followed using lead balls
dropped from different heights upon lead plates and
electric shocks at different intensities serving as the
wakening stimuli. They all reported that the deepest
sleep occurred during the first hour, and some
reported an additional period of fairly deep sleep that
occurred about an hour before awakening. Despite the
crudeness of the measures these data are still fairly
valid today.

The physiological experiments that followed were
made to relate sleep to the accumulation of acid wastes
in the blood; deficits of oxygen stores in brain cells; the
presence of a "hypnotoxin" that was supposed to be
formed during the waking hours and that which
ultimately reached a sleep-inducing concentration; and
the retraction of nerve endings of afferent nerve terminals from the dendrites of brain neurons. Pavlov
(1927) proposed that sleep merely represented the
spreading of the process of internal inhibition to the
entire cortex.

Because it was known that cerebral anemia brought
on unconsciousness, some sleep researchers proposed
that the alternation between sleeping and waking
reflected the rhythmical variation of blood flow
through the cortex. Many investigators agreed with
this hypothesis after observing diminished blood flow
through the brains of dogs which could be seen

through glass windows inserted in their skulls. However Shepard (1914) published a paper on his observations of two subjects that had been trephined.* These human subjects showed increased brain volume during sleep, and Shepard suggested that during sleep there was a vascular dilation, and increased blood circulation and blood supply during the period of least brain activity.

Kleitman, one of the leading investigators of sleep phenomena, proposed in 1929 that muscular fatigue resulting from constant maintenance of muscle tonus during waking hours caused a diminished flow of afferent impulses to the cerebral cortex. This was responsible for the functional break between the cerebral cortex and the lower centers of the CNS, bringing on the unconsciousness of sleep. But experimenters found that sectioning the dorsal white fiber columns of the spinal cord in animals had no such effect.

Ultimately brain studies showed that sleep centers could be identified in the brain, as pathological lesions in the central gray of the midbrain and thalamus apparently accounted for the chronic somnolence of sleeping sickness (*encephalitis lethargica*), and experimental lesions in the areas accounted for permanent somnolence and stupor in animals. Some authors stated that the activity of these centers promoted wakefulness; others said they promoted sleep.

Current Views of the Physiology of Sleep

The development of electronics and the refinements of biochemistry have made electrical measurements of brain activity more meaningful and provided new and fruitful insights into the neurochemistry of sleep.

Electroencephalographic Correlates of Sleep. Sleep, at least in higher animals, depends upon neuroelectric changes in the cerebral cortex. Animals without significant cortical development may not sleep at all. This argument is based upon observations of animals in the submammalian classes, such as birds and reptiles, which show states of torpor but do not seem to show the kinds of sleep activity shown by mammals. The development of the electroencephalograph (EEG) in the 1920s and 1930s—generally credited to Hans Berger (Brazier, 1961)—established EEG correlates for

*A trephine is an instrument that cuts a circular disc or button of bone that is removed from the skull. After appropriate treatment the hole is covered by the scalp. The brain volume can be estimated by palpating the depression in the scalp.

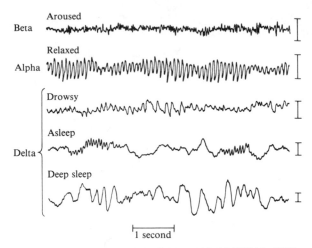

FIGURE 16   EEG RECORDS DURING AROUSAL AND SLEEP. Typical EEG records from normal humans during arousal (beta waves), quiet relaxation (alpha waves), and stages of sleep (delta waves). Delta waves are often classed into four levels rather than the three shown here. The vertical lines at the end of the tracings indicate a calibration of 50 μV. (From Penfield and Jasper, 1954.)

waking and sleep states. Recordings from the parietal or occipital lobes of a person at rest with his eyes closed show a rather rhythmic fluctuation of 8–12 Hz at a moderate amplitude, 20 to 30 μV, ALPHA RHYTHM (Figure 16). If the person is attentive to the features of the environment or tries to solve mental problems in arithmetic, the recording changes to a desynchronized condition with frequencies between 13 and 30 Hz at lower amplitudes, 5 to 10 μV, BETA RHYTHM. As a person relaxes and falls asleep, the recording progresses through four stages of increased synchrony and amplitude, 1 to 4 Hz at 30 to 150 μV, DELTA RHYTHM.

The delta rhythms correlate with a sleep state known as SLOW WAVE SLEEP (SWS or simply S-sleep), which is a rather profound, but dreamless, sleep. Typically after about 90 minutes of S-sleep, there is an abrupt change in the EEG record of the sleeping person: the EEG becomes desynchronized, with lower amplitudes resembling the EEG of an alert and active state. However, this state is actually a more profound sleep state than S-sleep. It is further characterized by moving eyeballs that correlate with dreaming, and reduced muscle tone. This condition has been called PARADOXICAL or RAPID EYE MOVEMENT (REM) sleep, or DEEP SLEEP (D-sleep). There are other behavioral and physiological correlates of D-sleep, one of which is the observed neuronal activity recorded in animals, consisting of bursts of phasic activity (100 to 200 μV spikes of 100 msec duration) in neurons located in the pons, lateral geniculate nucleus, and the occipital lobe. This activity is known as PGO SPIKES and is characteristic of D-sleep but may be found during S-sleep under certain circumstances. This phenomenon has not been observed in humans because their detection would require implantation of electrodes in the structures mentioned above.

Cats, dogs, and many other animals show the same EEG as humans: about 20 percent of sleep time in D-sleep as it alternates with S-sleep during the total sleeping period. Carnivores show about the same ratio, rodents show about 15 percent, ruminants (e.g., cattle) about 6.6 percent. Birds only show about 0.5 percent and reptiles show none; all of their sleep time is of the S-sleep variety (Jouvet, 1967). Whether or not fish sleep is a moot question.

The foregoing discussion has shown that it is unlikely that neurons get tired and run down; some neurons, like those responsible for PGO spikes, actually become

more active during deep sleep; and D-sleep is characterized by active processes as revealed by measurements of electrical activity of the cerebral cortex.

Are there "sleep" and "waking" centers in the brain? Experiments have established that wakefulness is not dependent upon sensory input to the cerebral cortex. Brain stem transections through the pons of cats eliminated all sensory input except smell and vision, yet this procedure led to an increase in wakefulness of from 70 to 90 percent compared to 30 to 40 percent for normal cats. In contrast, transections through the midbrain between the superior and inferior colliculi produced a somnolence for the few days the cats survived (Figure 17). Thus, a neural structure between the midcollicular and the midpontine region is important for wakefulness. Moreover, the midpontine lesion, which eliminated most sensory input but produced a state of insomnia, apparently cut off a neural structure that played a significant role in *inducing* sleep. It was even found that when thiopental (an anesthetic) was injected into blood vessels that were tied off so that only the caudal brain stem was affected, it caused sleeping cats to awaken (Jouvet, 1972). Thus,

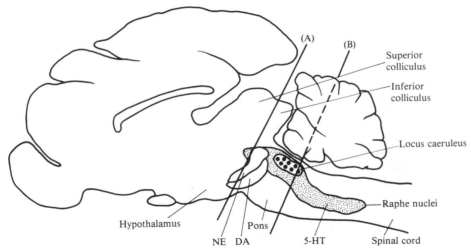

FIGURE 17 "SLEEP CENTERS" IN THE BRAIN STEM OF THE CAT. A sagittal view of the cat brain stem showing the sites of transection that affect sleep. The DA area is innervated by dopaminergic neurons that arise from the substantia nigra. (A) An intercollicular transection suppresses cortical activation by sensory stimulation and leads to somnolence for as long as the animal survives. (B) A transection through the midpontine area brings on cortical desynchronization (activation) and increases the daily amount of wake-

fulness. Thus, the raphe area caudal to the transection is important for the induction and maintenance of sleep. Otherwise normal sleeping cats are wakened when this area is suppressed by pentothal. The NE and DA areas between transection lines A and B are implicated in the maintenance of wakefulness. The caudal NE area is also implicated in the characteristics of D-sleep (EEG signs of arousal, suppression of muscle tone, rapid eye movements, and PGO waves). (Adapted from Jouvet, 1972.)

wakefulness appeared to be the result of suppression of a sleep center. A corollary of this finding is that sleep ought not to be considered as a result of diminished activity but rather as an active process in its own right. It should also be noted that other neural centers may play important roles in the sleep–waking cycles. For example, melatonin, which is secreted from the pineal gland, affects sleep; the dopaminergic pathway (arising from the substantia nigra) and the reticular formation are involved in the process of arousal; and stimulation of the midline nuclei of the thalamus and many other structures induces the cortical synchrony associated with sleep (Jouvet, 1967, 1972).

Serotonin-norepinephrine Interactions in Sleep and Wakefulness

Evidence for an NA Waking Center. As indicated above, brain stem transections at the midcollicular level produced a persistent somnolence, suggesting that the influence of a wakefulness center had been cut off from the cerebral cortex. In the rostral pons, there is a nucleus rich in norepinephrine (NE), the locus caeruleus (so named because of the presence of a blue pigment in this area). It is well known that amphetamine facilitates the release of NE and blocks its reuptake, resulting in strong arousal and sleeplessness. The amphetamine effect can be blocked with α-methyl-*p*-tyrosine, which blocks NE synthesis, supporting the role of NE in wakefulness (although a role for dopamine is not excluded). If the locus caeruleus is ablated, amphetamine no longer has a stimulating effect on wakefulness. If the ascending axons from the locus caeruleus—the dorsal noradrenergic bundle (DNB)—are severed, there is an increase in the duration of sleep with alternating S-sleep and D-sleep cycles. In contrast, electrical stimulation near the DNB leads to arousal. These data provide strong support for the hypothesis that the locus caeruleus is the noradrenergic waking center in the rostral pons.

Studies by Jones et al. (1968) showed differences in sleep-waking phenomena when brain dopamine (instead of NE) levels were reduced. They destroyed the substantia nigra in cats, which led to a 90 percent depletion of brain dopamine. Upon sensory stimulation, EEG evidence of arousal appeared even though the animals showed no overt behavioral arousal. This discrepancy may be explained by assuming that nigral lesions interfere with the initiation of movement (a symptom typically observed in patients with Parkinson's disease) as well as with the hypoactivity that frequently occurs when dopaminergic receptors are blocked by antischizophrenic drugs. Thus, dopamine deficits probably do not result in the unconsciousness of sleep but rather in deficits of motor expression. It should be pointed out, however, that nigral lesions do not adversely affect behavioral arousal in rats; there is even a report of an increase in activity in this species (Carlson, 1980).

Catecholamine Effects on D-Sleep. There is considerable evidence showing that CA neurons play a significant role in the initiation and manifestations of D-sleep. Jouvet (1974) summarized the neuropharmacological and neurochemical facts as follows:

1. Cats that have been pretreated with reserpine show a deficit of D-sleep. If these cats are treated with L-dopa (50 mg/kg), D-sleep reappears within 2–4 hours, whereas in cats not given L-dopa it takes 24 hours. Thus, refilling of CA pools appears necessary for the reappearance of D-sleep.

2. The administration of α-methyldopa (200 mg/kg) (which leads to the synthesis of α-methyl-NE, a false transmitter that reduces the release of NE), suppresses D-sleep in the cat for 12–16 hours and decreases waking.

3. Destruction of the caudal third of the locus caeruleus suppresses the motor inhibition associated with D-sleep, although PGO waves and the desynchronized EEG are still present. If the total locus caeruleus as well as the adjacent nucleus subcaeruleus is destroyed then all features of D-sleep are suppressed including PGO waves. The same phenomena occur when the neurotoxic substance 6-OHDA is injected into the laterodorsal pontine tegmentum, the site of the locus caeruleus. It was further suggested that the DNB that arises from the locus caeruleus is responsible for the EEG signs of cortical arousal, whereas fibers that issue from the nucleus subcaeruleus and form an intermediate pathway are responsible for the tonic feature, suppression of muscle tone; and phasic features such as PGO waves and rapid eye movements.

Thus a small number of neurons that issue from the locus caeruleus complex and synapse upon hundreds of thousands of cortical cells may be responsible for the major effects that characterize D-sleep.

Evidence for a Serotonergic Sleep Center. It was previously stated that midpontine transections of the cat brain stem led to increased wakefulness thus positing a sleep-inducing center caudal to the level of the cut. However, the early reports were not able to identify precisely the neural structures that were responsible for the waking effect (Jouvet, 1967). After the development of the fluorescence technique for identifying CNS adrenergic and serotonergic neurons (Falck et al., 1962), the serotonergic nature of the raphe nuclei was established and chemical studies could then parallel ablation techniques.

The nine nuclei of the raphe extend from the rostral medulla to the midbrain, making specific and total ablation of these cell groups quite difficult (Figure 1A). Nevertheless, Jouvet (1974) reported experiments with cats that showed that bilateral destruction of raphe nuclei led to almost permanent wakefulness, a sharp decline in brain 5-HT, and a desynchronized low voltage EEG. Smaller lesions caused a proportionately smaller drop in 5-HT and the sleep time was greater. With almost complete loss of the raphe nuclei, S-sleep did not exceed 10 to 15 percent of normal sleep duration and D-sleep was absent. However, PGO waves appeared about 3 hours after surgery for about 40 minutes but diminished by the third day to 10 minutes. These effects were not diminished by low doses of 5-HTP (5 mg/kg) because the conversion of the 5-HTP to 5-HT could not occur in degenerating neuron terminals. On the other hand, larger doses of 5-HTP (30–50 mg/kg) led to cortical synchronization even though the animals remained awake. This dissociation between the cortical synchrony and sleep (meaning that the former could exist without the latter) suggests that the large doses of 5-HTP themselves may have been responsible for the effect.

The rostral nuclei of the raphe complex were mainly responsible for the induction of S-sleep (and for serotonergic innervation of the teldiencephalon), whereas the intermediate nuclei seemed responsible for "priming" D-sleep. Furthermore, because the volume of the rostral group was greater than that of any of the others there was a significant correlation between the degree of destruction of the raphe system, the resulting insomnia, and the selective decrease of cerebral 5-HT. It should be noted that the topographic organization of the raphe nuclei pertaining to the duration of sleep does not seem to be congruent with the results of the transection experiments mentioned earlier. In other words, it is difficult to explain the wakefulness found after pontine transections when the major sleep-inducing centers appear to be rostral to the cut. Because the evidence strongly supports some role for the nuclei of the raphe, the explanation must include an understanding of the inputs (neuronal, hormonal, or both) to the raphe and the target sites of the serotonergic fibers emanating from the raphe. (See Jouvet, 1974, for speculations on this problem.)

Neurochemical Studies of Serotonin and Sleep. Jouvet (1974) recognized that although reserpine leads to a loss of neuron terminal 5-HT, it was not deemed suitable for 5-HT depletion studies on sleep, because it depleted stores of NE and DA as well. Consequently the more specific 5-HT-depleting drug PCPA was used. PCPA, which can serve as a preferred substrate for tryptophan hydroxylase, can block 5-HT synthesis and lower brain 5-HT by 90 percent. After a single injection of PCPA (400 mg/kg), there were neither EEG nor behavioral consequences for the first 18 to 24 hours, indicating that the drug itself had no observable effects. Soon after, however, there was an abrupt decrease in S- and D-sleep, with an almost complete insomnia that appeared after 30 to 40 hours and was accompanied by a high-frequency, low voltage EEG. At the same time, PGO activity (which is a constant feature of D-sleep but may occur in S-sleep just prior to the onset of D-sleep) appeared persistently during the drug-induced insomnia. This phenomenon also occurred after stereotaxic destruction of the raphe nuclei or after intraventricular administration of large doses of the 5-HT neurotoxin 5,6-dihydroxytryptamine. Forty hours after PCPA treatment, sleep patterns began to recover and were normal by 200 hours, a recovery pattern that was paralleled by a return to normal brain levels of 5-HT.

Because PCPA blocked the first stage of 5-HT synthesis, the effects of PCPA could be reversed by small doses of 5-HTP (2–5 mg/kg), which served as a direct precursor for 5-HT and bypassed the blocking action of PCPA. Given 30 hours after the PCPA injection, when insomnia in cats was maximal, a small dose of 5-HTP quantitatively and qualitatively restored S- and D-sleep for 6–8 hours. When a large dose of 5-HTP (30 to 50 mg/kg) was given, only EEG synchronization and sedation occurred for a few hours, followed by D-sleep 2–4 hours later. This suggested that after 5-HT synthesis was saturated, remaining amounts of 5-HTP seemed to interfere with the emergence of D-sleep.

Additional evidence supports a role for 5-HT in sleep. The hypersomnia (increased S- and D-sleep) caused by bilateral lesions in the dorsal NE bundle (DNB) was accompanied by an increase in the turnover rate of 5-HT; and pretreatment of cats with PCPA prevented the hypersomnia caused by DNB lesions (Jouvet and Pujol, 1974). Some authors tried to replicate these findings in rats. Two groups of investigators found that PCPA depleted brain 5-HT: however, although one group reported a 70 percent decrease in sleep, the other group found no significant change. Other variables such as prior sleep time, PCPA dose, environmental noise, and time of day of the tests, were examined, but they did not explain the differences (Seiden and Dykstra, 1977).

Effects of Prolonged Serotonin Depletion on Sleep and PGO Activity

An extensive study described by Henriksen et al. (1974) examined the effects of multiple doses of PCPA on sleep phenomena in cats. With daily administration of PCPA (150 mg/kg s.c.), the sleep changes that occurred were the same as those found after a single dose, that is, no effect for 12 to 24 hours, followed by a rapidly developing insomnia. However, after a number of doses, sleep patterns began to return so that S- and D-sleep were within 70 percent of normal by the eighth day of drug treatment. This is of special interest because throughout the recovery period 5-HT levels remained maximally depleted (90 percent). Figure 18 shows the changes that occurred in S- and D-sleep in a typical cat. It should be emphasized that with this dosage level of PCPA, the 5-HT levels in all assayed areas (cortex, midbrain, pons, medulla, and hypothalamus) were maximally depleted by the fifth day and remained so for as long as the drug was continued.

Another interesting finding in this type of experiment was that PGO waves paralleled the changes in brain 5-HT and not the loss of sleep time. More specifically, PGO waves began to change 16 to 24 hours after the first drug injection—days before the marked insomnia appeared. The first change was a sharp and progressive decrease of the PGO activity that is usually seen during S-sleep just prior to the onset of D-sleep, so that by the second drug day no PGO waves were seen until D-sleep occurred. At the same time, the PGO activity during D-sleep increased.

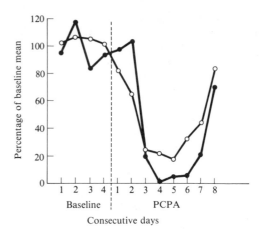

FIGURE 18 EFFECTS OF PCPA ON SLEEP. After establishing the baseline sleep levels in a representative cat for 4 days, PCPA (150 mg/kg, s.c.) was administered daily for 8 consecutive days. Sleep time abruptly declined to a minimum by days 3 and 4, but thereafter returned toward the baseline rate. (Solid circles represent D sleep, open circles S sleep.) (From Henriksen et al., 1974.)

By the third drug day, a reversal set in: PGO waves began to increase during S-sleep and decrease during D-sleep. Moreover, the increased PGO activity that occurred during S-sleep was distributed throughout the S-sleep intervals. When this effect was greatest, there occurred disruptions of the S-sleep pattern, that is, insomnia began to set in (days 3–6, Figure 18), and the PGO waves began to appear during these increasing periods of wakefulness. Ultimately, PGO activity occurred during all states with maximum PGO activity coinciding with the peak of insomnia. At this point the cats began to show some forms of "hallucinatory" activity. When brain recordings showed bursts of PGO waves the cats jerked their heads around, snarled, and jumped backward while hissing, suggesting that they feared or were attacking imaginary adversaries.

By the sixth or seventh day of drug treatment, the S-and D-sleep patterns began to return to near-normal values, but PGO activity was still present throughout all behavioral states. The "hallucinatory" episodes, however, began to subside in frequency and intensity. Still more gradually, PGO activity disappeared from the waking states and occurred predominantly in S-and D-sleep periods.

The PCPA treatments were terminated after 9 days, but brain and sleep monitoring continued. The sleep pattern quickly increased to baseline values. However, the PGO activity was very slow in returning to normal discharge rates and distribution, as it closely paralleled the recovery curves for 5-HT concentration. It took 15 to 20 days for PGO activity and 5-HT to return to normal.

The fact that almost normal sleep patterns return during prolonged PCPA treatment suggests some form of habituation to 5-HT depletion. Speculations about mechanisms other than habituation that could account for the reinstatement of sleep include both supersensitivity of transmitter-deprived 5-HT postsynaptic receptors to action from remnants of 5-HT pools and negative feedback after prolonged arousal associated with insomnia.

Interaction Between Serotonergic and Adrenergic Systems

To examine the effects of modifying CA systems (which are known to affect wakefulness) during states of insomnia, Jouvet (1974) injected α-methyl-p-tyrosine (200 mg/kg) in insomniac cats with rostral raphe lesions. This led to a quieting effect (less running around) and a sleep (synchronized) EEG that was maximum after 12 hours and lasted for 24 hours. Then there was a return to behavioral and EEG insomnia. This was interpreted to mean that 5-HT neurons exert a tonic inhibitory action directly or indirectly upon CA neurons (possibly in the locus caeruleus) at the onset of sleep. In other words, 5-HT neurons inhibit CA neurons. Without 5-HT, CA neurons become hyperactive and insomnia occurs. If the hyperactivity of the CA neurons is blocked by the CA synthesis inhibitor AMPT, sedation and EEG signs of sleep follow.

Apparently there are also inhibitory activities exerted by CA neurons upon 5-HT neurons. NE applied iontophoretically decreases firing rate of raphe cells (Couch, 1970); blockade of NE synthesis with AMPT or dopamine -β-hydroxylase inhibitors (Johnson et al., 1972) increased 5-HT turnover; and stimulating NE receptors with clonidine decreased 5-HT turnover (Lloyd and Bartholini, 1974). Lesions of the caudal part of the DNB (near the locus ceruleus) led to hypersomnia up to 300 percent for 3 to 8 days. This was accompanied by a decrease in forebrain NE and an increase in tryptophan and 5-HIAA in the teldiencephalon, the mesencephalon, and the spinal cord. The presence of tryptophan and 5-HIAA meant that there was an increased turnover of 5-HT (increased uptake of tryp-

tophan and increased synthesis and metabolism of 5-HT, leading to greater production of 5-HIAA). Thus, it appears that CA neurons normally suppress the activity of 5-HT neurons in the rostral raphe, an area rich with CA terminals.

Other CA–5-HT interactions are seen in the emergence of D-sleep. First, as described earlier, subtotal destruction of the serotonergic raphe nuclei led to a loss of all but 10 to 15 percent of normal S-sleep and D-sleep was totally absent. It was proposed that the loss of S-sleep can be attributed to the loss of rostral raphe groups whereas the loss of the intermediate groups accounts for the loss of D-sleep. Second, it was mentioned that large doses of 5-HTP seem to delay the emergence of D-sleep. A possible explanation of this is that the excess 5-HTP was taken up and decarboxylated within NE terminals, thus diminishing the release of NE that is necessary for D-sleep production. Everett (1974) has shown that 5-HTP at 200 or 400 mg/kg significantly reduces brain NE in mice. This is also borne out by the finding that depletion of NE with reserpine results in a deficit in D-sleep. It thus appears that CA–5-HT interactions control the emergence of D-sleep. The point of application of these interactions may be in the intermediate nuclei of the raphe, which are under the tonic control of CA neurons from the locus caeruleus.

Conclusions

From the foregoing it is clear that 5-HT plays a significant role in sleep. But precisely what role? The inhibition of PGO activity cannot be central because (at least in animals) it is a normal component just before and during D-sleep, the most profound sleep of all. Also we have seen that almost normal sleep can occur despite almost total (90 percent) 5-HT depletion that is clearly evidenced by the appearance of disinhibited PGO activity. Explanations for these inconsistencies (for example, supersensitivity of receptors and negative feedback on insomnia) are premature in the absence of supportive evidence.

Finally, there are reciprocal interactions between noradrenergic and serotonergic systems: the former being involved in wakefulness and D-sleep, the latter influencing S-sleep. S-sleep itself appears to be a determinant of D-sleep as there is no D-sleep without at least some S-sleep, the amount being about one-third the normal amount (Jouvet, 1974). It is not likely that this is the sole determinant of D-sleep. Questions remain about what modulates the NE–5-HT interactions, if indeed they are the principal systems controlling sleep–wakefulness cycles. Other factors, neuronal and hormonal, will probably emerge as answers to these questions (King, 1974).

Serotonin and Aggression

There is an extensive research literature that attempts to specify the role played by serotonergic systems in mediating various forms of aggressive behavior. As expected, the procedures involve the raising or lowering of brain 5-HT, by lesioning the 5-HT-bearing cells of the raphe nuclei or by chemical manipulation of serotonin synthesis or catabolism, and observing the effects upon elicited aggression. Other experiments have attempted to correlate aggressive behavior with changes in 5-HT turnover and to compare these changes with those of other neurotransmitters.

Aggression Defined

It is fair to say that the role of serotonin in aggression as elucidated by animal aggression paradigms has not been very consistently spelled out. One of the real problems in this research area, to begin with, is the definition of aggressive behavior. Moyer (1968), recognizing that aggression is not a unitary concept, attempted to operationally define various types of aggression and relate each of them to particular physiological substrates. He proposed that there are seven classes of aggression:

1. Predatory aggression (an attack on an object of prey).
2. Intermale aggression (fighting to establish dominance in mating functions).
3. Fear-induced aggression (reactions to threat or danger).
4. Irritable aggression (elicited by a wide range of stimuli, e.g., isolation, deprivation, pain, and directed to any of a number of available objects).
5. Territorial defense (attacks upon intruders).
6. Maternal aggression (attacks upon predators of the young).
7. Instrumental aggression (attacks upon objects that have been associated with fear or injury).

Physiological Substrates of Aggression

Many studies cited in Moyer's review have shown that each form of aggression has a particular neuro-anatomical and endocrine basis and that although there is some overlap among the classes, experimental manipulations will differentially affect the various types. For example, consider predatory aggression: Stimulation of the lateral hypothalamus of the cat will cause it to ignore the experimenter and attack a rat, but stimulation of the medial hypothalamus will cause the cat to ignore the rat and attack the experimenter. Stimulation of the lateral hypothalamus of a rat will not induce an attack on a mouse if the rat does not normally kill mice, but it does reduce the latency of the killing of a natural killer. Amygdalectomy (interruption of fibers running between the amygdala and hypothalamus) eliminates rat mouse-killing, and the same occurs by stimulating prepyriform cortex, the lateral olfactory stria, the olfactory bulbs, and some points in the midbrain. Frontal lobe lesions induce mouse-killing in nonkiller rats, but the topography of the killing is different in that normal killers bite once or twice through the back of the neck of the victim whereas killers with frontal lobe lesions are particularly vicious and ferocious, biting the mouse again and again even though the victim is dead. This observation suggested that this aggression is irritable rather than predatory aggression.

Examination of chemical substrates showed that testosterone is quite important in intermale aggression but of little importance on predatory aggression in rats. Cyclic food deprivation and competition over food will increase the percentage of killers among rats, but hypothalamic lesions that abolish feeding behavior in rats only temporarily inhibit predatory aggression, and nonkiller rats will not kill mice even if they are starved. Conversely, killer rats that are on ad lib food and water continually kill mice even when the mice are immediately withdrawn after the lethal attack.

From the viewpoint of eliciting stimuli, rats that kill mice will not generally kill rat pups (the rat pups are said to have a killer-inhibiting odor). Cats that attack rats during hypothalamic stimulation show reduced killing efforts the more the stimulus object differs from a rat (i.e., the object being a toy dog or a stuffed rat). Visual and tactile cues are important for cats in locating and biting rats, but olfaction is not important.

Thus, stimulation of the lateral hypothalamus elicits predatory behavior whereas amygdalectomy inhibits it. Gonadal hormones do not seem to be related to predatory behavior but are important for intermale aggression, and castration reduces irritable aggression.

Reproductive hormones are involved in maternal aggression but nothing is known of the neural basis of this behavior.

The intention of the examples given above was to illustrate the complexity of just one form of aggression, predatory aggression, in terms of its outward manifestations (topography), its physiological substrates (anatomical and neurochemical), and the sensory elements of the objects of prey. It is therefore, little wonder that some unifying aspect of these forms of behavior in which serotonin plays a significant role is not forthcoming.

Serotonergic Drugs and Aggression

Typically, mice that have been isolated in small cages (357 cm^2) for about 4 weeks pass through a hyperreactive stage to one of aggressiveness expressed as fierce and vicious attacks against other mice that have been introduced into the cage of the isolated mouse. In some tests two or more isolated mice are put together; in others a normal nonisolated mouse is added to the cage of an isolated mouse. When a drug such as PCPA that inhibits tryptophan hydroxylase and blocks serotonin synthesis was given to preisolated mice, intraspecies aggression among these mice was suppressed. But, after the use of another tryptophan hydroxylase inhibitor p-chloro-N-methylamphetamine, there was an increase in intraspecies fighting among preisolated mice.

In other studies with isolated mice, it was found that administering 5-HTP (200 mg/kg) along with a MAO inhibitor (pargyline) 1 hour prior to a test, attack behavior was suppressed without causing neuromuscular deficits. 5-HTP also suppressed predatory behavior in rats, an effect that was intensified by the peripheral decarboxylase inhibitor RO4-4602. However, 5-HTP did not alter predatory attacks upon rats by cats upon hypothalamic stimulation. This suggests that 5-HTP exerts effects that are antecedent to hypothalamic effects.

In isolation studies with rats, PCPA (400 mg/kg) was given 15 to 18 hours prior to the test. There was a 75 percent increase in attacks by the nondrugged resident rat against the PCPA-treated intruder. This could mean that PCPA diminishes the defense reactions of the intruder rat against the attacks of the resident rat.

In cats, PCPA generated strong defensive reactions (arching of the back and hissing) against nondrugged cats. In a group of macaque monkeys, PCPA (150 mg/kg given daily for 2 to 4 weeks) did not alter social activities, attacks, or threats, though there was a weight loss, ataxia, and other signs of debilitation (Miczek and Barry, 1976).

When pairs of rats were given foot shocks, they assumed upright postures, vocalized and sometimes grappled and bit one another (Ulrich, 1967; Ulrich and Azrin, 1962). If the animals were tested daily, one of them became the aggressor, the other the victim. Some investigators reported that PCPA-induced 5-HT depletions of 90 percent had no effect on this shock-induced aggression, whereas others reported an increase at roughly comparable size and frequency of doses. Conversely, PCA and fenfluramine, which also depletes 5-HT, were reported to decrease the aggressive–defensive reactions to foot shock; and chlordiazepoxide (15 mg/kg daily), which is purported to reduce 5-HT turnover, reliably reduced shock-induced aggression over 10 consecutive daily tests (Quenzer et al., 1974).

When pairs of reserpinized rats were given foot shocks, their aggressive defensive reactions were suppressed by 5-HTP or 5-HT (800 mg/kg in three injections) but these doses also suppressed locomotor activity. At lower doses (40 mg/kg), the suppressant effect was lost (Miczek and Barry, 1976).

Some investigators reported that PCPA increased mouse-killing (muricide) in rats, but in some cases the increase was small despite major decreases in brain 5-HT (80 to 90 percent). Also, p-chloroamphetamine (PCA), which decreased brain 5-HT by 60 percent, failed to produce muricide. On the other hand, Grant et al. (1972) reported that after dorsal and median raphe lesions, rats increased their attacks upon mice and reduced the latency of attack. The attacks increased and the latency decreased over a 30-day observation period and the end of the period was marked by a 70 percent depletion of forebrain 5-HT.

Valzelli (1974) examined the effects of isolation in rats and mice on behavior and brain neurochemistry. He observed, first of all, that only male mice show isolation-induced fighting, and that the response depended on the duration of the isolation and the strain used. Within some strains, 100 percent of the animals showed aggressiveness after 4 weeks of isolation whereas animals in other strains required 7 weeks. Still other strains showed no aggression even after 7 weeks. Among rats, only one of six groups (Wistar males) yielded 40 percent aggressors after 7 weeks of isolation.

In examining the effects of isolation on neurotransmitter activity Valzelli found that although brain levels of 5-HT, NE and DA did not change when mice were isolated, the turnover rates of 5-HT in aggressive mice were reduced compared to those in normal mice. Interestingly, the biochemical change occurred during the first or second day of isolation although the aggressive behavior developed more gradually reaching a maximum after 4 weeks of isolation. Moreover, the change in 5-HT turnover that did occur appeared only in those animals that eventually became aggressive, not in isolated females that did not become aggressive and not in members of strains not susceptible to isolation-induced aggression. With respect to other neurotransmitters, the aggressive mice also showed a decrease in NE turnover and an increase in DA turnover.

When rats were isolated, brain levels of neurotransmitters were similarly unchanged as in mice; however, changes in 5-HT turnover were not so easily correlated with their behavior. In the rat experiments, the isolated animals were tested for muricidal tendencies. The turnover of 5-HT was reduced in the muricidal rats, but the turnover rate was even more reduced in "indifferent rats" (rats that sat motionless and paid little or no attention to mice placed in their cage. Normal rats show curiosity by getting up and examining the intruder.) Other rats, designated as "friendly" because they exhibited maternal behavior and played with the mice, showed an increase in the 5-HT turnover rate. On the other hand, NE turnover was increased in muricidal and friendly rats but was unchanged in indifferent rats. There was no evidence that isolation changed other brain enzymes such as MAO and choline acetylase; nor were aspartic acid or glutamic acid concentrations altered.

In general the results of these experiments suggest that isolation induces a reduction in 5-HT turnover that is an antecedent for irritable aggressive behavior in mice and rats despite the paradoxical decrease in 5-HT turnover in indifferent rats. The changes in turnover in NE and DA are possibly secondary effects dependent upon the 5-HT changes (Chase, 1974; Everett, 1974).

Dominguez and Longo (1970) reported that PCPA had an immediate taming effect on rats with septal lesions. Septal lesions induce violent attack reactions in rats (and mice, but not in cats) when they are prodded with a stick or when attempts are made to pick them up. These attacks appear within hours after the animals recover from the surgical assault. The observation that PCPA subdues these attacks suggests that the septal syndrome results from a hyperserotoninism. The taming effect of PCPA occurs very rapidly however (within 30 minutes following drug administration), long before there is a significant 5-HT depletion; maximum depletion occurs in 2–3 days. Also, Welch and Welch (1968) reported an abolition of fighting in intact preisolated mice within 10 minutes of PCPA administration. The effect was accompanied by a slight drop in brain NE but not of 5-HT. This suggested that PCPA has taming effects independent of serotonin changes.

6-OHDA has cytotoxic effects on CA neurons; therefore, analogs to 6-OHDA have been developed that have damaging effects upon 5-HT cells. One of them, 5,6-dihydroxytryptamine (5,6-DHT), was administered intracisternally (75 μg) to nonkiller rats. It caused 47 percent of them to kill mice, which was concurrent with a 37 percent reduction of the rats' brain serotonin. Two injections (10 μg each) into the midbrain raphe caused the same 5-HT depletion with somewhat fewer (33 percent) killers.

LSD Effects on Aggression

LSD reduces serotonin turnover while increasing brain 5-HT, reducing 5-HIAA levels, and reducing 5-HT synthesis. These effects probably occur because LSD inhibits neuronal activity in the nuclei of the raphe. Thus, LSD may be presumed to have effects similar to those induced by other drugs that cause 5-HT depletion (e.g. PCPA, PCA, and fenfluramine). To some extent this is true; like PCPA, LSD and related compounds decreased isolation-induced aggression. But LSD increased shock-induced aggression, whereas PCA and fenfluramine decreased it and PCPA had no effect. Also, high doses of LSD (5.0 mg/kg, s.c.) given to pairs of rats induced the upright postures similar to those seen during shock-induced fighting episodes. However, doses of LSD (1.0 mg/kg, i.v.) given to juvenile rhesus monkeys caused them to assume prone postures followed by ataxic circling and then by unusual prolonged tameness (Miczek and Barry, 1976).

There have been reports that LSD promotes aggression and suicide in humans, but these anecdotal reports frequently fail to consider predrug personality characteristics, the drug-taking setting, and other drugs that may have been taken. Furthermore, the aggression may have been the consequence of drug-induced panic or delusions that the subject was being threatened or that he could perform superhuman feats that when attempted led to injury or fatal accidents. More objective reports about LSD effects from those humans who use the drug repeatedly provide a picture of euphoric feeling tone, bliss, and ecstasy, although apprehension, withdrawal, and paranoid rage reactions have been encountered, especially among individuals that are newcomers to the drug scene (Cohen, 1970). It may be that the drug-induced experiences of novices are different as they are a less selective group than repeated users and their reactions may be more typical and revealing.

It is more likely that acute amphetamine psychosis will provide a setting for drug-induced aggression in animals and men. Persistent use of this drug can lead to physical hyperactivity, suspicion, paranoia, and hallucinations that may gravitate toward acute terror attack and suicidal tendencies (Weinswig, 1973). It should be emphasized, however, that it is not likely that any drug is specific for inducing aggression apart from the predrug personality and the setting for the drug-taking experience (Ellinwood, 1974). There is probably no drug that promotes aggression more than ethanol, but there is abundant evidence that there are personality and situational antecedents for the aggression often released by this drug.

Summary

The foregoing section discussed the effects of serotonergic agonists and antagonists on behavior elicited during procedures intended to provoke aggression. When brain levels of 5-HT were depleted with PCPA, isolated-induced intraspecies aggression was suppressed; however, another 5-HT depletor increased the aggression. On the other hand, 5-HTP and 5-HT administered with a MAO inhibitor also suppressed isolation-induced fighting. The 5-HTP and 5-HT actions were presumed to be due to peripheral effects, but this is inconsistent with the finding that these effects were enhanced by a decarboxylase inhibitor. PCPA also suppressed what might be the counter-attacking ability of normal rats when confronted with attacking preisolated rats. In cats PCPA seemed to intensify defensive reactions, whereas in macaque monkeys there were no significant changes in social behavior, attacks, or threats. Predatory behavior (muricide) was increased by PCPA in some rat experiments but not in others.

The positive findings were supported by the results of another experiment that showed that 5-HTP suppressed muricidal activity in rats.

L-Dopa administration led to attack between pairs of rats if they had been pretreated with PCPA, but PCPA did not influence apomorphine-induced attacks between pairs of rats. Reserpinized rat pairs attacked each other when given foot shocks, but this was suppressed by large doses of 5-HTP or 5-HT, though the doses caused ataxia. With low doses, the effect was lost. In some experiments, shock-induced fighting in rat pairs was not altered by PCPA doses that caused 5-HT depletions of 90 percent, but other experiments showed an increase in attacks. However, PCA- and fenfluramine-induced 5-HT depletions decreased attacks caused by foot shocks. Rats with septal lesions showed vigorous attack behavior, which is suppressed by PCPA; PCPA also suppressed fighting between preisolated rats, but in these two cases the onset time of the suppression was too short to be explained by the usually long-delayed course of 5-HT depletion.

Destroying 5-HT neurons in rats with 5,6-DHT (i.c.) caused depletion of serotonin and an increase in muricide, a finding consistent with increased muricide following PCPA treatment and the suppression of muricide with 5-HTP, the 5-HT precursor. Valzelli (1974) reported that isolation caused reduced 5-HT turnover leading to the later appearance of aggression. This is consistent with an increased 5-HT turnover in friendly rats but not with the decreased turnover in indifferent rats.

Thus, we see instances of suppression of isolation-induced attacks associated with lowered brain 5-HT as well as after 5-HTP treatment, which should have increased brain 5-HT. On the other hand, PCPA increased muricide (sometimes), whereas 5-HTP suppressed it. PCPA did not affect shock-induced aggression whereas chlordiazepoxide and 5-HT depletors (PCA and fenfluramine) did reduce it. Instances of 5-HT depletion in humans (with reserpine) led to depression rather than aggression, but the catecholamines were also depleted. Because aggression can be elicited with the CA agonists (amphetamine, L-dopa, and apomorphine), interactions between 5-HT and the CAs are probably significant in the expression of the various forms of aggression.

LSD, which blocks 5-HT turnover, was found to have mixed effects on aggression. In rats it decreased isolation-induced aggression but increased shock-induced fighting. By itself, LSD caused upright posturing in rat pairs, but it led to prone positions, ataxia, and tameness in rhesus monkeys. LSD does not provoke aggression per se in humans, though aggression and self-injury may occur as secondary effects from drug-induced fright or panic. Thus, the effects of LSD on aggression depend upon the type of aggression and the animal species tested.

Finally, the foregoing evidence supports the idea that manipulation of the brain content of 5-HT alters the expression of aggression. The aggressions in animals are defined by the paradigms that were designed to elicit and measure them and are expressed in a variety of ways, each of which is probably associated with a different constellation of neural and physiological features. As we stated earlier, there is little wonder that no 5-HT effect can be isolated that can consistently serve to modulate the various forms of aggressive behavior. Thus, it is most likely that aggressive behavior (if such a generalization is at all justified), like any other complex behavior, is mediated by interacting neural systems, with multiple neurotransmitter systems being involved (Moyer, 1968). It is also likely that when 5-HT systems are manipulated, other neurotransmitter systems are altered as biological mechanisms redress physiological imbalances. So, although 5-HT does influence the expression of aggression, it appears that the effect is neither an exclusive nor a specific one; nor, for that matter, is it a very predictable one.

Serotonin and Sexual Behavior

Interest in the relationship between serotonin and sexual behavior may be said to have developed after Sheard (1969) and Tagliamonte et al. (1969) published findings that by depleting brain 5-HT with PCPA they caused an increase in sexual behavior in male rats. It is quite likely that this interest was related to the apparent search for a reliable aphrodisiac. Because of the wide range of 5-HT effects, a serotonergic compound has not ended that search, yet a considerable amount of research has attempted to clarify the role that serotonin might have in sexual behavior.

At the outset, one should be reminded of the enormous complexity of sexual behavior and the methodological problems associated with its study. First of all, interspecies differences abound in the details of courtship behavior, territorial considerations, breeding environments, aggression in the establishment of the dominant breeders, copulatory patterns, seasonal rhythms,

and so on. There is no doubt that rearing experiences and sexual experiences are important factors (consider the difficulties in breeding the giant Chinese panda in the United States). Furthermore the male-female ratio may have to be taken into account. In addition, there are decisions about whether to investigate sexual development or decline, or the display of mature sexual performance. In the latter case there are questions about which aspects of sexual activity are to be observed: overall sex drive as measured by frequency and latency of sexual encounters, the frequency and success of copulation and ejaculation in males, the receptivity of females, or the vigor with which females seek sexual contact with males, and homosexual behavior.

When studying hormonal factors, there are methodological problems in monitoring endogenous mechanisms prior to or during drug tests. These problems can be sidestepped by using adrenalectomized and ovariectomized females or castrated males and supplying the respective hormones (such as estradiol and progesterone to the female and testosterone for the male) at appropriate times. Coupled to these problems are other problems that arise when drugs are used. Ideally there should be neurochemical data to add to the behavioral data that is generated by drug tests. It is now possible to study changes in hormone-neurotransmitter interactions. There may be interspecies differences in reactions to chemical agents, which may call for differences in the timing and dosages of drug administration. Then, the behavioral effects of drugs must be compared to baseline rates of sexual activity. This requires patient observation of what must pass for control rates of sexual behavior for each animal species studied. Most studies in the pharmacology of sex employ rats or mice, but monkeys, cats, pigeons, and even certain species of fish have been observed. Assuming that the ultimate goal is the understanding of the effect of drugs on human sexuality, generalizations from findings from animal experiments to humans, because of the considerations discussed above, can be extended only with extreme caution (Meyerson et al., 1974, Miczek and Barry, 1976).

Neurotransmitter–Gonadotropin Relationships

Some Hormones of the Reproductive System. The substantial evidence showing monoaminergic influences on sexual behavior raises the issue about the relationships of neurotransmitters to the sex hormone system. The sex hormones and their precursors and metabolites make up an exceptionally complex system that governs sexual differentiation between males and females, sexual development during puberty and adolescence, courting behavior, sexual cycles, ovulation, spermatogenesis, copulation, pregnancy or brooding behavior, parturition, lactation or feeding the young by other means, and ultimately the decline of sexual behavior. Moreover, sex hormones govern many aspects of human secondary sexual characteristics such as bone structure, hair and fat distribution, pitch of the voice, and muscular development and growth. Furthermore, hormones determine many sex-differentiating behaviors such as competition for mates, territoriality, dominance, and defense of mates and offspring.

Many books on endocrine physiology can provide the details of sex hormone interactions, but our purposes will be met by a general description of the basic organization. Somewhat arbitrarily we may begin with the anterior hypothalamus, because the hypothalamic nuclei appear to be the junctional points for the multisynaptic neural inputs mediating olfactory, visual, auditory, tactile, and other types of cues that elicit sexual responses. For example, sexually exciting odors from the genitalia and urine of the female, sexual displays and mating calls from the male, soliciting behavior, and mounting behavior all provide sensory inputs to the hypothalamus directly or indirectly. There are additional inputs from the raphe nuclei, the limbic structures such as the amygdala and hippocampus, and the suprachiasmatic nucleus (the so-called "internal clock" that is governed in a significant way by the duration of daylight). Even the hormonal composition of the blood provides feedback information to the hypothalamus. All of the neural inputs that were mentioned account in some degree for the presence of adrenergic, cholinergic, and serotonergic axon terminals within the rostral and basal hypothalamus.

The neural inputs stimulate or inhibit the neuroeffector cells in the hypothalamus, which release various POLYPEPTIDES (molecules made up of a chain length of more than ten amino acids) into the capillary loops of the median eminence. The peptides, such as the gonadotropin-releasing hormone (GnRH), are then carried by the intricate portal system to the hormone synthesizing cells in the anterior pituitary gland (see Figure 12 in Chapter 3). GnRH causes the release of the luteinizing hormone (LH) [as well as the

follicle stimulating hormone (FSH)] into the bloodstream, and LH is circulated to the brain, sex organs, and other visceral structures. In the females, LH stimulates the ovaries, causing ovulation and the production of the hormones estradiol and progesterone. In the male, LH affects the testes, leading to the production of testosterone, whose principal effect is stimulating sperm production. In addition to these effects, estradiol from the ovaries acts back upon the pituitary gland to influence the release of LH, and testosterone has the same effect in the male. Additional feedback pathways have been traced to the hypothalamus and to the peptidergic neurons, which release GnRH and other hormone-releasing factors (Chapter 10).

Finally, the adrenal cortex, which is under the control of the peptide CRF (corticotropin releasing factor) and ACTH, also releases some sex hormones, principally testosterone, progesterone, and small amounts of estradiol. Other adrenocortical hormones, in addition to regulating such things as electrolyte and water balance, act back upon the hypothalmus and pituitary gland to regulate the release of CRF and ACTH.

Serotonergic Drugs and Sexual Behavior. Sheard (1969) and Taliamonte et al. (1969) found that reducing brain 5-HT levels with PCPA produced a long-lasting sexual excitation in male rats that was potentiated by pargyline* (a MAO inhibitor) and blocked by 5-HTP. The sexual excitation was characterized by an increased frequency of homosexual mounting with pelvic thrusting and penile erections. Of course, these observations were made among all-male populations. These sexual responses were also observed in later studies with castrated rats as well as with intact rats with or without testosterone treatment. The same effects were observed in rabbits (Tagliamonte et al., 1970) and cats (Ferguson et al., 1970).

Heterosexual copulation that was performed at low baseline rates by sexually sluggish male rats was increased by PCPA with or without pargyline, but PCPA did not increase the number of ejaculations in rats with high basal rates of sexual activity, although it did decrease their ejaculation latencies. However, although heterosexual copulation was induced in

---

*Tests were done with pargyline to see if enhancement of CA activity caused by blocking its catabolism would potentiate the effects of 5-HT depletion.

castrated males by testosterone, PCPA was found to be ineffective.

In female rats the lordosis response is an indication of sexual receptivity occurring during estrous when the ova are ready for fertilization. The response consists of the rat's crouching with the pelvis tilted upward, the tail also tilted upward and deviated to one side, and a flexion of the neck muscles to raise the head up and back. The response normally results from the action of estradiol and progesterone. In ovariectomized rats maintained on estradiol, a single dose of PCPA induced lordosis in the presence of a sexually active male in almost the same percentage as tests done with progesterone. Also, LSD (which can serve as a 5-HT agonist) inhibits lordosis. These data are supported by the finding that this effect disappeared after repeated dosing by LSD, a result that coincides with the well-known tolerance that rapidly develops for LSD. Furthermore, it was observed that soliciting behavior—the hopping and darting movements and ear wiggling in front of the male that are additional signs of sexual receptivity—was not evoked by serotonin-suppressing drugs. This suggests that other neurotransmitters are probably involved in sexual responsiveness (Meyerson et al., 1974; Marcyzinski, 1976; Miczek and Barry, 1976).

Other studies showed that the lordosis response can be elicited from ovariectomized females by intrahypothalamically administered 5-HT receptor blockers such as methysergide and cinanserin (Ward et al., 1975). The same effect could be elicited even from estrogen-treated males (Crowley et al., 1975). But these drugs had no effect when they were perfused into other subcortical structures. Methysergide also increased the number of ejaculations in copulation tests 3 hours after drug administration at a low dose (4–8 mg/kg, s.c.) but not at higher doses (13–18 mg/kg), which caused general stimulation. These results would support a central role for these drugs.

Depleting brain 5-HT with the neurotoxin 5,6-DHT also increased homosexual mounting and pelvic thrusting in male rats.

It was also shown that the sexual activity induced by 5-HT depletion could be reversed by i.v. injections of 5-HTP. Even without prior depletion of 5-HT, raising 5-HT levels with 5-HTP administration suppressed the copulatory behavior of normal rats in the presence of receptive females, an effect that was potentiated by RO4-4602 (a peripheral decarboxylase inhibitor), showing that 5-HTP had its effect by raising central

5-HT levels. Furthermore, MAO inhibitors suppressed copulatory activity in normal rats but not those that had been pretreated with PCPA (Gessa and Tagliamonte, 1974).

Other areas of research have shown that systemic injections of 5-HT or 5-HTP to immature rats at the critical period when a surge of LH release is necessary to induce ovulation will inhibit ovulation by blocking LH release. Also, blocking 5-HT synthesis with PCPA stimulates ovulation, and the intensity of the provoked ovulation is inversely proportional to the 5-HT level in the hypothalamus. It has been established that the 5-HT terminals in the median eminence are from cells of the dorsal raphe nucleus (Azmitia, 1978) and that electrical stimulation of the raphe inhibits ovulation in the rat. Thus, these 5-HT terminals are antagonists to the tuberoinfundibular DA neurons, which are believed to trigger the release of LHRH. And, finally, mapping studies have established that within the hypothalamus, the serotonergic receptors that are activated by high 5-HT levels and are responsible for the inhibition of ovulation are found exclusively in the median eminence (Marczynski, 1976; Kizer and Youngblood, 1978).

Summary

The foregoing data support the conclusion that serotonergic systems exert inhibitory influences on behavioral and physiological manifestations of sexual activity. However, there have been some negative reports concerning PCPA-induced sexuality. For example, in castrated rats copulation could be induced by testosterone but not by PCPA; and even though α-propyldopacetamide depleted brain 5-HT, it had no effect on lordosis.

Some investigators observed PCPA-induced homosexual, but not heterosexual, activity in rats and cats. This suggested that the hypersexuality was not the effect of an increased sex drive but rather was due to perceptual disturbances that prevented the male from distinguishing appropriate sex partners. This view is based on observations of PCPA-treated cats that showed bizarre behavior and pseudohallucinatory activity—abnormal rapid eye movements, staring at fixed points, and following moving objects not seen by the human observer (Marczynski, 1976; Seiden and Dykstra, 1977; Miczek and Barry, 1976). Nevertheless, the current consensus is that 5-HT systems play an inhibitory role in sexual phenomena.

Adrenergic versus Serotonergic Effects
on Sexual Behavior

As we have seen, a case can be made that CA and 5-HT systems interact to control sleep phenomena and aggression. The same probably holds for sexual behavior. Thus far it seems that serotonergic mechanisms normally inhibit sexual expression, an inhibition that is suppressed when 5-HT depletion or receptor blockade occurs. The evidence in support of a stimulating role for catecholamines on sexual behavior can be summarized as follows.

1. A tuberoinfundibular dopaminergic system projects to the median eminence and thus plays a role in the release of the gonadotropin-releasing hormone GnRH from the hypothalamus, which in turn influences the release of LH from the pituitary gland. This hormone has profound effects upon many male and female sexually related events. The activity of the peptidergic neurons is severely compromised if the monoaminergic neurotransmission is disturbed (Kizer and Youngblood, 1978). Radioactive sex hormones (estradiol and dihydrotestosterone) are taken up by CA cell bodies in the brain stem of rats. Both hormones may be taken up by the same CA nuclei; in other nuclei, the male and female hormones are differentiated. CA nerve terminals were also observed surrounding sex hormone target neurons in the midbrain and hypothalamus (Heritage et al., 1980).

2. MAO inhibitors such as pargyline potentiate the aphrodisiac effect of PCPA. The effect of the MAO inhibitor is probably due to the selective enhancement of CA activity because 5-HT is severely depleted by PCPA.

3. L-Dopa potentiates PCPA-induced homosexual mounting in male rats, and L-dopa with RO4-4602 by themselves also elicit the homosexual effect. There are also reports that Parkinsonian patients being treated with L-dopa experience aphrodisiac effects from the treatment (Davis, 1977).

4. The drug *p*-chloro-*N*-methylamphetamine, which inhibits 5-HT synthesis while releasing brain CAs, is more potent than PCPA in eliciting male-male mounting behavior. Also, this amphetamine analog has been reported to be beneficial in reversing impotence in male humans.

5. Small doses of apomorphine (0.5 mg/kg), a dopamine agonist, increased the number of rats showing mountings, intromissions, and ejaculations. These effects were more pronounced when two small doses were given 30 minutes apart. However, a large dose (5 mg/kg) caused marked stereotypic behavior that could have interfered with copulation.

6. Haloperidol, a dopamine receptor blocker, blocked the aphrodisiac effect of apomorphine, or L-dopa + RO4-4602. Haloperidol also blocked spontaneous copulatory activity in rats with high basal sexual activity.

7. L-Dopa in two small doses given 30 minutes apart to rats that were demonstrable copulators shortened ejaculatory latencies, the postejaculatory intervals, and the number of mounts and intromissions prior to ejaculation (Gessa and Tagliamonte, 1974).

All of the foregoing suggest that CA enhancement leads to increased sexual responsiveness. However, it should be noted that the summary reflects the fact that most of the studies have dealt with male sexuality and in a single species at that—the rat. In studies dealing with female sexual behavior, the evidence suggests that the role of the catecholamines is contrary to what one would expect. For example, in ovariectomized, estrogen-treated rats, *depletion* of CAs with α-methyl-*p*-tyrosine led to an increase in lordotic behavior, an effect that was also observed in estrogen-treated castrated males. That this effect was indeed related to CA depletion was shown when increased lordosis was prevented by additional treatment with L-dopa and RO4-4602. Furthermore, intracerebral administration of an adrenergic β-receptor blocker pindolol (LB-46) also increased lordosis both in female rats and estrogen-treated male rats, but an adrenergic α-receptor blocker (phentolamine) did not have this ef-

Pindolol (LB-46)

fect. Thus, whereas increasing CA activity quite clearly enhances male sexual activity, decreasing CA activity enhances female lordosis (Miczek and Barry, 1976). However, this paradoxical effect could be explained by assuming that CA depletion or receptor blockade, like a stress reaction, causes a release from the pituitary gland of ACTH, which stimulates the adrenal gland, thereby releasing NE and EPI as well as hormones from the adrenal cortex such as progesterone. These effects may account for the increase in some forms of sexual behavior.

Serotonin–Progesterone Interactions

The results of these experiments raise questions about the interactions between serotonin and sex hormones. For example, because PCPA elicits lordosis in estrogen-treated ovariectomized rats as readily as progesterone, the possibility exists that 5-HT depletion can substitute for progesterone by directly affecting mechanisms controlling sexual behavior. Alternatively, it is possible that 5-HT depletion causes the release of progesterone from the adrenal cortex, although lordosis occurs in adrenalectomized female rats treated with the 5-HT depletor reserpine or with the more specific 5-HT antagonists methysergide and PCPA. It is even possible that the effect proceeds in the opposite way, namely, progesterone decreases the activity of 5-HT-mediated, sexually related systems. Progesterone may also trigger a serotonergic system that acts synergistically with estrogen to induce lordotic responses. In any case, a 5-HT system would appear to have an inhibitory influence on sexual activity, and progesterone exerts an excitatory influence either as a direct effect or by suppressing the 5-HT-mediated inhibitory effect (Meyerson et al., 1974).

Can Serotonin Depletion Substitute for Progesterone? Experiments designed to investigate the manner by which serotonin depletion substitutes for progesterone in eliciting female mating behavior were reported by Zemlan (1978). He first showed that *p*-chloroamphetamine had a biphasic effect on lordosis. The measure of lordosis was expressed in the usual way as a lordosis quotient (LQ), which is the proportion of lordotic displays to mounts by vigorous males. At first (15 minutes postinjection) it suppressed hormone-primed lordosis to male mounts, and the same effect occurred with fenfluramine. But, beginning 3–5 days later, the frequency of lordotic behavior increased. The enhancement lasted for 10 days, at which time the rats were sacrificed for brain monoamine assays.

The biphasic effects were attributed to an initial short-term effect of PCA—releasing and blocking the reuptake of 5-HT—effects also shared by fenfluramine. The onset and duration of these short-term ef-

fects coincided with the suppression of female mating behavior. The long-term effect of PCA was that of a neurotoxin that damaged 5-HT terminals, causing a 5-HT depletion that was as much as 66 percent below baseline at day 10: this 5-HT depletion coincided with the enhancement of female mating responses. This enhancement could not be explained by the possible release of adrenal progesterone as the same effect was obtained when the release of adrenal hormones was blocked by dexamethasone. Thus, these data provided additional evidence that a 5-HT system suppresses female mating behavior in the rat.

Another observation bears on this problem. There are 5-HT terminals in the anterior hypothalamus—terminals that emanate from the serotonergic nuclei of the raphe (Saavedra et al., 1974). Also, radioactive estradiol was preferentially concentrated in the anterior hypothalamic area, and lesions in this area abolished female sexual behavior. Thus, the anterior hypothalamus seems to be a site where estradiol facilitates female mating behavior.

Furthermore, compared to the rest of the CNS, the mesencephalon has the highest uptake for [^{3}H]progesterone in the rat and guinea pig. Putting this all together led to the idea that the serotonergic system that terminates in the rich estrogen-binding area of the hypothalamus and suppresses female mating responses originates from a region that preferentially accumulates progesterone. To see whether there was a physiologically active system such as this, ovariectomized and adrenalectomized rats were given intracranial doses of progesterone, metycaine (a local anesthetic), and cholesterol (a steroid control), either in the ventral mesencephalon near areas B8 and B9 or in the dorsal mesencephalon near area B7 (see Figure 1). After 30, 90, and 180 minutes, the animals were tested for female mating behavior. The results of tests on the ventral mesencephalon showed that cholesterol was ineffective, but progesterone significantly enhanced estrogen-primed mating behavior, and metycaine had a similar, but smaller, effect. However, all injections in the dorsal raphe area were without effect (Zemlan, 1978).

The similarity of effect for progesterone and metycaine can mean that progesterone, like the anesthetic, blocked the ascending 5-HT fibers by which serotonin suppresses mating behavior. Thus, it can be reasonably concluded that the serotonergic system emanating from the ventral mesencephalon exerts inhibitory influences on mating behavior that can be blocked by progesterone.

The reasonableness of the above explanation should be considered along with a cautionary note reminding readers of the special conditions under which these experiments were undertaken. An extensive series of experiments on the mating behavior of the golden hamster have shown support for the preceding evidence even though there were significant differences in drug sensitivity. However, lordosis has been elicited in rats by amine depletors such as reserpine and tetrabenazine (which are less specific for 5-HT than PCPA) as well as by the dopamine receptor blockers pimozide and spiroperidol. However, the DA blocker haloperidol did not facilitate lordosis in the guinea pig, nor did pimozide facilitate lordosis in the hamster. One report described increases in lordosis in rats after PCPA that correlated with a depression of dopamine that preceded the PCPA-induced decline in serotonin, but the lordosis was not facilitated 24 hours after the PCPA administration when 5-HT levels were at their lowest. Furthermore, although the preceding accounts by Zemlan (1978) favored the interpretation that 5-HT systems suppress lordosis, similar effects are found with amphetamine, which probably acts as a dopamine agonist (Carter et al., 1978).

It may be concluded that progesterone seems to block the serotonergic fibers that ascend from the median raphe (B8 and B9) to the hypothalamus, where they normally have an inhibitory effect on the estrogenic activities located there. Thus, progesterone or 5-HT depletion can elicit female sexual responsiveness. There is also evidence that CA systems might be involved in the process, but their role is less clear.

From the foregoing we have seen that sexual behavior is the result of complicated neurochemical and hormonal interactions that are triggered by a variety of environmental stimuli. Neurochemical studies show that serotonergic systems are but one side of a multifaceted mechanism governing sexual behavior; thus manipulations of serotonergic systems can only provide a partial view of sexual function. These systems are indeed of substantial importance judging by serotonergic drug-induced changes that occur in the hormonal and behavioral aspects of sexuality. Catecholamines are also important in some aspects of sexuality and the evidence strongly suggests that whereas serotonergic effects are mainly inhibitory on sexual responsiveness, catecholaminergic systems are predominantly excitatory.

Summary

This chapter described the distribution of serotonergic systems in the CNS, serotonin synthesis and metabolism, and the unique characteristics of serotonin as a neurotransmitter. Whereas this system consists of a relatively sparse distribution of neural tracts emanating from the raphe nuclei of the pons and mesencephalon and ascend and descend in the neuraxis, the fibers ramify extensively so that virtually all neural and related structures come under its influence. The predominant effect of the serotonergic system is one of inhibition, and at least in some instances its role seems to be that of a neuromodulator controlling the amplitude of synaptic events mediated by other neurotransmitters such as the inhibitory effect of 5-HT on substance P which mediates pain. Thus, this system is designated as a trophotropic (inhibitory) system frequently working opposite an ergotrophic (excitatory) system which utilizes catecholamines as its neurotransmitter.

There are a number of drugs that can block 5-HT synthesis and metabolism, release and reuptake, in addition to those agents that mimic the action of 5-HT or block its receptor sites, or are neurotoxic and selectively destroy 5-HT neurons.

5-HT has been studied intensively to discern its role in many behavior categories. Evidence shows that it plays a significant role in the mediation of pain, sleep, aggression, and sexual behavior. Having no exclusive role in these phenomena serotonin rather interacts with other neurotransmitters in modulating the cyclic nature of sleep and sexual activity. Interestingly, 5-HT is found predominantly outside of neural tissue where it plays a significant role in the homeostasis of gastrointestinal, cardiovascular, and other organ systems.

Recommended Readings

Azmitia, E.C. (1978). The serotonin-producing neurons of the midbrain median and dorsal nuclei. In *Handbook of Psychopharmacology, Vol. 9* (L.L. Iversen, S.D. Iversen and S.H. Snyder, Eds.), pp. 233–314. Plenum Press, New York. An extensive review of the distribution of serotonergic systems in the brain.

Gillin, J.C., Stoff, D.M. and Wyatt, J. (1978). Transmethylation hypothesis: a review. In *Psychophar-*

macology: a Generation of Progress (M.A. Lipton, A. DiMascio and K.F. Killam, Eds.), pp. 1097–1112. Raven Press, New York. An excellent review about indoleamines used as therapeutic agents.

Green, A.R. and Grahame-Smith, D.G. (1975). 5-Hydroxytryptamine and other indoles in the central nervous system. In *Handbook of Psychopharmacology, Vol. 3* (L.L. Iversen, S.D. Iversen and S.H. Snyder, Eds.), pp. 169–245. Plenum Press, New York. A review of drugs that affect serotonergic systems in the brain.

Hartman, E. (1978). Effects of psychotropic drugs on sleep: the catecholamines and sleep. In *Psychopharmacology: a Generation of Progress* (M.A. Lipton, A. DiMascio and K.F. Killam, Eds.), pp. 711–728. Raven Press, New York. A review of recent neurochemical studies of sleep.

Hollister, L.E. (1978). Psychotomimetic drugs in man. In *Handbook of Psychopharmacology, Vol. 11* (L.L. Iversen, S.D. Iversen and S.H. Snyder, Eds.), pp. 389–424. Plenum Press, New York. A review of indoleamines used as therapeutic agents.

Mendelson, W.B., Gillin, J.C. and Wyatt, J.C. (1977). *Human Sleep and Its Disorders.* Plenum Press, New York. A lucid presentation of the effects of neurotransmitters and hormones on sleep. The studies discussed focus on normal sleep, narcolepsy, insomnia, and on sleep patterns associated with alcoholism and schizophrenia.

Meyerson, B.J. and Eliasson, M. (1977). Pharmacological and hormonal control of reproductive behavior. In *Handbook of Psychopharmacology, Vol. 8* (L.L. Iversen, S.D. Iversen and S.H. Snyder, Eds.), pp. 159–232. Plenum Press, New York. A comprehensive review that describes the effects of hormones and drugs on sexual development, adult sexual activity and parental behavior. The review discusses the diversity of sexual activity among species, the rationale and strategies for drug use in investigating sexual activity, and the many methodologies currently in practice.

Schultes, R.E. (1978). Plant and plant constituents as mind-altering agents throughout history. In *Handbook of Psychopharmacology, Vol. 11* (L.L. Iversen, S.D. Iversen and S.H. Snyder, Eds.), pp. 219–242. Plenum Press, New York. A brief historical account of mind-altering plant substances, with an extensive reference list.

Sexual Dimorphism (1981). *Science,* 211, 1263–1384. Nine major papers on the determinants of sex differences.

Shulgin, A.T. (1978). Psychotomimetic drugs: structure activity relationships. In *Handbook of Psychopharmacology, Vol. 11* (L.L. Iversen, S.D. Iversen and S.H. Snyder, Eds.), pp. 243–333. Plenum Press, New York. A review of the chemical structures and behavioral effects of many phantasticant drugs.

Wurtman, R.J. (1980). The pineal as a neuroendocrine transducer. In *Neuroendocrinology* (D.T. Krieger and J.C. Hughes, Eds.), pp. 102–108. Sinauer Associates, Sunderland, Mass. A recent review of pineal function by one of the active researchers on the subject.

CHAPTER NINE

Amino Acid Transmitters

Part I Inhibitory Amino Acid Transmitters

The chapters on the neurochemistry and psychopharmacology of acetylcholine and the biogenic amines easily lead to the impression that those transmitters play the major role in brain function. Indeed, the volume of research that has been conducted on the mechanisms of action of drugs that affect those transmitters is immense. Therefore, it may come as a surprise to learn that ACh and the biogenic amines constitute only a small proportion of the transmitters in the synaptic terminals of the CNS. For example, within the striatum (the brain region richest in dopamine terminals) only 15 percent of the nerve terminals appear to contain catecholamines (Snyder et al., 1973). Within the hypothalamus (the brain area richest in CA levels) only 5 percent of the terminals are catecholaminergic. Serotonin terminals are in even smaller proportion than NE, and ACh terminals account for no more than 10 percent of brain synapses. What then are the transmitters for the vast majority of synapses in the CNS, and what can we say about their relative importance in brain function? In this chapter we will discuss the transmitter properties of GABA, glycine, glutamic acid, aspartic acid, taurine, and histamine.

γ-Aminobutyric Acid

Identification

In 1950 Roberts and Frankel reported that γ-aminobutyric acid (GABA) could be found in brain extracts of many species, a finding soon confirmed by others working independently. By 1956 Roberts intimated that GABA might have a direct or indirect connection to conduction of nerve impulses. The same year Hayashi (1956) published a book describing experiments that he had done over many years on the excitatory or depressant effects of the amino acids, glutamate, and GABA; thus McLennan (1970) attributed the discovery of GABA as a neurotransmitter to Hayashi.

Also in 1956, reports at an international congress announced that GABA inhibited electrical activity in the brain; and in 1957 studies with convulsant drugs indicated that GABA had an inhibitory role in the CNS. Later studies established that GABA, obtained from brain extracts, inhibited action in the crayfish stretch receptor system; and, thereafter, studies on the role of GABA in epilepsy, schizophrenia, and mental retardation were undertaken (Roberts, 1974). In 1972 Iversen and Bloom (1972) reported that results from radioactive labeling experiments indicated that 20–40 percent of the terminals in various brain areas contained GABA and that quantitatively it was a major neurotransmitter in the brain.

Aprison and his co-workers (1968) identified glycine as also having inhibitory transmitter functions, and the research was on to seek out and identify similar substances in nerve terminals. The evidence that has been accumulated since that time clearly establishes GABA as an ubiquitous inhibitory neurotransmitter in the

CNS and other amino acids as neurotransmitters in many areas (McGeer et al., 1978).

Distribution

GABA is widely distributed in the nervous systems of vertebrate as well as invertebrate species. Although its presence in vertebrates is almost exclusively confined to the brain and spinal cord there have been reports of GABA receptors located in peripheral sympathetic ganglia (Iversen, 1978). The distribution of GABA in monkey, rabbit, and rat brains described by Fahn and Côté (1968) and other investigators, revealed that there are regional differences in GABA concentrations within the CNS. The highest concentrations were found in the substantia nigra, globus pallidus, and other brain areas rich in cell bodies, whereas lowest concentrations were found in white matter (Table I). Nevertheless GABA is more extensively and more evenly distributed in brain tissue than ACh or the monoamines (Roberts, 1978; Fonnum and Storm-Mathisen, 1978).

The tissue and subcellular distribution of GABA has

TABLE I   Distribution of γ-Aminobutyric Acid in the Brain

Brain area	GABA (μmol/g wet wt.)		
	Rhesus monkey[1]	Rabbit[2]	Rat[2]
Substantia nigra	9.70	8.50	10.07
Globus pallidus	9.54	6.43	7.67
Hypothalamus	6.19	5.33	7.68
Inferior colliculus	4.70	3.06	5.06
Dentate nucleus	4.30	4.09	—
Superior colliculus	4.19	4.93	7.67
Oculomotor nucleus	—	4.52	—
Putamen	3.62	3.48[3]	3.58[3]
Pontine tegmentum	3.34	1.82	3.34
Caudate nucleus	3.20	3.48[3]	3.58[3]
Hippocampus	—	2.39	3.58
Occipital cortex	2.68	—	—
Medullary tegmentum	2.27	2.76	2.11
Frontal cortex	2.10	2.10	2.86
Motor cortex	2.09	—	—
Cerebellar cortex	2.03	1.80	3.01

[1]Data from Fahn and Côté, 1968.
[2]Data from Okada et al., 1971.
[3]Caudate nucleus and putamen fused together.

(From Fonnum and Storm-Mathisen, 1978)

been successfully identified by immunocytochemical techniques which use antibodies of glutamate decarboxylase (GAD, the synthesizing enzyme for GABA). The presence of GAD correlates well with GABA content; therefore, the presence of GAD can be used as a marker for GABA. Electron microscopic analysis showed that GAD was highly localized in synaptic terminals close to synaptic vesicles (Roberts, 1978). The same techniques were used to define the regional localization of this transmitter.

Synthesis and Catabolism

Glucose Catabolism. A clear understanding of GABA synthesis and catabolism requires a familiarization with glucose catabolism as some of the enzymatic steps are shared by both processes. Glucose is the principal energy source for the brain and its catabolism largely takes place within mitochondria which are liberally distributed within cells, but are more highly concentrated where energy transfers occur at higher rates. In nerve cells, these points are synaptic junctions and nodes of Ranvier, where action potentials are generated in myelinated axons.

The first step in glucose catabolism (glycolysis) is the conversion of glucose into pyruvic acid and occurs under anaerobic conditions (without molecular oxygen) (Figure 1). No less than ten enzymes and a number of cofactors are needed for this process, even though it yields relatively small amounts of energy in the form of ATP. When the available oxygen stores in the blood are reduced (such as in muscles after prolonged physical exertion), pyruvic acid is further catabolized to lactic acid, which is ultimately discharged into the bloodstream. It is the accumulation of lactic acid in muscle tissue that accounts for the pain associated with extreme fatigue. In the brain, even when it is at rest and well oxygenated, about 13 percent of pyruvate is converted to this substance (Maker et al., 1976).

The Tricarboxylic Acid Cycle and Oxidative Phosphorylation. If sufficient supplies of oxygen are available, most pyruvic acid is oxidized to acetic acid, which rapidly combines with coenzyme A to form acetyl coenzyme A. Acetyl CoA enters a series of chemical transformations known as the tricarboxylic acid cycle (Figure 2) or the Krebs cycle (in honor of Hans Krebs, who with his discoveries in 1937 was among the first of many investigators to contribute to

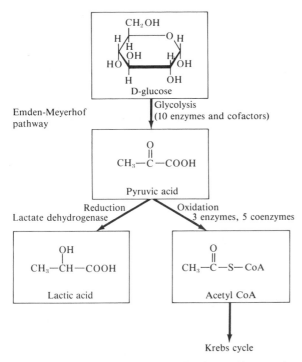

Emden-Meyerhof pathway

FIGURE 1 GLUCOSE CATABOLISM. Glucose is anaerobically catabolized via the Emden-Meyerhof pathway to pyruvic acid, and then reduced to lactic acid. With sufficient oxygen, pyruvic acid can be oxidized to acetyl CoA, which then enters the Krebs cycle for energy mobilization. The intermediate and end products are shown in un-ionized form, although at normal intracellular pH these compounds exist largely as anions. Thus, we say pyruvic acid or pyruvate.

the final full understanding of this process during the mid 1950s). Acetyl groups, which can be derived from amino acids and lipids as well as from glucose and other carbohydrates, contribute to the formation of acetyl CoA. Acetyl CoA combines with oxaloacetic acid (in its ionic state, oxaloacetate) to from citric acid (citrate), which is converted to isocitrate, and so on. Ultimately, oxaloacetic acid is formed again and interacts with more acetyl CoA to start the process all over again. This cyclic process releases the respiration byproduct CO_2 and hydrogen ions which are fed into an electron transport system and oxidized to form water. This latter process, which is known as oxidative phosphorylation, yields large amounts of ATP and a byproduct of respiration, H_2O. It is this aerobic process that supplies energy for neuronal, as well as for all cellular activities.

Each oxidized mole (180 grams) of glucose yields 304,000 calories during the formation of ATP from ADP and inorganic phosphate (P_i). This energy is made available when ATP is converted to ADP and is about 45 percent of the total energy (673,000 calories) that would result from complete oxidation of 180 grams of glucose. (Therefore, the organic process has about the same efficiency as a modern oil- or coal-fired power station.) Some of the energy is used to transport the fuel to the cells and for fueling the metabolic machinery. Thus, large amounts of energy are made available, but in a gradual way—step by step to avoid sudden and possibly disruptive accumulations of energy—for the operation of the cells of the organism. It is now a generally accepted fact that these processes occur in mitochondria in all tissues of higher organisms, in most aerobic microorganisms, and even in many plant tissues (Lehninger, 1975).

The GABA Shunt and GABA Synthesis. We will now consider the special features of the Krebs cycle that are instrumental for GABA synthesis and catabolism. The immediate substrate for GABA is glutamic acid (glutamate) which is a nonessential amino acid. ("Nonessential" in this sense means only that it need not be obtained from food as it can be readily synthesized by almost any form of life.) Glutamic acid can be formed from the amino acid glutamine via the enzyme glutaminase, or by the principal route of transamination of α-ketoglutarate (obtained from the Krebs cycle) with the amine group supplied by ammonia (NH_3) which is a byproduct of GABA catabolism.

GABA is formed by the α-decarboxylation of glutamic acid by L-glutamic acid decarboxylase, a synthesizing enzyme that requires vitamin B_6 for its activity (Figure 3). This enzyme is found in soluble form almost exclusively in axon terminals rather than being bound to mitochondria. Therefore, GABA synthesis seems to be confined to axon terminals where GABA exists in the cytoplasm or bound to vesicles.

It is not known exactly what proportion of glutamic acid goes into GABA synthesis as glutamic acid plays a role in many physiological processes. However, it has been tentatively established that approximately 8–10 percent of the carbon atoms going through the Krebs cycle are shunted to glutamate, GABA, and its principal metabolite (Iversen, 1978). This agrees well with earlier estimates by Balasz et al. (1970), who showed that GABA flux in guinea pig brain slices was about 8

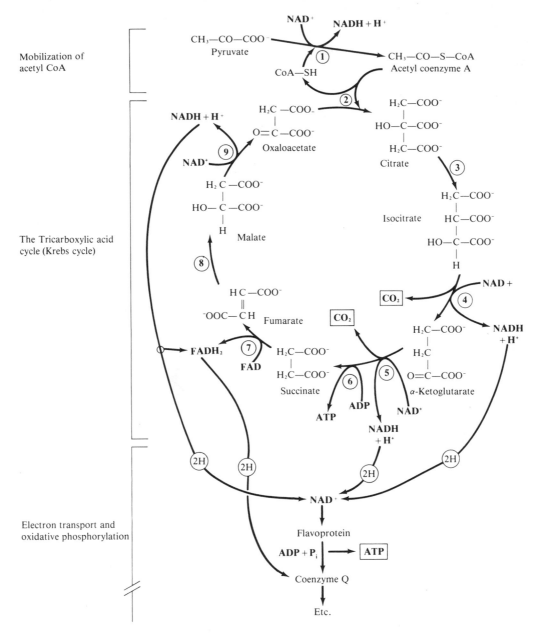

FIGURE 2   RESPIRATION PROCESS. In neurons, metabolites derived primarily from carbohydrates lead to the production of acetyl CoA. Acetyl CoA enters the Krebs cycle to interact with oxaloacetate to form citrate, isocitrate and so forth. This process results in the production of CO_2 and four pairs of hydrogen atoms. The hydrogen atoms provide the electrons for oxidative phosphorylation leading to the pro- duction of ATP and H_2O. All of the intermediates of the Krebs cycle are shown in their anionic state. NAD^+ is a cofactor at step 1 where pyruvate is converted to acetyl CoA, and at steps 4, 5, and 9. FAD is a cofactor at step 7. A single mitochondrion may contain as many as 15,000 of these res- piratory units, each of which contains a dozen or more separate enzymes.

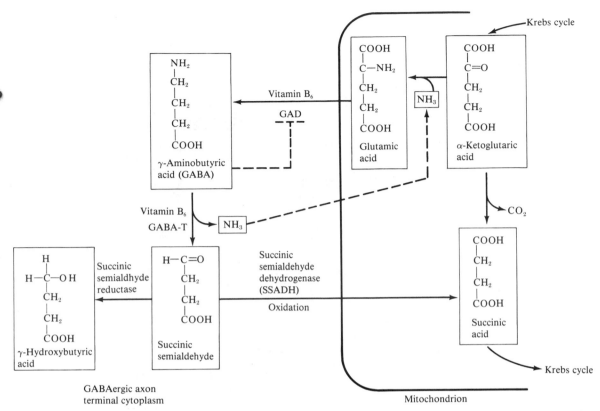

FIGURE 3   THE GABA "SHUNT." A bypass from the Krebs cycle provides the precursor glutamate for the synthesis of GABA. GABA-T converts GABA to succinic semialdehyde, most of which is oxidized to form succinic acid which reenters the Krebs cycle; however, small amounts of succinic semialdehyde are reduced to form γ-hydroxybutyric acid. Ammonia, a byproduct of GABA catabolism is utilized in the production of glutamate. GAD is subject to endproduct inhibition.

percent of the total tricarboxylic acid flux. It has also been shown that GAD is inhibited by the endproduct of its activity—GABA (i.e. when GABA concentrations reach 100 mM, GAD activity ceases.)

Catabolism. The catabolic pathway for GABA is also shown in Figure 3. GABA is catabolized by transamination (the amine group is transferred to α-ketoglutarate) by the vitamin B$_6$–dependent enzyme GABA:α-ketoglutarate aminotransferase (GABA-T) forming succinic semialdehyde (SSA) and an ammonia byproduct. In this reaction, α-ketoglutarate combines with ammonia to form glutamic acid thereby providing a continuous supply of the GABA precursor. Succinic semialdehyde is either oxidized or reduced, depending on the ratio of certain cofactors and the presence of succinic semialdehyde dehydrogenase (SSADH). The availability and activity of SSADH is so high that SSA is always oxidized to form succinic acid, which then enters the Krebs cycle within the mitochondria. Indeed, SSADH concentration is so high that SSA is rarely present in neural tissue despite active metabolism of GABA. It is possible that SSA can be *reduced* to form γ-hydroxybutyric acid, which, as was mentioned in Chapter 7, blocks the activity of dopaminergic neurons.

GABA-T and SSADH are always found together bound to mitochondria, but mitochondria bearing GABA-T are found in places other than axon terminals. They are also found in postsynaptic structures and in glial cells (Figure 4). Within axon terminals GABA catabolism via GABA-T is presumed to main-

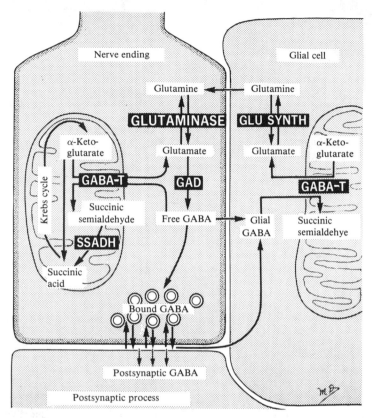

FIGURE 4 GABAERGIC SYNAPSE. Glutamate, derived from glutamine or the GABA shunt, provides the substrate for GABA synthesis which takes place via GAD in the cytoplasm of nerve endings. GABA catabolism takes place via GABA-T in the pre- and postsynaptic cytoplasm and is converted to succinic semialdehyde and succinic acid which reenter the Krebs cycle. The byproduct ammonia is utilized in the production of more glutamate. GABA is readily taken up by glia where it is acted upon by GABA-T to produce succinic acid and glutamate. The glutamate is acted upon by glutamine synthetase to form glutamine, which can be transferred to nerve endings where it can be acted upon by glutaminase to form substrate glutamate. (From McGeer et al., 1978.)

tain appropriate concentrations of GABA for synaptic activity. In postsynaptic structures GABA-T is instrumental in terminating synaptic action of GABA. Synaptic GABA can also be taken up by glia where the action of GABA-T also leads to the formation of glutamate from α-ketoglutarate and NH_3. However, glutamate cannot be converted to GABA within glia because they lack the enzyme GAD. Rather, glutamate is converted to glutamine by the enzyme glutamine synthetase. This enzyme is highly concentrated in glia but is absent in neurons (Martinez-Hernandez et al., 1977). Glutamine can then be transported across glial membranes and taken up by axon terminals. Within the terminals glutamine is converted by glutaminase to glutamate.

In summary, GABA is produced from glutamate that is obtained from glutamine or the GABA shunt. Glutamate is acted upon by cytoplasmic GAD in axon terminals. GABA is metabolized by GABA-T to form succinic semialdehyde and succinic acid which returns to the Krebs cycle while at the same time releasing ammonia to be taken up by mitochondrial α-ketoglutarate to form new sources of glutamate. GABA can also be taken up by glia where it is also metabolized by GABA-T. In glia, glutamate is converted to glutamine which can be transported to axon terminals where glutaminase acts on it to provide an additional source of glutamate.

GABA Release and Recapture

In vitro studies show that GABA is released from brain slices or synaptosomes upon electrical stimulation, but it is not certain that the efflux is from vesicles. Studies using radioactive GABA or its precursor pyruvic acid have revealed that GABA release is Ca^{2+}-dependent as GABAergic synapses are nonfunctional in a Ca^{2+}-free environment. Also newly synthesized GABA has a higher turnover rate than stored GABA and is preferentially released, which is typical for other transmitters as well. It has also been shown that GABA is taken up into synaptic terminals by a high affinity, Na^+-dependent transport system and is selectively accumulated in inhibitory neurons that use GABA as their neurotransmitter. Thus, like other transmitters, the termination of synaptic action of GABA may be effected by an efficient recapture mechanism. However, diffusion out of the synaptic cleft may also play a role in the cessation of transmitter action. This notion is supported by the fact that GABA is rather efficiently taken up and metabolized by glia, Schwann cells, and surrounding tissue. This nonneural GABA is not released by electrical stimulation.

GABA Receptors

The identification of GABA receptors has been aided by the finding that they exist in peripheral sympathetic ganglia. This makes it convenient to investigate isolated membrane reactions to GABA agonists. Subsequent studies have shown that the reactions of these receptors are similar to those in the CNS. A second approach to the identification of GABA receptors has been to measure the binding of [³H]GABA and GABAergic drugs to brain membrane preparations and to correlate the binding rates to physiological responses to the drugs. In general the biochemical findings were in good agreement with the physiological results. However, the GABA receptor has not been chemically identified (Iversen, 1978). GABA receptors have been difficult to isolate because there is no known high-affinity ligand (such as α-bungarotoxin for the nicotinic cholinergic receptor) with which to label them. GABA itself is not suitable because there are a number of metabolizing enzymes that also have a high affinity for GABA (Roberts, 1975).

GABA receptors on muscle membranes in crustacea

$$HN = \overset{\overset{\displaystyle NH_2}{|}}{C} - NH - CH_2 - CH_2 - COOH$$

β-Guanidinopropionic acid

seem to be concentrated opposite inhibitory nerve terminals. Also, there seem to be presynaptic autoreceptors that are on GABA terminals that differ pharmacologically from postsynaptic receptors, even though both show ionic conductance increases in response to GABA. The drug β-guanidinopropionic acid duplicates the action of GABA on presynaptic receptors, but it combines with and blocks the postsynaptic receptor without changing ionic conductance. This suggests that there are at least two types of GABA receptors (Kravitz, 1967).

The Distinctiveness of GABA and Glutamic Acid Uptake Systems. The K_m value for the high-affinity uptake of glutamic acid is similar to that for GABA, and glutamic acid is also a neurotransmitter as well as a precursor for GABA. Therefore, GABA might compete with glutamic acid for uptake into neurons, and vice versa. An experiment by Snyder and co-workers indicated that GABA in high concentration (as high as 1.0 μM) failed to reduce the uptake of glutamic acid into cerebral cortical or spinal cord homogenates and that glutamic acid had little affinity for the GABA uptake system. These results implied that, despite the chemical similarity and the metabolic interdependence between GABA and glutamic acid, the receptors for the uptake systems for these two transmitters were quite distinct.

GABA: An Inhibitory Transmitter

The neural inhibitory action of GABA seems to be its predominant characteristic, but not its exclusive one. Support for this idea stems from early findings by Florey (1954), who isolated a mammalian brain substance that blocked the discharge of the afferent stretch receptor neuron in the crayfish. Because the substance seemed to have an inhibitory action, he named it Factor I. Later, he and his colleagues (Bazemor et al., 1957) found that GABA was a principal constituent of Factor I, even though all active preparations of Factor I did not contain GABA. Still later it was discovered that GABA concentrations in inhibitory axons and cell bodies of the lobster nervous system are much higher than in excitatory axons and cell bodies. The ratio of the former to the latter is on the order of 100:1.

Much research on amino acid transmitters has been done on nerve–muscle preparations of crustaceans such as lobsters and crayfish. The exoskeletal muscles of these animals have a dual innervation of excitatory and inhibitory neurons, and for certain muscles there is only one large axon of each type. These neuron–muscle units can be easily dissected free, and detailed chemical analysis can be accomplished in nerves of known function.

Iontophoretic studies have shown that GABA inhibits the firing of neurons in the mammalian CNS in practically every area tested. For example, the Purkinje cells of the cerebellum provide the total neural outflow from the cerebellum, and this outflow is known to be inhibitory. Deiter's nucleus is the lateral vestibular nucleus in the brain stem that receives one of the direct inputs from Purkinje cell axons. If GABA is iontophoretically applied to Deiter's nucleus, hyperpolarizing potential changes occur.

Postsynaptic Inhibition. GABA seems to be involved in two types of inhibitory processes: postsynaptic inhibition and presynaptic inhibition. GABA can induce postsynaptic inhibition by the usual process of hyperpolarizing the postsynaptic membrane. Hyperpolarization occurs either by an influx of Cl^- or an efflux of K^+. Stimulation-induced release of GABA or GABA applied iontophoretically to a nerve–muscle preparation changes the permeability of chloride. Therefore, altering the chloride concentration of the surrounding medium can block the hyperpolarizing effect of GABA. On the other hand, altering the K^+ concentration of the medium has no effect on GABA-induced hyperpolarization. This indicates that Cl^- flux causes the hyperpolarizing effect.

Presynaptic Inhibition. Another form of inhibition mediated by GABA is presynaptic inhibition. This type of inhibition is commonly found in sensory systems and serves to modulate sensory input. The mechanism of action was described earlier (see Figure 7 in Chapter 5). Briefly, GABAergic neurons form axoaxonic synapses upon sensory axon terminals and slightly depolarize them. When a sensory nerve impulse reaches the slightly depolarized terminals there is a smaller influx of Ca^{2+} and a smaller amount of transmitter is released resulting in a smaller excitatory effect upon the postsynaptic

membrane. Thus, the GABAergic neurons indirectly reduce the sensory input into the CNS.

Presynaptic inhibition can be blocked by bicuculline which has a stimulating effect on sensory input. It is not known whether the drug blocks the release of GABA or blocks the GABA receptors. But, this finding supports the notion that GABAergic neurons are *depolarizing* sensory axon terminals. Thus, although GABA increases Cl^- conductance, it is acting as an excitatory transmitter causing membrane depolarization (Takeuchi and Takeuchi, 1966). Can increased Cl^- conductance be responsible for both GABA-induced hyperpolarization and depolarization? The answer may rest upon the relative concentration of intracellular and extracellular chloride. Thus, a GABA-induced increase of Cl^- conductance would lead to hyperpolarization if there were a cellular Cl^- influx and depolarization if there were a cellular efflux (Nicoll, 1978a).

Presynaptic inhibition seems to be the major effect of GABA in the spinal cord, although postsynaptic inhibition is its dominant role in the brain stem and cortex. Postsynaptic inhibition in the spinal cord is not antagonized by bicuculline; this observation is explained by the presence of glycine as the postsynaptic inhibitor in that region (Snyder, 1975a).

GABA and Cortical Neurons

From a review by Kelly and Beart (1975) of extracellular recording studies on the effects of GABA on cortical neurons, the following facts emerge:

1. The spike discharges of cortical neurons are quickly blocked upon iontophoretic application of GABA, but the effect quickly dissipates.
2. GABA seems to be very potent in this regard, only 20 nA are required for the iontophoretic currents to block spontaneously firing neurons or those stimulated by excitatory substances such as acetylcholine.
3. Only the frequency of discharge is affected; the shape and amplitude of the spike are not altered as they are by local anesthetics such as procaine.
4. The action of GABA appears to be directed to receptors on the postsynaptic membrane in supraspinal regions, as presynaptic inhibition is a process relegated for the most part to the spinal cord.
5. These GABAergic inhibitory processes, however, are ineffective in blocking seizure activity induced by repetitive stimulation or topical applications of

penicillin. These synaptic events are presumably too intense to be overcome by the conductance changes induced by GABA.

6. A number of other amino acids are fairly potent inhibitors of cortical neurons; and the monoamine neurotransmitters, as well as histamine and its metabolite imidazoleacetic acid, are also capable of inhibition of neural discharge. Consequently, GABA should not be thought of as the sole inhibitory transmitter in the CNS, even though GABA seems to be the most plentiful and the most potent.

A number of studies have established that GABA is probably the major inhibitory transmitter in the CNS. For example, Krnjević et al. (1966) wanted to show that synaptically induced inhibition in cortical neurons was the same as that induced by iontophoretic applications of GABA. Their approach was to try to block both types of inhibition with drugs that were known to block adrenergic, cholinergic, and other transmitters. Results indicated that strychnine, brucine, tetanus toxin, picrotoxin, pentylentetrazol, thiosemicarbazide, morphine, atropine, dihydro-β-erythroidine, tubocurarine, dimethyltubocurarine, gallamine, nicotine, dibenamine, phenoxybenzamine, and dichloroisoproterenol failed to alter the inhibitory effects induced by either method. This finding strongly supported the idea that GABA interacts with receptors that are distinct from those that react to other transmitters.

Later studies showed that strychnine blocked neuronal depression induced by acetylcholine, norepinephrine, serotonin, histamine, and glycine, but not that induced by GABA. Also, strychnine was found to have virtually no effect on cortical inhibition, but does have potent effects in the spinal cord. These results clearly indicate that a unique inhibitory process exists in the cerebral cortex and support the view that GABA is probably the most widespread inhibitory transmitter in the cererbral hemispheres (Kelly and Beart, 1975).

Drugs That Affect GABA Synapses

One of the techniques that permits the identification of GABAergic drugs is the GABA receptor binding assay. This technique determines a drug's ability to bind specifically to GABA receptors in brain membrane preparations (Goldstein, 1976b). The validity of the procedure was established when a high correlation was found between binding and physiological effects.

Iversen (1978) has used this technique to identify GABA agonists and antagonists.

Drugs That Block GABA Synthesis

The synthesis of GABA may be retarded or blocked by interfering with the synthesizing enzyme GAD. Thus far only compounds that are pyridoxal (vitamin B_6) antagonists are known to have any effect on this process and these are obviously not specific for GAD because there are a number of pyridoxal-dependent enzymes apart from GAD, one of them being GABA-T. A few of such drugs are thiosemicarbazide (TSC), isoniazid, allylglycine, L-glutamate-γ-hydrazide, and 3-mercaptopropionic acid. The latter two compounds have a structural similarity to the natural substrate glutamate and perhaps for that reason seem to yield a more specific inhibition of GAD. 3-Mercaptopropionic acid is a particularly useful research tool for the *in vivo* inhibition of GABA synthesis. Systemic administration of a moderate dose of this drug to rats significantly inhibited brain GAD activity and produced increased running; at higher doses convulsions occurred, the onset of which correlated well with the time course of the inhibition of brain GAD but not with the resulting decrease in brain GABA concentration (Iversen, 1978).

A number of studies reported that pyridoxine has a protective action against convulsant drugs that inhibit GAD activity (Tapia, 1975). This finding suggests that pyridoxine blocks the action of drugs having antagonist actions against other B_6 compounds. There are some vitamin B_6 antagonists that have a greater affinity for GABA-T than for GAD. Thus, by blocking the GABA-metabolizing enzyme, there can be significant increase in brain GABA: as much as 500 to 1000

Thiosemicarbazide

Isoniazid

Allylglycine

L-Glutamate-γ-hydrazide

3-Mercaptopropionic acid

percent. On the other hand, in a vitamin B_6 deficiency, GABA levels are depressed because GAD has a lower affinity for the vitamin than does GABA-T. It is fair to say that the inhibition of GAD activity, the chemistry of vitamin B_6, and seizure activity will require much more study before a clear understanding emerges.

Drugs That Block GABA Release

Pentylenetetrazol is a well-known CNS stimulant and convulsant. For a time it was widely used in con-

Pentylenetetrazol (Metrazol)

vulsant therapy for psychiatric depression, but this treatment has largely given way to the effective results obtained by the use of antidepressant drugs. It is still used as a diagnostic aid in epilepsy. The drug is injected intravenously in subconvulsive doses alone or in combination with flashing lights, which will often activate epileptogenic foci that can be detected by simultaneous electroencephalographic (EEG) recording. Eccles et al. (1963) found that pentylenetetrazol had no effect on presynaptic or postsynaptic inhibition, and studies by Costa et al. (1975) showed that the drug reduces the efficiency of GABA-mediated transmission. Nicoll and Padjen (1976) reported that it blocked postsynaptic receptors in the frog spinal cord, and Iversen (1978) cites studies that purport to show that pentylenetetrazol blocks the stimulus-evoked release of GABA from brain slice preparations. However, this latter conclusion should be regarded as being quite tentative.

Tetanus toxin causes acute convulsions and appears to do so by blocking GABA and glycine release. The toxin appears to bind to gangliosides, which are lipid–carbohydrate structures found in synaptic membranes. It has been proposed that the role of gangliosides in synaptic function is binding and release of the calcium ions that are essential for neurotransmitter release. The binding of tetanus toxin to the ganglioside thus may interfere with Ca^{2+} transport, thereby blocking GABA (and glycine) release (Dunn and Bondy, 1974; Suzuki, 1975).

Drugs That Stimulate or Block GABA Receptors

3-Aminopropane sulfonic acid has been found to be more than three times more potent than GABA in depolarizing GABAergic receptors in the sympathetic ganglia in the rat and in the spinal cord of the toad (Iversen, 1978).* Muscimol, which is a degradation product of ibotenic acid from the mushroom *Amanita muscaria*, is a potent GABA agonist and has the ability to inhibit CNS neurons. These substances attract flies and make them stuperous—hence the "fly" (muscaria) *Amanita*. In eighteenth century Europe the mushroom was used to make a substance called "fly agaric" to kill flies. Muscimol is a good research tool because it penetrates the CNS and has central muscle-relaxing properties. When given to human volunteers at relatively high doses, it causes an intoxication characterized by hyperthermia (elevated body temperature), pupil dilatation, elevation of mood, difficulties in concentration, palinopia (endless repetitions of visions seen minutes before), anorexia (loss of appetite), ataxia, catalepsy and hallucinations. These effects are similar to those experienced after ingestion of psychedelic drugs such as LSD. Muscimol and ibotenic acid, by serving as GABA agonists, affect other transmitters. (For example, they inhibit the release of serotonin and increase the release of norepinephrine and dopamine. It is believed that the blockade of serotonin release is mainly responsible for the symptoms described above.) The intoxicating property of the mushrooms was known long ago by primitive tribesmen of Siberia, and it has also been suggested that the ancient marauding Vikings were induced to occasional fits of savage madness by ingesting the mushroom (Schultes, 1970). Other poisonous mushrooms (e.g., *Amanita phalloides*) have other types of poisonous substances that can be fatal. The toxins of these fungi primarily destroy liver and kidney tissue (Litten, 1975).

3-Aminopropane sulfonic acid

Muscimol

Ibotenic acid

---

*The effect of GABA here is one of depolarization, not of hyperpolarization as one would expect of this inhibitory transmitter (Iversen, 1978).

A recent report described a structural analog to muscimol—tetrahydroisooxazolo-[5,4-c]pyridine-3-ol (THIP)—that is less toxic than muscimol and has potent analgesic properties equal to those of morphine (Krogsgaard-Larsen, et al., 1977). However, it differs from morphine in that it has virtually no addiction potential and its analgesic effect is not blocked by the morphine antagonist naloxone (Maugh, 1981). It is possible that this substance, like muscimol, may interact in some way with GABA receptors to provide its analgesic action.

A GABA analog ((β-chlorophenyl)-GABA = lioresal = Baclofen) has been found to depress the firing rate of spinal interneurons and cerebellar Purkinje cells. However, it has a low affinity for binding to GABA receptors (Iversen, 1978), it does not activate GABA receptors on cortical neurons, and it does not affect GABA transport. Its mode of action may be in its ability to block the effect of substance P, and it is used as a muscle relaxant (McGeer et al., 1978).

Two GABA antagonists are picrotoxin and bicuculline. Picrotoxin is obtained from the seeds of *Animirta cocculus*, a shrub found in the East Indies. The active ingredient is picrotoxinin. Picrotoxin is

Lioresal   Picrotoxin

classed as a powerful CNS stimulant, but its mode of action was deduced after Eccles et al. (1963) demonstrated that it blocked presynaptic inhibition. This finding, plus the observation that picrotoxin and GABA were mutually antagonistic in invertebrate preparations, led to the presumption that GABA plays a significant role in presynaptic inhibition, and therein possibly lay the explanation for picrotoxin's central excitatory effect. With the clarification of the role of GABA in the CNS, the action of picrotoxin was explained. However, it was later noted that although picrotoxin was physiologically active as a GABA antagonist it was inactive in a GABA binding assay. This raised questions about the precise mode of action of this compound (Tapia, 1975). More recently this contradiction became more understandable when evidence showed that picrotoxin seemed to inter-

tere with the chloride conductance channel, which presumably is distinct from the GABA recognition site (Olson et al., 1978).

Early uses for picrotoxin were confined to the treatment of poisoning by CNS depressants such as barbiturates, but there are now better means of managing that problem. Picrotoxin, for the most part, is now used as a research tool.

Bicuculline is a potent convulsant alkaloid derived from *Dicentra cucullaria* and other related plants. The threshold dose for eliciting convulsions in the cat is 0.3 to 0.5 mg/kg. It is somewhat more specific than picrotoxin in its inhibitory action on GABA at several sites in the mammalian CNS and the crayfish stretch receptor. Because it effectively blocks the electrical and GABA-induced inhibition of Deiter's cells in the brain stem, it provides strong support for the notion that GABA is the inhibitory transmitter that is released by the Purkinje cells upon Deiter's nucleus. Bicuculline effectively blocks synaptic and GABA-induced inhibition of cortical neurons, but neither picrotoxin nor strychnine has this effect.

Bicuculline does not block spinal inhibitory processes that are sensitive to strychnine (a glycine antagonist), but it is, like picrotoxin, effective in blocking spinal inhibitions that have the characteristics of presynaptic inhibition. This again suggests that GABA is the transmitter for spinal presynaptic inhibition (Ryall, 1975).

A number of studies have shown that GABA does not pass the blood brain barrier, but systemic administration of bicuculline or picrotoxin will block the inhibitory effect of iontophoretically applied GABA in certain neurons (Tapia, 1975). Thus, although it would appear that bicuculline clearly is an effective GABA antagonist, there are numerous reports that raise questions about the reliability of bicuculline effects. For example, Roberts (1975) cites studies that reported that in measures of ion conductance neither bicuculline nor picrotoxin were competitive antagonists of GABA action on postsynaptic membranes of crustacean neuromuscular junctions. Neither did bicuculline block neurally evoked inhibition at the neuromuscular junction of the hermit crab (a locus that is sensitive to applied GABA). Kelly and Beart (1975) proposed that the difficulty may be due to the relative insolubility of bicuculline and the consequent problem of getting sufficient concentrations of the alkaloid within a micropipette for reliable iontophoretic studies. Bicuculline methochloride is more soluble than bicuculline and is

Bicuculline   Bicuculline methochloride

almost as potent as GABA with respect to its binding properties. However, it is less potent as a convulsant than bicuculline when administered systemically, but more potent when given intraventricularly. Moreover, the compound has a tendency to increase cell excitability, which is also true to some extent for other putative GABA receptor blockers. Consequently, studies based upon the antagonistic properties of bicuculline must be interpreted with some caution.

Although picrotoxin and bicuculline seem to block the function of GABA receptors, it is not clear just how this effect comes about. As was mentioned earlier, neither of those drugs is a competitive inhibitor of GABA binding to postsynaptic receptors, hence neither is, strictly speaking, a receptor blocker. Indeed, there are no known specific receptor blockers; instead there are drugs that appear either to facilitate or impede receptor responsiveness (Mao and Costa, 1978).

It has been known for some time that topical applications of penicillin to the cerebral cortex will induce an epileptic focus and will even produce seizures in humans when systemically administered in large doses, especially when the blood brain barrier has been breached by trauma or infection. Penicillin, which is structurally related to GABA and bicuculline, also blocks presynaptic inhibition in amphibian and cat spinal cords as well as GABA-induced inhibition of Renshaw cells in the cat. However, GABA does not show its normal inhibitory effect on the cortical cells of an epileptogenic focus induced by penicillin (Tapia, 1975; Ryall, 1975).

There are a number of other substances that have been found to be weak GABA antagonists, for example, d-tubocurarine, morphine, and the morphine antagonist naloxone (Tapia, 1975; Ryall, 1975; Kelly and Beart, 1975; Iversen, 1978).

From the foregoing it is logical that GABA itself

should have anticonvulsant properties. Tapia (1975) cites a number of studies that support this view. In spite of its limited permeability through the blood brain barrier, GABA had anticonvulsant effects in some human epileptics. Intravenous GABA had anticonvulsant effects in dogs subjected to electrical stimulation of the motor cortex; and intravenous and intraperitoneal injections of GABA in rats had anticonvulsant effects on seizures induced by pentylenetetrazol and thiosemicarbazide, a pyridoxal phosphate (vitamin B_6) antagonist that blocks GAD activity. As there are a number of highly effective antiepileptic agents, GABA is of little value for this purpose.

Pyridoxal phosphate (of the Vitamin B_6 complex)

Drugs That Block GABA Uptake

From a clinical standpoint, there is a great need to potentiate the action of GABA as a possible way of relieving the symptoms of diseases such as Huntington's chorea, epilepsy, Parkinson's disease, and schizophrenia—diseases that may be traced to observed deficits in GABA and GAD activity (Barbeau, 1978; Roberts, 1972, 1975; Tapia, 1975; Mao and Costa, 1978). It is not possible to achieve GABA potentiation by systemic administration of GABA because it does not readily penetrate the blood brain barrier; and even if one could use instead a barrier-passing GABAmimetic substance, it probably would not be desirable to do so. This is because GABA acts on many neurons that do not have a natural input from GABA-releasing neurons. Therefore, a nonspecific flooding of the CNS with GABAmimetics could result in neurophysiological chaos. It would therefore be more appropriate to potentiate GABAergic mechanisms by amplifying existing GABA synapses, either by increasing GABA release or by interrupting the inactivating reuptake systems with substances that have no GABAmimetic or GABA antagonist properties of their own. The latter strategy is the one employed through the use of the tricyclic antidepressant drugs such as imipramine and desmethylimipramine (DMI), which block the reuptake of catecholamines and are effective in treating psychiatric depression. In 1975 Roberts held that substances that mimic GABA and were clinically useful did not exist. More recently, a number of compounds that are structurally related to GABA (such as 2-hydroxy GABA, 4-methyl GABA, and nipecotic acid) have been found to be fairly potent in blocking the reuptake of GABA in brain slices or snyaptosomes. Some other nonrelated compounds have the same properties, but these compounds are not highly specific and evidence is still lacking that these compounds are clinically effective for potentiating synaptic activity of amino acids (Iversen, 1978).

$$H_2N-CH_2-CH_2-\overset{\overset{\displaystyle OH}{|}}{CH}-COOH$$

2-Hydroxy GABA

$$H_2N-\overset{\overset{\displaystyle CH_3}{|}}{CH}-CH_2-CH_2-COOH$$

4-Methyl GABA

Nipecotic acid

Drugs That Block GABA Catabolism

Aminooxyacetic acid (AOAA) blocks the catabolism of GABA by antagonizing the action of GABA-T. It does so by serving as an antagonist to pyridoxal phosphate. As mentioned previously, effective blockade of GABA-T with AOAA can raise brain GABA levels as much as 500 percent. Another GABA-T antagonist, ethanolamine-O-sulfate (EOS), forms an irreversible inhibitor-enzyme complex that can raise brain GABA levels as high as 1000 percent and maintain elevation over several days. However, the compound has no clinical utility because it must be administered directly into the brain or cerebral spinal fluid because it does not readily pass the blood brain barrier. Gottesfeld et al. (1972) provided direct evidence that AOAA enhances the inhibitory action of GABA by demonstrating that within 1 hour of an intraperitoneal injection of AOAA cortical neurons in the cat were significantly more sensitive to iontophoretically applied GABA and that the duration of inhibition due to synaptically released GABA was also prolonged by AOAA. Furthermore, the collection of GABA after neural stimulation from the surface of the cortex and from the fourth ventricle was facilitated by pretreating the animals with AOAA (Kelly and Beart, 1975).

It would be supposed that raising GABA levels by using GABA-T antagonists should block convulsant

$$H_2N-O-CH_2-\overset{\overset{\displaystyle O}{\|}}{C}-OH$$

Aminooxyacetic acid

$$H_2N-CH_2-CH_2-O-SO_3H$$

Ethanolamine-O-sulfate

drugs that are GAD antagonists or GABA receptor blockers. GABA-T antagonists do block convulsant drugs, but the effect is a complex one. First, AOAA protects rats from convulsions elicited by electroshock, but the anticonvulsant effect lasts only for a few hours, whereas the increase in brain GABA lasts much longer. One possible explanation for this is that the increased brain level of GABA is due to an increase in glial GABA and that this is not related to anticonvulsant activity. A related explanation stems from the fact that AOAA, especially at high doses, also blocks neuronal GAD activity because this enzyme is also B_6 dependent. (EOS does not block GAD at high doses.) GAD activity generates newly synthesized GABA, and the release of this GABA causes a tonic GABAergic inhibition that controls the activity of other neurons. Thus, high rates of AOAA reduce GAD activity, thereby lessening GABA synthesis and release and reducing inhibitory tone. At the same time, GABA metabolism may be blocked in glia, contributing to the increase in brain GABA levels, but this GABA is not available for synaptic release. Thus, although AOAA can block GABA-T and increase synaptic GABA with anticonvulsant effects, AOAA can (if the dose is excessive) block neuronal GAD as well as GABA-T activity, thereby producing higher sensitivity of neurons and convulsions (Mao and Costa, 1978). Finally, it is worth mentioning that sodium-n-dipropylacetic acid is a specific GABA-T inhibitor that is widely used to control epileptic conditions that are resistant to traditional anticonvulsants.

$$\begin{matrix} CH_3-CH_2-CH_2 \\ CH_3-CH_2-CH_2 \end{matrix} CH-\overset{\overset{\displaystyle O}{\|}}{C}-ONa$$

Sodium-n-dipropylacetic acid (Epilim)

The Role of GABA in the Action of the Benzodiazepines

The drugs known as the benzodiazepines include diazepam, chlordiazepoxide, oxazepam, flunitrazepam, and many other related compounds. This class of compounds has many properties, including muscle relaxant and anticonvulsant effects. In high doses they cause ataxia. These drugs have been extensively investigated, with an important goal being the delineation of the role of neurotransmitters in their mode of action. It turns out that virtually all of the monoamines and acetylcholine seem to be affected by these drugs, and in the last few years GABA has assumed a large role in the explanation of the wide range of effects.

Diazepam (Valium)

Chlordiazepoxide (Librium)

Oxazepam (Serax)

Flunitrazepam

A point of departure in the investigations of the role of GABA was to consider the main therapeutic and side effects of these drugs and to relate these effects to the known functions of GABA (Haefely et al., 1975). The obvious connection was with the anticonvulsant, muscle relaxant, and ataxic effects of the drugs and the inhibitory role played by GABA. To investigate this hypothesis, a number of studies have been done to examine the effects of the benzodiazepines on the activities that specifically depend on GABA. In one study two of the benzodiazepines were compared with anticonvulsant drugs (such as AOAA) in their ability to block convulsions induced in mice by thiosemicarbazide (TSC), 3-mercaptopropionic acid, and bicuculline. Thiosemicarbazide was injected subcutaneously (20 mg/kg) in mice: a dose that normally causes convulsions and kills all animals in 80 minutes. Flunitrazepam and diazepam were both much more potent in blocking TSC effects than phenobarbital, AOAA, diphenylhydantoin (Dilantin) a drug structurally similar to barbiturates, and n-dipropylacetic acid in measures of survival rates (Figure 5). Similar results were found when 3-mercaptopropionic acid and

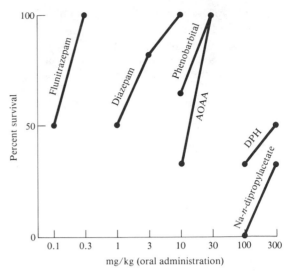

FIGURE 5 TSC-INDUCED MORTALITY PREVENTION by benzodiazepines and other drugs. TSC (thiosemicarbazide) blocks GABA synthesis and at 20 mg/kg is lethal to mice. Flunitrazepam and diazepam were more potent than other anticonvulsant drugs in blocking the lethal effects of TSC. See text for details. (From Haefely et al., 1975.)

Phenobarbital   Diphenylhydantoin (Dilantin)

bicuculline were used as the convulsants, but the effect of the benzodiazepines was diminished when strychnine (a glycine antagonist) was used to induce convulsions. The benzodiazepines also enhanced presynaptic inhibition in the spinal cord, the mechanism that controls muscle relaxation. Also diazepam inhibited the spontaneous firing of Purkinje cells in the cerebellum by potentiating GABA effects upon the Purkinje cells, and it potentiated the inhibitory action of GABA in several other brain areas. Thus, the benzodiazepines act as GABAmimetic agents. However, it was not known until recently how this effect occurs. This will be discussed in Chapter 11.

Role of GABA in Behavioral Inhibition

The experiment discussed in the preceding section

demonstrated that reducing GABA synthesis (with thiosemicarbazide) could produce lethal convulsions in mice and that the benzodiazepines could antagonize these effects, apparently by exerting a GABAmimetic action. Thus, it would appear that the inhibitory effects of GABA that occur at the cellular level also control convulsive behavior. In this instance, the parallel effects are easily explained, because EEG studies show that convulsive behavior accompanies a high-voltage discharge from the brain that is associated with unrestrained cellular activity.

However, there are other forms of inhibitory behavior whose neurotransmitter substrates are more difficult to identify. For example, there is (1) novelty-induced inhibition, that is, reduced eating when novel foods are offered or when ordinary foods are offered in novel containers or in a novel environment; (2) punishment-induced inhibition, that is, decreased responding for food reinforcement when some responses are paired with shocks; (3) nonreward-induced inhibition, that is, reduced responding when reward contingencies are decreased [for example, after a shift from CRF (continuous reinforcement) to a FR (fixed ratio) schedule or when food rewards are permanently terminated (extinction)].

Soubrie et al (1979) investigated the role of GABA in these forms of behavioral-inhibition by treating rats with the GABA antagonist picrotoxin. The effect of the drug on novelty-induced inhibition was evaluated by comparing the degree of responding of animals subjected to novelty while receiving infraconvulsant doses (0, 0.5, or 1.0 mg/kg) of picrotoxin with the degree of responding of animals receiving the same drug treatment while not subjected to novelty. Similar comparisons were made for punishment and nonreward-induced inhibition.

The experimenters found that picrotoxin magnified the response suppression induced by novelty, punishment, nonreward, or bitter taste. They also found that the drug inhibited water drinking in unfamiliar surroundings more during the first 5 minutes than during the last 5 minutes of the 10-minute test, a finding that suggested that there was satiety and/or less "neophobia" during the second half of the test. The data also showed that (1) the drug, although reducing punished responding, had no effect on nonpunished responding; (2) it depressed food or water intake when novelty was a factor, but failed to produce this effect in animals that were experienced with respect to the in-

gested substances; and (3) it reduced lever-pressing for food when there was a shift from CRF to FR-4, but had no effect on animals well adapted to an FR-4 schedule. These findings showed that it was unlikely that nonspecific depressant actions of the drug were significant.

These results indicate that some intervening system is involved in behavioral suppression because the picrotoxin-induced depression of GABA systems enhances behavioral suppression. GABA systems in themselves are most certainly inhibitory; therefore, drug-induced suppression of the GABA system should have a releasing action on GABA-influenced behavior if the GABA system acts directly. However, if GABA inhibits a secondary behavior-suppressing system, then blocking the GABA system should release the action of the secondary behavior-suppressing system. This would account for the enhancement of the behavior-depressant action of novelty, punishment, and so forth by picrotoxin. In other words, picrotoxin inhibits an inhibitory system, thus releasing a secondary behavior-suppressing system.

It will be seen in the discussion of anxiolytic drugs in Chapter 11 that the intervening system postulated above is probably a serotonergic system that is acted upon by GABAergic neurons (Figure 5 in Chapter 8). A growing body of evidence supports the view that the benzodiazepines induce a GABA-inhibitory input upon the serotonergic raphe system. This system seems to play a role in suppressing behavior that has nonreward or punishing consequences. The GABA system seems to inhibit the serotonergic system, thus releasing behavior suppressed by punishment, nonreward, and even satiety. Such a neural arrangement supports the findings by Soubrie et al. (1979) that show that blockade of the GABA system enhances behavior suppression. Finally, it is important to note that in this experiment the low doses of picrotoxin did not have suppressant effects on behavior per se; rather, it only increased the inhibition of behavior under the control of aversive events. More study is needed to clarify this selectivity.

Ethanol Effects on GABA-Mediated Activity

There is evidence that ethanol (ethyl alcohol) alleviates anxiety and potentiates spinal presynaptic inhibition—activities that are mediated by GABA inhibitory systems. Also bicuculline, a GABA antagonist, diminishes the behavioral aspects of alcohol

$$CH_3—CH_2—OH$$

Ethanol

intoxication, whereas AOAA, an inhibitor of GABA catabolism, increases them. In view of these findings, Nestoros (1980) investigated the possibility that ethanol, like the benzodiazepines, could selectively induce GABA-mediated inhibition.

Nestoros used a multibarreled microelectrode to release ethanol and the inhibitory transmitters GABA, dopamine, serotonin, and glycine on cortical cells of cats. The results showed that ethanol potentiated the GABA-induced inhibition of cell firing, that it antagonized dopamine- and serotonin-induced inhibition, and that it either had no effect or antagonized glycine-induced inhibition. All the actions of ethanol occurred within 10 seconds of its release and were fully reversible within 1–3 minutes after release was dis-

TABLE II Some Drugs That Affect GABA Action

Drug	Mechanism of action	Major effects
Synthesis blockers		
Allylglycine		
Isoniazid	Vitamin B_6 antagonists	Convulsant
3-Mercaptopropionic acid	and GAD inhibitors	
Theosemicarbazide		
Release blockers		
Pentylenetetrazol	Inhibit stimulus-induced	Convulsant
Tetanus toxin	GABA release	
GABA uptake pump inhibitors		
2-Hydroxy GABA		Convulsant at high doses
Imipramine		Antidepressant
4-Methyl GABA	Block GABA uptake	Convulsant at high doses
Nipecotic acid		Convulsant at high doses
Catabolism blockers		
Aminooxyacetic acid		Sedative, anticonvulsant
Ethanolamine-O-sulfate	Vitamin B_6 antagonists	Anticonvulsant if given IVT
3-Hydrazinopropionic acid	and GABA-T inhibitors	Sedative
Sodium-n-dipropylacetate		Anticonvulsant
GABA antagonists		
Bicuculline		
Bicuculline methochloride	GABA receptor blockers	Convulsant
Picrotoxin (indirect)	Blocks Cl^- ionophores	CNS stimulant
GABA agonists		
γ-Hydroxybutyrate	Stimulate GABA receptors (?)	Weak sedative
Lioresal		Muscle relaxant
Muscimol	Stimulate GABA receptors	Psychotomimetic
THIP		Analgesic
Indirect GABA agonists		
Chlordiazepoxide		
Diazepam		
Flunitrazepam	Facilitate GABA effects	Anxiolytic and
Oxazepam		anticonvulsant
Ethanol		CNS depressant

continued. Similar effects were obtained when ethanol was administered intravenously while cortical cells were being electrically stimulated or iontophoretically treated with GABA.

Was the effect caused by blockade of GABA uptake, induction of GABA release, or a direct effect on postsynaptic receptors? The evidence indicated that the most likely site of action was the postsynaptic membrane. Because the glycine-induced inhibition was unaffected or antagonized by ethanol, it is unlikely that ethanol acted directly upon the Cl^- channels. Also, because ethanol could potentiate GABA-mediated inhibition in doses that alone had no inhibitory effect, it is unlikely that ethanol is a direct GABA agonist. Rather, it appears that ethanol potentiates GABA by acting upon a regulatory site located on or near the GABA receptor binding site. This is similar to the action of the benzodiazepines (see Chapter 11), but ethanol does not bind to the benzodiazepine binding sites.

These findings are significant with respect to the causes and treatment of alcoholism because the most-often prescribed antianxiety drugs (the benzodiazepines) enhance GABA-mediated activity, and anxiety is implicated in the cause of alcoholism. Also, because long-term ethanol intake decreases brain GABA concentration long-term users of ethanol show a tolerance to ethanol. This requires ingestion of greater amounts of ethanol to obtain the GABA potentiation for the needed antianxiety effect or to counteract the GABA depletion that results in tremulousness, or in severe cases, disastrous convulsive withdrawal effects.

Table II summarizes the mechanism of action and the physiological effects of most of the GABAergic drugs that have been discussed.

Glycine

By 1965 a number of laboratories had reported that glycine as well as a number of other amino acids had inhibitory or excitatory properties on neurons in the CNS. The investigators at that time felt that these were nonspecific effects, but Aprison and Werman (1965) suggested that for glycine these effects could be designated as nonspecific only if the inhibited neurons were not innervated by glycine-secreting presynaptic elements. In other words, if glycine inhibited a certain neuron that was innervated by a glycine-secreting presynaptic element, then glycine might well be a specific neurotransmitter.

It was considered to be a formidable task to establish glycine as a transmitter because glycine is the simplest amino acid and has many biological functions. Nevertheless, Aprison and his co-workers set out to see whether glycine was present in presynaptic neurons of cells that reacted to glycine, whether glycine reproduced the membrane changes that could be elicited by synaptic activation, and whether glycine could be collected from the extracellular fluid in response to synaptic activation. Their studies focused on the excitatory and inhibitory transmitters in the lumbosacral spinal cord of the cat. It was known that inhibition in the cord is mediated through short axon interneurons in the gray matter. Thus, it was reasonable to assume that a suspected transmitter like glycine would be more abundant in the gray matter than in the white matter (Aprison, 1978).

Distribution of Glycine

By using a number of micromethods for chemical identification the investigators found that GABA and glycine had a pattern of distribution in the spinal cord that was consistent with their suspected roles as neurotransmitters. Figure 6 shows the areas of the spinal cord with their respective concentrations of GABA and glycine. The dorsal gray and ventral gray areas have the greatest concentrations of these compounds. This observation strongly suggests that GABA and glycine are associated with the interneurons of these areas. Moreover, anoxia of the lumbosacral cord of cats (a condition that is obtained by clamping the thoracic aorta and that selectively destroys interneurons in the central and ventral gray matter) caused a significant decrease in glycine concentration but not in that of GABA (Davidoff et al., 1967). This latter finding was reinforced by the additional finding that cell counts showed that the number of remaining small (20 μm) neurons correlated highly (r = 0.71; p < 0.05) with glycine content.

Within the spinal cord of the cat, the glycine content in the ventral gray of the cervical and lumbar enlargement was higher than in midthoracic cord, whereas in the snake and fish (animals without limbs) glycine was uniformly distributed along the spinal cord. Thus, glycine seems to be associated with the inhibition of motoneurons that are more numerous in the spinal enlargements (Ljungdahl and Hökfelt, 1973). Investigators examined other brain areas of vertebrates and found glycine in high concentrations in medulla and

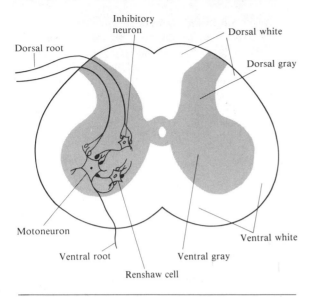

Tissue	Contents*	
	Glycine	GABA
Dorsal white	3.04 ± 0.26	0.43 ± 0.05
Dorsal gray	5.65 ± 0.18	2.18 ± 0.25
Ventral gray	7.08 ± 0.31	1.04 ± 0.10
Ventral white	4.39 ± 0.26	0.44 ± 0.06
Dorsal root	0.64 ± 0.04	0.06 ± 0.01
Ventral root	0.64 ± 0.00	0.08 ± 0.01

*μM/g + Standard Error of the Mean (S.E.M)

FIGURE 6 SPINAL CORD OF A CAT at the seventh lumbar segment. Some synapses are shown in the ventral gray matter. The open axon terminals are excitatory; the closed ones are inhibitory. When stimulated, inhibitory interneurons and Renshaw cells inhibit the firing rates of motoneurons. The table shows the tissue content of glycine and GABA (mean ±SEM) in the indicated areas. (After Aprison, 1978.)

pons—concentrations that were higher than anywhere else in the brain (Aprison et al., 1968). This is not surprising because the medulla and pons are the areas containing motoneurons from which emerge the cranial nerves that innervate the muscles of mastication (the trigeminal nerve), the lateral rectus muscle (the abducens nerve), the facial muscles (the facial nerve), the muscles of the pharynx, larynx, and esophagus (the glossopharyngeal, the vagus, and the cranial branch of the spinal accessory nerve), and the tongue (the hypo-

glossal nerve). No doubt glycine-mediated inhibition plays a vital role in the intricate muscular activities associated with eating, facial expression, eye movements, and speech.

It is of some interest that autoradiographic studies showed that radioactive grains of glycine were found in nerve terminals having flat vesicles but not in those having round vesicles (Ljungdahl and Hökfelt, 1973). This supports the hypothesis that flat vesicles are associated with inhibitory neuron terminals and round vesicles with excitatory terminals (see Chapter 4). It was also found that glycine was taken up by glia, probably as part of an inactivation process.

Transmitters versus Metabolic Glycine

Glycine as well as other amino acids subserve a variety of metabolic functions in addition to any suspected transmitter role. Thus, it was deemed necessary to differentiate between the metabolic and transmitter pools. Snyder et al. (1973) and Snyder (1975a) reported a series of investigations designed to identify selectively transmitter pools of amino acids. Their procedures were based on the premise that amino acids serving as transmitters should, like other transmitters, be associated with high-affinity uptake systems that facilitate the rapid removal of the transmitter from the synaptic cleft. Consequently, synaptosome fractions from brain and spinal cord were incubated with a variety of radioactive amino acids in various concentrations to evaluate both low- and high-affinity systems. They found that glycine was taken up and localized in the synaptosomal fractions, a finding that was supported by additional autoradiographic evidence. Furthermore, the uptake of nontransmitter amino acids in cortical tissue indicated a single low-affinity glycine uptake system ($K_m = 760\ \mu M$). But in the spinal cord and brain stem, there were distinct high- ($K_m = 26\ \mu M$) and low- ($K_m = 923\ \mu M$) affinity systems. This is strong evidence that glycine probably plays only a metabolic role in the cortex, whereas in the spinal cord and brain stem, glycine has a dual function, one of them being as a neurotransmitter.

Glycine Synthesis and Metabolism

Unlike the monoamines and acetylcholine, glycine is available for incorporation in axon terminals in a preformed state. Glycine is a nonessential amino acid, meaning that it need not come from dietary protein because it can be synthesized in most animals, includ-

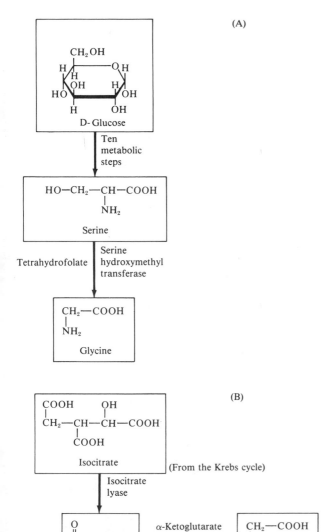

FIGURE 7 SYNTHESIS OF GLYCINE. (A) Some of the steps of glycine synthesis from glucose. (B) The synthesis from isocitrate.

ing man. Consequently, it is not known how important glycine synthesis is for the maintenance of appropriate levels of spinal cord glycine. Furthermore, there are no drugs that can selectively alter synthesis or metabolism of glycine for any neurophysiological purpose.

Briefly, then, glycine is synthesized in mitochondria in conjunction with glycolysis and the Krebs cycle (Figure 7). One of its precursors is serine, an amino acid that is synthesized from glucose. Glycine is formed by the action of the enzyme serine hydroxymethyltransferase (SHMT), which requires the coenzyme tetrahydrofolate (FH_4), a derivative of the vitamin folic acid. The glucose-serine-glycine pathway is not the only one for glycine synthesis. Another synthetic pathway may be via glyoxylate. Glyoxylate is formed from isocitrate from the Krebs cycle by the action of isocitrate lyase. Then glyoxylate is transaminated by glycine-α-ketoglutarate transaminase to form glycine. These reactions are both reversible.

Nothing much is known about the degradative process for glycine in the CNS, except that it is thought to involve FH_4 and four proteins, including SHMT, and that it also occurs in the mitrochondria by a process known as the GLYCINE-CLEAVAGE SYSTEM (GCS). The end product is 5,10-methyline FH_4.

Figure 8 shows a representation of a glycinergic synapse with four glycine compartments. Mitochondrial glycine (G_{mito}) is the site of synthesis by SHMT and of catabolism by the GCS. After release from the mitochondria, glycine is distributed either to the metabolic compartment (G_{metab}) or to the functional compartment (G_{func}), which is the suggested depot for transmitter glycine. The free compartment (G_F) is glycine released into the synaptic cleft. Free glycine hyperpolarizes the postsynaptic membrane by causing Cl^- influx and/or K^+ efflux. Free glycine is then recaptured by the presynaptic terminal or diffuses from the cleft and is taken up by glia or other neurons.

Related to these processes is the question of whether or not vesicles are associated with glycine, and for that matter, with any other amino acid transmitter. There is little evidence either for or against the presence of vesicles. The difficulty in visualizing them is presumably due to the diffusion of the small molecules of amino acids from vesicles into the surrounding media during the procedures (tissue homogenization, centrifugation, and washing) used in the attempts to label the amino acids in the vesicles.

Glycine Release

There is evidence (reviewed by Johnston, 1975) that a spontaneous efflux of glycine from the rat cerebral cortex and spinal cord occurs via a carrier-mediated facilitated diffusion. It is supposed that this release is for metabolic glycine. The release of glycine that is elicited

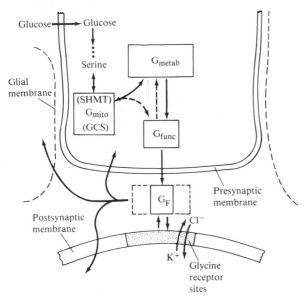

FIGURE 8 MODEL OF A GLYCINERGIC SYNAPSE. Glycine is synthesized in the mitochondrial compartment (G_{mito}); it is released into the metabolic compartment (G_{metab}) where it participates in peptide and protein synthesis; the functional compartment (G_{func}) is the source of synaptic glycine; and free glycine (G_F) is found in the synaptic cleft. SHMT, serine hydroxymethyltransferase; GCS, glycine cleavage system. (From Aprison and Daly, 1975.)

by peripheral nerve stimulation, electrical stimulation, or by increased extracellular potassium is diminished by the absence of calcium ions, and this is characteristic of a transmitter release mechanism. However, other investigators reported an inability to elicit glycine release by stimulation of the dorsal roots of the frog spinal cord. In this case it is possible that the release of glycine was too small above basal levels to be detected. It is also possible that released amino acids were taken up rapidly by axon terminals or glia, or effectively bound to postsynaptic receptors (Ryall, 1975). More experiments, especially on higher species, are necessary to resolve these issues.

Sodium Requirements for Uptake of Amino Acid Transmitters

The low-affinity uptake system can function in the absence of special sodium requirements. However, the high-affinity system is highly dependent upon sodium ions, because during membrane transport an exchange

takes place between glycine and sodium ions on a one-to-one basis. If the surrounding medium is sodium free, the high-affinity uptake systems of the amino acid transmitters are almost completely inhibited; a sodium-free medium completely inhibited the uptake of glutamic acid and aspartic acid in both the cerebral cortex and the spinal cord, of proline in the cerebral cortex, and of glycine in the spinal cord. Thus, it appears that glutamic acid and aspartic acid play distinctive neurotransmitter roles in the cerebral cortex and the spinal cord, whereas glycine has a transmitter role that is confined to the spinal cord and brain stem. This conclusion is supported by the additional finding that depolarization of central nervous tissue slices selectively released glutamic and aspartic acids, glycine, and proline, whereas other amino acids such as phenylalanine, lysine, alanine, leucine, and serine were not released.

Glycine Is an Inhibitory Transmitter

That glycine is a postsynaptic inhibitory neurotransmitter has been amply demonstrated by iontophoretic studies of motoneurons in the spinal cord. Iontophoretic application of glycine increases the membrane potential (hyperpolarization) and decreases membrane resistance. The hyperpolarization is rapid in onset and quickly reversible (within 12 seconds after glycine iontophoresis is turned off). The degree of hyperpolarization is related to the iontophoretic current. Glycine reduces spike amplitude and that of EPSPs and IPSPs and increases Cl^- permeability in a dose-related fashion. All of these effects are similar to those that are elicited by stimulating inhibitory interneurons.

To demonstrate that glycine is released upon stimulation of inhibitory neurons, the isolated amphibian spinal cord was studied. Stimulation of the dorsal (sensory) roots caused a release of [^{14}C]glycine but not of [^{14}C]insulin, which was used as a control label. The amount of glycine in the tissue bath was measured before stimulation, during stimulation, and after stimulation. There was an increase in radioactivity during stimulation, and similar results were obtained from slices of spinal cord from the rat and synaptosomes from the medulla and spinal cord. However, the results were somewhat unpredictable, probably because of the rapid and efficient uptake system for glycine. More consistency would probably be forthcoming if a specific glycine uptake inhibitor could be found and utilized (Ryall, 1975).

The Glycine Receptor

The glycine receptor has been identified by the high affinity of [3H]strychnine for membrane fractions upon which glycine is normally bound to produce postsynaptic inhibition. The distribution of specific strychnine binding parallels the regional distribution of endogenous glycine, with the greatest amount in the spinal cord and the second highest amount in the medulla. The midbrain concentration is 35 percent of spinal cord binding activity, and the hypothalamus and thalamus displayed 29 percent and 21 percent of cord binding activity, respectively. There was none in the cerebellum, hippocampus, corpus striatum, or cerebral cortex (Snyder et al., 1973). Other studies have shown that the highest specific strychnine binding occurs in subcellular fractions enriched in synaptic membranes, a fact consistent with the localization of the binding sites on postsynaptic glycine receptors. Because strychnine has no appreciable effect on glycine uptake, it is doubtful that strychnine binds to the presynaptic receptors of this uptake system.

Drugs That Affect Glycine Synapses

Strychnine. There are very few drugs that exert any action on glycine synapses. There are no specific substances that affect glycine synthesis and glycine uptake. However, as we previously noted, tetanus toxin blocks the release of GABA and glycine by interacting with synaptic gangliosides. Tetanus toxin will even block the release of glycine (and other amino acids) from synaptosomes obtained from rats that had been given an intramuscular injection of the toxin 15 hours before death (Aprison, 1978).

The only drug that significantly modifies glycinergic activity is strychnine, a compound that has a long history in medicine and research. It is an alkaloid derived from the seeds of a tree native to India, *Strychnos nux vomica*. The alkaloid brucine is also found in *S. nux vomica*. Brucine is a compound that is chemically and physiologically similar to strychnine, but less potent. Nux vomica, as strychnine was known

in old pharmacopoeias, has been erroneously translated as "emetic nut." However, strychnine is not an emetic, and *vomica* means "depression" or "cavity", which is a feature of the strychnos seed. In the sixteenth century, nux vomica was used as a poison for rats and other animal pests in Germany, and its use in modern times in "rat biscuits" has been responsible for some accidental poisonings of children (Esplin and Zablocka, 1965).

Early studies showed that strychnine was a potent convulsant and had its greatest effect on the antigravity muscles, causing them to display symmetrical extensor thrusts. These thrusting movements could be elicited by almost any sensory stimulus—tactile, auditory, visual, and so forth. These convulsions were also found in spinal animals, suggesting that the principal effects were spinal in character. At high doses, strychnine caused excitation in the cerebral cortex and the medulla, but not in the cerebellum; nor was it effective when applied directly on skeletal muscles. The effects of strychnine can be strikingly demonstrated by injecting a subconvulsive dose in a mouse. The mouse seems to act normally in a quiet environment, but a loud clap of the hands will cause it to jump about wildly.

The Mechanism of Action of Strychnine. In 1953 Bradley et al. rejected the idea that strychnine enhanced all central excitatory synaptic action when they found that the drug was relatively ineffective on monosynaptic reflexes in comparison with the large facilitation of polysynaptic reflexes. That finding, together with other data (which was by no means conclusive), led them to speculate that strychnine competed with the inhibitory transmitter of spinal interneurons at postsynaptic sites—a view that later proved to be correct (Ryall, 1975).

About 15 years later, renewed interest in inhibitory transmitters led to iontophoretic studies that elucidated the mechanism of action of strychnine. The drug was found to inhibit the depressant action of glycine and to a lesser extent the depressant action of a wide variety of other amino acids (but not GABA, except at very high doses) on spinal interneurons. There were many inconsistencies among the many reports about these phenomena and these inconsistencies were mostly due to differences in procedure. For example, a question arose as to whether strychnine was a competitive or noncompetitive antagonist of glycine. The implication of this argument is that if strychnine is a non-

Strychnine

Brucine

competitive glycine antagonist it occupies the receptor sites and cannot be displaced no matter how great the glycine concentration. Figure 9 illustrates the results of an experiment by Curtis et al. (1971), showing the effect of glycine alone (control) and in combination with strychnine on the inhibition of firing rates in spinal interneurons. Both glycine and strychnine were applied

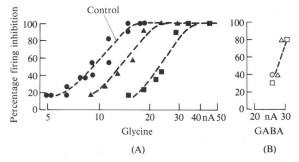

FIGURE 9 SPECIFICITY AND COMPETITIVE ANTAGONISM OF GLYCINE by strychnine on a spinal interneuron. (A) The curves show the inhibition of the firing rate of a spinal interneuron as a function of increased iontophoretic applications of glycine alone or in combination with strychnine. The abscissa shows the ejection current of glycine. Strychnine was administered by currents of 5 nA (triangles) or 10 nA (squares). The control group is plotted with circles. (B) No significant effect is seen when strychnine is combined with GABA. (From Curtis et al., 1971.)

iontophoretically via a multibarreled electrode. When glycine was applied by itself, the S-shaped curve indicated that the inhibition of the firing rate increased as the iontophoretic current increased until the inhibition was complete (100 percent). When strychnine was added, the dose–response curves were shifted to the right, the distance depending upon the iontophoretic current of strychnine (5 or 10 nA). This means that in the presence of strychnine more glycine was needed to get the same inhibitory effect. The parallel displacement of the dose–response curves, plus the fact that a maximum glycine-induced inhibition can still be obtained in the presence of strychnine, means that glycine competes with strychnine and that the strychnine can be displaced from the receptor sites providing enough glycine is available to do so.

If strychnine were a noncompetitive glycine antagonist, then the glycine-strychnine curve would not be displaced from the glycine-alone curve but would merely reach an asymptote at a lower level of the glycine inhibitory effect (see Chapter 1). This would indicate that strychnine cannot be displaced by glycine from receptor sites.

Figure 9B shows the effect of strychnine and GABA combinations. It can be seen that strychnine has virtually no effect on GABA-induced inhibition because the three curves overlap. These results again show that postsynaptic inhibition in the spinal cord is mediated largely by glycine, with GABA probably playing a role only in presynaptic inhibition.

Benzodiazepine Effects on Glycine Receptors. As we discussed earlier, the benzodiazepines have a wide range of effects, including anticonvulsant activity and the ability to induce skeletal muscle relaxation. These effects were attributed to a GABAmimetic action. The benzodiazepines, especially diazepam, have also been reported to have a glycinemimetic action that enhances muscle-relaxing effects. Young et al. (1974) found that diazepam was very potent in its ability to inhibit strychnine binding to glycine receptor sites, a potency that was equal to glycine itself. Snyder and Enna (1975) and Snyder (1975b) reported that the ED 50 binding affinity of diazepam for glycine receptor sites was commensurate with the concentration necessary for therepeutic efficacy in cats. Moreover, it was shown that potency tests of different benzodiazepines in inhibiting [³H]strychnine binding closely correlated with their potency in a human bioassay that was based on the minimal dose at which 50 percent of tested human subjects reported subjective anxiolytic effects. Because there appeared to be a significant relationship between anxiolytic activity of these drugs and their affinity for the glycine receptor, it was suggested by some investigators that glycine may play a significant role in the control of anxiety (Costa et al., 1975).

Young et al. (1974) also examined the chemical structure of 21 benzodiazepines and found that the compounds that could interact best with glycine were more potent, whereas the compounds that could interact least were less potent in inhibiting strychnine binding and in tests that predicted human responses to the drugs. These findings are vitiated by the finding that the anxiolytic effect of oxazepam was not selectively antagonized by strychnine (Stein et al., 1975). Moreover, the binding experiments rest upon the assumption that strychnine binds very specifically to glycine receptors—an assumption that may not be justified. It has been reported that strychnine binds at sites different from glycine receptors while exerting significant effects on neuronal and muscular membranes. Further electrophysiological evidence failed to support the notion that benzodiazepines either activate or block glycine receptors, because the drugs neither induced glycine-mediated inhibition nor blocked it. And although benzodiazepines were strong protectors against convulsions induced by GABA antagonists such as picrotoxin and bicuculline, they were weak protectors against strychnine-induced convulsions (Costa et al., 1975; Haefely, 1978). Other evidence has shown that neither glycine nor strychnine displaced [^{3}H]diazepam binding (Squires and Braestrup, 1977).

Summary

There are a number of substances that have strych-

nine-like effects, but none of them are as potent as strychnine. Also, strychnine does not suppress all spinal postsynaptic inhibition, nor are all glycine-sensitive receptors responsive to strychnine. This latter observation suggests that there are multiple forms of glycine receptors—a suggestion in keeping with characteristics of most other neurotransmitter receptors. There are some compounds that seem to potentiate the inhibitory action of glycine, presumably by blocking amino acid reuptake, but how potent and specific these effects are is not clear (Ryall, 1975; Aprison and Daly, 1975).

Part II Excitatory Amino Acid Transmitters

The two candidates for excitatory amino acid transmitters in the CNS are the nonessential protein amino acids, glutamic acid and aspartic acid. During the 1950s they were suspected to be neurotransmitters because virtually all neurons in the CNS could be depolarized by them. Glutamic acid concentration in the brain is higher than that of any other amino acid, yet, at the same time, this universality of action and general and generous distribution in the CNS made it seem unlikely that this compound was appropriate for neurotransmitters because this pattern of action and availability lacked the specificity of the cholinergic and monoaminergic systems. Moreover, some of the important criteria for the identity of a neurotransmitter could not be met by these compounds. For example, metabolizing enzymes could not be identified or were absent from synaptic sites; and synthesis, storage and release criteria were difficult to establish because these substances have a general physiological role to play in practically all tissues. An additional problem, aside from glutamic acid serving as a precursor to GABA, is that these glutamic and aspartic acids have a very similar structure. There is hardly a reaction involving one compound that cannot also occur with the other. It has even been shown that glutamate and aspartate

compete with each other in uptake systems and that there are no known selective inhibitors of the uptake of either one (Snyder, 1975a; Johnston, 1975). Nevertheless, these observations are not sufficient to rule out a transmitter role for these substances or prove that it exists (Cotman and Hamberger, 1978).

Identity of Glutamate and Aspartate as Neurotransmitters

One of the arguments in favor of glutamate being a neurotransmitter is that it is an excitatory motor transmitter in the neuromuscular junction of crustaceans and insects, whereas the putative transmitter for sensory neurons of crustaceans and insects is acetylcholine. This argument is held to be valid even though in vertebrates, the situation is just the opposite—the motor transmitter is acetylcholine and the transmitter for sensory neurons is presumably glutamate (Roberts and Hammerschlag, 1976).

Stimulating the motor nerve caused a release of glutamate in the locust and several varieties of crustaceans, and the release was proportional to the frequency of the stimulation and the concentration of Ca^{2+} in the bathing fluid. Also, glutamate was found to be the most effective of a number of compounds in eliciting muscle contractions in crustaceans and insects. Furthermore, after iontophoretic application, glutamate was found to be localized in specific patches on postsynaptic membranes of crayfish. It was also ob-

$$COOH—CH_2—CH_2—CH—COOH$$
$$\underset{NH_2}{|}$$

Glutamic acid

$$COOH—CH_2—CH—COOH$$
$$\underset{NH_2}{|}$$

Aspartic acid

served that prolonged administration of glutamate led to desensitization of the muscle to glutamate and to the natural transmitter released from the presynaptic terminals (if it were something else), whereas the action of GABA (the likely inhibitory transmitter) was unaffected. Electron microscopic autoradiographic studies showed glutamate uptake in neuromuscular preparations of the cockroach, and the rate of uptake at that site was greater than at any other tissue site. Also, the rate of uptake was increased by nerve stimulation. This provides a mechanism for transport-mediated termination of glutamate action. Thus, there is little doubt that the transmitter action in this case was well established.

With respect to vertebrate systems, synaptosomes derived from cortical tissue revealed a specific Na^+-dependent high-affinity, and a low-affinity system for the binding of glutamate and aspartate (the high-affinity K_m = 2–3 $\times$ 10^{-5} M and the low-affinity K_m = 0.5–1.0 $\times$ 10^{-3} M). These findings support the view that these substances have a dual role in the CNS (Snyder, 1975). Moreover, high-affinity uptake decreases after certain brain lesions which suggests the existence of glutamatergic and aspartatergic tracts in the brain (McGeer et al., 1978). However, due to the absence of suitable staining techniques, the mapping of long fiber pathways that utilize these putative transmitters has at present not been possible, even if they do exist. Consequently, one can only establish the presence of glutamate and aspartate systems where they are more easily accessible in neural structures such as the brain stem and spinal cord.

Distribution of Glutamate and Aspartate. Examination of the bipolar neurons of sensory ganglia of the spinal cord and brain stem reveals that there is a higher concentration of glutamate in the cell body and centrally directed axon than in the peripheral branch and that there are high concentrations in the gray matter of the spinal cord and sensory nuclei of the brain stem where the sensory branches of the cranial nerves terminate. There is additional evidence based on the action of agonist and antagonist drugs (see later) that glutamate plays a transmitter role in the cuneate nucleus of the brain stem, which receives impulses mediating tactile and proprioceptive signals from the spinal cord, as well as in the sensory relay nuclei of the thalamus. Thus, glutamate (and possibly aspartate) appears to be

the transmitter of primary afferent excitation (McLennan, 1975). However, as Snyder (1975a) points out, one would expect the levels of the sensory afferent transmitter to fall after lesions of the dorsal root, but glutamic acid levels were unchanged after that procedure. Instead, a peptide known as substance P (see Chapter 10) was severely depleted from the dorsal gray after section of the dorsal root.

It has been discovered that the granule cells of the cerebellum (cells that are more numerous than any other cell type in the CNS) seem to have glutamate as their neurotransmitter. It has been possible in the hamster to deplete granule cells selectively by inoculating the brain of newborn hamsters with a unique virus that destroys granule cell precursors. This results in adult hamsters whose cerebella show a perfectly normal uptake of most amino acids, although the uptake of glutamate and aspartate is diminished by 70 and 80 percent, respectively. This does not indicate whether glutamate or aspartate is the natural transmitter, but whereas the endogenous levels of most amino acids are normal, the level of glutamate is depleted by about 40 percent. This evidence points to glutamate as the transmitter for granule cells, which neurophysiological evidence clearly shows serves an excitatory function (Young et al., 1974).

Finally, when brain slices were labeled with a variety of radioactive amino acids and then depolarized by an excess of potassium in the bath medium, there was a selective release of glutamic acid, aspartic acid, GABA, and glycine from spinal cord, but not of other amino acids.

From the foregoing one can conclude that glutamate is a very abundant amino acid in the CNS; the highest concentrations appear in the cerebral cortex and caudate nucleus, in granule cells of the cerebellum, in hippocampal mossy fibers, and in the gray matter of the spinal cord (with a slightly higher concentration in the dorsal than in the ventral gray). Aspartate is also evenly distributed in the CNS, with highest concentrations in spinal cord gray (Johnston, 1975; Snyder, 1975; McGeer et al., 1978).

With respect to subcellular distribution, the neurotransmitter amino acids do not seem to be associated with any particular subcellular particle and appear to exist as cytoplasmic constituents. This, of course, may be due to disruption of a specific subcellular distribution during fractionation procedures. However, synaptic vesicles from rat brain homogenates containing amino acid transmitters have been detected by some investigators (Johnston, 1975).

Synthesis and Metabolism of Glutamate and Aspartate. The synthesis of these closely related amino acids is simple and appears to be identical in all forms of life. Glutamic acid is formed from ammonia and α-ketoglutarate, an intermediate in the Krebs cycle. This reaction requires the enzyme α-ketoglutarate transaminase with a vitamin B_6 cofactor and the cofactor NADPH, which is the reduced form of nicotinamide adenine dinucleotide phosphate (NADP$^+$, a phosphorylated form of NAD$^+$) (see Equation 1 in Figure 10). The reverse of this reaction requires glutamic acid dehydrogenase (L-GD). Glutamate can also be taken up by glia, where it can be converted to glutamine via the enzyme glutamine synthetase (Equation 2 in Figure 10). Glutamine can then be transferred to glutamatergic neurons where it can be converted to glutamate via the enzyme glutaminase (Equation 3 in Figure 10).* The relationship between glutamate neurons and glia is shown in Figure 11. The catabolism

*However, glutaminase has not yet been found in glutamate nerve endings. (Personal communication, E.G. McGeer, 1982.)

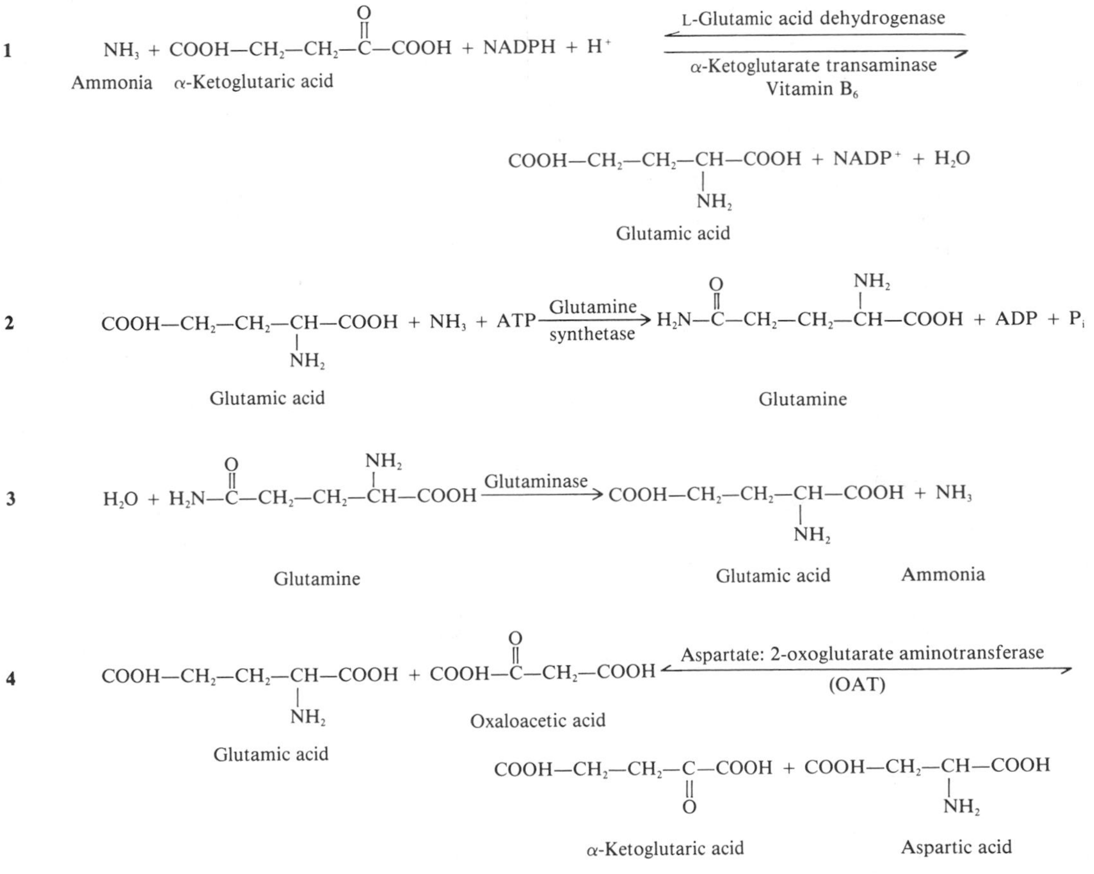

1   $NH_3 + COOH-CH_2-CH_2-\overset{O}{\overset{\|}{C}}-COOH + NADPH + H^+$

Ammonia α-Ketoglutaric acid

L-Glutamic acid dehydrogenase
α-Ketoglutarate transaminase
Vitamin B_6

$COOH-CH_2-CH_2-\underset{\underset{NH_2}{|}}{CH}-COOH + NADP^+ + H_2O$

Glutamic acid

2   $COOH-CH_2-CH_2-\underset{\underset{NH_2}{|}}{CH}-COOH + NH_3 + ATP \xrightarrow[\text{synthetase}]{\text{Glutamine}} H_2N-\overset{O}{\overset{\|}{C}}-CH_2-CH_2-\underset{\underset{NH_2}{|}}{\overset{NH_2}{}}CH-COOH + ADP + P_i$

Glutamic acid   Glutamine

3   $H_2O + H_2N-\overset{O}{\overset{\|}{C}}-CH_2-CH_2-\underset{\underset{NH_2}{|}}{\overset{NH_2}{}}CH-COOH \xrightarrow{\text{Glutaminase}} COOH-CH_2-CH_2-\underset{\underset{NH_2}{|}}{CH}-COOH + NH_3$

Glutamine   Glutamic acid   Ammonia

4   $COOH-CH_2-CH_2-\underset{\underset{NH_2}{|}}{CH}-COOH + COOH-\overset{O}{\overset{\|}{C}}-CH_2-COOH \xleftarrow{}$

Glutamic acid   Oxaloacetic acid

Aspartate: 2-oxoglutarate aminotransferase
(OAT)

$COOH-CH_2-CH_2-\overset{}{\underset{\underset{O}{\|}}{C}}-COOH + COOH-CH_2-\underset{\underset{NH_2}{|}}{CH}-COOH$

α-Ketoglutaric acid   Aspartic acid

FIGURE 10   GLUTAMIC AND ASPARTIC ACID SYNTHESIS AND CATABOLISM. Glutamic acid can be derived from α-ketoglutarate (Equation 1). Synaptically released glutamic acid can be taken up by adjacent glia and converted to glutamine (Equation 2). Glutamine can be transported to neurons where it is converted to glutamic acid (Equation 3). Aspartic acid is derived from glutamic acid and oxaloacetic acid, with α-ketoglutaric acid as a byproduct (Equation 4).

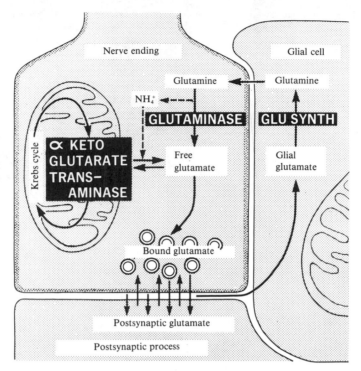

FIGURE 11 GLUTAMATERGIC SYNAPSE. Glutamate is derived from α-ketoglutarate from the Krebs cycle, or from glutamine via the enzyme glutaminase. Glia can take up synaptic glutamate where it is converted to glutamine. Glutamine can be transferred to neurons where it is converted to glutamate (possibly by glutaminase). (From McGeer et al., 1978.)

of glutamate consists of the reversal of the synthetic process shown in Equation 1 of Figure 10. It requires the enzyme α-ketoglutarate transaminase.

Newly synthesized glutamate in the hippocampus is preferentially released and most (70 percent) of releasable glutamate is derived from glutamine. The rest is from glucose catabolism. In response to nerve terminal depolarization, glutamate synthesis increases by way of increased uptake of glutamine and increased glutaminase activity. Glutaminase activity is governed by end product inhibition: when glutamate levels fall, glutaminase activity increases (Cotman and Hamberger, 1978).

Aspartic acid synthesis and catabolism occurs by reversible transamination: from glutamic acid and oxaloacetic acid to form α-ketoglutaric acid and aspartic acid (Equation 4 in Figure 10). These reactions require the enzyme aspartate: 2-oxoglutarate aminotransferase (OAT). Other possible catabolic routes are described by Johnston (1975), but none of these are believed to be of any significance in limiting the synaptic action of aspartate or glutamate. Rather, as in similar cases, reuptake seems to be the most significant method by which this is accomplished. As mentioned earlier, there are high- and low-affinity uptake systems for these amino acids, with the high–affinity, sodium–dependent system being specific for the transmitter pools. These metabolic events, which occur in mitochondria, are dependent upon the Krebs cycle, reminding us that these metabolic events are not exclusive for stores of transmitter amino acids, but that the amino acids in question play other significant physiological roles in such processes as peptide, protein, enzyme and hormone construction, and fatty acid synthesis.

Amino Acid Transmitter Function in the Spinal Cord

Roberts and Hammerschlag (1976) summarized the putative role of amino acids in spinal cord function

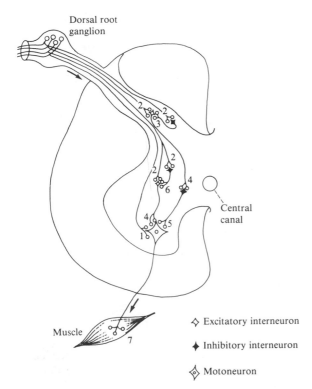

Dorsal root
ganglion

Central
canal

Muscle

◇ Excitatory interneuron

✦ Inhibitory interneuron

◈ Motoneuron

FIGURE 12   SPINAL CORD LOCI of amino acid transmitter action. The synapses occur within cell groups in the
gray matter of the spinal cord. 1 and 2, glutamic acid; 3,
GABA; 4, aspartic acid; 5, glycine; 6, glycine or GABA; 7,
acetylcholine. (From Roberts and Hammerschlag, 1976.)

layer of the hippocampus, it was found that glutamate
was released by electrical or chemical depolarization in a
normal calcium medium (2 mM free Ca^{2+}), but the effect was markedly reduced in a Ca^{2+}-free medium.
Subcellular release originated from synaptosomes in a
Ca^{2+}-dependent manner. Iontophoretically and *extra-
cellularly* applied glutamate had a powerful excitatory
effect on hippocampal neurons. *Intracellularly* applied
glutamate has no such effect. The excitatory effect is
accompanied by membrane depolarization brought on
by increased Na^+ conductance (Cotman and Hamberger, 1978).

Drugs That Affect Glutamic
and Aspartic Acid Systems

Many of the experiments that tested the action of
drugs on amino acid-induced neuron excitation were
done on brain slices, and single neurons in the spinal
cord and brain stem in amphibia and mammals. In
many cases the drug effects were similar for both
glutamate and aspartate systems, this being especially
true for antagonistic agents.

Amino Acid Agonists. A number of glutamate analogs have been compared with glutamate with respect
to their ability to stimulate spinal interneurons. Some
of these studies utilized microiontophoretic techniques
and therein lay some serious difficulties in making
valid comparisons among the substances tested. The
potencies of the tested substances were compared by
observing the magnitudes of the ejecting currents that
were required to elicit similar neural excitations. The
assumptions that underlie comparisons of this sort are
first, that the same electrode must be used for all tests
because the diameter of the opening determines the
number of molecules that will be ejected by a given
current. Second, the number of molecules increases
with time after the start of an application; and third,
the same area of membrane must be stimulated for all
tests. Clearly, when multiple tests must be done, these
conditions cannot be met. Moreover, even if these conditions could be met, high ejection currents cause large
amounts of a given compound to be ejected, resulting
in diffusion and causing a greater membrane area to be
affected. Thus, the validity of comparisons made
under these conditions is suspect (McLennan, 1975).
Unless supporting studies are done utilizing other procedures (such as measuring the effects of drug in a
superfusing medium), the potency of would-be glu-

(Figure 12). They suggested that glutamate is the chief
afferent excitatory transmitter liberated by the terminals of the dorsal root fibers—most of which end in
the dorsal horn gray, where polysynaptic pathways
have their origin (site 2). Other endings form monosynaptic contacts with motor neurons (site 1). The dorsal gray is characterized by the presence of numerous
interneurons. Some have presynaptic inhibition as the
mode of action (site 3). Some of these interneurons
may exert excitatory influences on motor neurons and
have aspartate as the neurotransmitter (site 4). Glycine
is secreted by others to exert inhibitory postsynaptic effect (site 5).

Mechanism of Action of Glutamate

In studies of the role of glutamate in the molecular

tamic acid agonists cannot be assessed with confidence.

Along with glutamate and aspartate themselves, a number of their analogs have been tried as amino acid transmitter agonists. However, as mentioned earlier, they are relatively unspecific. Among these are kainic acid, N-methyl-DL-glutamic acid, and β-N-oxalyl-L-α,β-diaminopropionic acid. These substances show some specificity for glutamate receptors. N-Methyl-D-aspartic acid shows some preference for aspartate receptors, whereas DL-homocysteic acid, quisqualic acid, and ibotenic acid seem to affect both glutamate and aspartate receptors.

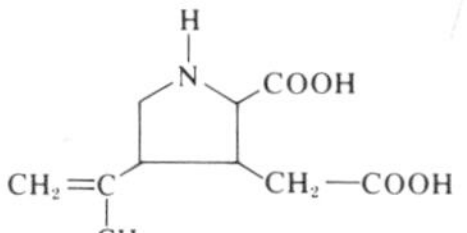

Kainic acid

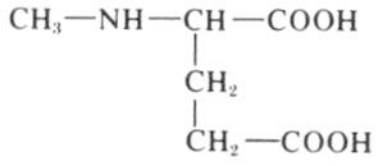

N-Methyl-DL-glutamic acid

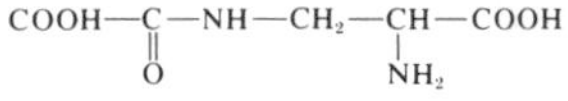

β-N-Oxalyl-L-α, β-diaminopropionic acid

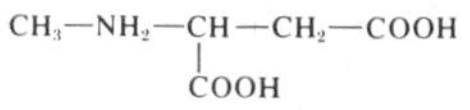

N-Methyl-D-aspartic acid

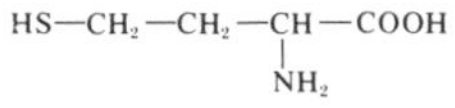

DL-Homocysteic acid

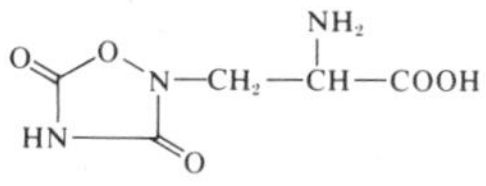

Quisqualic acid

In the 1940s, glutamate was used in attempts to control petit mal and psychomotor epilepsy, but the results were not significant. Also glutamate was used at that time in the treatment of mental retardation because it had been shown to increase maze performance in rats. However, control studies showed that the positive effects were transient and trivial and were ascribed to the nutritional benefit that might have accrued from the amino acid treatment.

In the 1960s and 1970s, a number of studies showed that systemically administered glutamate damaged retinal and hypothalamic cells and at higher doses caused seizures in immature animals. In mature animals, the same effects were caused by intraventricular administration of glutamate and aspartate. It appeared that the intense depolarizing effects of these excitatory transmitters were responsible for the toxic effects. Microinjections of glutamate into various brain areas caused destruction of certain neurons while sparing others in the lesion area, suggesting that the toxic effect was directed upon those cells that were subject to excitation by glutamate. These findings were partly responsible for the elimination of monosodium glutamate (MSG) from baby food preparations. This substance is a flavor enhancer and is deemed to be safe for mature nervous systems. However, the abundant use of MSG in Chinese cooking has resulted in what is known as the "Chinese restaurant syndrome," which is characterized by burning sensations, facial pressure, and chest pains in individuals deemed sensitive to the effects of glutamate.

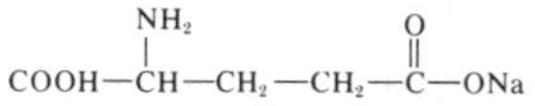

Monosodium glutamate

Microinjection of the amino acid transmitter analogs were also found to have toxic effects, leading to the destruction of neural tissue. Despite the difficulty in assessing relative potency when using microinjection procedures, the order of potency of the toxic effects was found to be kainic acid > N-methyl-DL-aspartic acid > L-glutamic acid > DL-homocysteic acid. Electron microscopic examination showed that the damage started at dendrites and other postsynaptic sites, with no early effects in presynaptic elements. This would suggest that postsynaptic receptors are the sites for the initial effect, which presumably is overstimulation and which then leads to cell damage (McGeer et al., 1978).

Amino Acid Antagonists. A few drugs are found to have some selectivity as antagonists of amino acid-induced excitation: D-lysergic acid diethylamide (LSD), L-methionine-DL-sulfoximine, 2-methoxyaporphine, L-glutamic acid diethylester (GDEE), and 1-hydroxy-3-aminopyrrolid-2-one (HAP). GDEE seems to have the greatest specificity because it is quite effective in blocking the effect of glutamate applied electrophoretically while leaving the neuronal response to other amino acids and ACh relatively unaffected. The blockade of aspartate-induced excitation was also observed but not to the same degree. Because GDEE,

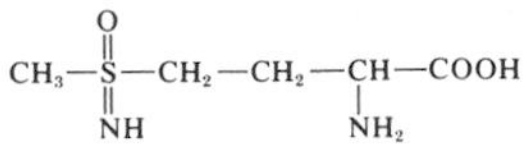

L-Methionine-DL-sulfoximine

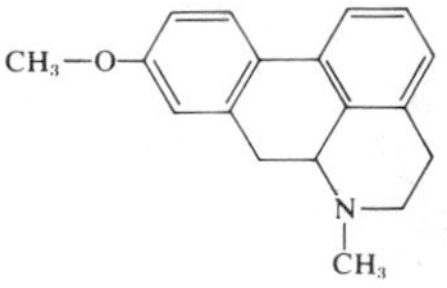

2-Methoxyaporphine

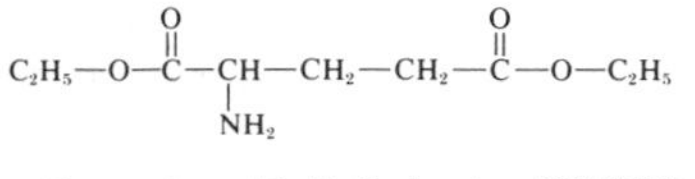

L-Glutamic acid diethyl ester (GDEE)

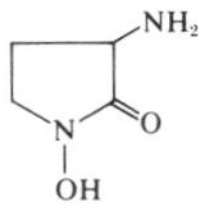

1-Hydroxy-3-aminopyrrolid-2-one (HAP)

p-hydroxymercuribenzoate, and p-chloromercuri-phenylsulfonate (PCMP) (McLennan, 1975). How-

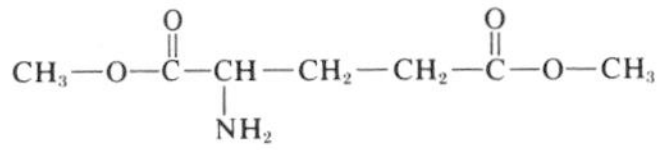

L-Glutamic acid dimethyl ester (GDME)

p-Hydroxymercuribenzoate

p-Chloromercuriphenylsulfonate

methionine sulfoximine, and HAP have structures similar to that of glutamate, it is presumed that they compete with glutamate for its receptor sites. This view is supported by the fact that (1) the excitatory action of ACh is relatively unaffected by these compounds; (2) the spontaneous activity of neurons are unaffected, ruling out some nonspecific depressant effect; (3) the action of HAP is not reduced by strychnine nor bicuculline, drugs that antagonize glycine and GABA, respectively. Thus, HAP does not appear to mimic glycine or GABA.

Glutamate and Aspartate Uptake Antagonists. Among the glutamate agonists mentioned earlier β-N-oxalyl-L-α,β-diaminopropionate seems to block glutamate uptake, and the same is true for DL-homocysteic acid. Also, folic acid is a nonspecific uptake blocker for glutamate and aspartate. Three other com-

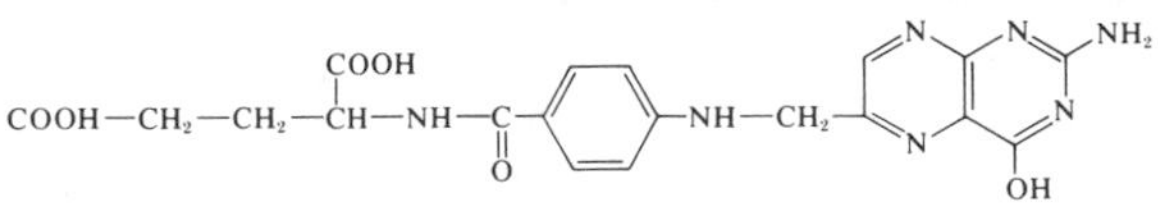

Folic acid

pounds have been identified as blockers of the high-affinity uptake system for glutamate and aspartate, with the consequence that the excitatory properties of these amino acids are enhanced. The blockade of the receptor is competitive for L-glutamic acid dimethyl ester (GDME) and noncompetitive for the mercurials

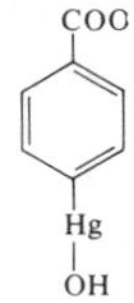

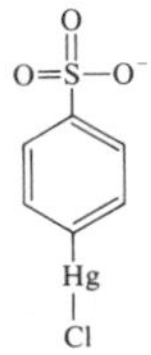

ever, Johnston (1975) reported that GDME has a direct excitatory action and that PCMP is not specific. What uptake studies show is that the reuptake processes for the amino acid transmitters is significant for limiting the neurotransmitter action as well as for supplying glutamate for metabolic purposes in the many intracellular compartments. However, no pharmacologically useful glutamate uptake inhibitor is known at present.

Kainic Acid as a Glutamate Receptor Toxin. Kainic acid is a glutamate analog that is several orders of magnitude more potent than glutamate as a neuronal depolarizer. Potent depolarizers damage neurons, and their neurotoxicity is correlated with their neuroexcitatory action. The granule cells of the cerebellum have glutamate as their transmitter. Consequently, Herndon and Coyle (1977) performed experiments based on the hypothesis that the cerebellar neurons normally receiving a glutamate input would be severely damaged by kainic acid. After injecting 2 μg of kainic acid into the cerebellums of rats and hamsters, they sacrificed the animals after various intervals and examined the cerebellums for damage in those cells that received an input from the granule cells. Control animals were similarly treated with a nonneurotoxic analog of glutamate.

Some damage was found in cerebellums removed 30 min. after drug injection, and after 1 hour all cells (Purkinje cells, basket cells, stellate cells, and Golgi II cells) were involved. Cerebellums taken 24 hours after drug injection showed disintegration of Purkinje cells as well as widespread damage to other cells. However, the granule cells showed only a temporary swelling after 1 or 2 hours but appeared unaffected after that. What is of particular interest here is the fact that the cell damage was highly selective for certain cell types, namely, those that received inputs of glutamate. When injected into the striatum, kainic acid caused a loss of neurons having glutamate receptors and caused biochemical changes characteristically associated with Huntington's chorea. Thus, this disease may be the result of selective system degeneration that is the consequence of metabolic errors that produce neurotoxic transmitter agents. Furthermore, kainic acid can be used to show regional variation in kainic acid binding that may be indicative of differences in the distribution of glutamate receptors (Table III).

TABLE III   Distribution of Specific [³H]Kainic Acid Binding in the Rat Brain

Brain area	Specific binding (counts per min/mg protein)	Number of experiments
Striatum	273 ± 9	6
Cerebellum	106 ± 11	6
Cerebral cortex	141 ± 13	5
Hippocampus	151 ± 8	5
Midbrain	52 ± 8	5
Thalamus	74 ± 8	5
Medulla-pons	49 ± 7	4

(From Simon et al., 1976)

Taurine

Identity and Distribution

Taurine is one of the few sulfur-containing amino acids that is found in relatively high concentrations in the CNS of mammals. The highest regional concentration in cats is in the lateral geniculate nucleus and the retina. In the retina, taurine appears to mediate the lateral inhibition that is the function of some amacrine cells. Also, when cats are fed a diet free of taurine for 3

months or longer, they develop a severe plasma deficiency of taurine and the retinal concentrations are reduced by up to 80 percent, accompanied by degeneration of the photoreceptors. Overall the greatest concentration of taurine is in heart tissue, and it is found in the nervous system of invertebrates as well. In the rat brain, the greatest concentration is in the olfactory bulb, and high levels exist in the cerebellum, cerebral cortex, and the striatum. (For concentrations in the cat brain, see Table IV.)

TABLE IV   Concentration of Taurine in the Cat Brain

Region	Concentration mol/g
Pituitary	8.08
Pineal	5.20
Cortex	2.10
Caudate	2.90
Thalamus	2.31
Lateral geniculate	4.30
Medial geniculate	1.70
Hypothalamus	1.81
Cerebellum	2.71
Pons	2.10
Medulla	1.70
Spinal cord	1.70
Heart (rabbit)	10.80

(From Guidotti et al., 1972)

Synthesis and Catabolism

Taurine is synthesized from cysteinesulfinic acid, and it is metabolized to isethionic acid (Figure 13). Uptake occurs via low– and high–affinity systems, but it is uncertain whether the high–affinity uptake system serves to recapture taurine to replenish a neurotransmitter pool. Studies of subcellular distribution tentatively indicate that only 17 percent of the taurine in whole rat brain is in the synaptosomal fraction, but almost 67 percent of the synthesizing enzyme cysteine-sulfinic acid decarboxylase (CAD) is found in this fraction (McGeer et al., 1978).

Release and Mechanisms of Action

Labeled taurine is released from brain cortical slices by electrical stimulation and from synaptosomes by high potassium concentrations. The release is Ca^{2+} dependent. Stimulation of the midbrain reticular formation in the cat resulted in the release of taurine in the

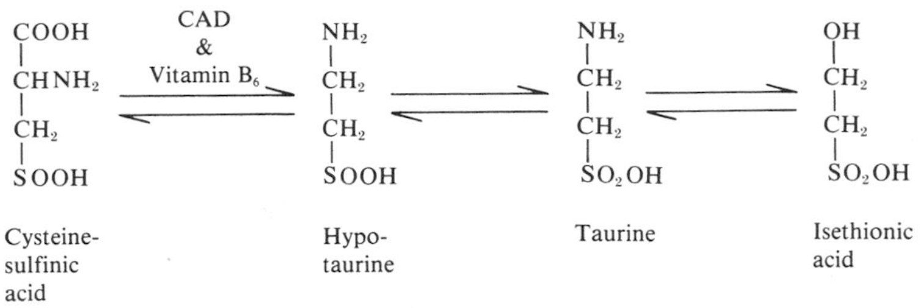

FIGURE 13 SYNTHESIS AND CATABOLISM OF TAURINE.

cerebral cortex. Taurine receptors are similar in some respects to glycine receptors because the depressive action of taurine and glycine in the retina and spinal cord is blocked by strychnine but not by the GABA receptor antagonist bicuculline. The depressive action of taurine on neural excitation is comparable in potency to that of GABA in certain supraspinal regions, but the potency of taurine inhibition of cortical, thalamic, and cerebellar neurons is less than that of GABA, and in these latter areas the inhibitory effect is blocked by both strychnine and bicuculline. Taurine has been found to block chemically induced convulsions in experimental animals (mice, cats, rats, and baboons). Tests also have been done on human epileptics. Positive, but mild, effects have been reported, and failure to find more dramatic results have been attributed to the inability of taurine to pass the blood brain barrier in significant amounts (McGeer et al., 1978). The wide distribution of taurine in the CNS is probably of some significance to CNS function, but its role and the possibility of pharmacological intervention with it must wait for further developments (Roberts and Hammerschlag, 1976; Cooper et al., 1978).

Histamine

Identity and Distribution in the CNS

Histamine, though not itself an amino acid, is derived from histidine which is. Histamine has been intensively investigated as a possible neurotransmitter in the CNS. It has a nonuniform distribution in the brain. It is associated with the synaptosomal fraction of brain homogenates. The specific enzymes for its synthesis and metabolism have been identified in the brain. Neurons respond to histamine. It stimulates adenylate cyclase activity that can be blocked by specific antagonists. Endogenous histamine can be released from brain slices by depolarizing nerve cells. In adult mammals the whole brain concentration of histamine is between 50 and 70 ng/gr wet weight. Its concentration in the monkey and human brain is shown in Table V, the greatest concentration is found in the hypothalamus (Brownstein et al., 1974).

Histamine exists in two pools in the brain, one neuronal, the other nonneuronal. The nonneuronal pool is found in MAST CELLS which are connective tissue cells containing heparin (a blood-clotting element), and in some animals, small amounts of serotonin and dopamine. Mast cells are especially numerous in the blood vessels of the MENINGES (the membranes covering the brain). The neuronal pool of histamine is found in axon terminals, and much of it is attached to synaptic vesicles. Each of the brain pools can be selectively released by appropriate chemical agents. Neuronal histamine is released by reserpine and high levels of potassium-induced depolarization. However, it is not known if there is a high affinity uptake system.

A histaminergic pathway seems to exist in the medial forebrain bundle (MFB) because MFB lesions in the rat lead to a decrease in the activity of the histamine-synthesizing enzyme (histidine decarboxylase) in brain areas rostral to the lesion. This is not a secondary effect because the change does not occur when 6-OHDA and 5,6-DHT lesions interrupt catecholamine and serotonin fibers in the MFB. Thus, a histaminergic pathway may arise from the brain stem to project to the hypothalamus and the telencephalon.

Synthesis and Catabolism

The synthesis and catabolism of histamine are illustrated in Figure 14. The amino acid precursor is histidine, which is decarboxylated by the vitamin B_6-requiring enzyme histidine decarboxylase. Synthesis by this enzyme is blocked by α-methylhistidine but not by dopa decarboxylase inhibitors such as α-methyldopa. Also, as mentioned earlier, the serotonin neurotoxin,

TABLE V Regional Localization of Histamine and Histidine in the Monkey Brain and of Histamine in Human Brain

	Monkey[1]		Human[2]
	Histidine mg/100 mg protein	Histamine ng/100 mg protein	Histamine ng/g tissue
Postcentral gyrus			
Cerebral cortex	9.4	47	105
White matter	12.1	54	—
Corpus callosum	16.3	52	—
Limbic cortex			
Olfactory bulb	8.7	74	213
Hippocampus	12.1	46	109
Amygdala	16.4	69	95
Septal nuclei	16.1	127	—
Pituitary, posterior	15.8	449	—
Pituitary, anterior	19.2	84	—
Pineal	10.3	1465	—
Hypothalamus			
Supraoptic nucleus	24.7	2059	—
Paraventricular nucleus	15.6	709	Ant: 630
Median eminence	25.5	1142	—
Infundibulum	41.7	521	—
Preoptic nucleus	16.9	616	Middle: 1068
Ventromedial nucleus	22.8	1701	—
Ventrolateral nucleus	23.2	1578	—
Mammillary bodies	14.9	2619	Post: 1381
Thalamus			
Anterior nucleus	18.2	264	139
Dorsal	11.8	151	118
Extrapyramidal nuclei			
Caudate	18.4	77	91
Putamen	13.4	63	102
Midbrain			
Substantia nigra	21	271	215
Superior colliculus	9.7	71	259
Inferior colliculus	6.9	117	320
Interpeduncular nucleus	14.3	22	—
Red nucleus	23.2	161	225
Raphe nucleus	29.3	301	—
Central gray	26.6	361	—
Cerebellum and lower brain stem			
Pons	8.3	86	109
Cerebellar cortex	11.4	15	40
Dentate nucleus	8.3	68	122

[1]Data from Taylor et al., 1972
[2]Data from Lipinski et al, 1973.

(From McGeer et al., 1978)

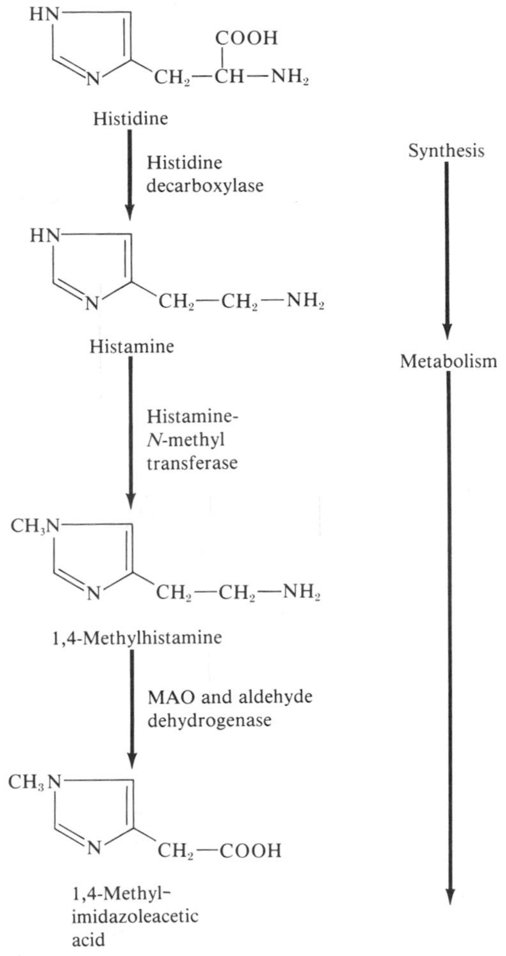

Histidine

Histidine
decarboxylase

Histamine

Histamine-
N-methyl
transferase

1,4-Methylhistamine

MAO and aldehyde
dehydrogenase

1,4-Methyl-
imidazoleacetic
acid

Synthesis

Metabolism

FIGURE 14 SYNTHESIS AND CATABOLISM OF HISTAMINE.

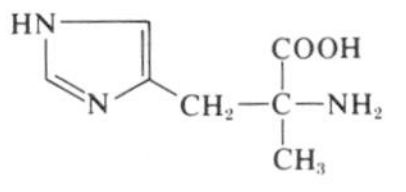

α-Methyl histidine

5,6-DHT and 6-OHDA, in concentrations that lowered dopa decarboxylase and 5-HTP decarboxylase by 50 percent, had no effect on histidine decarboxylase activity. These findings indicate that histidine decarboxylase is specific for histidine. The absence of a correlation between histamine levels and levels of the enzyme is added support for the existence of a neuronal and a nonneuronal pool of histamine.

Histamine is catabolized in two steps, first by histamine-N-methyltransferase (HNMT) to form 1,4-methylhistamine, then by MAO and aldehyde dehydrogenase to form 1,4-methylimidazoleacetic acid.

Pharmacology of Peripheral Histamine

Histamine in mast cells in peripheral tissues acts on smooth muscle of the viscera and vascular system. When this tissue is damaged or responds in an allergic reaction, histamine is released (along with other substances), causing capillary dilatation and venous constriction. There are two types of histamine receptors in peripheral tissue: H_1 receptors respond to allergic reactions, whereas gastric secretion is mediated via H_2 receptors.

Each receptor type is affected by a different array of agonist and antagonists drugs. Diphenhydramine (Benadryl) and chlorpheniramine (Chlortrimeton) are typical H_1 antagonists and are found in many antihistamine preparations that are used for the relief of allergy symptoms. These drugs have been of substantial benefit for allergy sufferers. Most antihistaminics, and especially methapyrilene, have mild hypnotic effects and are used to combat insomnia, a practice of questionable value. Diphenhydramine is also found in motion-sickness remedies (Douglas, 1975). Currently, one of the most effective drugs for the treatment of peptic ulcer and other conditions accompanied by excessive secretion of hydrochloric acid into the stomach is cimetidine (Tagamet), which is an H_2 receptor blocker and thus inhibits the release of HCl.

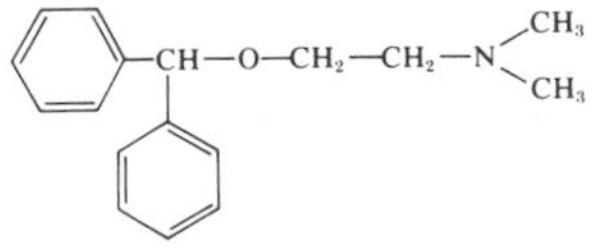

Diphenhydramine (Benadryl)

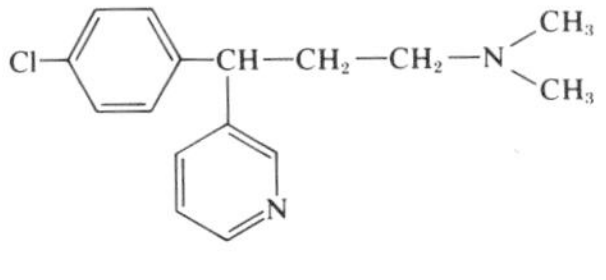

Chlorpheniramine (Chlortrimeton)

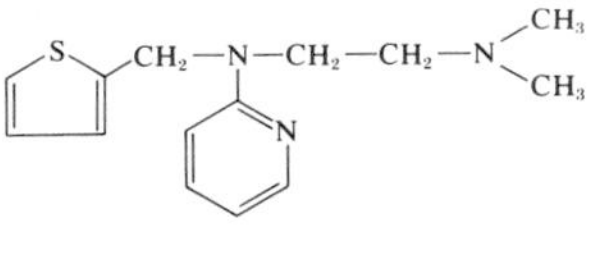

Methapyrilene

$$CH_3-NH-\overset{\overset{\displaystyle NCN}{||}}{C}-NH-CH_2-CH_2-S-CH_2$$

Cimetidine (Tagamet)

Central Effects of Histamine

Although histamine does not pass the blood brain barrier, preloading an animal with histidine has been used to raise brain levels of histamine. A wide variety of effects result because histidine raises concentrations of other neural stimulants and inhibitors as well, and reduces the brain levels of other amino acids by inhibiting their membrane transport into the brain. Histidine also depresses the firing of neurons in the medulla more markedly even than histamine. A variety of autonomic effects occur after intraventricular injections of histamine—increased blood pressure and heart rate, hypothermia, increased water intake, emesis, and decreased urine flow; such injections produce arousal reactions in cats and rabbits.

Metabolites of histamine are also active within the CNS. For example, injection of imidazoleacetic acid in mice caused hyperactivity, ataxia, catalepsy and loss of righting reflexes. It also potentiated the effects of pentylenetetrazol, picrotoxin, and strychnine—all blockers of the inhibitory actions of GABA and glycine. Some metabolites are more, some are less active depending upon how they penetrate the brain. They, too, have a variety of effects, but it is unknown how specific these effects are. It has been suggested that histamine plays a role in the extrapyramidal motor system, in morphine tolerance, pain perception, the release of vasopressin and prolactin from the pituitary gland, and in schizophrenia (Green et al., 1978). However, the results of these studies are quite tentative.

Conclusion

This chapter points out that acetylcholine and the biogenic amines make up only a small fraction of the neurotransmitter substances that are thought to be necessary for synaptic action among the billions of cells of the central nervous system. This conclusion is supported by the identification of the transmitter role of some amino acids among most of these synapses. It is proposed that GABA is the major transmitter among 30 to 40 percent of brain synapses and that its function is principally inhibitory (Bloom and Iversen, 1971).

Also, it is estimated that within the brain stem and spinal cord glycine accounts for 25 to 40 percent of the transmitters in these areas and that the function of glycine is also inhibitory (Iversen and Bloom, 1972). Glutamate and aspartate are shown to have widespread excitatory effects in the CNS, and other amines such as taurine, histamine, and related substances are implicated in the modulation of neural circuitry.

So far few drugs have been developed that have specific actions on one or another of the amino acid transmitters, and those drugs that have been found are mainly useful in controlling general neural excitability. Thus, they are used in the prevention of epilepsy in its various forms and in controlling muscle tone. It will also be seen later that GABA systems exert inhibitory actions upon other transmitter systems, for example, upon the serotonergic system that seems to account for the anxiety-reducing functions of certain drugs. These features will be discussed more fully in Chapter 11.

It would be tempting to develop hypotheses about the specific role played by each neurotransmitter and each neuromodulator, and some authors have attempted this. The task is easier when examining sensorimotor systems but very difficult when examining global behavior patterns. However, it has been proposed that an individual with a paucity or defective function of horizontal GABA neurons in the motor cortex might be more susceptible to the occurrence of grand mal seizures; or if such a problem existed in the region of the globus pallidus, postural control would be defective. Also, a person with an inadequate GABA system in the region of the hypothalamus dealing with food intake might show symptoms of hyperphagia or anorexia nervosa. Abnormalities of GABA neurons in the dorsal horn of the spinal cord might result in inordinately greater sensitivity to tactile and thermal stimulation and inadequate spatial and temporal discrimination of the stimuli. If there were functional defects in GABAergic systems in the retina, there might be faulty visual perception and integration (Roberts, 1974).

It is true that there is some evidence that a GABA deficiency is associated with Huntington's chorea (Chapter 11); there is a marked pathology consisting of a selective, degenerative loss of GABA-containing neurons in the corpus striatum and a loss of GAD, the GABA-synthesizing enzyme. However, attempts to treat this disease with drugs purported to have GABA-mimetic action (imidazoleacetic acid, lioresal, and

HC══C─CH₂─COOH
HN   N
  C
  H

Imidazole acetic acid

muscimol) or GABA catabolism inhibitors such as sodium *n*-dipropyl acetate, have been disappointing. It was even shown that binding sites for GABA were not significantly decreased in these patients, which indicated that there was an adequate population of receptors for these drugs (Iversen, 1978; Barbeau, 1978).

The major difficulty is that these transmitter agents, as well as the others described in the previous chapters, interact in many intricate ways to mediate motor activity, ingestive behaviors, perceptual processes, and mood so that many avenues have yet to be investigated to complete our understanding of the problems in these areas.

Recommended Readings

Aprison, M.H. (1978). Glycine as a neurotransmitter. In *Psychopharmacology: A Generation of Progress* (M.A. Lipton, A. DiMascio and K.F. Killam, Eds.), pp. 333–346. Raven Press, New York. A thorough review with an extensive reference list.

Fonnum, F. (1978). *Amino Acids as Chemical Trans-mitters*. Plenum Press, New York. The proceedings of a conference on amino acid transmitters. This volume contains 51 research papers which cover virtually every aspect of the subject.

Fonnum, F. and Storm-Mathisen, J. (1978). Localization of GABAergic neurons in the CNS. In *Handbook of Psychopharmacology, Vol. 9* (L.L. Iversen, S.D. Iversen and S.H. Snyder, Eds.), pp. 357–401. Plenum Press, New York. A detailed description of the distribution and morphology of GABAergic neurons in the mammalian brain, and the methods used to establish these findings.

Green, J.P., Johnson, C.L. and Weinstein, H. (1978). Histamine as a neurotransmitter. In *Psychopharmacology: A Generation of Progress* (M.A. Lipton, A. DiMascio and K.F. Killam, Eds.), pp. 319–332. Raven Press, New York. An excellent review and thorough reference list.

Iversen, L.L., Iversen, S.D. and Snyder, S.H. (Eds.) (1975). *Handbook of Psychopharmacology, Vol. 4 Amino Acid Transmitters*. Plenum Press, New York. Seven reviews by leading authors of the subject.

Roberts, E., Chase, T. and Tower, D.B. (Eds.) (1975). *GABA and Nervous System Function*. Raven Press, New York. A large collection of review articles on the functional significance of GABA.

CHAPTER TEN

Peptides as Neurotransmitters

It has been known for some time that neurons in the paraventricular and the supraoptic nuclei of the hypothalamus send axons to the posterior pituitary gland and that these axons contain the hormones oxytocin and vasopressin (or antidiuretic hormone). The hormones are released into the blood vessels of the posterior pituitary and enter the general blood circulation. The hormones are thus carried to their target organs in the body to control lactation, blood pressure, uterine contraction, and kidney function. A variety of hormones are secreted into the bloodstream from the anterior pituitary gland: adrenocorticotropic hormone (ACTH), thyrotropin, gonadotropins, somatotropin, and others. These hormones control metabolism, sexual cycles and responses to sexual stimulation, maternal behavior, growth, and responses to stress. As there is no significant neural input to the anterior pituitary gland how is the release of these substances controlled?

Ovulation occurs in some mammals, such as rabbits, only after coitus. It was presumed that the sexual excitement caused ovulation by the release of the luteinizing hormone from the anterior pituitary gland. In 1937, Geoffrey Wingfield Harris showed that ovulation could be induced in the rabbit by electrically stimulating the hypothalamo-hypophyseal stalk; and Spatz (1951) demonstrated that hypophysectomy (removal of the pituitary gland) in rabbits within one hour after coitus blocks ovulation. On the other hand, ovulation can be induced by electrical stimulation of the spinal cord or the median eminence, but it does not occur by stimulating the pituitary directly, nor if the spinal cord

is sectioned thereby blocking sensory input to the brain. In 1955, Harris reported that if the pituitary is severed from its stalk and transplanted to any site other than the immediate vicinity of the hypothalamus, it never reaches the state of full functional activity. However, normal activity is achieved if the severed gland is replaced into the sella turcica (the bone cavity normally occupied by the gland) or placed under the hypothalamus where it could be revascularized by the portal blood vessels. Thus, Harris demonstrated that it was likely that the hypothalamus that overlies the pituitary gland secretes releasing and inhibiting hormones into the portal blood vessels which carry these hormones from the hypothalamus to the anterior pituitary (see Figure 11 in Chapter 3).

This idea was zealously followed up by Roger Guillemin and Andrew Schally, who competed to identify these hypothalamic hormones (Wade, 1978a, 1978b, and 1978c). Their task was extremely difficult because these hormones are present in only nanogram amounts. They had to obtain hypothalami from hundreds of thousands of freshly slaughtered swine and sheep to obtain kilograms of tissue, from which they obtained a few milligrams of partially purified hormone.*

Guillemin, Schally and their coworkers worked 20

---

*Guillemin estimated that the cost of isolating the first milligram of pure thyrotropin releasing hormone from 300,000 sheep hypothalami was two to five times more than the cost of transporting a kilogram of moon rock to Earth by the Apollo 13 mission. This cost was met mainly by the National Institutes of Health and Veterans Administration (Meites, 1977).

years to isolate and analyze enough hormone to determine the structure of the thyrotropin releasing hormone (TRH). Their work was aided by the discovery and development of a new method of analysis—radioimmunoassay—which enabled the detection of substances that are found in small amounts such as the hypothalamic peptide hormones. Rosalyn Yalow was credited with the development of this technique, and in 1977 she, Guillemin and Schally shared the Nobel Prize in Medicine (Yalow, 1978).

As a result of their work, it is now feasible to isolate and identify many of the regulating hormones important to health, and to create synthetic analogs to be used in the therapy of hormone pathology. At the present time, most of the hypothalamic releasing and inhibiting hormones have been identified as peptides (short chains of amino acids), and their mode of action has been clarified (Schally et al., 1973; Schally, 1978).

Furthermore, after the structures of these hypothalamic peptides were known, experiments using radioimmunoassay revealed that the hormones were found not only in the hypothalamus and pituitary gland, but throughout the brain, in areas quite remote from the hypothalamic–endocrine system. For example, TRH is scattered throughout the rat brain, even in the vicinity of the spinal motoneurons. It is interesting that this TRH does not come from hypothalamic neurons, because a chronic separation of the hypothalamus from the rest of the brain has little effect on TRH in other parts of the brain (Brownstein, 1978).

There is ample evidence that TRH plays a neurotransmitter role in addition to (and possibly unrelated to) its neuroendocrine role; the same is true to an equal or lesser degree for other hypothalamic peptide hormones. In this chapter, we will discuss some of the research that shows that peptides have widespread neurotransmitter activity in the CNS. One important group of these peptides is the endorphins, which have opiate-like characteristics in attenuating pain. These peptides are discussed in Chapter 13 which deals with pain and analgesic drugs.

Thyrotropin Releasing Hormone

Thyrotropin releasing hormone is found in the hypothalamus and controls the release of thyrotropin (thyroid stimulating hormone, TSH) from the pituitary gland. The ratio of release of TRH to TSH is 1 to 100,000. Thyrotropin, in turn, regulates the release of hormones from the thyroid gland. TRH is a tripeptide

Thyrotropin releasing hormone (TRH)

amide consisting of three amino acids (glutamine, histidine, and proline) in equimolar ratios (Guillemin and Burgus, 1972). Within the hypothalamus, the highest concentration of TRH is found in the median eminence, in relation to the portal veins that transport the hormone to the anterior pituitary gland. Other hypothalamic areas containing the hormone include the dorsomedial nucleus and its lateral perifornical region, the parvocellular part of the paraventricular nucleus, the ventromedial nucleus, and the bordering zona incerta (Figure 12 in Chapter 3).

Examination of the effects of the TRH on CNS function and behavior was prompted by the discovery that as much as 80 percent of the TRH in the brain is located outside the hypothalamus. Relatively large amounts of TRH have been found in the forebrain, the posterior diencephalon, and the posterior cortex (Winokur and Utiger, 1974), in the nuclei of the occulomotor and trigeminal (facial) and hypoglossal nerves, and in the ventral horn of the spinal cord (Hökfelt et al., 1974b; Snyder, 1980b). The extrahypothalamic TRH is apparently synthesized *in situ* and is not dependent on hypothalamic secretion (Jackson and Reichlin, 1977). Diverse localization of TRH within the brain would indicate a function other than as a releasing hormone.

Immunohistochemically identified TRH has been found to be restricted primarily to nerve terminals (Hökfelt et al., 1978), where in adult rats as much as one half of all TRH is stored in synaptosomes (Barnea, 1978). In brain homogenates, Winokur et al. (1977) found that at $37\,^{\circ}C$, virtually all exogenous TRH was inactivated by enzymes, whereas the endogenous TRH was, for the most part, not destroyed. This would imply that the endogenous substance was protected, perhaps by being bound to a membrane or by being enclosed in vesicles. Indeed, it is now generally believed that TRH is enclosed in synaptic vesicles and is released by a Ca^{2+}-dependent mechanism (Cooper et al., 1978). In addition, stereospecific, high-affinity binding sites for TRH have been found in various sites of rat brain, although, as is frequently the case, high receptor density does not correlate well with localization of the tripeptide (Burt and Snyder, 1975).

TRH, as well as the peptide substance P, have been found to be co-localized in descending 5-HT terminals, especially in those terminals innervating the ventral and lateral gray matter of the spinal cord of the rat. These peptides were not found in descending CA terminals, since intraventricular injection of 6-OHDA failed to affect spinal localization. On the other hand, intraventricular injection of the 5-HT neurotoxin 5,7-DHT resulted in a virtual disappearance of spinal 5-HT, TRH and substance P; whereas two other peptides, met-enkephalin and somatostatin, were unchanged. Furthermore, there was no depletion of substance P in the brain following 5,7-DHT treatment, suggesting that spinal 5-HT neurons may be unique in their peptide content. Also, in agreement with the findings of Hökfelt et al. (1974b), 5-HT, TRH and substance P-labelled fibers could be seen most strikingly localized around somatic motor neurons (Gilbert et al., 1982).

Effects on Motor Activity and Autonomic Responses

Behavioral evidence also stimulated the inquiry into CNS actions distinct from pituitary regulation. To begin with, pituitary-released thyroid stimulating hormone (TSH) (whose release is under the control of TRH) and the thyroid hormone triiodothyronine (T_3), potentiated the antidepressant effects of imipramine in depressed patients (Wilson et al., 1970; Prange et al., 1970). In animal studies TRH antagonized the sedative effects of alcohol or barbiturates (Prange et al., 1974). In addition, TRH (i.p.) potentiated the stimulant action of L-dopa in pargyline-treated rats (Plotnikoff et al., 1974)—a test used to screen for putative antidepressant drugs. Pargyline (a MAO inhibitor) is needed in this test to prevent the destruction of L-dopa by MAO. But, whether TRH acted directly or via the activity of TSH and T_3 was not known. Evidence that TRH has CNS activity apart from its neuroendocrine function was demonstrated by repeating the TRH potentiation of L-dopa stimulation after either hypophysectomy (removal of the pituitary) or thyroidectomy.

When administered systemically, TRH alone increased motor activity which is characterized by frequent tremors, tail raising, mild sniffing, grooming, preening, and other excitatory behaviors that resemble the effects of d-amphetamine (Miyamoto and Nagawa, 1977; Vogel et al., 1979). Further comparison of the two drugs showed that TRH and d-amphetamine both depress food intake and produce a dose-related decrease in bar-pressing on an FR-30 schedule of food reinforcement. Neither drug had an effect on shuttle box avoidance in the doses tested. However, the drugs' effects were distinctive when bar-pressing for low rates of electrical stimulation of the lateral hypothalamus was examined: TRH decreased the rate of responding whereas d-amphetamine increased bar pressing for brain self-stimulation. Further distinction between the two drugs was demonstrated by intracisternal pretreatment with 6-hydroxydopamine (6-OHDA), a catecholamine neurotoxic agent. The 6-OHDA-induced destruction of catecholamine neurons antagonized both the anorexia and the locomotor stimulant effects of amphetamine, whereas TRH-induced anorexia was enhanced by 6-OHDA pretreatment and the locomotor stimulation produced by TRH was unaffected. These results demonstrate that the behavioral effects of TRH are quite distinct from those of d-amphetamine and that in contrast to the catecholamine-mediated action of amphetamine, TRH activity does not depend on catecholamines to the same extent.

The similarities and differences between amphetamine and TRH provide an example of the danger of classifying psychoactive substances on the basis of a single, presumably dominant, effect. The ability of a drug to act as a "stimulant" is clearly dependent upon (1) the behavior examined, (2) the existing level of arousal of the organism, and (3) previous drug history. Also, the ability of 6-OHDA to enhance the anorexic effect but not alter the motor activity after TRH reminds us that the neurochemical substrates underlying behaviors are distinct and that each behavior may result from a balance among various neurotransmitters.

The neurochemical basis for the increased motor activity by TRH has not been clearly elucidated. Although Vogel et al. (1979) have shown that 6-OHDA pretreatment does not alter TRH-induced activity, Miyamoto and Nagawa (1977) found that microinjection of either dopamine (DA) or TRH into nucleus accumbens increased motor activity. The relationship of the effect of the DA system was demonstrated by antagonizing the intraaccumbens TRH injection by systemic pretreatment with the DA receptor antagonist, haloperidol. Also, the locomotor hyperactivity induced by i.p. injection of either TRH or DA was significantly suppressed by bilateral intraaccumbens injection of haloperidol.

Microinjection of TRH into the caudate nucleus (the site of termination of the DA-containing nigrostriatal fibers) did not produce an increase in motor activity, although mild sniffing, grooming, and preening did occur. These results suggest that TRH-stimulated locomotor activity is mediated by the DA fibers originating in the midbrain (interpeduncular nucleus) and terminating in nucleus accumbens (mesolimbic pathway), although other TRH-induced behaviors may be mediated by nigrostriatal function. The hypothesized significance of nucleus accumbens to the motor effects is appealing because we know that high concentrations of TRH are found in this area of the brain. However, it is impossible to determine from these experiments whether TRH has a direct action on the DA fibers or whether it works by modifying other neurons that end on DA cells in the nucleus accumbens.

Other investigators (Wei et al., 1975) found that injecting TRH into other brain sites (such as periaqueductal gray, medial hypothalamus, and medial preoptic area) produced shaking, lacrimation, paw tremor, and intense shivering. They noticed the similarity of these behavioral effects to the morphine abstinence syndrome. By discrete injections of TRH into various brain areas, they found that in those areas of the brain of morphine-dependent rats where naloxone precipitated withdrawal shaking, TRH also induced shaking. Martin et al. (1977) found that TRH enhanced the shaking behavior elicited by morphine withdrawal and that TRH-induced shaking is blocked by morphine. However, apomorphine (a dopamine agonist), chlorpromazine (a neuroleptic drug that blocks DA receptors), and Δ^9-tetrahydrocannabinol (the active ingredient in marijuana) also inhibited the TRH-induced shaking, indicating that the antagonism was not specific. In addition, it is clear that TRH does not directly alter stereospecific binding of morphine to brain in vivo or in vitro. Although TRH does not have effects on pain, it does antagonize morphine-induced hypothermia.

Intracerebral injection of TRH into rabbits produced a dose-dependent hyperthermia that was associated with hyperactiviy (Horita and Carino, 1975). In contrast, others have found i.c.v. (intracerebroventricular)-administered TRH produced a significant fall in body temperature in cats (Myers et al., 1977). Although these apparently contradictory results may be attributed to species variability or differences in injection site, in rats the TRH-induced change in body temperature was dependent on environmental temperature. At 4 °C, TRH caused hypothermia, at 22 °C no change in body temperature occurred, and at 31 °C, TRH caused hyperthermia (Prasad et al., 1978). These authors believe that TRH and a TRH metabolite have opposite effects on body temperature, which sum to produce the net change. Environmental temperature may have an effect on the activity of the TRH degrading enzymes and thus may alter the balance between TRH and its metabolite. The influence of the metabolites on other TRH-induced behaviors will have to be examined more fully.

Mechanisms of Action

In general, there has been very little research on the transmembrane effects and molecular mechanism of action of TRH. In frog spinal motor neurons, TRH produced a long-duration depolarization of small magnitude that was accompanied by an increase in membrane conductance and excitability. Blocking synaptic transmission either with magnesium ions or tetrodotoxin reduced the size of the TRH-induced depolarization by 10–40 percent. This result suggests that TRH produces depolarization by both direct (acting on the cell depolarized) and indirect (relying on synaptic activity) means. Other experiments using intracellular recording suggested that TRH increases conductance of Na^+. Experiments with various analogs of TRH demonstrated a structural specificity for the peptide-induced depolarization: the 1-methylhistidine-TRH analog was devoid of activity, whereas the 3-methylhistidine-TRH analog was about ten times more potent than TRH. Interestingly, the structural requirements for membrane depolarization are quite similar to those for TRH-induced shaking (Wei et al., 1975), and membrane-depolarizing potency parallels thyrotropin releasing activity.

In brain, however, the majority of neurons that are responsive to TRH show a depression of firing rate (Renaud, 1978). Although initially this neuronal depression may seem contrary to the known TRH stimulant action on behavior, inhibition of an inhibitory neuronal pathway may indeed permit unantagonized excitation to occur. Other evidence raises the possibility that TRH may act as an excitatory transmitter on one cell type and as an inhibitory transmitter on another. For instance, Yarbrough (1976) found that

TRH, although having no effect alone, is capable of potentiating the excitatory effect of iontophoretically applied acetylcholine in neurons of the somatosensory cortex. Other reports show that cells in the septum, hypothalamus, and cerebral cortex do not respond in the same way (Winokur and Beckman, 1978). Nevertheless, the demonstration that atropine (a muscarinic cholinergic receptor antagonist) can reduce the TRH antagonism of barbiturate-induced sleep suggests that cholinergic mechanisms may contribute to some of the behavioral effects of TRH (Breese et al., 1975).

Several investigators have shown no change in brain levels of DA, NE, or 5-HT after systemic treatment with TRH over a period of several days. However, an increased metabolism of DA and NE (Rastogi, 1979) and an increased release of [^{3}H]DA and [^{3}H]NE from rat brain synaptosomes (Horst and Spirt, 1974) demonstrate an increased turnover of catecholamines following TRH treatment. In addition, the activity of tyrosine hydroxylase (the rate-limiting enzyme in the synthesis of catecholamines) was increased in some brain areas (e.g., cerebral cortex and brain stem) after acute (Marek and Haubrich, 1977) and chronic (Agarwal, 1977) TRH administration. The increase in synthesis to match demand is probably the basis for the inability to detect a change in the absolute levels of DA and NE. TRH-induced increase in CA turnover is supported by fluorescent histochemical studies (Constantinidis et al., 1974), which showed that TRH alone produced no change in NE fluorescence but accentuated the loss of green fluorescence in NE terminals of α-methyl-p-tyrosine (AMPT)-treated rats. These results show that when synthesis of new NE is inhibited by AMPT, TRH accelerates the release of previously synthesized NE.

It is still not clear whether TRH acts directly on DA-containing cells or whether it acts by means of cells impinging on CA neurons. For example, it is well established that GABA-containing neurons originating in striatum and ending in substantia nigra provide an inhibitory control on the DA nigrostriatal pathway. Thus, if TRH inhibits GABA cells, enhanced release of DA might be expected to occur. In this regard, several GABA agonists have been found to antagonize selected actions of TRH (Cott et al., 1976). Furthermore, inhibition of GABA metabolism by aminooxyacetic acid (thus raising GABA levels) antagonizes the TRH-induced reduction of ethanol-induced sleep.

(Compare these results with the effects of ethanol on GABA systems in Chapter 9.)

Clinical Effects of TRH

The ability of TRH to increase CA turnover and increase locomotor activity fits well with the biogenic amine hypothesis of depression (Chapter 12) and prompted testing of TRH as an antidepressant drug. One commonly used test is the L-dopa test, which assesses the motor response of aggregated mice that are pretreated with the MAO inhibitor pargyline (40 mg/kg orally) and then given a single i.p. injection containing the test substance (e.g., TRH) and a fixed dose of L-dopa (100 mg/kg). TRH potentiated the stimulant action of L-dopa even after hypophysectomy or thyroidectomy, procedures that eliminate the normal endocrine action of TRH. These results, along with the finding that TRH antagonized the sedative effect of a variety of depressant drugs, suggested that TRH might be therapeutically useful in treating depression. However, despite several encouraging reports, TRH has not proved to be an effective antidepressant (Prange et al., 1978a). For instance, in a DOUBLE-BLIND CROSSOVER STUDY* of ten women with unipolar depression, TRH (i.v.) produced a rapid, partial, brief, beneficial effect (Prange and Wilson, 1972). Both observer and self-rating measures showed that the patients improved by about 50 percent within a few hours of treatment.

In a second study (Lakke et al., 1974), the effectiveness of TRH (and its L-dopa-potentiating action) was evaluated for the treatment of Parkinson's disease, a motor disorder known to be related to loss of DA cells. Although no improvement of motor symptoms followed TRH administration, the patients reported a sense of well-being and optimism and showed reduced depression scores on a self-administered test.

In contrast, TRH was ineffective in alleviating depression associated with alcoholism (Prange et al., 1979). Results with schizophrenic patients are similarly variable. In three studies, TRH had no effect on behavior of schizophrenic patients; in three other studies, TRH reduced the symptoms of apathy and social withdrawal; two other studies showed a worsen-

*A study in which neither patient nor evaluator knows whether the patient has received drug or placebo. After several trials those receiving drug are given the placebo and those receiving placebo are treated with drug.

H—Ala—Gly—Cys—Lys—Asn—Phe—Phe—Try—Lys—Thr—Phe—Thr—Ser—Cys—OH

Somatostatin (SRIF)

ing of depression, especially in paranoid schizophrenic patients. These results suggest that TRH may be effective in a subpopulation of depressed patients, perhaps those that show a neuroendocrine abnormality. Much more research is required before any conclusions are reached.

Somatostatin

Somatostatin is a peptide containing 14 amino acids, with a disulfide bond between the cysteine residues. It is the somatotropin release inhibiting factor (SRIF) known for inhibition of growth hormone release from the pituitary. SRIF is also found in the pancreatic islets, where it inhibits release of both glucagon and insulin, and in the stomach. It is another of the hypothalamic hormones that are apparently more widespread in the nervous system than was assumed previously. In fact, like TRH, more than two-thirds of the total brain SRIF is found outside the hypothalamus.

Distribution

The largest concentration of SRIF (located by radioimmunoassay) within the hypothalamus is in the external layer of the median eminence near the portal vessels. However, somatostatin has also been found to be scattered throughout the hypothalamus. Hökfelt et al. (1974a) found rather large concentrations in the ventromedial and arcuate nuclei and smaller amounts in the anterior and preoptic areas of the hypothalamus. Various researchers have had very conflicting results in locating SRIF, especially in regions where concentrations are very small. One simple reason for this was suggested by Epelbaum et al. (1977a), who found that concentrations vary with time of day; but other factors, such as cross-reactivity of the antibody used, may also be involved. SRIF has been found in the amygdala, the amount being roughly one-third that found in the hypothalamus; it was evenly distributed between the corticomedial and basolateral areas. Small, but consistent, amounts have been found in the parietal cortex, pons, medulla, spinal cord, and septal region (Epelbaum et al., 1977a; Kobayashi et al., 1977).

Somatostatin often appears in immunohistochemical studies as small dots on fibers and fiber networks,

indicating axons or chains of neurons and terminals. It has been determined, in fact, that over 70 percent of the somatostatin present in the CNS is localized in nerve terminals. However, although the terminals have been located, finding the cell bodies from which they came can prove difficult. Petrusz et al. (1977) found nerve cells in the thalamus that were completely embedded in SRIF fibers and had coarse terminal-like structures surrounding cell bodies and dendrites. Terminals have also been found surrounding dendrites of large neurons in the neocortex and pyramidal cells in the hippocampus.

To investigate somatostatinergic pathways originating in the medial basal hypothalamus or preoptic area, Epelbaum et al. (1977b) made selective lesions in these areas and measured the content of somatostatin in other regions of the brain. Bilateral anterior hypothalamic or ventromedial preoptic lesions reduced somatostatin content in the median eminence to less than 10 percent of control levels but did not have an effect on amygdala or cortex. Combined preoptic and ventromedial nucleus lesions also had no effect on somatostatin levels in amygdala or cortex; even extensive knife cuts separating the hypothalamus from the remainder of the CNS did not modify extrahypothalamic somatostatin. Thus, their results suggest an anterior hypothalamic–preoptic somatostatin-containing pathway to the median eminence, although extrahypothalamic somatostatin is not derived from hypothalamus. It has already been shown that somatostatin can be released from cerebral cortical slices in a calcium-dependent manner by depolarization (Havlicek and Friesen, 1979). Therefore, it is possible that somatostatin has a neurotransmitter or neuromodulator role apart from its function in hypothalamic control of the pituitary.

Physiological Effects

SRIF is known to inhibit growth hormone release. Therefore, it would not be surprising if SRIF had inhibitory functions in its role as a transmitter or modulator. Iontophoretic SRIF application decreased firing rates in responsive cells in the cerebral and cerebellar cortex and the hypothalamus of rats (Renaud and Martin, 1975; Renaud et al., 1975). This depression was rapid in both onset and termination. Electrical stimulation of cells in the ventromedial and arcuate hypothalamic nuclei caused release of growth hormone in guinea pigs. This could be completely inhibited by i.v. application of SRIF, indicating an inhibitory action on the cells that secrete growth hormone releasing factor in the hypothalamus (Hökfelt et al., 1974a). These results are in contrast to those described by Havlicek and Friesen (1979). In order to avoid the complications of anesthesia, this latter group used microiontophoretic application of SRIF in unanesthetized rabbits. They found that 35 of 60 neurons tested in somatosensory cortex showed a dramatic increase in firing. Subthreshold stimulation by somatostatin showed a potentiation of excitation by glutamate. In none of their tests were cells inhibited. Although the technique and the species were different from those used by Renaud et al. (1975), such dramatically different results are difficult to interpret.

SRIF has been shown to affect ACh turnover in rat brains. Intraventricular (i.v.t.) administration caused increased ACh turnover in the hippocampus, brain stem, and diencephalon, indicating a connection with cholinergic systems (Malthe-Sorenssen et al., 1978). It may also interact with catecholamine systems. Herchl et al. (1977) found that i.v.t. SRIF causes an increase in cAMP levels in the hippocampus of rat brains; an increase that is gone within 15 minutes. The elevated cAMP was accompanied by seizures, tremor, and motor excitation. Pretreatment with the noradrenergic β-blocker sotalol abolished the cAMP increase but did not alter the behavioral effects. Similar cAMP increases, also antagonized by sotalol, were noted in the cortex. The SRIF-induced increase in cAMP in the neostriatum, however, was not antagonized by the β-blocker. Apparently, SRIF-induced cAMP accumulation is mediated by β-noradrenergic action in the hippocampus and areas of the cortex, whereas the increase in neostriatum may be mediated by DA or another transmitter that is not blocked by sotalol.

Behavioral Effects

In addition to the behavioral effects previously mentioned, administration of SRIF has been found to cause decreased spontaneous motor activity, sedation, and occasional catalepsy. In contrast to TRH, systemically administered SRIF enhances pentobarbital-induced sleeping time and hypothermia in rodents (Prange et al., 1978a). However, the results of all the experiments utilizing systemic administration of SRIF must be interpreted carefully, as peripheral actions of SRIF can secondarily alter brain function. Also, the passage of SRIF from systemic circulation through the blood brain barrier has not been demonstrated.

When examined in the pargyline–L-dopa test, SRIF surprisingly potentiated the behaviorally stimulating effect of L-dopa. These results were similar to those found for TRH (Plotnikoff et al., 1974).

An even more dramatic demonstration of somatostatin-induced excitation was described by Havlicek and Friesen (1979). In a series of experiments, Havlicek and co-workers microinjected somatostatin into the ventricles (supracortically) and into the amygdala, hippocampus, and striatum. In each case, no sedative effects were noted. Through several stages, the somatostatin-treated animals demonstrated excessive grooming and exploring, tonic–clonic seizure activity, and, finally, stuporous immobility. At even very small doses, clear signs of motor incoordination were apparent, particularly after infusions into amygdala or striatum. Following high doses of somatostatin, motor incoordination developed into hemiplegia-in-extension, general rigidity of all body muscles. Following intraventricular infusion, 33 percent of the animals developed seizures. In some cases grand mal seizures followed administration of only 100 picograms of somatostatin.

Somatostatin has also been found to increase eating and reduce slow-wave sleep while virtually eliminating the REM stage of sleep. As with most of the peptides described in this chapter, investigations into the behavioral effects must be considered to be in the preliminary stages. In general, mapping peptide pathways, identifying subcellular localization, confirming peptide structure, and purifying the peptide will precede examination of its effects on behavior.

Melanocyte Stimulating Hormone (MSH)

The earliest research on the pituitary hormone MSH almost exclusively involved its role in the regulation of color adaptation in cold-blooded vertebrates. More recently it has become clear that in mammals several physiological stimuli modify MSH secretion and that the peptide may have actions on the CNS.

There are two primary forms of MSH—α- and β-MSH—each having a parent precursor molecule. α-MSH is identical to the amino acid sequence 1-13 of ACTH, whereas β-MSH probably comes from cleav-

ACTH (4-10)

$$CH_3—C—Ser—Tyr—Ser—Met—Glu—His—Phe—Arg—Trp—Gly—Lys—Pro—Val—NH_2$$
$$|$$
$$O$$

α-Melanocyte stimulating hormone (MSH)

age of β-lipotropin (Lowry and Scott, 1977). The relationship of β-MSH to β-lipotropin will be discussed in Chapter 13; our present emphasis is on α-MSH.

Distribution and Release

MSH is found in highest concentration in the pituitary. Release of α-MSH from pituitary is regulated by a Ca^{2+}-dependent stimulation-secretion coupling mechanism much like the release mechanism of neurotransmitters. At this time it is not clear which of the neurotransmitters act on α-MSH-containing cells under physiological conditions. Because α-MSH release is modified by many interoceptive and exteroceptive stimuli, such as light, stress, vaginal stimulation, suckling, and dehydration, it is possible that several neurotransmitters modulate such release.

α-MSH in the Brain

Although originally thought to exist solely in the pituitary, it has been demonstrated that this hormone exists in nerve terminals in the hypothalamus and other brain areas including thalamus, brain stem, cerebral cortex, and cerebellum (Oliver et al., 1977). Thus, the presence of α-MSH in brain and its localization in nerve endings suggests that the peptide may have a role in brain function. However, far more research is required before a transmitter function for the peptide can be assumed. For instance, the site of synthesis of brain α-MSH is not clear. Although hypophysectomy does not eliminate brain α-MSH, it is possible that portions of the pituitary that remain synthesize α-MSH and transport it to the brain by blood or CSF. Further investigation will undoubtedly focus on the effects of α-MSH on brain neurotransmitters and electrophysiological responses within discrete brain areas.

Physiological Effects of α-MSH

The most pronounced effect of α-MSH on brain electrical activity is the increase seen in the somatosensory cortical evoked response in human subjects after infusion of α-MSH (Kastin et al., 1975a). Similar changes in the EEG have been reported for other species such as rat, rabbit, and frog. Intraperitoneal

α-MSH also increased cAMP levels in occipital cortex by 65 percent, whereas other cortical areas did not demonstrate a change (Spirtes et al., 1978). These phenomena may or may not be related.

Behavioral Effects of α-MSH

α-MSH apparently has some striking behavioral effects. The most significant behavioral effects indicate a role for ACTH, α-MSH, and related peptides in adaptive behavior. In general, the entire class of peptides and fragments are examined in an attempt to uncover a structure–activity relationship. The clearest demonstration of behavioral effects is the resistance to extinction of a conditioned avoidance response (e.g., pole climbing) (Van Wimersma Greidanus, 1979). Under normal conditions, a rat will learn to avoid a signaled foot shock by climbing an available pole. When the experimenter eliminates the shock, the rat gradually discontinues the pole-climbing response, that is, it learns that avoiding the shock is no longer necessary. When ACTH or α-MSH is administered subcutaneously, the rat is much slower to discontinue the response.

Kastin et al. (1975b) have shown a similar reduced extinction rate for rats in an appetitive task (e.g., running a T-maze for food reward). These investigators have identified several variables that alter the effect of α-MSH on the behavior. For instance, α-MSH increases general motor activity in animals, thus increasing the probability of responding in some experimental tests. Also, when testing involves the use of electric shock, α-MSH tends to facilitate avoidance learning in low-shock, but not high-shock conditions. The stress-induced release of endogenous α-MSH may play a part in the latter case. The peripheral actions of the peptides, particularly ACTH, must be considered when evaluating experimental results. ACTH has strong effects on the adrenal gland, which in turn releases glucocorticoids, which per se may have an effect on behavior. Finally, the age of the animal used may be a significant variable in measuring α-MSH action. α-MSH administered to animals for several days immediately after birth has profound effects on behavior that persist into adulthood. α-MSH given to somewhat older animals has a much less dramatic and short-lived action.

Attempts to localize the action of α-MSH in brain involve the implantation of crystalline ACTH (1–10)* and other ACTH fragments into discrete brain areas. When the drugs are implanted in limbic midbrain structures, a reduced rate of extinction in conditioned pole climbing occurs. Within the limbic midbrain, selected lesions in the parafascicular nuclei prevent the inhibitory effects of ACTH (4–10)* and α-MSH on extinction of pole climbing (Van Wimersma Greidanus, 1977).

Further evidence for limbic midbrain structures as a site of action for the peptides comes from EEG studies. Urban et al. (1974) demonstrated in rats that ACTH (4–10) produces a frequency shift in theta activity (4–7 Hz) in the hippocampus and thalamus following stimulation of the reticular formation. The authors suggest that the peptide may facilitate transmission in these brain strutures and hence increase the animal's arousal, resulting in further motivational strength of environmental stimuli. No direct test of this hypothesis has confirmed the hypothetical model. However, in several studies with human subjects, α-MSH alters performance as a result of enhanced attention or arousal. In one experiment, human subjects were given a visual retention test in which the subject was instructed to reproduce geometric forms shown briefly a few seconds earlier. After receiving α-MSH, the subjects performed significantly better. The finding that α-MSH did not improve performance on a memory test where attention was less critical suggests that its beneficial effects involve attention rather than memory. These results fit very well with the α-MSH-induced increase in cortical evoked responses mentioned earlier.

When extensive lesion studies (Van Wimersma Greidanus et al., 1975a, 1975b) were done to obtain information on the CNS site of action of the peptides, several brain structures, including parafascicular area, rostal septum, and anterodorsal hippocampus, were found to be essential for the effects of ACTH or α-MSH on the extinction behavior. Each of these areas at various times has been implicated in the modifica-

*The hormone, ACTH 1-10, contains the same first 10 amino acids as α-MSH, and ACTH 4-10 consists of the amino acid sequence 4 through 10. Each of these amino acid sequences has actions similar to those of α-MSH (see Figure 5 in Chapter 13).

tion of learning and motivation. Such a diffuse site of action is not surprising when complex behaviors are examined. Rarely are behaviors regulated by a single locus of neural action; generally the neural substrate is a functional structure such that each of many units must contribute to the production of behavior. For these reasons, as well as because techniques for modifying brain activity are still quite crude, the role of α-MSH and the related peptides in CNS function is still very unclear.

$$\underset{\rule{4.5em}{0.4pt}}{\text{Cys—Tyr—Phe—Gln—Asn—Cys}}\text{—Pro—Arg—Gly—NH}_2$$

Vasopressin (ADH)

Vasopressin

Distribution and Physiological Effects

This hormone contains nine amino acid residues, but because the cysteine residues combine to form cystine, it is classified as an octapeptide. It is formed in the cell bodies of the paraventricular and supraoptic nucleus and transported down to and stored in the axons and terminals in the posterior pituitary gland. Peripherally, vasopressin facilitates distal tubular water reabsorption in the kidney. For this reason it is also known as the antidiuretic hormone (ADH). At high nonphysiological doses, it increases blood pressure; hence its alternative name, vasopressin. Secretion of vasopressin is stimulated by dehydration, saline loading, or any stimulus that requires conservation of body water. Increased amounts of urine follow inhibition of vasopressin release.

The hypothalamic axons transporting vasopressin are known to give off recurrent collaterals to the vasopressin and oxytocin cell bodies of the supraoptic nucleus and the median eminence. Investigators have speculated that these collaterals are involved in the prolonged recurrent inhibition resulting from stimulation of the posterior pituitary. Investigators have also proposed that vasopressin is an inhibitory transmitter because local application inhibits supraoptic neurons in rats. However, because homozygous Brattleboro rats, completely lacking in vasopressin, have normal supraoptic recurrent inhibition, an alternate inhibitory transmitter is suspected. That transmitter might be GABA. The possibility of two substances—vasopressin and an inhibitory transmitter—being released from these neurons is supported in part by the discovery of two types of vesicles in the neuron terminals (Cooper et al., 1978; Nicoll, 1975).

Behavioral Effects

In addition to actions in the hypothalamus, vasopressin also has central behavioral effects. The major effect involves memory consolidation. Van Wimersma Greidanus et al. (1975a, 1975b) and Van Wimersma Greidanus, (1979) found that intracerebral vasopressin analogs prolong extinction time for active and passive avoidance behaviors in rats. Application of lysine-8-vasopressin (LVP) to the posterior thalamus, especially the parafascicular nuclei, resulted in the preservation of avoidance responses; i.v.t. administration gave the same result. Length of preservation was dose dependent. Although bilateral sectioning of the parafascicular nuclei abolished the inhibition of extinction caused by α-MSH, it merely lessened LVP-induced prolongation. However, bilateral septal lesions did abolish the LVP-induced enhancement of avoidance response preservation. Van Wimersma Greidanus and co-workers concluded that vasopressin in the septal region is part of a larger limbic midbrain circuit involved with memory consolidation and retrieval, as many substances (α-MSH and LVP, for example) have similar effects on memory but operate on different areas of the brain.

In another experiment, these investigators found that i.v.t. (but not intravenous) administration of antiserum to arginine-8-vasopressin (the rat's natural vasopressin), which prevents the action of the natural hormone, drastically reduced memory of learned passive avoidance behaviors when retention was tested 6 hours or more after treatment and acquisition of the response. The effect was most pronounced at 24–48 hours after the learning sessions. Following the learning trial, control rats (untreated) waited an average of 300 seconds before entering a chamber in which they had previously received a severe electric shock. Rats treated with antiserum entered within 35 seconds, apparently "forgetting" that they had been shocked in that chamber previously. If tested within 6 hours of treatment and learning, the antiserum-treated rats responded like controls and waited approximately 300 seconds to enter the chamber. That is, animals treated with anti-vasopressin demonstrated passive avoidance for 6 hours following the learning trial; this result shows that they were able to acquire the response. Therefore, the antiserum must have acted on the memory process rather than on the learning process. However, administration of anti-vasopressin just prior to the retention session (but after the learning trial) also disrupted passive avoidance. This suggests that vasopressin is not only important for storage of information and memory but also for retrieval of information already stored (Van Wimersma Greidanus and De Wied, 1976).

Vasopressin increases norepinephrine utilization in limbic–midbrain areas, such as septum, dentate gyrus, parafascicular nucleus, dorsal raphe nucleus, and locus caeruleus (Kovacs et al., 1979). Selective destruction of the dorsal noradrenergic bundle, which originates in locus caeruleus, prevents the facilitative action of vasopressin on a passive avoidance response. However, injection of vasopressin into locus caeruleus did not alter memory consolidation. Utilizing the technique of discrete microinjection and selective sectioning, these investigators concluded that vasopressin interacts presynaptically with norepinephrine-containing nerve terminals. The finding of a distinctive pattern of catecholamine disappearance in specific brain regions in Brattleboro rats and in rats treated with vasopressin, as compared with control rats, also supports the importance of CA to the CNS action of vasopressin. Certainly a better understanding of the interaction of vasopressin and CNS neurotransmitters will be developed as research in this field continues.

Other studies suggesting a role for vasopressin in memory storage involve animals who have a low level of endogenous vasopressin. Brattleboro rats (lacking vasopressin) demonstrate slower learning and show more rapid passive avoidance extinction than normal rats. These deficits can be reversed by vasopressin treatment. Hypophysectomized rats, which lack pituitary-supplied vasopressin, have extremely rapid avoidance extinction that can be prolonged by administration of arginine-8-vasopressin (Bohus, et al., 1975).

The effect of vasopressin on human memory also has been tested. Oliveros et al. (1978) have shown that the ingestion of vasopressin in doses of from 10 to 30 units per day produced a dramatic improvement in the memory of patients suffering from posttraumatic amnesia. Legros et al. (1978) studied the effects of vasopressin on memory tests in patients 50–65 years of age: a group selected because it was shown that the levels of a peptide normally associated with vasopressin is significantly reduced in that age group.

After 3 days of administration of lysine-vasopressin, an improvement in certain attention and memory tests and a few changes in mood tests occurred. Furthermore, several drugs that act on central cholinergic neurons and that release vasopressin, such as nicotine and choline, improve consolidation of memory. Based on the research with human subjects, it appears that peptide treatment has potential as therapy for memory disorders. Certainly far more research in this area is required before a firm conclusion about its usefulness can be made and before the dangers of side effects will be outweighed by the potential benefits.

Vasopressin and Catecholamines

Demonstration of vasopressin interaction with other neurotransmitters has been described (Telegdy and Kovacs, 1979). For instance, α-methyl-p-tyrosine (AMPT), which inhibits the synthesis of catecholamines, reduces the learning of a conditioned avoidance response (jumping to a platform at the buzzer to avoid foot shock). Pretreatment with vasopressin was shown to prevent the AMPT-induced decrement in learning. Although vasopressin is known to delay extinction under similar conditions and AMPT facilitates extinction, vasopressin was not able to counteract this memory effect of AMPT.

Angiotensin-II

Angiotensin-II (AT-II) is an octapeptide hormone that was for many years thought to be mainly a peripherally acting substance—a potent vasoconstrictor involved in peripheral modulation of blood pressure. It has since been discovered to have profound central effects, most importantly a centrally mediated pressor response and a dipsogenic action (an induction of drinking behavior). AT-II is known to be formed in the blood. Renin from the kidneys cleaves AT-I from a circulating α_2-globulin. A converting enzyme from the lung then cleaves off two amino acids to form AT-II.

H—Asp—Arg—Val—Tyr—Ile—His—Pro—Phe—OH
Angiotensin-II

Distribution of Angiotensin-II

The areas within the brain that are most responsive to AT-II are the area postrema, the neurohypophysis, the subfornical organ, and the organum vasculosum—all of which lie outside the blood brain barrier.

Although AT-II is found within the brain, it is not clear whether peripherally administered AT-II penetrates the blood brain barrier. Autoradiographic studies showed the spread of labeled AT-II into the CNS after peripheral administration. However, polyacrylamide gel studies (Schelling et al., 1976) showed that only radioactive fragments of AT-II accumulated in the brain. Nevertheless, it is possible that the fragments may have been made within the brain by the AT-II degradative enzyme angiotensinase. Also, the sudden high increase in systemic blood pressure following peripherally administered AT-II may have forced the peptide through the brain capillaries, a situation that is unlikely under normal physiological conditions.

Many responsive sites inside the blood brain barrier have been found. It is possible that AT-II is formed locally in the brain in the same manner as in the bloodstream, as all components of the "renin-angiotensin system" are present in the brain (Phillips, 1978). Most angiotensin in the brain is in the form of AT-I, which is generally located in areas reciprocal to those of renin. Presumably, stimuli are able to release AT-I so that it can be acted upon to form AT-II. Renin activity, incidentally, is generally localized to synaptosomes. An interesting note is that drinking induced by i.p. injections of renin can be blocked by i.v.t. administration, but not by peripheral administration, of SQ 20,881 (a converting enzyme inhibitor). Because SQ 20,881 cannot enter the brain, central synthesis of AT-II is suggested (Nicoll, 1975).

Sirrett et al. (1977) have discovered AT-II binding receptors in the rat brain. Binding to the receptors was demonstrated to be specific by displacing binding by 80 percent with AT-II agonists and antagonists. This specific binding was essentially reversible, saturable, and occurred with high affinity. Over 90 percent of the binding was associated with particulate matter. It was mainly localized to the midbrain, thalamus, septum, hypothalamus, and medulla, although low levels of binding occurred in the cortex, hippocampus, and striatum. Of all areas examined, the lateral septum had the highest binding activity. Highest binding activity in the medulla is in the area postrema, an area known to be involved in AT-II effects.

Physiological Effects of Angiotensin-II

Electrophysiological techniques have shown cells in several areas of the brain to be specifically sensitive to application of AT-II. Microiontophoretic application of AT-II stimulated cells in the subfornical organ in a dose-related manner (Phillips, 1978). The action could be antagonized by the AT-II analog saralasin, which is known to be an AT-II blocker. Other investigators have reported AT-II-sensitive neurons in the periventricular area and the supraoptic nucleus but not in cortex or hippocampus. Unfortunately, most of the areas identified with the receptor binding assay by Sirett have not as yet been systematically examined with refined electrophysiological techniques.

Autoradiographic techniques were used by Swanson et al. (1978) to localize brain sites involved in AT-II's effect on drinking behavior and to follow efferent pathways from these sites. They discovered that the caudal half of the medial preoptic area and the rostral part of the anterior area of the hypothalamus were the sites involved with the dipsogenic effect in rats. Previous studies have shown the subfornical organ, the organum vasculosum, areas of the thalamus, the periaqueductal gray matter, and various regions of the septum to be active sites for AT-II-induced drinking. Swanson, however, found that in rats no drinking was induced unless the labeled AT-II leaked from the subfornical organ through the third ventricle into the caudal section of the medial preoptic area and the adjacent rostral part of the anterior area. In many other areas studied, the effect was the same—drinking occurred apparently only if there was ventricular leakage to the caudal medial preoptic area or if the site was near this region and AT-II could diffuse through the tissue. Thus, based on these results, the medial preoptic area may be an important site of AT-II action.

The argument has been made, however, that the most significant site of action of AT-II is not the preoptic area but is the subfornical organ or the organum vasculosum (both located in the anterior wall of the third ventricle). Evidence to support this view is summarized by Phillips (1978). The subfornical organ (SFO) and organum vasculosum (OV) are apparently the most sensitive sites to the dipsogenic action of AT-II, having thresholds of 0.1 picogram (10^{-13} grams) and 50 femtograms (5×10^{-14} grams), respectively. Sectioning the SFO reduced (but did not abolish) the dipsogenic effect of AT-II administered intraventricularly or directly into the preoptic area. Microiontophoretic application of AT-II into SFO demonstrated the presence of cells specifically sensitive to the peptide. Based on these results, the idea of multiple sites of AT-II must be entertained. Phillips suggests that separate blood-side and CSF-side receptors may also exist.

Dipsogenic Response to Angiotensin-II

Administration of AT-II to the dipsogenic areas has been shown to cause drinking behavior even in animals previously water loaded. AT-II applications to nearby regions either resulted in no increase or decreased drinking behavior. The drinking response is quite specific; starved rats will drink instead of eat after AT-II administration, and animals even drink water heavily adulterated with quinine if it is the only fluid available. Application of other peptides (e.g., bradykinin, vasopressin, or AT-II derivatives) has had no effect. Once started, angiotensin-induced drinking usually continues throughout the drug infusion and stops as soon as the infusion is ended. In rats, AT-I and renin cause drinking, but this can be blocked by the converting enzyme inhibitor, SQ 20,881, supporting the notion that AT-II is the active peptide (Severs and Daniels-Severs, 1973).

Some interaction between AT-II and known neurotransmitters has been identified. Although carbachol (a cholinergic agonist) is capable of eliciting drinking in rats and AT-II has been found to release ACh from cerebral cortical tissue, atropine (an ACh antagonist) does not modify the dipsogenic effect of angiotensin. In contrast, catecholamine neurons may interact with AT-II in the brain. Briefly summarized (Fitzsimons, 1975), the evidence for CA involvement includes the following observations: (1) AT-II releases norepinephrine or prevents its reuptake. (2) Distribution of AT-II and NE in the brain is similar. (3) Destroying CA neurons with 6-OHDA attenuates AT-II-induced drinking but does not alter carbachol-induced drinking. (4) The dopamine antagonist haloperidol prevents AT-II-induced drinking but does not alter carbachol-induced water intake. Furthermore, neither α- nor β-adrenergic blockers alter fluid intake following AT-II administration. (5) Intraventricularly administered DA causes some drinking. Based on these results from a variety of laboratories, one might suspect a relationship between AT-II and catecholamine (especially DA) systems.

Pressor Response and Angiotensin-II

Bickerton and Buckley (1961) designed the first dramatic demonstration that AT-II produces an increase in blood pressure by an action within the brain.

They cross-perfused blood from an intact dog to one in which the head was vascularly isolated although the neural connections were intact. The recipient dog showed a rise in arterial blood pressure.

Various brain regions have been associated with the central pressor response to AT-II. Spread of AT-II into the midbrain through the lateral ventricles of a cat has been shown to initiate peripheral blood pressure increases. Sectioning the subnuclealis medialis drastically inhibited the pressor response, whereas sectioning other midbrain areas did not (Buckley et al., 1977). Thus, there is apparently a specific active midbrain site for pressor activity.

The area postrema of the medulla may also be involved, although results from several groups are contradictory. Sectioning the area postrema abolishes the pressor activity of i.v.t.-administered AT-II in dogs, whereas injection of AT-II directly into the area postrema causes a pressor response. (However, similar experiments in rats yielded opposite results; Phillips and Hoffman, 1977.) Local cooling of the area postrema reversibly reduces the AT-II response. A degree of specificity may be shown by the fact that ablation of the area postrema reduces the pressor response to AT-II but not to NE. Various regions of the hypothalamus have also been shown to be active sites for pressor action in dogs, cats, and rats. However, the evidence is not very convincing, as all studies could have had problems with ventricular leakage to other sites (Nicoll, 1975; Severs and Daniels-Severs, 1973).

The central pressor effect of AT-II may also involve the sympathetic nervous system: an increase in blood pressure may be brought about following vasopressin release and increased sympathetic activity (Severs et al., 1970). AT-II is known to release vasopressin, and the pressor response has been shown to correspond to increased sympathetic output in nearly every animal studied. Hypophysectomy, which eliminates the release of vasopressin, reduces the pressor response to AT-II by 45 percent. In rats that are genetically incapable of producing vasopressin, AT-II produces only a small pressor response (Hutchinson et al., 1976). In addition, AT-II is one of the most potent endogenous ganglion stimulators known. AT-II administration to superior cervical ganglion cells (part of the sympathetic chain ganglia) of cats *in vitro* rapidly depolarized the postsynaptic membranes, leading to repetitive firing at doses of 5 μM. Preganglionic denervation did not block the AT-II effect. Responsive receptors are apparently not cholinergic, as the responses were not antagonized by *d*-tubocurarine or atropine in concentrations high enough to block nicotinic and muscarinic receptors. It would appear that there are specific postsynaptic AT-II receptors in the sympathetic nervous system. Apparently Na^+ flow is involved in the depolarization of the responsive cells, as responses were not changed significantly in K^+- or Cl^--free solutions, whereas low Na^+ reduced the response, and lack of Na^+ in the solution totally inhibited depolarization (Dun et al., 1978).

AT-II clearly has very great effects on the nervous system, and its role as a neuromodulator has good support. It is very likely that it influences the excitability of neurons in several areas of the brain. Such a widespread action may provide a sustained influence on a number of neural systems and may potentially bring about a prolonged and harmonious response to environmental change. Thus, dehydration, loss of electrolytes, and fall in blood pressure stimulate plasma renin-angiotensin. Plasma AT-II stimulates vaso–constriction and release of hormones and CA from the adrenal gland. In the CNS, angiotensin may simultaneously increase drinking, release ADH, increase sympathetic nervous system activity, and elevate blood pressure. In this way, both systems (central and peripheral) respond in concert to severe changes in internal milieu, thus ensuring survival of the organism (Ganten and Speck, 1978).

Arg—Pro—Lys—Pro—Gln—Gln—Phe—Phe—Gly—Leu—Met—NH$_2$
Substance P (SP)

Substance P

Substance P (SP) is an undecapeptide (having 11 amino acids) and was discovered half a century ago by von Euler and Gaddum (1931) when they were studying the tissue distribution of acetylcholine. They isolated a substance found in brain and intestine of horses that caused hypotension when injected intravenously and caused contraction when directly applied to rabbit intestine. Because the substance did not act like any other known neurochemical, they labeled the unique powder extract "Substance P" (P referring to powder).

It took 40 years before the substance was chemically identified because of scarcity of the material, its unstable nature, and contamination by other peptides. The availability of synthetic SP and an extremely sensitive and specific radioimmunoassay stimulated a renewed effort to elucidate the role of substance P in the CNS (Nicoll, 1975; Phillis, 1977).

Distribution of Substance P in the Central Nervous System

SP was found to have an extensive and uneven distribution in the CNS of several species, suggesting a possible neurotransmitter function. SP has been identified in 15 to 20 brain areas, including the substantia nigra (site of the greatest concentration), the hypothalamus, the amygdala, the interstitial nucleus of the stria terminalis, the habenula, the interpeduncular nucleus, periaquaductal gray, the mesencephalic tegmental nucleus dorsalis, and some nuclei of the raphe (Hökfelt et al., 1978). Their results suggest that the SP system may be as extensive as the catecholamine system, albeit the CA system represents only about 1 percent of all brain neurons.

SP is apparently concentrated in nerve endings, where it has been localized immunohistochemically in the synaptic vesicles (Pickel et al., 1977). Mayer et al. (1979) have demonstrated binding of SP to phosphatidylserine, a major phospholipid in neural membranes. Such binding may represent a storage mechanism for SP. The release of SP from the phosphatide could be brought about by a competitive mechanism involving another compound or an ion at the binding site of SP. A saturable, high affinity, specific binding of [^{3}H]SP to synaptic membranes was reported by Nakata et al. (1978). They found that specific binding occurred to synaptic membranes in various areas of the brain generally correlated with endogenous SP levels. This suggests that SP acts as a neurotransmitter in discrete areas of the brain.

A large amount of data indicates that SP serves a neurotransmitter function which mediates sensory input. Immunofluorescent studies have shown that SP is localized in about 20 percent of the cell bodies of the dorsal (spinal) and the trigeminal ganglia. These small-type cells give rise to the thin unmyelinated axons associated with the transmission of impulses arising from painful stimuli. Cells with SP are also found in the substantia gelatinosa, and in the descending tract of the trigeminal nerve and its nucleus. SP concentration is 50 to 10 times greater in dorsal root than in ventral root fibers (Nicoll, 1975). Within the spinal cord, substance P is concentrated within lamina I and II (Rexed, 1954) of the dorsal horn gray at levels 5 to 10

times greater than in ventral gray (Figure 1). Lamina I and II consist of the posteromarginal nucleus and the substantia gelatinosa, respectively. All these systems are associated with nociceptive stimuli (Hökfelt et al., 1975b).

Sectioning of the dorsal root (medial to the dorsal ganglion) virtually depletes SP from that section of dorsal horn gray; thus, it is clear that the afferent fibers contain SP. However, the small amounts of SP in the rest of the spinal cord gray (about 10 percent of that in lamina I and II) is left unchanged, indicating there is some intrinsic SP in the spinal cord. Also, after sectioning peripheral nerves, the distal stump (the part separated from the cell body) contains only 10 to 30 percent of its normal SP concentration, whereas the proximal stump with the attached cell body increased in SP concentration by as much as 600 percent. This suggests that SP is produced in perikarya of the dorsal ganglia and migrates (probably by fast axoplasmic flow) centrally and peripherally (Nicoll, 1975). Peripheral flow is further suggested by the finding that after ligation of the sciatic nerve of the cat, there were a number of swollen unmyelinated fibers central to the ligation. SP is also found in the putative pain receptors of the skin, the free nerve endings (Hökfelt et al., 1975a, 1975b).

Unfortunately, the synthesis pathway of SP has not been completely uncovered, and the mechanism of inactivation has also been difficult to identify. Because ^{125}I-labeled SP was not accumulated in tissue slices prepared from spinal cord or brain, reuptake into the nerve terminal is probably not the way SP action terminates. An inactivating enzyme was reported by several groups and has been extracted and partially purified (Benuck and Marks, 1975). Generation of antibody to the enzyme will enable its localization in the nervous system and evaluation of its functional significance.

Another important criterion that must be met by a putative neurotransmitter is that of release under appropriate conditions. SP has been found to be released into a bath containing a rat spinal cord during electrical stimulation of the dorsal roots (afferent fibers carrying sensory information into the spinal cord) (Otsuka and Konishi, 1976). When the same preparation contained a low Ca^{2+}–high Mg^{2+} medium (to prevent transmitter release), the same stimulation of dorsal roots produced no release of SP. Depolarization of rat hypothalamus slices by the addition of high K^+ (55

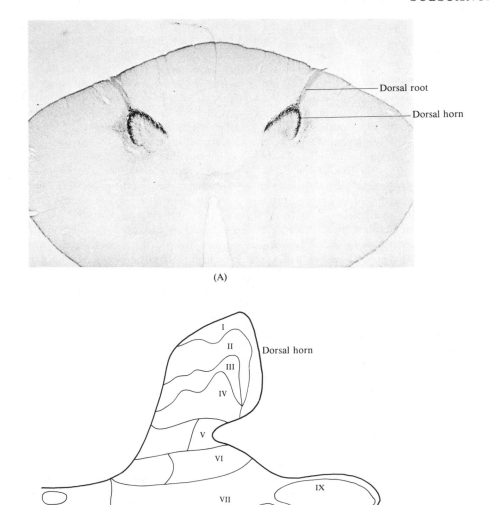

(A)

(B)

FIGURE 1   LOCALIZATION OF SUBSTANCE P IN THE SPINAL CORD. (A) Monkey tissue. The dark-stained area identifying SP was obtained by treating the tissue with specific antibodies labeled with a dark-staining chemical. The stain is present only in laminae I and II in the dorsal horns, which receive input from peripheral pain fibers. (From Iversen, 1979, and by courtesy of Stephen Hunt.) (B) Human tissue. An enlarged view of the gray matter on one side of the cervical spinal cord showing Rexed's laminae, the various nuclear groups in the gray matter. Neurons in laminae I and II project to laminae V and VI to synapse upon cells forming the lateral spinothalamic tract that ascends, mostly contralaterally, to higher centers in the brain stem.

mM) also produced a large increase of SP in the medium (Iversen et al., 1976).

Electrophysiological Effects

The characteristics of SP described thus far are highly suggestive of a neurotransmitter function in the CNS. Because SP has potent effects on the electrical activity of nerve cells, the possible functions of this brain peptide are being actively pursued. One of the impediments to a rapid answer to many questions regarding the actions of SP is the lack of a specific antagonist. Although the muscle relaxant lioresal (Baclofen) antagonized the action of SP on neurons in the spinal cord and brain, the drug also inhibited the effects of L-glutamate and acetylcholine (Saito et al., 1975; Phillis, 1976b). Later studies indicate that instead of blocking SP, lioresal probably has a direct inhibitory action on neurons of the spinal cord (Phillis, 1977).

In general, SP excites nerve cells both in brain and spinal cord. The depolarizing effect persists in the presence of elevated Mg^{2+} or lowered Ca^{2+} (which prevents presynaptic release of neurotransmitters). Because of this and other evidence it is likely that SP acts postsynaptically rather than by releasing another endogenous substance (Phillis, 1977). When pure SP and synthetic SP-like substances were tested, it was found that spinal motoneurons were depolarized by very small amounts of the peptide. Their potency was 500 times that of the excitatory amino acid, glutamate. Excitatory effects were also found following microiontophoretic applications of SP on the Betz cells of motor cortex and on cells in the cuneate nucleus of the medulla, which receives inputs from primary afferent neurons. The excitatory effects at these sites were frequently slow in onset and long in duration, characteristics that have prompted Krnjević (1977) to suggest that SP is likely to be a modulator of nerve activity rather than a neurotransmitter that typically has a rapid onset and short duration.

Substance P and Pain

A close relationship between SP depolarization and the transmisson of pain was demonstrated by Henry (1977). Single cells in the dorsal horn of the spinal cord of anesthetized cats were classified on the basis of their responses to natural peripheral stimulation such as touch, pressure, or noxious heat. When SP was applied to these cells, it either had an excitatory effect or produced no change at all. In one series in which 57 units were tested, all units that were excited by SP were also excited by noxious heat but not by the other peripheral stimuli. However, some units that were activated by noxious heat were unaffected by SP. Whether this observation is due to insufficient application of SP or due to the cells' location beyond the first afferent (possibly SP) synapse is not clear at present.

Other studies showed that removal of tooth pulp, which contains only pain-sensitive sensory fibers, leads to degeneration of nerve terminals containing SP in the trigeminal nucleus of the brain stem, where pain fibers from the teeth terminate. Serotonin is also associated with pain phenomena. In general, the release of serotonin contributes to analgesia, and serotonin depletion is associated with lower pain thresholds. However, the experiments reporting these findings may be confounded by the additional finding that reducing serotonin turnover is associated with diminished fear and indifference to punishment (see Chapter 11). Nevertheless, SP seems to be a co-transmitter in serotonin nerve terminals in the amygdala, periaquaductal gray, raphe nuclei, and the substantia nigra. Some of the serotonergic pathways that arise in the raphe and descend to the spinal cord elicit analgesia, and some of the cells in the raphe contain both serotonin and SP. Thus these two substances may interact to regulate pain perception (Snyder, 1980b).

Further support for SP modification of pain transmission comes from a report (Yaksh et al., 1979) that showed that selectively depleting the stores of SP by 55 percent causes a prolonged increase in thermal and chemical pain thresholds but no apparent change in response to mechanical stimuli. The intrathecal injection of capsaicin,* a tissue irritant, in the spinal subarachnoid space rapidly liberates most releasable stores of SP from the nerve terminals and then induces

Capsaicin

*Capsaicin is the pungent principal obtained from various species of *Capsicum*, pepper plants. This substance is used as a gastric stimulant when taken internally, and as a counterirritant when applied externally.

a prolonged and possibly permanent depletion of SP from neurons. Although the animals initially show contracture of the caudal portions of the body, they rapidly regain motor coordination within a few minutes. Twenty-four hours after SP depletion, no abnormality in motor function can be detected; they are able to climb a vertical wire mesh, exhibit normal righting and stepping reflexes, respond normally by orienting to light touch, and demonstrate no ataxia in the rotarod test. Nevertheless, the animals show profound analgesia when tested with aversive heat stimuli (tail-flick test and hot plate test) or chemical stimuli (phenylquinone-induced writhing test). The finding that the opiate antagonist naloxone did not block the analgesic effect suggests that capsaicin-induced analgesia is independent of endogenous opiate systems.

Nevertheless, a relationship between SP and the endogenous opiate-like peptides has been demonstrated. A striking similarity between the anatomical distribution of opiate-like peptides and SP exists (Jessell and Iversen, 1977; Hökfelt et al., 1977). Also, when morphine or an endogenous opiate-like peptide was added to the incubation medium, the depolarization-induced release of SP from tissue slices prepared from spinal cord or brain stem was inhibited. If SP is indeed a transmitter in primary afferent pathways carrying pain information, then opiate-induced analgesia may occur by inhibition of the SP neurons. Support for this hypothesis comes from research data that show that a high extracellular potassium level induced release of SP. This release was inhibited by an analog of enkephalin, which is an endogenous opiate-like substance. The mechanism for this effect is shown in Figure 2. In this model, enkephalins from terminals of local inhibitory neurons are released upon the terminals of small-diameter primary afferent neurons that transmit pain signals to the spinal cord. Enkephalins (or exogenous morphine) depolarize the primary afferent nerve terminals, thereby decreasing the amplitude of incoming action potentials and decreasing Ca^{2+} influx into the terminal. This results in decreased neurotransmitter release upon the spinothalamic projection neurons with a consequent loss of transmission of pain signals to the brain and analgesia (Mudge et al., 1979). It should be noted, however, that enkephalin binding sites exist on the postsynaptic cell bodies of spinothalamic neurons as well (see Chapter 13).

Within the brain, the effects of SP on pain responses are more complex. Naloxone-reversible analgesia

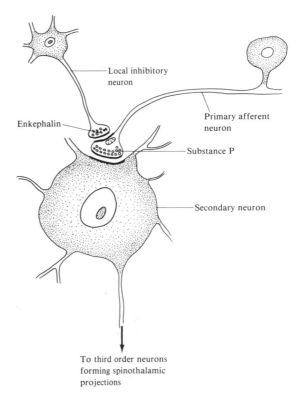

FIGURE 2   OPIATE-INDUCED INHIBITION OF SUBSTANCE P RELEASE. A local inhibitory neuron releases enkephalin (an endogenous opiate-like peptide) upon the presynaptic terminal of a primary afferent axon containing SP. The axon transmits nociceptive information into the spinal cord. Enkephalin reduces the release of SP, thereby attenuating the transmission of pain impulses to the brain.

following SP injections into the periaqueductal gray has been reported, whereas hyperalgesia occurred under other experimental situations. The discrepancies can be resolved by proposing a dual action for SP in brain (Frederickson et al., 1978). This group found that intraventricular administration of low doses of SP produced analgesia that could be blocked by opiate antagonists. Because SP does not bind to opiate receptors, it is likely that SP releases endogenous opiate peptides. At higher doses of SP, hyperalgesia occurred when naloxone was administered, a result consistent with the idea that higher SP concentrations produce postsynaptic excitatory activity that counteracts the inhibitory activity of the endogenous opiates. Thus, no simple model of SP action (like the one in Figure 2 for spinal cord) in brain can be proposed at present.

Effects of Substance P on Motor Behavior

Because SP is found in high concentrations in substantia nigra (SN) and an SP-containing pathway from striatum to SN has been identified, it is not surprising that SP effects on behaviors associated with these brain regions have been investigated. For instance, posttrial electrical stimulation of the SN leads to amnesia for avoidance learning. Under similar conditions, injection of SP into SN (by way of a permanently implanted cannula) immediately after an avoidance learning trial, produced a drastic retrograde amnesia for the event (Huston and Staubli, 1978).

The relationship of the nigrostriatal pathway to the extrapyramidal motor system (Chapter 6) has prompted investigators to examine the effects of SP on motor behavior. Intraventricular infusion or bilateral injection of SP into the ventral tegmentum increases spontaneous activity (Rondeau et al., 1978), increases exploratory activity, and potentiates amphetamine-induced activation (Stinus et al., 1978). Unfortunately, results are not consistent, and other laboratories have demonstrated a behavioral depression and antagonism of amphetamine's stimulant action. Very probably these results are due to differences in dose administered, method of administration, experimental design, or species; further experiments will be needed to clarify the action of SP (Rondeau et al., 1978).

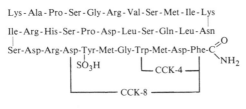

Cholecystokinin-33

Cholecystokinin

Another peptide having a probable neurotransmitter function is a variant of cholecystokinin (CCK). A substance released from endocrine cells in the upper intestine during meals, CCK stimulates gall bladder contraction. This substance has five main components one of which has 33 amino acids, CCK-33, and serves as a precursor for an octapeptide (CCK-8) and a tetrapeptide (CCK-4) which are purported to be neurotransmitters, each perhaps in different neurons.

Distribution

CCK-8 seems to be the major CCK entity in the brain and receptor binding studies reveal binding affinity in distinctive brain areas for CCK-8 and CCK-4. However, it has not been fully established where each of the transmitter candidates are located in the nervous system. Consequently, the transmitters will be referred to simply as CCK unless the specific variant is known.

CCK is located in peripheral and central nerves. CCK nerves are especially concentrated in the cerebral cortex, the hippocampus, the amygdaloid nuclei, the hypothalamus, and most abundantly in the periaquaductal gray. CCK is in relatively small supply in the neocortex but because the neocortex is so large in humans the total there (1-2 mg) far exceeds the weight of any other peptide.

Within the neurons CCK is more concentrated in axon terminals than cell bodies, and upon tissue fractionation it is predominantly in the synaptosomal vesicular fraction. CCK, like substance P, is found in primary sensory neurons of the spinal cord, and thus may be involved in the pain modulating activities in these areas. CCK-4 neurons have been identified as acting upon the pancreatic islet cells that release insulin and glucagon. Administration of picomolar concentrations of CCK-4 upon the pancreatic cells have a dramatic effect upon the release of these hormones, whereas CCK-8 is almost entirely without effect in this function. These peptides have no effect upon the exocrine tissue of the pancreas. CCK-8 is found coexisting with dopamine in the same neurons that project from the midbrain to the limbic system, but not in dopamine neurons that project from the substantia nigra to the caudate nucleus. This is still another case where two transmitters occupy the same neuron.

Synthesis

Synthesis studies of CCK in the cerebral cortex indicate that radioactive methionine is first incorporated into a large CCK polypeptide that is subsequently cleaved into smaller variants. It was also shown that CCK is rapidly synthesized in large amounts suggesting it has an active role in the brain.

Release and Deactivation

Depolarizing superfused brain slices produced a

Ca^{2+}-dependent release of CCK, which is characteristic of neurotransmitters. With respect to transmitter deactivation, the rapid synthesis of CCK suggests that reuptake is not significant, and that enzymic degradation is probably the mechanism of action. However, data are lacking in this regard.

Functional Significance

Application of low concentration of CCK show that it has rapid and potent excitatory effects on neuronal membranes of the hippocampus and the cerebral cortex. Intraventricular administration of as little as 0.01 picomole/minute of CCK-8 suppressed feeding behavior in sheep, and a low dose of CCK-8 injected intraperitoneally caused satiety in previously hungry rats. The effective dose for i.p. injection was smaller than that for intraventricular administration. Thus, CCK-8 appears to subserve a satiety mechanism when it is released from the gut during meals. However, CCK-8 and CCK-33 do not pass the blood brain barrier easily, and the gut does not release CCK in amounts that approximate the high exogenous doses necessary for this effect. Furthermore, the satiety effect of CCK disappears with vagotomy (sectioning the vagus nerve). It seems that the CCK effect is mediated in the periphery by a mechanism yet to be understood (Snyder, 1980b; Rehfeld, 1980).

Cholecystokinin, like serotonin, is found in the gut as well as in the brain. Though it has many characteristics of a neurotransmitter, the full extent of its activities must await the development of useful analogs and sensitive and reliable CCK assays.

Prostaglandins

Before concluding discussion of the peptide neurotransmitters, at least brief mention should be made of the prostaglandins (PGs), a group of substances that probably have a transmitter role. The PGs are acidic lipids that are synthesized via multienzyme systems from fatty acids in membranes and from lipid droplets in the cytoplasm. They are so named because one of them was found in human seminal fluid by von Euler in 1935 and it was thought at the time that prostaglandin was secreted solely by the prostate gland.

Instead, PGs are formed in many organs, including the brain, and are normal constituents of the cerebrospinal fluid. They are released from the cerebral cortex by direct electrical stimulation or by stimulation of afferent nerves. Release from any special part of the brain has not been associated with stimulation of some well-defined pathway, but release from the cerebellum follows electrical stimulation of the reticular formation. ACTH promotes PG release from the adrenal cortex, and release from the CNS has been found after administration of convulsant drugs such as picrotoxin, pentylenetetrazol, and strychnine.

Iontophoretic administration of some PGs blocks the response of cerebellar Purkinje cells to NE or to stimulation of the NE pathway to the cerebellum but not the response of Purkinje cells to inhibitory pathways or to inhibitory substances including cAMP. It may be that PGs that are released from cells receiving adrenergic stimulation block the NE-sensitive adenylate cyclase and thus prevent an increase in intracellular cAMP. This arrangement could act as a negative feedback system for modulating local synaptic activity (Cooper et al., 1978). But in other cases, PGs seem to mimic hormone action by elevating intracellular cAMP concentration.

Functionally, PGs play a role in inflammation, fever, and perception of pain, and it is thought that the synthesis of PGs is inhibited by drugs such as aspirin and indomethacin, thus explaining their therapeutic effects.

Conclusion

The peptide transmitters are among the latest substances proposed to play a neurotransmitter or a neuromodulator role in the CNS, but they have by no means closed the list. The list of putative neurotransmitters continues to grow as more sophisticated techniques are developed to detect and identify them (see Chapter 4).

This list includes the peptide bradykinin, which induces not only bradycardia but also causes the release of an antidiuretic substance by direct action on the CNS. Bradykinin has analgesic effects and also lowers endogenous levels of brain norepinephrine and depresses NE uptake.

We discussed the melanocyte stimulating hormone, which controls skin color in amphibia but in mammals increases the resistance to extinction of a conditioned avoidance response. It also seems to improve some forms of memory, alters the EEG, and effects many other psychological and physiological processes.

Prolactin is suggested as a neurotransmitter because, in addition to its promotion of lactation, it influences parental behavior and behavior associated with migration in birds. It initiates premigratory hyperphagia and nocturnal migratory activity. Implanted in the hypo-thalamus of virgin rats, it enhances nest building and pup licking and retrieving. Also it appears to control the emission of the maternal pheromone that attracts neonatal rats to their mothers, and it is related to nest building in pregnant rabbits (Prange et al., 1978b).

A peptide known as SLEEP FACTOR DELTA has been proposed to account for the fact that something in the cerebrospinal fluid taken from a sleep-deprived dog in-duces sleep when injected into the ventricles of a nor-mal recipient dog, and in rats it induces sleep and a decrease in locomotor activity (Nicoll, 1975).

From the foregoing it appears quite likely that these substances are either bona fide neurotransmitters or neuromodulators that need not even be synthesized by neurons. They could reach neurons by humoral path-ways to regulate both synaptic transmission and mem-brane excitability of neurons either by themselves or by interaction with other neuroactive substances. Thus, the peptide that inhibits the melanocyte stimulating hormone has been shown to increase striatal dopamine synthesis; and bradykinin, as mentioned earlier, lowers brain NE levels and blocks NE uptake. It has also been proposed that many peptide hormones are involved in the formation of "second messenger" cAMP (Nicoll, 1975).

The group of peptides known as enkephalins are regarded as endogenous opiate-like substances, and thus are of great interest for understanding the action of opium derivatives (such as morphine and heroin) and other related narcotic analgesics. This subject is discussed at length in Chapter 13.

Recommended Readings

Ajmone Marsan, C. and Traczyk, W.Z. (Eds.) (1980). *Neuropeptides and Neural Transmission*. Interna-tional Brain Research Organization Monograph Series, Vol. 7. Raven Press, New York. Reviews on the current status of the nature and function of neuropep-tides as they relate to neurotransmission.

Barker, J.L. and Smith, T.G. (Eds.) (1980). *The Role of Peptides in Neuronal Function*. Marcel Dekker, New York. A compendium of review articles by leading authors in the field.

Bloom, F.E. (1981). Neuropeptides. *Scientific American*, 245, 4, 148–168. A concise review of recent data, and interesting speculations about the neuro-transmitter role of some peptide hormones.

Krieger, D.T. and Hughes, J.C. (Eds.) (1980). *Neuroendocrinology*. Sinauer Associates, Sunderland, Mass. A collection of excellent papers by leading authors on the relationships among neural and endo-crine functions.

Martin, J.B., Reichlin, S. and Bick, K.L. (Eds.) (1981). *Neurosecretion and Brain Peptides: Implica-tions for Brain Function and Neurological Disease, Advances in Biochemical Psychopharmacology, Vol. 28*. Raven Press, New York. A recent collection of review articles covering the synthesis, anatomic distribution, and function of neuropeptides especially as they relate to neurologic disease.

Snyder, S.H. (1980b). Brain peptides as neurotransmit-ters. *Science* 209: 967–983. A short but comprehensive review that emphasizes recent developments.

CHAPTER ELEVEN

Anxiolytic Drugs

Between birth and death every individual must constantly attempt to adjust to his or her social, physical, and personal environment. Humans are beset by circumstances and confrontations, and they must constantly make behavioral adjustments to promote well-being and to avoid pain and suffering. As a corollary to the above, it has been said that life is unfair—i.e., life's vicissitudes are not shared equally by all. Moreover, some individuals seem to better able than others to continue the struggle against adversity, a condition that may be related in significant part to one's genetic inheritance. This reality has been a dominant feature of our total existence, and we almost certainly inherited our ability to cope with adversity from our subhuman forebears. Thus it is possible to study the physiological and behavioral phenomena associated with that struggle in other animals, and to relate the findings usefully to human cases.

Maladjustment seems to be a frequent occurrence in individuals who have diminished or inadequate resources and who are overwhelmed by circumstances beyond their control. At this point therapeutic, or at least ameliorative, measures need to be considered. The history of mental illness goes back to prehistoric times and therapeutic measures were attempted even then (Davison and Neale, 1978). Early cultures were replete with customs and taboos which, judging by their persistence, provided some prophylaxis and help in coping with the conflicts inherent in human existence and in making life more tolerable and secure.

Anxiety

Sigmund Freud called attempts to deal with the problem of anxiety "the most difficult task that has been set [before] us." Anxiety seems to arise from problems of adjustment and thereafter contributes to them (Lader, 1978b). Anxiety has a number of antecedents, concomitants, and consequences. There are genetic and situational antecedents; there are physiological and psychological manifestations that can be normal or abnormal; the avoidance of anxiety can serve as an incentive for improved adaptation, but high levels of anxiety can disrupt performance and can lead to somatic pathology. Anxiety in its more extreme forms has come to be regarded as the *sine qua non* of a number of forms of mental illness, and drugs that are designed to blunt or reverse the consequences of anxiety are known as ANXIOLYTIC COMPOUNDS.

Sources of Anxiety

One way to study mental illness is to use the epidemiological approach, which attempts to establish the relationships of various factors that determine the frequency and distribution of the illness. Since life-changing events are instrumental in causing anxiety and mental illness, a number of investigators have catalogued events that occurred to mentally ill patients within a year or two prior to the onset of their illnesses (Rahe and Arthur, 1978). Table 1 is a list taken from the studies of Rahe (1975), and Dohrenwend and Dohrenwend (1974a, 1974b). The list is divided into five categories: health, work, financial, home and family, and personal and social (Rahe, 1979). Even this partial list emphasizes the variety and ubiquity of anxiety-provoking events to which we are all potentially exposed. This provides an appreciation of the

TABLE I Life-changing Events as Sources of Anxiety

Health

1. Illness or injury   2. Change in eating habits   3. Change in sleeping habits   4. Onset of menopause   5. Unable to get treatment for illness or injury   6. Major dental work

Work

1. Change to new type of work   2. Change in work hours or conditions   3. More responsibilities at work   4. Fewer responsibilities at work   5. Promotion, demotion, or transfer   6. Trouble with boss or coworkers   7. Trouble with those under your supervision   8. Promotion not forthcoming   9. Started business or new profession   10. Suffered business loss or failure   11. Retired, laid off, or fired   12. Returned to work after long absence

Financial

1. Taken on a major purchase—TV set, car, freezer   2. Taken on a mortgage loan on home, business, property   3. Foreclosure on mortgage or loan   4. Sudden increase or decrease in income   5. Credit rating difficulties   6. Unprofitable investments   7. Expected wage increase not forthcoming   8. Went on welfare, or off welfare

Home and family

1. Change in residence   2. Move to a different town   3. Separation from family members   4. Inability to make anticipated move   5. Remodeled home   6. Death of spouse   7. Death of a child   8. Death of a parent   9. Death of a brother or sister   10. Death of a close friend   11. Married, separated, or divorced   12. Trouble with in-laws   13. Pregnancy and birth   14. Pregnancy and abortion   15. Miscarriage or stillbirth   16. Inability to have children   17. Marital infidelity   18. Relative joining the household   19. Child leaving home   20. Loss of home through fire or other disaster

Personal and social

1. Major personal achievement   2. Change in lifestyle for self, children, friends   3. Change of school or college   4. Change in religious beliefs or affiliation   5. Change in social activities—leaving clubs, loss of friends, etc.   6. Graduated from school, college, training program   7. Did not graduate from school, college   8. Started a love affair   9. Became engaged   10. Engagement broken   11. Girlfriend or boyfriend problems   12. Loss or damage to personal property   13. An accident   14. Death of a pet   15. Enter Armed Services   16. Discharged from Armed Services (honorable or dishonorable)   17. Assaulted or robbed   18. Accused of a felony   19. Convicted of a crime   20. Went to jail   21. Didn't get out of jail when expected   22. Lost driver's license

---

(After Rahe, 1979)

magnitude of the problem and the need for assistance in dealing with it.

Fear versus Anxiety

Fear has been designated as the psychological, somatic, and autonomic responses to physical threat that is accurately apprehended, such as a physical attack, an anticipated accident, and environmental dangers. Anxiety, on the other hand, is supposed to represent the same reactions when the threat is more symbolic, such as the withdrawal of love or a threat to one's self esteem. Another distinction is that fear is rational, can lead to rapid action in the face of threat, and can motivate the learning and performance of skills such as safe driving or writing examinations. Of men in aerial combat, 50 percent reported that mild fear had a beneficial effect and 37 percent thought they performed their duties better even when they were very afraid (cited in Marks, 1969). Anxiety, in contrast, often carries the connotation of abnormality or irrationality because the source of the anxiety reaction is frequently unknown, and the reaction is disruptive, handicapping, and destructive.

It does not seem that any useful purpose would be served here by maintaining these distinctions, because anxiety, at least to a given point, has also been given a useful role. The aversiveness of anxiety can motivate behaviors that lead to the avoidance of anxiety-provoking situations and indeed can serve as an important force in character formation and personality development. The anxiety invoked by parental disapproval can often motivate good work or study habits, the results of which can be reinforcing enough to perpetuate the habits for their own sake. Under extreme conditions this sequence of events can lead to a compulsive devotion to achievement at the expense of social development, mental health, and even physical health. Thus, it seems that fear and anxiety can be both adaptive or maladaptive and that our principal concern is to block or ameliorate the causes or effects of extreme or disabling levels of these states.

The Somatic and Autonomic Components of Emotion

The reader, well aware of the aversiveness of anxiety, may not appreciate that many of the concomitants of this state are similar to those of emotional states that are regarded as pleasant and sought after such as humor, excitement (sexual or physical), joy, and love. First, there is a cognitive aspect of emotion, which means that the quality of it depends upon the setting and the expectations that are part of it. Thus, pratfalls arouse us and are deemed funny, whereas aggression also arouses us but is perceived as threatening. It is also clear that there are somatic and autonomic aspects of all emotions, including fear and anxiety. A sexual encounter with a loved one is accompanied by a rapid heart rate and breathing, increased blood pressure, high arousal, and perspiration, but these effects plus many others are also found in persons experiencing fear or anxiety. Strong fear is accompanied by a pounding heart, trembling, exaggerated startle, dryness of the throat and mouth, a sinking feeling in the stomach, nausea, perspiration, urge to urinate or defecate, irritability, crying, difficulty in breathing, paralyzing weakness of the limbs, faintness, and falling. Chronic fear can lead to feelings of fatigue, depression, slowing of movements and mental processes, restlessness, aggression, loss of appetite, insomnia and nightmares. Other physiological changes include pallor, sweating, pilomotor erection, pupil dilation, tachycardia, hypertension, rapid breathing, increased secretion of adrenalin, increased availability of glucose and red blood cells, and a rerouting of the circulation to somatic musculature and away from the gastrointestinal tract.

Many attempts have been made to equate a given emotional feeling or experience with a specific number or constellation of the somatic and physiological effects enumerated above, but these have achieved limited success. Furthermore, efforts to pinpoint specific brain areas as mediating particular emotional reactions have not been very edifying. To be sure, the arousal mediated by the reticular formation, the mediation of emotional responses by the hypothalamus, the inhibitory influences of the cerebral cortex, and the strange aberrations resulting from surgical assaults upon the limbic structures, all have produced their share of interesting conjectures, but we have yet to obtain, nor perhaps can we expect to obtain, an anatomically based distinctiveness between different emotional patterns (Kemper, 1978).

Neurochemical Determinants of Emotion

There have been a number of attempts to distinguish between emotional states based upon differential rates of release of the neurotransmitters norepinephrine and epinephrine (Schildkraut and Kety, 1967). These investigations were reasonable because of the significant role in emotion played by the catecholamine-mediated sympathetic division of the autonomic nervous system. However, early positive claims were not confirmed. Later studies compared catecholamine levels in anxious patients. The catecholamine levels in blood plasma correlated with anxiety ratings but not with ratings of depression. Studies on the effects of infused catecholamines and emotional reports from anxious patients and normals showed little in the way of a systematic relationship, probably because of prior learned associations between psychological feelings and sympathomimetic symptoms induced by the drug (heart palpitations, etc.), and the anxiety engendered by the experimental setting (Lader, 1978b).

The Theoretical Concept of Emotion

The preceding observations impose a conservative view that forces a recognition of all aspects of the emotional experience in the formulation of theories of emotion in general, and of anxiety in particular. Incorporation of ideas by Lader (1978b) results in the following theory:

External stimuli impinge on the organism. The stimuli can be physical (e.g., trauma or noise), social (e.g., poor living conditions), or psychological (e.g., marital discord). Internal stimuli are also important (e.g., thoughts, needs). Internal and external stimuli are evaluated as possible threats to the organism. These are influenced by the organism's genetic endowment and past experiences. If there is a potential advantage or disadvantage, activity in the CNS results in arousal and an affect is experienced: danger results in fear; obnoxious stimuli result in disgust. The CNS arousal is accompanied by widespread autonomic changes that are felt by the subject (pounding heart, trembling limbs) and contribute to the perceptual aspects of the emotion and help to sustain it. Behavioral responses occur and efforts at various levels of vigor lead to additional sensations (stemming from fatigue, increased heart rate, and breathlessness) that contribute to the emotional percept.

If this concept of anxiety is reasonably correct, it is quite remarkable that emotions with so many ramifications can be rather selectively manipulated by chemical agents of relatively simple design that are characteristic of anxiolytic drugs.

Early Anxiolytic Drugs

The principal characteristic of early anxiolytic drugs, as one might expect, was CNS depression, and even today this is a major feature of drugs in this class (once commonly known as anodynes, i.e., something that calms, soothes, or comforts). In addition to sedative and anxiolytic properties, the early drugs have soporific and hypnotic effects. These properties are also characteristic of contemporary anxiolytic compounds or their analogs. For this reason, there is a justifiable argument against referring to these compounds as anxiolytics or tranquilizers because none of them are that specific. Nevertheless, with this caveat in mind, we shall refer to these compounds as anxiolytics only because that is our major interest and we shall consider the other effects as ancillary properties or side effects. Those compounds that are used almost exclusively as hypnotics will not be considered here in any detail.

Alcohol

No doubt the earliest drug in common use as an anodyne was ethanol or ethyl alcohol. The substance commonly referred to as alcohol is the product of fermentation of sugar in solution by yeast. Yeasts are quite common in the air where plants are grown, and it is small wonder that alcohol was produced when crushed grapes or berries in water were left standing in a warm place. This easily explains the existence of alcohol as far back as 6400 BC; and mead, which is made from honey, is regarded as the oldest alcoholic beverage and is said to have existed in the paleolithic age, about 8000 BC (Blum and Associates, 1969). Although proof would be hard to establish, it is unlikely that the pervasiveness of the use of alcoholic beverages is explained by thirst quenching, taste, or nutritional factors alone. Rather it was the added character of the beverages induced by their alcohol content that made them so desirable.

In the Middle Ages the Arabs introduced the technique of distillation, enabling alcohol to be concen-

trated at high levels. This then became another beverage in common use, one variant coming to be known as whisky (from the Gaelic "usquebaugh," meaning "water of life".) It is easy to imagine that if alcohol were discovered today it would be hailed as a wonder drug with its anxiolytic, soporific, hypnotic, analgesic, astringent, antibactericidal, and solvent properties. Even as a food, although deficient in amino acids, vitamins, and minerals, it has the shortest metabolic pathway and hence provides the fastest source of calories among known foods. Were it not for its abuse potential, its relatively high toxicity, and its relatively short duration of effect, it would truly deserve the high esteem connoted by the name "whisky." Yet, despite heroic research efforts, the mechanisms of action and the causes for alcohol's toxic effects on the CNS and other organs are now just beginning to be understood (see Chapter 9). Still alcohol is used as a beverage in one form or another in almost every country in the world, with the exception of those embracing the Moslem religion and culture. Used in moderation, alcoholic beverages produce relaxation, elevation of mood, increased appetite, and release of inhibition caused by social constraints. In the late nineteenth and early twentieth centuries in America, alcohol was a prime ingredient in a wide assortment of nostrums such as nerve tonics, vegetable compounds, and elixirs, whose major benefits were conferred even upon the ladies of the Women's Christian Temperance Union, because the proof of the compound was equal to that of a fairly good sherry. It is thus easy to see why under increased tension and anxiety one can resort to alcohol to a point of chronic or acute danger.

Bromides

Bromide compounds had a high popularity a century ago as CNS depressants. According to Sharpless (1970), these compounds were discovered to be effective against epilepsy, although the rationale for their use was based upon an argument that today seems ludicrous. Potassium bromide earlier had been used to reduce sexual drive, and because some forms of epilepsy were thought to be related to masturbation, a certain Dr. Locock utilized the compound in 1857 for the treatment of epilepsy and found it effective in 13 out of 14 cases. In the latter half of the nineteenth century, bromides were used on an enormous scale, and in the 1870s it was reported that in London a single hospital dispensed several tons annually as sedatives and anticonvulsants. Until recently bromides were found in nostrums, nerve tonics, and headache remedies (e.g., Bromoseltzer), but their use has been largely discontinued because of the toxicity of bromides.

Bromide intoxication occurs because bromides are excreted slowly by the kidneys—plasma half-life being about 12 days. Thus, if taken on a regular basis, dangerous levels can be attained in a few weeks. The symptoms include impaired thought and memory, drowsiness, dizziness, irritability, and emotional disturbances. These symptoms frequently induced the user to increase the dose, with dire consequences— delirium, delusions, hallucinations, mania, and ultimately, lethargy and coma. The symptoms were accompanied by neurological signs that suggested acute alcoholism, paresis, tabes dorsalis, encephalitis, cerebral tumor, multiple sclerosis, and other maladies. Bromism was also accompanied by a repulsive looking skin eruption and gastrointestinal disturbances.

Once diagnosed on the basis of serum bromide levels, the therapy consisted of the administration of NaCl at relatively high doses (6 grams/day in divided doses). The intoxication occurs because the kidney preferentially reabsorbs bromide and excretes chloride, thus causing an increasing buildup of bromide in the blood while the urine reflects a higher chloride-to-bromide ratio. Raising the chloride level in the blood apparently hastens the excretion of the bromide ion, and this process can be accelerated by the additional use of drugs that increase the excretion of halides from the blood. Fortunately, bromides have been banned from over-the-counter preparations, and no bromide compounds are currently listed in the Physicians Desk Reference, an annual publication that lists drugs in current use. Thus, bromide poisoning is no longer observed.

Belladonna Alkaloids

The belladonna alkaloids are of historical interest because of their use over many centuries. The most familiar drugs in this class are atropine and scopolamine (see Chapter 6). These compounds are anticholinergic drugs that block muscarinic receptors. Of the two, scopolamine is the more potent in CNS depression. It has not been used as a sedative or anxiolytic drug by itself in modern times, but it has been and continues to be used in preanesthetic medication.

In addition to its CNS effects (drowsiness, euphoria, and amnesia), it also blocks secretions in the nasopharynx that might be induced by anesthetic inhalants. When scopolamine is administered alone or supplemented with barbiturates or opiates, a patient approaches and tolerates surgical procedures under local anesthesia, sometimes appearing fully awake but in a state of quiet and repose. When the procedures are complete, the patient hardly remembers that they ever started, and hours are condensed into minutes. These effects are difficult to explain physiologically.

Narcotic Analgesics (Opiates)

These drugs (which are the alkaloid derivatives of the poppy plant) and their synthetic and semisynthetic derivatives were known before recorded history. These substances have had and continue to have widespread clinical utility, primarily for their analgesic effects. They are also potent gastrointestinal inhibiting agents, and in the days when food contamination and dysentery were commonplace they may have been of lifesaving importance. These effects and their mechanisms are discussed thoroughly in Chapter 13. Opiates are mentioned here because of the associated strong psychological effects that were recognized as far back as 4000 BC, when the Sumerians had an ideograph for the poppy plant that was composed of *hul* ("joy") and *gil* ("plant") (Jaffe, 1975). In the eighteenth century, opium smoking became common in the Orient and the practice was widespread among Oriental laborers in America during the next two centuries. In Europe, the practice of ingesting laudanum (a 10 percent tincture of opium with about 1 percent morphine) was widespread. The invention of the hypodermic needle and, subsequently, the injection of morphine, heroin, and other derivatives created a population of addicts with attendant physiological and social problems (see Chapter 13).

Psychologically opiates produce drowsiness, changes in mood, and mental clouding. Patients suffering from pain, discomfort, tension, and worry experience euphoria with as little as 5 to 10 mg of morphine. To normal individuals who are free of pain, the effect is not always pleasant; rather, the effect is dysphoria or mild anxiety, restlessness, and nausea. (The subjective effects—both euphoria and dysphoria—increase with increased doses.)

Coupled to the fact that tolerance and physical dependence is associated with opiate use, it is not difficult to appreciate how easily one can become addicted to a drug that seems to alleviate psychological stress and to replace boredom, frustration, worry, anxiety, and fear with feelings of peace, repose, and surcease of all cares, even those that are related to immediate needs for survival. It is no wonder then that opiate addiction is prevalent, but not exclusively, among the poor and uneducated, the economically disadvantaged, and the racially oppressed. It is also a fact that physicians and nurses, for whom supplies of opiates are easily available, frequently succumb to the use of opiates to alleviate the anxieties brought on by the pressures of their occupations. In one study cited by Jaffe (1975), 15 percent of known narcotic addicts had medical professions, a percentage many times higher than that in the general population. Fortunately for them, however, their drugs were pure, their self-injection procedures were sterile, and their doses were more likely to be controlled. Under those conditions, opiate use could continue for decades without serious deleterious physical effects, but it is clear that the responsibilities of medical practice are not optimized by these attempts at self-therapy.

Thus, although many other substances had been tried over the ages on the mentally ill (see Caldwell, 1970, for a review) for the most part, ethanol, belladonna alkaloids, opiates, and bromides were the drugs in greatest use for the relief of fear and tension until about the 1930s. At about that time, there was a developing awareness of concepts of anxiety, probably initiated by Freud's book *The Problem of Anxiety* (1936), which was first published in the 1920s but was not translated into English until approximately some 10 years later. Before that there were no formalized concepts of the role of fear and anxiety in behavior nor of their consequences of maladaptation, psychosomatic manifestations, and compulsive, phobic, and hysterical symptoms. Even in World War I, soldiers who were incapacited by their experiences were referred to as being shell-shocked or as suffering from battle fatigue. In 1935 Thorner published a paper that was entitled "The Psycho-Pharmacology of Sodium Amytal" and that described the use of drugs in psychiatric practice to reduce tension and anxiety. This may have been the first use of the term "psychopharmacology" in the psychiatric literature (Caldwell, 1970, p. 10). During World War II and the Korean War, a significant role was played by psychiatry in the effort to treat soldiers incapacitated by the rigors of combat. New techniques were introduced in an effort to hasten the return of these soldiers to duty. Among these techniques was the use of drugs such as amytal and thiopental, which could facilitate treatment during the psychiatric interview. These developments were described in the notable book *Men Under Stress* by Grinker and Spiegel (1945). In retrospect it seems that this was the beginning of specific treatment of recognized anxiety states by the use of drugs.

The Barbiturates

History

In 1864 Adolph von Baeyer (or Bayer), who was later instrumental in forming the great Bayer chemical firm in Germany, synthesized barbituric acid (malonylurea) from malonic acid (the acid from apples) and urea. The name of the compound is said to have been derived from the fact that on the day of the experiment the inventor visited a tavern frequented by artillery officers who were celebrating the Day of St. Barbara, their patron saint. Combining Barbara with urea signified the celebration of the two events (Sharpless, 1970).

Barbituric acid itself was not a central nervous depressant, but when substitutions were made for the hydrogens in position 5 (Figure 1), compounds having hypnotic potency were found. In 1903 Fischer and von Mering introduced to medicine diethylbarbituric acid, formed by replacing the hydrogens in position 5 with ethyl groups. The compound was called barbital, and its trade name became Veronal. The name is said to be related to von Mering's presence in Verona, where he was visiting when he first heard that Fischer had synthesized the compound. Another version of the story has it that the drug was named after Verona because of the peace and solace that is associated with this Italian town. (A more prosaic example is "Miltown," a tranquilizer of the 1950s named after a town in New Jersey.) Barbital became very popular in medicine as a drug that facilitated sleep and had anxiolytic properties in the daytime. Although still regarded as an excellent hypnotic, it has been supplanted in recent years by compounds having a shorter duration of action.

In 1912 two independent teams of researchers introduced phenobarbital (Luminal). This was a drug with excellent sedative and anticonvulsant properties. Interestingly, these two effects seemed to be independent of each other because the sedative effect could be

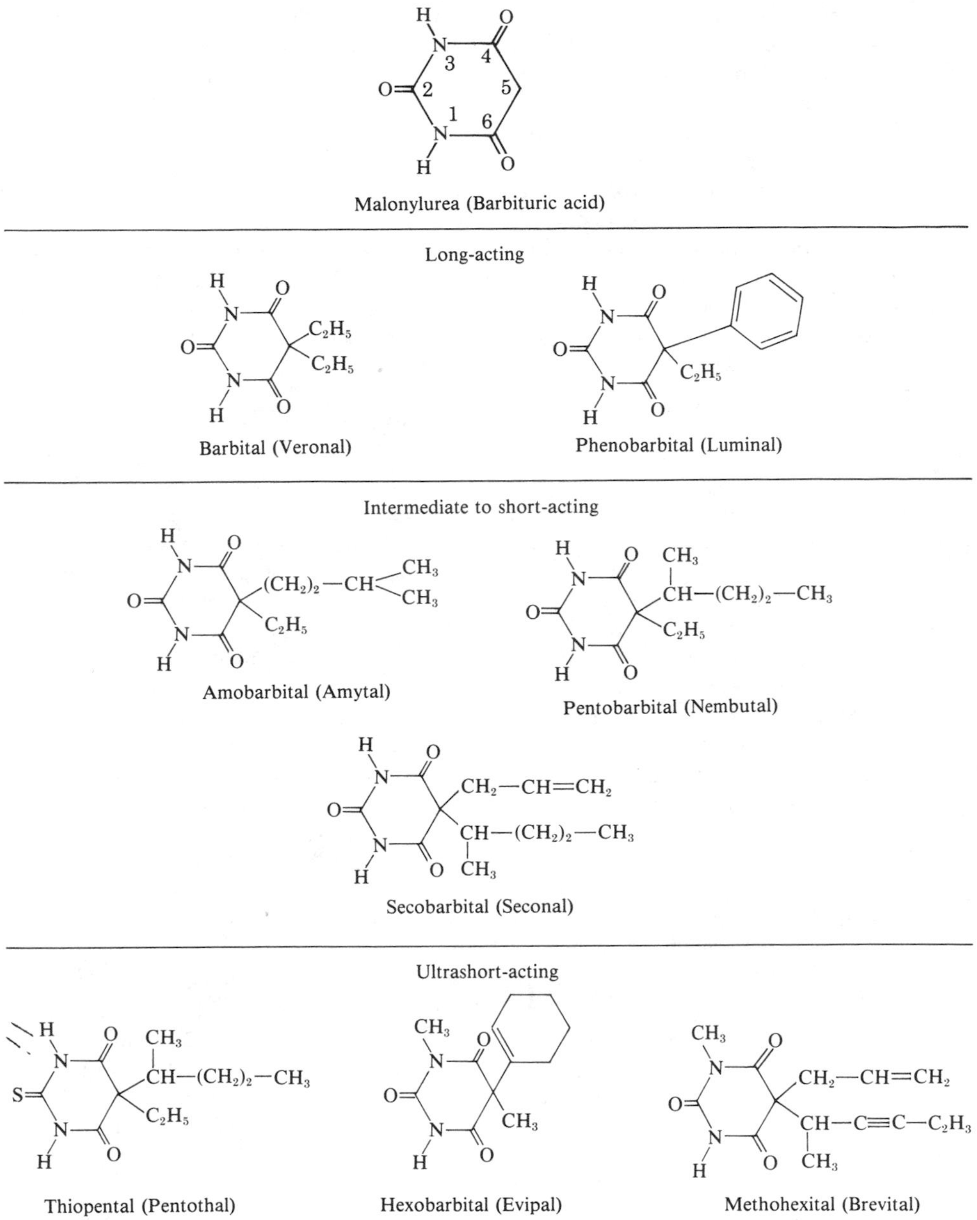

Malonylurea (Barbituric acid)

Long-acting

Barbital (Veronal)

Phenobarbital (Luminal)

Intermediate to short-acting

Amobarbital (Amytal)

Pentobarbital (Nembutal)

Secobarbital (Seconal)

Ultrashort-acting

Thiopental (Pentothal)

Hexobarbital (Evipal)

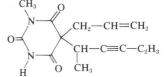

Methohexital (Brevital)

FIGURE 1 CHEMICAL STRUCTURES OF BARBITURATES.

reversed with amphetamine while not disturbing the anticonvulsant activity.

Over the years, 2500 different barbiturates were synthesized, many of which were tested for their clinical usefulness. About 50 barbiturates were marketed, but 5 or 6 of these seem to fulfill most needs (Figure 1). One of the goals of barbiturate research was to find compounds with shorter durations of action. This led to the discovery of amobarbital in 1923 and of pentobarbital and secobarbital in 1930. All three of these compounds were found to be useful for inducing sleep and, in smaller doses, to provide relief from mental stress. The fact that they differed in their duration of action provided considerable versatility in this class of drugs.

The barbiturates were also useful as anticonvulsants. The drugs with rapid onset and short duration of action were given intravenously to terminate acutely generated convulsions (e.g., by drugs such as strychnine or by brain injury), whereas phenobarbital, given orally twice a day, was used to keep chronic seizure activity in abeyance. In the latter case, other more specific anticonvulsants have been introduced to supplement or replace barbiturates.

In the 1930s the ultra-short-acting barbiturates were introduced as intravenous anesthetics. The first was hexobarbital; this was followed by thiopental and methohexital (Price, 1975). Thiopental is one of a few barbiturates in which a sulfur atom replaces oxygen at position 2; this is the only difference between it and pentobarbital (Figure 1). Thiopental seemed to be the drug with the greatest popularity, which continues to the present day. An intravenous injection of a single small dose can result in anesthesia within seconds after infusion begins. The patient quietly falls asleep, sometimes in the middle of a sentence. There is no excitement or vomiting, no salivation, and quiet respiration, and there is rapid recovery after small doses. The drug must be slowly infused over 15 or 30 seconds because a single large dose can result in anesthesia that is too deep, with the risk of respiratory arrest. However, because the duration of action of thiopental is short—about 5 minutes—prolonged surgical procedures require supplementation by inhalant anesthetics.

Onset and Duration of Action of Barbiturates

Up to this point we have emphasized that important differences exist among the barbiturates with respect to the onset and duration of their action. These differences can be explained in terms of the lipid solubility, rates of ionization, plasma protein binding, metabolism, and excretion of the various barbiturate compounds (see Chapter 1). One of the best illustrations of these principles is a comparison of the actions of thiopental and pentobarbital, whose chemical structures are very similar but whose onset-duration characteristics are very different.

Pentobarbital is approximately equal in potency to thiopental because the same brain concentration of each drug is necessary for anesthesia. But no dose of

pentobarbital has been found that will mimic the ultrashort duration of action of thiopental. If a dose of pentobarbital equal to an anesthetic dose of thiopental is injected, no anesthesia will result. By raising the dose of pentobarbital, any level of anesthesia can be attained, but the onset of anesthesia will be much slower than for thiopental and the duration will be long (an hour or more).

Explanations were sought for the onset-duration differences between pentobarbital and thiopental. Initially, thiopental was thought to be metabolized at a very high rate, because it rapidly disappeared from the blood without being found in the urine. Later it was discovered that the drug was taken up by fat deposits; a whole dose was found there after a few hours. This led to the suggestion that the high lipid solubility of the drug explained the rapid onset and short duration of its action. Lipid solubility is expressed as a ratio between the amount of a substance that dissolves in an organic solvent compared with the amount that dissolves in water. Thiopental has a ratio (the partition coefficient) of 3.30 compared to a partition coefficient of 0.05 for pentobarbital. It is easy to see why lipoprotein cell membranes are more easily penetrated by thiopental than by pentobarbital—which explains the rapid onset of the effects. The plasma level of the drug immediately begins to fall as the drug distributes rapidly to other tissues such as muscle and fat, and the drug moves rapidly out of the brain to establish equilibrium with the falling plasma levels. This accounts for the short duration of action. Studies have shown that the brain reaches its peak drug concentration within 30 seconds after intravenous administration of thiopental, whereas muscle and skin require from 15 to 30 minutes and fat requires about 2 hours to become saturated. By 30 minutes, the brain may give up as much as 90 percent of its peak concentration (Sharpless, 1970). In contrast, pentobarbital, being much less lipid soluble, enters the brain very slowly—so slowly, in fact, that by the time the drug in the brain has reached equilibrium with the plasma level, the plasma level already has begun to fall because of the drug's metabolism and excretion. Thus, at low doses, no anesthesia occurs.

Thiopental shows a *larger* amount of ionization than pentobarbital and also shows more plasma protein binding. Ionization blocks membrane transport because ionized molecules are lipid insoluble, and molecules bound to plasma proteins are not easily transported. Yet because of the great difference in lipid solubility, thiopental is the faster-acting barbiturate. (See Chapter 3 for further discussion of membrane transport.)

Thiopental is largely metabolized in the liver, and its metabolites are excreted in the urine. However, metabolism occurs rather slowly (10 to 15 percent per hour), much too slowly to account for its short duration of action. Therefore, the rapid shift of thiopental to other tissue compartments and its rapid removal from the brain probably accounts for the ultrashort duration of action.

Finally, one can compare thiopental and pentobarbital with barbital. The latter drug has a partition coefficient of 0.002 (less than that of thiopental by a factor of 1650) and thus is so lipid insoluble that, even after an intravenous injection of this drug, many minutes elapse before any effects are seen. Consequently, barbital is not an effective anesthetic or hypnotic agent, but serves well as a long-acting sedative.

Synaptic Effects of Barbiturates

The biochemical effects of barbiturates have been studied in great detail. Barbiturates not only depress the actions of neurons but also those of skeletal and smooth muscles of the viscera, of cardiac muscle, of the nonneurogenic aspects of respiration, and of the kidney (Sharpless, 1970; Harvey, 1975). Early investigations showed that during barbiturate anesthesia there was an inhibition of oxidative metabolism within neurons that was thought to be responsible for the depression in function. However, the question was raised as to whether this was the cause for a decrease in nerve impulse traffic or the result of it. Neither of these alternatives appeared to be correct because it was also found that inhibition of oxidative metabolism does not occur with all barbiturates, and although other drugs such as salicylates also produce this effect, they lack hypnotic potency.

Neuroelectric Studies. Later experiments showed that barbiturates render postsynaptic membranes insensitive to the depolarizing effects of neurotransmitters and artificial stimuli, and this effect applies to neuronal and nonneuronal membranes alike. It has also been suggested on the basis of *in vitro* studies that barbiturates as well as other anesthetics have an effect on membranes that is described as "electrical membrane stabilization," referring to a reduction of membrane conductance to physiological or artificial stimuli with little or no alteration of the membrane resting potential. This effect is postulated to be the result of drug-induced changes in the membrane macromolecules, causing the membrane to swell and block the physiological action pertaining to the conduction of nerve impulses. However, it was not known whether the drug concentrations achieved in the *in vitro* preparations to obtain these effects were reached during actual anesthesia. Moreover, that this is not a generalized effect of barbiturates is supported by the fact that some higher CNS functions are depressed by barbiturate doses that have little effect on more primitive brain functions and at peripheral organs. Thus, it seems that barbiturates at different doses have more discrete and specific effects on neuronal elements (Haefely, 1977).

Barker and Gainer (1973) investigated the problem of whether anesthesia was due to a decrease in excitatory synaptic events or to an increase in inhibitory synaptic events. They studied the effects of barbiturates on nerve–muscle preparations from several molluscan and crustacean species from which EPSPs and IPSPs could be readily measured. The activities of the nerve or muscle membranes were measured from inserted electrodes while the tissue was perfused with saline or drugs dissolved in the saline and electrically stimulated to evoke postsynaptic potentials. They found that pentobarbital reversibly antagonized the EPSPs in lobster muscle fibers but did not affect the IPSPs. Under control conditions, the EPSPs ranged from 5 to 7.5 mV, whereas in the presence of pentobarbital at anesthetic concentrations ($2 \times 10^{-4}\,M$), EPSPs decreased to 2 to 3.5 mV without any significant change in IPSPs. Washing the preparation for 10 minutes restored the EPSPs to their original range of amplitudes. Similarly, pentobarbital selectively and reversibly antagonized the Na^+-dependent depolarization of lobster muscle fibers by the excitatory transmitter glutamate but did not affect the action of Cl^--dependent inhibitory transmitter GABA. Similar results were obtained in snail preparations, with pentobarbital consistently depressing EPSP Na^+-dependent effects while leaving hyperpolarizing inhibitory effects unchanged. It was also found that ACh-induced depolarizations were selectively reduced by the following anesthetics and anticonvulsants, with their indicated relative potencies: diphenylhydantoin $\cong$ pentobarbital > chloralose > chloroform > urethane > ethanol. It was concluded that these phenomena may be generalizable to include selective depression of all transmitter-coupled sodium conductances, with preservation of all transmitter-coupled chloride and potassium conductances. Furthermore, the fact that there is a close correspondence to the drug doses that produce the experimental effects and the plasma concentrations during anesthesia and anticonvulsive therapy suggests that similar mechanisms are responsible.

Site of Barbiturate Action

The next question to be addressed was the identification of the site of action of pentobarbital's synaptic effect. The depression of postsynaptic excitatory effects could occur because of a block of presynaptic transmitter release, and this in turn could be due to a blockade of the action potential invasion into presynaptic terminals or to the blockade of Ca^{2+} entry, and so on. Or the depression may be the result of changes on the postsynaptic membrane. This latter view seemed more reasonable because the barbiturate-induced depression is selective for excitatory neurotransmitters and not for the inhibitory ones, suggesting that the presynaptic transmitter release mechanisms are functional. Nicoll and Iwamoto (1978) set out to answer these questions by studying the effects of barbiturates on synaptic transmission through the ganglia of the sympathetic trunk of the bullfrog. The preganglionic fibers were electrically stimulated and record-

ings were made of membrane changes in the preganglionic nerve trunks and the postsynaptic ganglion cells. The preparation was installed in a chamber that was constantly perfused with a Ringer solution at the appropriate pH and containing appropriate salts, oxygen, etc. By opening a stopcock the drug was allowed to flow into the chamber. Stimulus intensity was adjusted to just elicit EPSPs and IPSPs.

The preganglionic trunk contains B and C fibers, which are responsible for different postsynaptic responses. Both of these fibers release ACh and together lead to a postsynaptic response characterized by a fast EPSP followed by a slow IPSP and concluding with a slow EPSP (see Figure 5 in Chapter 7). The B fiber is responsible for inducing the EPSPs, but the receptors are nicotinic and muscarinic for the fast and slow EPSP, respectively. The slow IPSP response is generated by small unmyelinated C fibers and is also mediated via muscarinic receptors and a dopaminergic interneuron. It was first established that presynaptic action potentials always preceded postsynaptic EPSPs. Figure 2 shows that in tests with pentobarbital the impulse transmission through the ganglion (postsynaptic) was more sensitive to the drug than was axonal conduction (presynaptic) through the presynaptic B fibers. Whereas pentobarbital at 0.1 mM suppressed the amplitude of the postsynaptic fast EPSP by 50 percent, a 20-fold increase in pentobarbital concentration

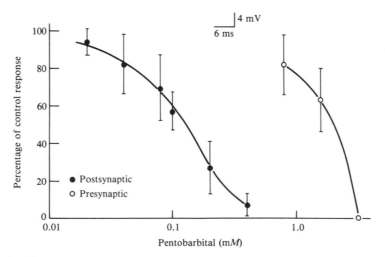

FIGURE 2 PENTOBARBITAL-INDUCED SENSITIVITY of axonal (presynaptic) conduction compared to ganglionic (postsynaptic) transmission. Values are expressed as a percentage of control amplitude. Each point represents the average ($\pm$SD) of 4 to 9 preparations. (From Nicoll and Iwamoto, 1978.)

was needed to produce a 50 percent decrease in the presynaptic action potential. Figure 3 shows the changes in the synaptic response after a stimulus (1.5-second train, 60 Hz). At 0.1 mM pentobarbital, the fast EPSP was depressed by 50 percent, whereas the slow IPSP and EPSP were not noticeably altered. At 0.4 mM, however, the fast EPSP was reduced by 87 percent, the slow IPSP was slightly increased, and the slow EPSP was decreased by 17 percent. The concentrations that were able to block the slow EPSPs by 50 percent approached the concentrations that blocked the presynaptic action potentials. Accordingly, this was at least partly responsible for the decline in the slow EPSPs.

The foregoing experiments appear to show that the fast EPSP, which reflects a change in sodium conductance, is significantly blocked by the action of pentobarbital, and much higher doses of the drug are required to alter, even slightly, the slow IPSP and EPSP. To explain these phenomena, the idea has been put forward that barbiturates might be acting upon specific proteins associated with membrane channels concerned with sodium conductance but not with channels associated with other ionic conductances. The barbiturates may act on membrane lipids surrounding sodium channels, causing the lipids to swell and thus hinder channel function. Or the sodium channels may be less well-protected or rigid than other

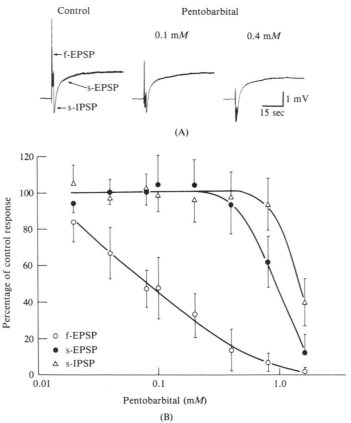

FIGURE 3 (A) PENTOBARBITAL-INDUCED SENSITIVITY of fast (f) and slow (s) synaptic potentials. The stimuli were 60 Hz, 1.5-second trains. Note that the responses are recorded over a 60-second period. The responses were recorded for pentobarbital after the depression had stabilized (20 minutes for 0.1 mM and 27 minutes for 0.4 mM). (B) Group data show that 0.1 mM pentobarbital reduced the fast EPSP 50 percent whereas the concentration of pentobarbital had to be increased 10-fold to block the slow potentials. Each point represents the average (±SD) of 3 to 11 preparations. Responses were recorded after their size had reached a stable value (20 to 45 minutes). (From Nicoll and Iwamoto, 1978).

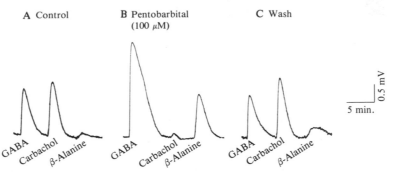

A Control **B** Pentobarbital (100 μM) **C** Wash

FIGURE 4 GANGLION DEPOLARIZATION BY CAR-BACHOL, GABA, AND β-ALANINE. Pentobarbital (100 μM) blocks the carbachol response but augments the GABA and β-alanine responses. Carbachol (20 μM) was applied for 15 seconds, GABA (40 μM) for 10 seconds, and β-alanine (120 μM) for 30 seconds. (From Nicoll, 1978c).

channels. Further research will be addressed to these questions (Nicoll, 1979).

Additional experiments investigated the effects of pentobarbital on chemical stimulation of bullfrog sympathetic ganglia. It was known that the ganglia can be depolarized by GABA and by β-alanine, which weakly mimics GABA. The mechanism of action involves the increase in Cl^- conductance. The ganglion can also be depolarized by carbachol, which has a potent Na^+-dependent nicotinic effect. Figure 4 shows the effects of GABA, carbachol, and β-alanine on the ganglion response with and without the presence of pentobarbital. In A, GABA and carbachol significantly depolarized the ganglion whereas the response to β-alanine was weak. In B, pentobarbital (100 μM) increased the depolarization of the GABA- and β-alanine-treated ganglion whereas the same treatment produced a significant suppression of the carbachol effect. In C, washing the preparation free of pentobarbitol restored the original GABA, carbachol, and β-alanine effects (Nicoll, 1978c).

These experiments give strong support to the notion that the mechanism of action of barbiturates is related to their complex effects on synaptic activity. In particular, the effect is accompanied by a depression of excitatory Na^+-dependent depolarization of the postsynaptic membrane. In addition, there is an enhancement of inhibitory Cl^--dependent postsynaptic activity that is dose dependent. For example, barbiturates prolong presynaptic inhibition in the spinal cord as well as in the nuclei of the dorsal columns (N. gracilis and cuneatus). In the latter structures, postsynaptic inhibition is also prolonged. Similar effects on post-synaptic inhibition occur in the olfactory bulb and on recurrent inhibition in the hippocampus. All of these inhibitory synaptic events are probably mediated by GABA. Even the isolated frog motoneurons are hyperpolarized by pentobarbital, and because the effect is blocked by picrotoxin and bicuculline, GABA receptors are probably involved. It also appears that the same transmitter (e.g., ACh) can be blocked by barbiturates when it acts as an excitatory transmitter and that it is unaffected when acting as an inhibitory transmitter. This effect has also been demonstrated for other neurotransmitters. Evidence shows that the excitatory effects of amino acids, serotonin, and norepinephrine are all depressed by barbiturates, yet the inhibitory effects of serotonin, norepinephrine, dopamine, and GABA are not reduced by moderate amounts of barbiturates. These data clearly showed that pentobarbital enhanced inhibition by increasing the depolarizing effects of GABA and β-alanine, which reflects increased Cl^- conductance, whereas the Na^+-mediated carbachol effect was substantially diminished. Nicoll (1979) has pointed out that these effects cannot be explained by blockade of GABA uptake; rather, the enhancement of the GABA response is more compatible with an increased affinity of the GABA receptor. However, biochemical studies show that barbiturates (as well as the GABA antagonist picrotoxin) fail to modify GABA binding on membranes in the CNS. On the other hand, because of the specific interaction between barbiturates and picrotoxin, it does appear that these two substances compete for a common site; and, again, this might be a protein associated with the chloride channel. Picrotoxin might block chloride conductance, and barbiturates would prolong it once the receptors were activated by GABA. Interestingly, if the chloride channel is the site of action of barbiturates and picrotoxin, then the chloride channels associated with the glycine receptor must be different from those associated with the GABA receptor because barbiturates and picrotoxin do not seem to affect glycine-mediated response.

Thus, although all the details are not yet known, it seems fairly reasonable to assume that barbiturates exert their neurodepressant action by rendering postsynaptic membranes unresponsive to Na^+-dependent excitatory transmitter action, combined with a dose-dependent enhancement of Cl^--dependent postsynaptic inhibitory effects (Haefely, 1978; Nicoll, 1978b). In a later discussion of the benzodiazepines, we will encounter a related model involving the enhancement of GABAergic effects by a drug receptor.

General Central Nervous System Effects of Barbiturates

With fair agreement about the synaptic effects of barbiturates, we can now examine the general effects that barbiturates exert on the CNS. Because excitatory synaptic events are suppressed and inhibitory effects are either unaffected or enhanced, it is not surprising

that the overall effect of these drugs is one of depression. Nevertheless, one should consider the possibility that regional effects of the drugs may be responsible for some of their action. This is especially important because barbiturates have a variety of effects—hypnotic, anesthetic, anticonvulsant, anxiolytic, euphoric—and some barbiturates are even convulsants (Nicoll, 1978b).

The Role of the Reticular Activating System

The consensus among investigators seems to be that barbiturates do not exert selective neurochemical actions on specific parts of the CNS such as on a "sleep center" or on the hypothalamus or on the cerebral cortex; nor do they act via one or more particular neurotransmitters or unique receptor substances. On the other hand, there is evidence that the common response to barbiturates in neurons of the reticular activating system (RAS) may account in large part for the most prominent effects of these drugs. The reticular formation is an amorphous cluster of small neurons with few distinct nuclear groupings in the brain stem; it forms multisynaptic connections to rostral and caudal centers (Figure 5). Functionally it serves to gate sensory inputs, to modulate neural transmission to caudal centers for control of spinal effector

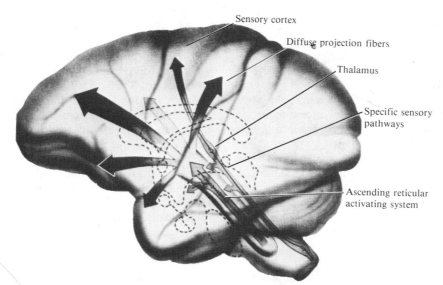

Sensory cortex

Diffuse projection fibers

Thalamus

Specific sensory pathways

Ascending reticular activating system

FIGURE 5 ASCENDING RETICULAR ACTIVATING SYSTEM (ARAS) of the monkey brain. Reticular formation, consisting of a multineuronal, multisynaptic central core of

the medulla, pons, and midbrain, receives collaterals from specific sensory pathways and projects diffusely upon the cortex. (From Lindsley, 1958.)

mechanisms and visceral functions, and to modulate neural transmission in rostral-coursing tracts that influence "a spectrum of states of consciousness from deep coma through a series of sleeping states to maximal vigilance" (Scheibel and Scheibel, 1967).

Within the RAS there are two mutually antagonistic structures: one in the midbrain, which has an activating function on cortical structures; and a medullary center, which has a negative feedback influence on the midbrain center. Electroencephalograph (EEG) studies show that direct electrical stimulation of the former center leads to a low-voltage, desynchronized, high-frequency EEG pattern in cortical structures that is associated with high levels of arousal and attention. Stimulation of the medullary center yields a synchronous, high-voltage EEG pattern that is associated with relaxation, drowsiness, and sleep. These two systems are in a dynamic equilibrium, each tending to counterbalance the other.

When barbiturates are administered in small doses, there is an initial increase in the energy of the high-frequency (25–35 Hz) pattern. The frequency subsequently declines to 15–25 Hz, which is associated with clouding of consciousness and occasionally with euphoria. With increasing doses, large-amplitude slow waves (5–12 Hz) appear superimposed upon the high-frequency waves at about the time the patient loses contact with the environment, although he can be aroused by strong stimuli. Increasing the dose still more leads to slow waves (1–4 Hz) and spindle waves (short bursts of 10–12 Hz) that are characteristic of deep sleep and a failure to respond to moderate noxious stimuli. With still higher doses, deep anesthesia occurs, with a flattening of the EEG; and finally, at extremely high doses, respiratory and cardiac depression increases and there is death with no electrical activity at all. These results are supported by many animal studies. For example, Magni et al. (1961) found that intracarotid injections of thiopental perfused the midbrain and led to the irregular slow waves of an EEG associated with sleep, whereas intervertebral injections that depressed the medulla led to an EEG activation (low voltage–high frequency). Thus, the depression of one RAS center led to the heightened expression of the other.

It is now possible to relate these findings and propose that the midbrain center of the RAS serves to activate cortical centers, whereas the medullary center suppresses it; and the equilibrium between these two

centers can be altered even by small doses of barbiturates. If the medullary system is affected first, there will be activation and euphoria; if the midbrain system is affected, the result will be relaxation, drowsiness, or sleep. Thus, although the direct effect of barbiturates on neural tissues are roughly the same throughout the nervous system, the unique characteristics and location of the RAS, i.e., athwart the principal ascending and descending systems of the brain stem, bestows upon it a special role in producing the prominent effects of barbiturates.

Behavioral Pharmacology of Barbiturates

Behavioral studies of barbiturates in animals and humans are numerous, and many reviews have been published (Efron, 1968; Thompson et al., 1970; McMillan and Leander, 1976; Iversen and Iversen, 1981). Consequently, we will only try to summarize the overall findings of these studies. First, however, it must be acknowledged that the bulk of behavioral research on drug effects for more than two decades has utilized the techniques of operant conditioning developed by Skinner and his many followers. The details of these procedures have been reviewed in Chapter 2.

Schedule Effects of Barbiturates

The first example illustrates the method and reflects the precision that can be obtained when drugs are imposed during different schedules of reinforcement. In this study by Morse (1962), a food-deprived pigeon was trained to peck at an illuminated key to obtain a food reward. The bird was subjected to a repeating multiple schedule such that in the presence of a blue light the animal first had to peck 30 times to obtain the reinforcement (food). This is a fixed ratio 30, or FR-30 schedule. After the reinforcement, the blue light was replaced by a red light, and the bird received reinforcement after the first peck following a 5-minute interval. This is a fixed interval-5 minute, or FI-5 min, schedule. Figure 6 shows the behavioral responses of a well-trained bird in this experiment. At first there was a short, almost perpendicular rise of the response-recording pen as the pigeon quickly made 30 pecking responses. The short diagonal pen stroke at the end of the rise indicates a reinforcement. Then the light color changed, indicating that the schedule was altered. The pigeon ceased pecking for about 3 minutes, as though it knew that food would not be forthcoming for

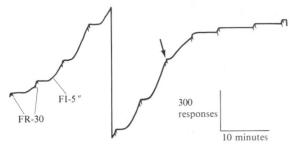

FIGURE 6 CUMULATIVE RESPONSE CURVE. The schedule is a multiple fixed ratio (30)/fixed interval (5 minutes) schedule. Reinforcements are marked by short diagonal strokes. Sodium pentobarbital (3 mg) was administered intramuscularly to the pigeon at the point by the arrow (body weight, 430 grams). (From Morse, 1962.)

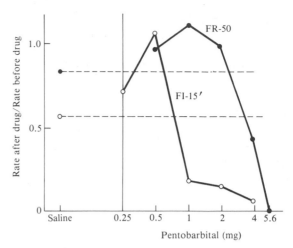

FIGURE 7 PENTOBARBITAL EFFECTS ON PECKING BEHAVIOR OF PIGEONS. Each point represents the mean of the ratios for the same four birds at each dosage. The rate of responding under the FI schedule is decreased at lower doses than those required to decrease rates under the FR schedule. Note that saline also had an effect. (From Dews, 1955.)

awhile, then began pecking at an accelerated rate as if it anticipated a reinforcement sooner and sooner. The reinforcement after 5 minutes returned the schedule to the FR-30 condition and so on. Pentobarbital (3 mg, body weight, 430 grams) was injected intramuscularly at the time indicated by the arrow. It is clearly seen that the drug had little if any effect on the FR component but severely depressed the response rate during the FI component. This would pretty much rule out the idea that the drug either depressed the overall functioning of the bird or depressed its hunger because responding on the FR part of the schedule would have been just as vulnerable to these factors as the FI component, but it was not. Why the FI-controlled performance was differentially affected by the drug is subject to considerable conjecture, which we will not engage in now; but the essence of the experiment is clear, namely, that the stimulus and response conditions were clearly specified and that hypothetical interpretive internal states, such as anxiety, hunger, fatigue, and boredom, are minimized or ignored.

Related experiments have shown that FI response rates increase between pentobarbital doses of 0.5 to 1.0 mg/kg and then decrease, whereas FR rates increase over a much wider range of doses (up to about 8 mg/kg), including doses that decreased FI rates (Figure 7). The topography of the response pattern shows that the increased FR rate resulted from decreases in postreinforcement pauses rather than from decreased interresponse intervals. In general, barbiturates yield inverted U-shaped dose–effect curves, i.e., low doses increase response rates whereas high doses decrease them.

This effect is found in different schedules of reinforcement and with different reinforcers, especially when the baseline response rate is low. This latter point is noteworthy, as it can be generally stated that the response-increasing effect of many drugs (and barbiturates, in particular) is in large part determined by the pre-drug control response rate (McMillan and Leander, 1976). Why these effects occur invite much speculation. The effect may occur simply because, if the control rate is low to begin with, a rate-increasing effect can easily become manifest; whereas, if the control rate is high for some intrinsic reason, an increase in rate becomes more difficult to achieve because of the constraints of the physiological limitations of the animal or of the mechanical limitations of the response mechanism. However, it is difficult to assess these limitations and it would be wrong to assume that these factors arbitrarily account for rate effects.

Response-Rate Effects on Barbiturates

The following experiment illustrates the effect of barbiturates on response rates: Pigeons were trained to peck an illuminated disk for food on a FR-33 or an FR-330 schedule. The FR-33 schedule induced a response rate of 155/min, whereas a FR-330 schedule induced a rate of only 80/min. Intuitively one could expect the opposite, on the grounds that the bird reinforced once after 330 responses would work faster to obtain as much food as could be obtained after only 33 responses. When these pigeons received 5.2 mg of amobarbital, the birds on the FR-33 schedule showed little change in response rate, but the birds on the FR-330 schedule almost doubled their rate (to 140/min) and almost equaled the rate of the other birds (Figure 8). When both groups received 10 mg of the drug, the rate for the FR-33 birds dropped much lower than that for the birds on the FR-330 schedule. What this result and similar results using other schedules seem to mean is that the environment that is less eventful (fewer reinforcements in FR-330) is less subject to the effects of high doses of barbiturates; or, possibly, behavior requiring 330 responses for one reinforcement has more conditioned behavior that is less subject to depression by the drug than the FR-33 schedule with less conditioned behavior (Morse, 1962).

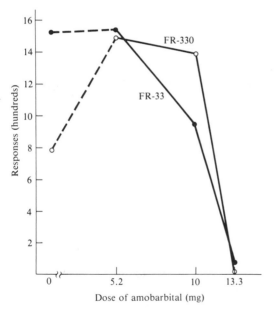

FIGURE 8 DOSE–EFFECT CURVES FOR AMOBARBITAL at two values of fixed ratio (FR) reinforcement. Each drug point represents the average number of responses in a 10-minute session starting 15 minutes after drug injection. Note that after 10 mg of the drug, the curve for FR-33 is depressed below its control value, and the curve for FR-330 is elevated above its control value as well as above the FR-33 curve. (From Morse, 1962).

But these interpretations are subservient to the finding that barbiturates cannot be categorized simply as depressant drugs, because the above examples show that the interactions among the dosage, the schedules of reinforcement, and the history of responding are mainly responsible for either the pattern or the rise and fall in the response rate.

The interaction between drug effects and baseline response rates is an important consideration in interpreting results in other experiments. Geller and Seifter (1960) introduced a conflict procedure to evaluate the efficacy of anxiolytic drugs. The experimental design utilized a multiple VI-2 min/CRF schedule with the following features. Rats were trained to lever-press on a VI-2 min schedule for liquid food reward. After 15 minutes, a tone of 3 minutes duration signaled a change to a CRF (continuous reinforcement) schedule during which every lever-press was followed by reinforcement. However, reinforcements during the CRF segment were accompanied by foot shocks that were sufficiently annoying to suppress responding to very low levels. When these animals were given pentobarbital (5.0 mg/kg), the response rate during the VI segment was only slightly decreased, but the rate during the 3-minute CRF segment increased from 4 to 18, a 350 percent increase (Geller, 1962). Later the question was raised as to whether the drug-induced increase in the CRF response rate was a reflection of anxiolytic properties of the drug as Geller proposed or merely the effect of the drug on a low response rate. Various strategies were used to answer this question, but in the main they consisted of studying the effects of barbiturates and other anxiolytic agents on equal response rates that were maintained under both punishment and nonpunishment contingencies. In general, the results were that the drugs increased the response rates of punished behavior over and above that which would be increased on the basis of a low baseline rate alone, and it was concluded that the punishment situation modified the usual rate-dependent effects of the drugs (McMillan, 1975; McMillan and Leander, 1976; Cook and Davidson, 1973).

Effects of Barbiturates on Negative Reinforcement

Reinforcement is defined as a condition in which the consequence of a response tends to change the probability that the response will recur. Positive reinforcement is exemplified by the offering of food after a lever-press; and negative reinforcement involves the termination of an aversive stimulus by a response such as pressing a lever to terminate a shock (escape). Barbiturates have been found to have small effects on responses in negative reinforcement paradigms. For example, in a discriminated avoidance paradigm, rats that are warned by a tone or a light change to avoid shock by running to the opposite side of a shuttle box or climbing a pole are not significantly affected by pentobarbital, secobarbital, barbital, and phenobarbital unless the drugs are administered in doses that cause ataxia.

In continuous or nondiscriminated avoidance schedules, animals must, for example, respond (usually by pressing a lever) to postpone for 40 seconds the onset of a 5-second shock. If there are no responses, the 5-second shock repeats every 20 seconds. There are no external cues indicating to the rat that a response to avoid the shock is due. Rather, it is some kind of "internal clock" that presumably initiates the response. A well-trained rat should theoretically respond as close to the end of the 40-second period as possible to minimize effort and avoid most shocks. If it should occur, the shock itself can also be terminated by lever-press (an escape response). Phenobarbital, hexobarbital, and pentobarbital disrupt the response rate in that fewer responses are made and more shocks are taken. Doubling the dose that significantly depressed the avoidance rate also yielded failures of escape responding, i.e., the animals failed to turn off the shock before the shock turned off by itself after 5 seconds. Thus, moderate doses depress avoidance behavior whereas doses that are more likely to be toxic will depress escape responses as well. It is proposed that the difference in drug effects between discriminated and nondiscriminated avoidance experiments depends upon differences in the strength of stimulus control and that responses under strong stimulus control are affected less by the drugs. This is based on the assumption that external warning lights or sounds are stronger stimuli than internal time cues (McMillan and Leander, 1976).

Effects of Barbiturates on Conditioned Suppression

In this paradigm, first described by Estes and Skinner (1941), food- and water-deprived animals are trained to lever-press on a variable-interval schedule for water rewards. The rewards come after variable time intervals of 30 seconds to 4 minutes, with an average of 1 minute (VI-1 min). During an experimental session, the animal is intermittently presented with a conditioned stimulus (CS) (a buzzer or clicker) for 3 minutes; the CS is terminated by foot shock. The effect of this is a suppression of bar-pressing behavior during the presentation of the CS (Figure 9). During the suppression of bar-pressing, the animal assumes a crouching or "freezing" posture, it frequently urinates and defecates with malodorous loose feces. There is piloerection and frequent vocalizations. These responses are associated with intense fear and anxiety, hence the response if referred to as a CONDITIONED EMOTIONAL RESPONSE (CER) (Hunt and Brady, 1951). One good feature of this procedure is that the slope of the cumulative response curve when the CS is not sounded provides a baseline rate of responding, or when a drug is administered, it provides an independent measure of the drug's effect on the animal's general activity level. Several doses of barbiturates alleviate the physical symptoms and increase the response rate during the CS (Brady, 1968). However, there are some inconsistencies when different anti-anxiety agents such as barbiturates, chlordiazepoxide, and ethanol are used in CER paradigms and whether

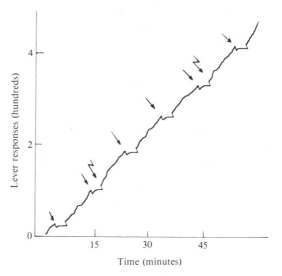

FIGURE 9 CUMULATIVE RESPONSE CURVE OF CONDITIONED SUPPRESSION. The record is from a well-trained rat. The short offset sections mark the duration of the 3-minute clicker (conditioned stimulus). The straight arrows indicate clicker onset and the broken arrows indicate shock on the two trials in which it was administered. No shock was administered on the four trials without the broken arrows (conditioned suppression). (From Brady, 1956.)

they are used in acute versus chronic treatments. Moreover, the results of CER experiments are sometimes inconsistent with Geller paradigm studies. (For discussion of the theoretical implications of these differences, see Bignami, 1978.)

The effect of barbiturates on another form of the conditioned suppression paradigm is illustrated by the studies of Kelleher and Morse (1964). Pigeons were trained to peck a transilluminated disk under a FR-30 schedule for food reinforcements when the disk was illuminated by orange light. After 5 reinforcements (150 responses), the color of the disk was changed to white. During this segment, the FR-30 schedule was still in effect, but the first 10 responses in each 30-response section caused a brief (0.035 sec) shock applied by a gold wire implanted in the tail region of the bird. This segment continued until there had been five food reinforcements or until 3 minutes had elapsed. After a few tests, the birds pecked vigorously during the orange light (nonpunishment segment) and suppressed responses during the white light (punishment segment).

Figure 10 shows that pentobarbital (10 mg/kg) had the effect of increasing the response rate during the white light to one that was almost equal to the rate occurring during the orange light. In another experiment in which the white-light condition was maintained continuously, the birds responded hardly at all, but pentobarbital restored high pecking rates. This indicated that the drug effect in the first experiment was not due to some interaction between the orange- and white-light condition. In addressing the question of whether the drug effect is specific for punished behavior, the authors point out that when chlorpromazine was given in a nonpunishment–punishment experiment, the response rate in the nonpunishment segment increased, but responding was not restored during the punishment segment. The same effect was found using amphetamine. Thus, the barbiturates seem to have some specific effect that causes the release of behavior that has been suppressed by punishment.

The effects of barbiturates have been studied on a wide variety of behaviors, learning and memory, sensory discrimination, state-dependent effects, drug discrimination effects, and so on. Our emphasis here has been on those experimental designs that might illuminate the mechanism of action of the barbiturates that are effective antianxiety agents. The reader is thus referred to the reviews cited earlier in this section for studies dealing with the other matters.

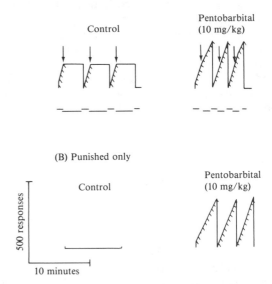

FIGURE 10 PENTOBARBITAL EFFECTS ON RESPONDING SUPPRESSED BY PUNISHMENT. Each frame shows a complete control session followed by a complete drug session for a single bird. Pentobarbital was given intramuscularly 15 minutes before beginning the drug session. (A) Upper displacement of the bottom record indicates the nonpunishment components when a FR-30 schedule of positive reinforcement with an orange stimulus was in effect. The termination of the nonpunishment components is indicated by the small arrows. During the punishment components, (downward displacement of the bottom record) a FR-30 schedule was accompanied by a white stimulus. Each of the first 10 responses of each ratio (30-response section) produced a brief (35 msec) electric shock of 6 mA. The termination of each punishment component is indicated by the resetting of the pen to the bottom of the record. (B) The punishment procedure was in effect throughout each session in the presence of the white stimulus. Note that pentobarbital attenuates the suppression of responding by punishment under both procedures. (From Kelleher and Morse, 1964.)

Barbiturate Abuse and Toxicology

It is almost a truism that any substance that can induce euphoria, allay anxiety, and promote sleep has a high abuse potential. This is especially true for barbiturates. Because of the development of tolerance to its effects and the life-threatening aspects associated with overdosing or sudden withdrawal after prolonged use, barbiturates present major toxicological problems.

Fort (1970) and Cohen (1969) estimated that at least

10 billion doses of barbiturates were produced in the United States annually, enough for 40–50 doses for every man, woman, and child in the country. A significant percentage of this production is diverted into black market channels, where it finds its way into the hands of the drug abusers. The abuse of barbiturates and related drugs occurs at all ages and in all classes, but occurs slightly more often in women than men. Abusers are typically Caucasians between 30 and 50 years old and are members of the middle and upper classes. They, like alcoholics, frequently mask their addiction by adhering to acceptable social norms of behavior, and this facilitates the acquisition of multiple prescriptions and refills from numerous physicians who try to ameliorate their neurotic complaints. Younger people and teenagers tend to use the drugs occasionally to obtain an intoxicated state with feelings of improved performance, euphoria, excitement, and exhilaration. In violent subcultures, the drugs, paradoxically perhaps, lead to increased violence, especially among the young. The drug is sometimes injected intravenously to provide an opiate-like rush of warmth and drowsiness, a practice of considerable danger because of the possibilities of overdosage. Frequently barbiturates are used to counterbalance the effects of stimulant drugs, and vice versa, or to relieve psychotic symptoms such as hallucinations and intense anxiety. Unfortunately, another class of barbiturate abusers is found among medical personnel (physicians, nurses, and pharmacists), who, because of the easy availability of these substances, frequently come to rely on them as hypnotics or as sedatives in time of stress (Berger and Tinklenberg, 1977).

Barbiturate Toxicity, Tolerance, Physical Dependence, and Withdrawal Effects

Aside from the inadvisability of treating chronic insomnia or anxiety states symptomatically with drugs, barbiturate toxicity, tolerance, drug dependence, and withdrawal effects present serious dangers to chronic users of these substances and to those who self-medicate or use the drugs for frivolous purposes.

It is estimated that there are 1500 deaths annually and six or seven times as many sublethal poisonings in the United States directly involving barbiturates taken alone or in combination with other CNS depressants such as alcohol. Moreover, there are significant risks associated with sublethal doses that cause drowsiness, decreased mental acuity, and decreased coordination

and that contribute to accident proneness. Other toxic effects include impaired judgment, confusion, decreased emotional control, euphoria, or depression. Neurological signs include slurred speech, ataxia, and nystagmus. After ingestion of large toxic amounts, there is deep stupor, coma, or death. There are no fast-acting antidotes to the toxic effects of barbiturates, and because pulmonary, cardiovascular, and renal functions are all depressed, the rapidity with which life-threatening events can overtake the patient require immediate intensive emergency room efforts to support vital functions. In contrast, overdoses of opiates can readily be reversed by opiate antagonists such as naloxone. Thus potentially dangerous situations can be more easily averted (Berger and Tinklenberg, 1977).

Tolerance to barbiturates is a well-recognized phenomenon, and it is directly related to drug dependence. DRUG TOLERANCE is defined as a progressively decreased responsiveness to a drug. Thus, a person seeking a drug's effects must increase the dosage with continued use. DRUG DEPENDENCE, on the other hand, is a condition in which an individual requires the drug to function normally. This condition becomes evident when the drug is withheld, and withdrawal effects or an abstinence syndrome ensues, which can be terminated by readministration of the drug. The relationship between drug tolerance and drug dependence emerges when tolerance leads to increased drug intake, which then results in the abstinence syndrome when the drug is suddenly withheld. The term "drug dependence" as used here (and sometimes referred to as addiction) is to be differentiated from "drug dependence" that is defined as the desire to use drugs for their hedonic effects. In the hedonic sense, one can be dependent upon television, and the removal of this mode of diversion can make one irritable and unhappy. But abstinence from watching television is not very likely to be directly responsible for life-threatening physiological effects. This type of dependence is better known as PSYCHIC DEPENDENCE or HABITUATION (Harris and Balster, 1970).

Tolerance to barbiturates is of three types: drug disposition tolerance, pharmacodynamic tolerance, and acute tolerance. DRUG DISPOSITION TOLERANCE results from the drug-induced induction of metabolizing enzymes in the liver. When more enzymes are available, the drug is metabolized at higher rates, thus requiring higher intake to maintain appropriate plasma and tissue levels for effective drug activity. Evidence for this mechanism is found when some animals are pretreated with pentobarbital or secobarbital for a few days and then injected with a hypnotic dose of the drug. These animals will sleep less than animals that are not pretreated, yet the blood plasma levels at the time of awakening for both groups are the same. This shows that the drug is metabolized faster in the animals of the pretreated group because the waking plasma level occurs earlier in the pretreated group.

Cross tolerance is conferred upon other substances because the enzymes involved in barbiturate biotransformation are not solely specific for barbiturates and frequently result in more rapid detoxification of other more or less related substances. Some barbiturates are not greatly affected by liver enzymes but are largely excreted unchanged by the kidney. Thus, drug disposition tolerance is of little effect here. It is estimated that 65–90 percent of injected barbital is removed from the blood by renal clearance, whereas only 30 percent of phenobarbital is cleared this way.

TISSUE TOLERANCE or PHARMACODYNAMIC TOLERANCE also occurs with barbiturates. This type of tolerance refers to the fact that the blood plasma level of barbiturates may remain the same after repeated doses of the same strength, but the drug effects may be significantly lower or even absent. Parenthetically, it should be noted that while drug disposition and tissue tolerance lead to reduced drug effects, the size of the lethal dose is not altered (Sharpless, 1970; Harvey, 1975). This is explained by the fact that tolerance does not occur to all of the effects of barbiturates. Whereas tolerance to the sedative effect does increase, the respiratory centers do not become tolerant to the presence of the drugs. Thus, if a person increases barbiturate doses to maintain a wanted state of sedation, he increases the risk that the blood levels of the drug may reach the lethal level as far as the respiratory centers are concerned.

Explanations for tissue tolerance are somewhat tentative, but a few possibilities seem reasonable. One is that the drug–receptor interaction induces effects that are antagonized or compensated by changes that occur in other biochemical pathways, or there may be changes in the drug receptors themselves—either changing their number or their sensitivity to the drug. There is a sizable body of evidence in support of these hypotheses, but more work is needed for a generally acceptable view (Goldstein et al., 1974).

Finally barbiturates exhibit an ACUTE TOLERANCE effect or TACHYPHYLAXIS. This is illustrated by the finding that the plasma concentration at the time of awakening from a single barbiturate dose depends directly upon the dose of administration. That is, the larger the dose of administration, the higher the plasma concentration at the time of recovery of consciousness. Thus, the CNS appears resistant to the drug effects even after a single dose (Sharpless, 1970; Harvey, 1975).

The onset of drug tolerance is determined in large part by the doses and the persistence of use, but for many years it was not known what a safe barbiturate regimen was with respect to tolerance and dependence. As early as 1905, Kress reported withdrawal symptoms following abstinence after sustained use of barbital (Veronal). However, it was not until 1950 that Isbell and his co-workers reported results of controlled studies on the parameters of barbiturate tolerance and dependence (Isbell, 1950; Isbell et al., 1950; Fraser et al., 1958). Their research was accomplished at the U.S. Public Health Service Hospital for drug addicts in Lexington, Kentucky. It involved giving human subjects, who were long-term prisoners, large doses of barbiturates for extended periods (92 to 140 days) and then abruptly withdrawing the drugs. The Lexington investigators conducted similar experiments with dogs.

Their general findings, as reported by Essig (1970), were that one dose of 0.4 to 0.7 grams of secobarbital or pentobarbital or 0.9 to 1.2 grams of amobarbital led to drug intoxication. The five subjects tested showed peak sedative effects 30 minutes after secobarbital injection, 45 minutes after pentobarbital injection, and 90 minutes after amobarbital injection. After 2 hours the effect declined, and after 4 hours the subjects seemed fully awake. But this was followed by difficulty in thinking, dysarthria (poorly articulated speech), coarse tremor of the hands, and depressed superficial reflexes. Some became boisterous and silly; others became quiet and depressed.

The five volunteers then were given either of the three drugs in gradually increasing doses every 12 hours over a period of 92 to 140 days. The doses started at 0.2 gram and increased to 1.3 to 1.8 grams for secobarbital and pentobarbital, and 3.0 to 3.8 grams of amobarbital. These doses caused a continuous mild intoxication in most instances; these men were confused to the point of not being able to do ordinary tasks, they were unkempt, their living quarters were untidy, they were irritable, quarrelsome, and aggressive. They staggered, frequently fell, and occasionally did so hard enough to injure themselves. During this period their pulse rate increased about 10 beats per minute, but most vital signs and blood chemistry appeared normal.

After the last dose of the drug, there was an interval of 12 to 16 hours when the subjects seemed to "sober up." Then they became anxious and weak with increasing severity until at 24 to 36 hours they could hardly stand or walk unassisted. Their blood pressure dropped, causing them to feel faint on standing. There was tremulousness, muscular fasciculations, anorexia, vomiting, abdominal distress, mydriasis, hyperreflexia, insomnia, weight loss, and increased startle responses to auditory and visual stimuli.

What was more significant was the appearance of generalized convulsions and/or the onset of a reversible psychosis. It was noted that the time course for the

onset of convulsions was quite variable—some occurred between the thirtieth and thirty-ninth hour after withdrawal—and the latest convulsion occurred as late as the one hundred fifteenth hour of abstinence. Other investigators found abstinence convulsions as early as 16 hours after abstinence and as late as the eighth day. Wikler (1968) studied the effects of barbiturate withdrawal after daily treatment of increasing doses for 6 weeks or more. His results are summarized in Table 2.

The psychotic episodes began between the third and fifth day and lasted as long as 9 days. These symptoms were similar to those of alcohol-induced delirium tremens and were characterized by agitation, insomnia, confusion, disorientation of time and place, delusions, and auditory and visual hallucinations. Body temperature was elevated; rapid pulse rate and the appearance of exhaustion was evident. The delirium

TABLE II Barbiturate Abstinence Syndrome

Clinical phenomenon	Incidence[1]	Time of onset[2]	Duration	Remarks
Apprehension	100%	1st day	3–14 days	Vague uneasiness, or fear of impending catastrophe.
Muscular weakness	100%	1st day	3–14 days	Evident on mildest exertion.
Tremors	100%	1st day	3–14 days	Coarse, rhythmic, nonpatterned, evident during voluntary movement, subside at rest.
Postural faintness	100%	1st day	3–14 days	Evident on sitting or standing suddenly. Associated with marked fall in systolic and diastolic blood pressure and pronounced tachycardia
Anorexia	100%	1st day	3–14 days	Usually associated with repeated vomiting.
Twitches	100%	1st day	3–? days	Myoclonic muscular contractions; or spasmodic jerking of one or more extremities. Sometimes bizarre patterned movements.
Seizures	80%	2nd–3rd day	8 days	Up to a total of 4 grand mal episodes, with loss of consciousness and postconvulsive stupor.
Psychoses	60%	3rd–8th day	3–14 days	Usually resemble "delirium tremens"; occasionally resemble schizophrenic or Korsakoff syndromes; acute panic states may occur.

[1]Data are based on 19 cases of experimental addiction to barbiturates. Four developed seizures without subsequent psychoses, one exhibited delirium without antecedent seizures. Three escaped both seizures and delirium.
[2]After abrupt withdrawal of secobarbital or pentobarbital following chronic intoxication at dose levels of 0.8 to 2.2 gm/day taken orally for 6 weeks or more.

(From Wikler, 1968)

tended to occur after the convulsions, and either pattern could occur alone or together. These were the life-threatening aspects of the abstinence syndrome.

Diagnosis and Treatment of Barbiturate Abuse

Phenobarbital is frequently used in the diagnosis and treatment of barbiturate abuse. A suspected patient is given an oral dose of 60 mg of the drug and the reaction indicates the degree of barbiturate tolerance that has developed. If the patient, 1 hour after ingestion, is asleep or grossly intoxicated, the tolerance level is minimal and withdrawal symptoms will be mild. If the patient is comfortable, has normal speech, has no ataxia, and shows only a fine lateral nystagmus, the tolerance level is moderate, and withdrawal symptoms can be prevented with 200–300 mg of phenobarbital per day. A patient with strong or high levels of tolerance will show no response to the 60-mg test dose and may even show withdrawal effects. These patients require 300–500 mg of phenobarbital daily to prevent withdrawal symptoms. After establishing the level of tolerance that has developed, the phenobarbital dose is gradually reduced by approximately 30 mg every other day until the patient is drug free. This treatment is supplemented by psychotherapy to forestall a return to drug abuse.

Clinical Use of Barbiturates

Despite the grim aspects of barbiturate use described in the preceding section, barbiturates continue to be used to treat epilepsy, to alleviate anxiety, and to promote sleep. When used judiciously by the oral route, some are quite effective, and users are relatively safe from the dangers of both overdose and addiction. The drug most commonly used to manage some forms of epilepsy and neurotic anxiety is phenobarbital, a drug with a slow onset and a long duration of action. These features make it difficult to obtain a quick subjective "high," thereby lessening the drug's abuse potential; and its long duration of action reduces its potential for severe withdrawal symptoms. Secobarbital and pentobarbital are frequently prescribed for episodes of insomnia. They are inexpensive and fairly effective. A study done by the Lexington researchers showed that patients that had taken twice the usual sleeping dose every night for a year showed no withdrawal symptoms when the drug was abruptly withdrawn (Adams, 1958). But if these compounds are taken at a dose four or five times the usual daily dose for more than a

month, severe life-threatening withdrawal symptoms can be expected to occur within 2 or 3 days after drug discontinuation (Baldessarini, 1977). These compounds, because of their relatively rapid onset and short duration of action, do have an abuse potential, are frequently used as suicidal agents, or are accidentally ingested with alcohol, with dire consequences.

Barbiturates: Summary

The barbiturates are a class of chemical agents having a long history of use for the treatment of anxiety, insomnia, and epilepsy, with some forms being used for surgical anesthesia. The distinguishing feature between their modes of action can be traced to their lipid solubility and mode and time course of deactivation. Their effects have been shown to be related to the ability of the drugs to depress excitatory postsynaptic potentials (EPSPs) and at fairly high doses to affect or enhance inhibitory postsynaptic potentials (IPSPs). Numerous animal experiments seem to illustrate anxiety-reducing effects of these drugs and support the results found in clinical data. Unfortunately, some barbiturates have a high abuse potential and frequently are the instruments of suicide, unintentional self-poisoning, and drug addiction, with its consequent dangers of injury or death following abrupt abstinence. Consequently these drugs, although clinically useful in many instances, have given way to other drugs that are somewhat safer.

The Propanediols

Mephenesin Carbamate

In the 1940s, chemists at Wallace Laboratories were attempting to modify a phenylglycol ether (a disinfectant) to produce a compound that would kill certain bacteria that are resistant to penicillin. In the course of their work, they came upon the compound mephenesin carbamate (2-hydroxy-3-(tolyloxy) propyl carbamate), a compound that has been known since 1908 (Figure 11). When the Wallace researchers tested it in animals, the drug was found to produce profound muscle relaxation and a sleeplike condition from which the animals could easily be aroused. Larger doses produced ataxia and paralysis from which there was complete recovery.

The mechanism of action was different from that of curare in that the drug did not block the action of acetylcholine at the neuromuscular junction; rather it

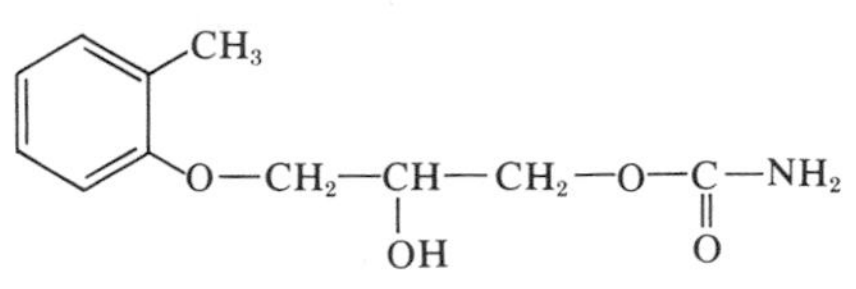

Mephenesin carbamate
(Tolseram)

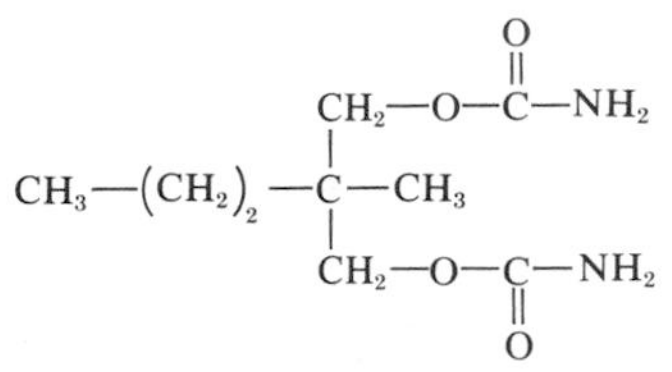

Meprobamate
(Miltown)

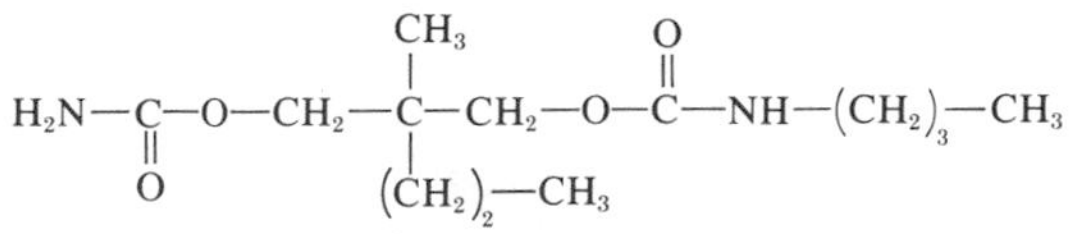

Tybamate
(Solacin)

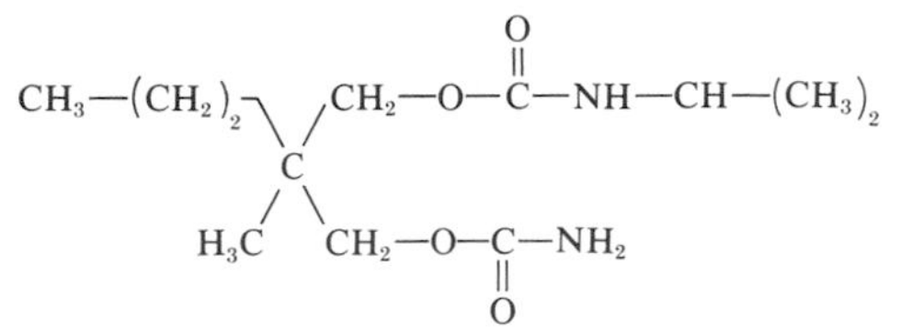

Carisoprodol
(Soma)

FIGURE 11 CHEMICAL STRUCTURES OF SOME PROPANEDIOLS.

acted "within the central nervous system by depressing conductivity in the interneurons." Mephenesin carbamate had a specificity for the polysynaptic neuronal chains involved in spinal reflexes—the more interneurons, the more the depression; and whereas curare caused paralysis of the muscles of respiration, mephenesin carbamate did not do so because the phrenic nerve innervates the diaphragm with no interneurons interposed in the circuit. Mephenesin carbamate, unlike the barbiturates, did not affect the polysynaptic chains in the reticular formation that function in EEG arousal, thus conscious awareness was not significantly affected. The drug also antagonized the effects of strychnine, a glycine receptor blocker. This suggested that the drug is a glycine agonist, increasing spinal interneuronal inhibitory action.

Mephenesin carbamate was introduced as a drug for psychiatric patients and used rather extensively in the late 1940s before the discovery and use of reserpine, chlorpromazine, and other antipsychotic drugs. There were reports that it allayed anxiety without clouding consciousness; that it had a sedative effect in manic-depressive psychosis; that in a deteriorated negativistic schizophrenic it resulted in communication for the first time in years; and that an agitated patient became calm and communicative under the drug. However, the drug was found in practice to be impractical because it was rapidly metabolized in the liver, thus shortening its duration of action and requiring frequent administration or high doses. This led the Wallace researchers to alter the mephenesin carbamate molecule to correct these shortcomings, with the result that meprobamate (MPB) was developed by Ludwig and Piech (1951) (Berger and Ludwig, 1964). For this reason, as well as the then concurrent development of other antipsychotic agents, mephenesin carbamate came to be dropped from the list of useful drugs.

Meprobamate

Pharmacological Effects. Meprobamate (2-methyl-2-propyl-1,3-propanediol dicarbamate; Miltown, named after Milltown, New Jersey, a town near Wallace Laboratories) has muscle relaxant qualities similar to those of mephenesin carbamate but with a slower induction period. The effect is sustained longer, and MPB is more effective when administered orally. It is also more effective than mephenesin carbamate in protecting mice from convulsions and death induced by pentylenetetrazol, strychnine, or electric shock.

Behavioral Effects. MPB had a marked tranquilizing action when tested on monkeys; they lost their fear, hostility, and aggressiveness and became friendly. Yet, they seemed alert and fully in touch with the environment. The sedative effect of MPB on cats and mice was never preceded by the excitement found with barbiturates. MPB (50 or 100 mg/kg) affected neither spontaneous nor coordinated activity in rats whereas amobarbital (20 to 60 mg/kg) significantly affected both. A fearful, catatonic dog became normal and friendly after MPB injection, but not after phenobarbital or reserpine injection. Electric shock-induced or isolation-induced fighting was suppressed in mice by MPB at doses that caused no motor impairment; however, pentobarbital had no effect on the fighting but increased motor agitation. MPB facilitated exploration and acquisition of a maze habit in rats and permitted good retention, whereas pentobarbital had the opposite effect. The drug also counteracted the aggressiveness, irritability, and startle responses of rats with bilateral septal lesions.

In operant conditioning experiments, MPB had effects similar to those of barbiturates with respect to behavior suppressed by punishment (Geller, 1962). In a multiple VI-120/CRF schedule, rats were trained to bar-press for food rewards during both segments, but during the CRF segment (signaled by a 1850-Hz tone) each response that was rewarded with food was also followed by a brief foot shock. Under no-drug conditions, bar-pressing was surpressed during the CRF (punished) segment, but 1 hour after MPB (120 mg/kg) the number of punished responses was substantially increased (Figure 12). A similar effect was obtained with squirrel monkeys using the same dose of MPB (Cook and Catania, 1964).

Electrophysiological Effects. In the brains of animals and man, significant differences were seen between the effects of MPB and those of barbiturates; but what was most significant were the data that appeared to show that MPB could induce a tranquil state without the suppression of the reticular formation that occurred with barbiturates, suggesting that MPB had a uniquely selective action on the CNS in controlling anxiety states. For example, F.M. Berger, the director of the drug's development wrote that because the barbiturates have nonselective actions, they produce significant impairment of intellectual performance, coordination, and perception in doses that may have an anxiolytic effect. He also pointed out that the hypnotic and confusion-producing effects of the barbiturates seriously compromise their usefulness in psychiatry, whereas meprobamate does not suffer from these limitations. Also data were presented that appeared to show a clear superiority of meprobamate (400 mg) over secobarbital (50 mg) on performance tasks such

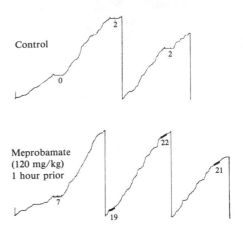

FIGURE 12 MEPROBAMATE EFFECTS ON SHOCK-SUPPRESSED RESPONSES. The numbers indicate the frequency of responses during the CRF/shock periods (3-minute duration) that are separated by 15 minutes of the VI-120 sec schedule. Indications of food rewards during the VI segments are not shown. (From Geller, 1962.)

as tapping speed and pursuit rotor activity; on "mental speed and accuracy" tests such as serial addition tasks; and self ratings of alertness or drowsiness. He emphasized that meprobamate had little or no effect when given to normal subjects, and is primarily effective in patients suffering from anxiety and irritability. In clinically effective doses it does not affect motor, sensory or intellectual performance (Berger, 1962).

The above argument was quite compelling in light of the known abuse potential of the barbiturates in treating anxiety states. In retrospect, it is clear that with arbitrary doses of any drug, one can prove whatever one wants to prove, and the validity of such comparisons would not be acceptable today. In fairness, perhaps, these kinds of errors occurred two decades ago because of the state of the art and the costs and time involved in dose-response studies with clinical patients. In any event, MPB, after being duly licensed, was widely prescribed and sold. "Miltown" became a household word, and in the 1950s and 1960s MPB became one of the most widely used drugs in the world.* Congeners of MPB were developed; among

*In the listing *Psychotropic Drugs and Related Compounds,* Second Edition (1972) prepared by the National Institute of Mental Health (E. Usdin and D.H. Efron, eds.), there were 193 trade names for meprobamate used by foreign drug companies or foreign affiliates of U.S. firms. Almost every nation in the world was represented. Some interesting examples are Calmadin, Edenal, Harmonia, Pan-tranquil, Pensive, Anastress, and Tranquilate.

them were tybamate (Solacin; 2-methyl-2-propyltrimethylene butylcarbamate carbamate), another anxiolytic agent not significantly different from MPB, and carisoprodal (Soma; *N*-isopropyl-2-methyl-2-propyl-1,3-propanediol dicarbamate), which is used primarily as a muscle relaxant (Figure 11). Before long, studies revealed that the uniqueness of MPB was more imagined than real; and numerous reports appeared showing that the drug could be dangerous in that withdrawal symptoms could be life threatening, lethal overdoses could occur, and mixing it with alcohol could be fatal. Moreover, a consensus developed that the mode of action of MPB was not significantly different from that of the barbiturates because there was cross tolerance between MPB and most other CNS depressant drugs (Jarvik, 1970).

At the present time MPB is regarded as having a narrow margin between therapeutic and lethal doses, and MPB is associated with many cases of physical dependence. Also, tolerance can occur rapidly and withdrawal symptoms can be severe. Because withdrawal symptoms can be managed by the substitution of short-acting barbiturates, the similarity in the mode of action of these substances is well established. The MPB congener tybamate requires repeated doses; in some patients it is erratically absorbed, leading to irregular effectiveness (Tinklenberg, 1977). Baldessarini (1977) emphasizes that addiction to meprobamate is well known and can occur after prolonged doses not much greater than the upper limits of recommended doses. The therapeutic range is 1200 to 2400 mg/day; physical withdrawal signs can follow discontinuation of doses as low as 1200 mg/day, and severe signs of withdrawal and seizures can be expected at doses above 3200 mg/day. Therefore, MPB carried an unacceptable risk of addiction and fatality on overdosage. Most physicians no longer prescribe this drug unless the patient has shown a favorable response to safe dosages. In 1970 the Bureau of Narcotics and Dangerous Drugs of the U.S. Government included meprobamate in its list of controlled substances in recognition of its possible danger and abuse potential.

The Benzodiazepines

History of Development

It would be reasonable to assume that the commercial success of a drug can serve as a stimulus to competing members of the pharmaceutical industry to design a similar drug, if not a better one. This was the case with meprobamate, which arrived during the psychopharmacological ferment of the 1950s. The drive to find a competing drug was certainly there, and this drive was no doubt accelerated when the shortcomings of MPB began to appear. This probably led to the development of the benzodiazepines. What was needed was an antianxiety agent that was safe (i.e., free from addictive properties and the ability to cause CNS and respiratory depression and toxic overdose) and effective (i.e., effective in allaying anxiety at doses that were benign in most other respects). Indeed, Leo H. Sternbach, who directed the chemical development of the benzodiazepines, wrote in the introduction of a chapter on benzodiazepine chemistry, "Our interest in tranquilizers started in the mid-fifties shortly after the first representatives of this group of drugs [presumably referring to meprobamate] proved to be of remarkable clinical value. Since we were chemists at heart, we planned to attack this problem completely empirically, considering mainly the chemically attractive features of such an approach. We decided to select a relatively unexplored class of compounds and to prepare novel members belonging to this group, in the hope that some of these products might exhibit the desired pharmacological properties" (Sternbach, 1973). They started work in 1955, and the compounds that were selected for study were some of those that Sternbach had synthesized at the University of Cracow in Poland as a postdoctoral research assistant in the 1930s. These compounds were now selected because they were easily available and were expected to lend themselves to many variations and transformations. The hope was to find reaction products to which could be added side chains that were known to impart biological activity.

However, according to Tinklenberg (1977), the sequence of events went something like this. Sternbach, 20 years after his Cracow experience and now a medicinal chemist at Roche Laboratories, decided to screen the drugs he had synthesized in Poland for biological activity. He first discovered that the compounds were not heptoxdiazines as he had thought, but quinazolone 3-oxides. Sternbach then synthesized 40 derivatives and found that all but one of these were pharmacologically inert. The last one was not tested; instead it was labeled RO-5-0690 and shelved because of other research priorities. In May 1957, during a cleanup of the laboratory, one of Sternbach's chemists turned up the compound and suggested that it be tested. It was given to the Roche pharmacologist team headed by Lowell O. Randall, who subjected the compound to a battery of tests and discovered that it had a number of clinically important properties. RO-5-0690 turned out to be what was first called methaminodiazepoxide and, shortly after, chlordiazepoxide (Figure 13).

Randall and his colleagues (1960) first announced that it had potent sedative, muscle relaxant, taming, and anticonvulsant activity. Soon afterward it was reported that the drug, now given the trade name Librium (from "equilibrium"), had potent antianxiety effects in humans. Others showed that Librium acted almost as a psychostimulant because of the feelings of well-being that led to an increase in social activity, verbal productivity, and appetite, and reduction of anxious depression. The anticonvulsant properties were demonstrated by the drug's ability to increase the threshold to pentylenetetrazol-induced convulsions (Randall and Kappell, 1973).

Within a year, a more potent congener was

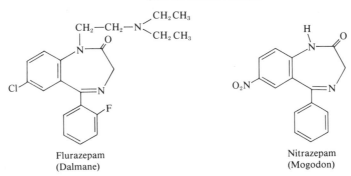

FIGURE 13 CHEMICAL STRUCTURES OF SOME BENZODIAZEPINES.

developed, diazepam (Valium) (Randall et al., 1961). This was followed by oxazepam (Serax), which is a metabolite of diazepam and differed from it essentially by having a shorter plasma half-life than either chlordiazepoxide or diazepam. Nitrazepam (Mogodon) appeared in 1965, and it, like flurazepam (Dalmane), which appeared in 1970, was found to have marked hypnotic properties. The most recent (1969) addition to this class of commercially successful antianxiety agents is clorazepate (Tranxene).

When these drugs ultimately became known to physicians, their popularity was almost instantaneous and their commercial success was assured. Valium and Librium have been among the most prescribed of all kinds of drugs. In 1972 these two substances together accounted for an estimated 49 percent of all psychoactive drug prescriptions in the United States (Blackwell, 1973). Over 100 million prescriptions for these two drugs are filled annually, at a cost of over 500 million dollars. This includes 3 million refills written for Valium each month. In 1977 the newest benzodiazepine (clorazepate, which was claimed to have fewer side effects but to be equal in effectiveness to diazepam) was reported to be selling in the United States at a rate of about 188,000 prescriptions per month (Shader and Greenblatt, 1977). The popularity of these drugs peaked in 1973; then, because of adverse publicity, there was a drop of about 20 million prescriptions per annum over the next five years (Rickles, 1980).

Predictably, the appearance of the benzodiazepines led to a veritable flood of reports of animal experiments, which probably numbered in the thousands and centered on the range and mode of action of these drugs: how they compare with earlier drugs such as the barbiturates and meprobamate in terms of effects, safety, tolerance, and dependence; and how they affect psychological variables other than anxiety, seizures, and muscle tension. Bearing in mind that benzodiazepine effects are not exclusive for this class of drugs, a partial listing of the effects found for the benzodiazepines would include antianxiety effects without sedation, muscle relaxant, and anticonvulsant activity; taming of wild animals and aggressive zoo animals without undue sedation; reduced aggression; increased food consumption; hypothermic effects; prolongation of thiopental-induced hypnosis and the effects of other barbiturates; suppressed rage in animals with septal lesions; reduced defensive hostility and increased socia-

bility of cats; marked muscle relaxation at doses that did not interfere with muscle coordination in cats (the cats hung limply with limbs fully extended when suspended by the scruff of the neck, yet they reacted normally by landing on their feet when dropped from a height); blocking of decerebrate rigidity; increase of behavior suppressed by punishment; increase of response rates for food rewards even at doses that produced ataxia; and nontransfer of stereotypic behavior (i.e., when benzodiazepines were administered during a frustrating insoluble problem, the resulting stereotyped behavior in rats did not transfer to a subsequent soluble problem) (Sternbach et al., 1964; Feldman, 1962; 1968).

By the end of 1966, there were already well over 2300 papers published in the world scientific literature describing the therapeutic (clinical) use of the benzodiazepines. The studies of effects on normal subjects showed that at reasonable doses there were virtually no effects on mental tasks and motor performance whereas the tasks were significantly compromised by ethanol at a dose approximately equal to 3 ounces of whiskey for 150 pounds of body weight. Feelings of well-being and friendliness were seen in male student volunteers. Diazepam caused some apathy, boredom, and lethargy but did not interfere with a motor task. High doses caused ataxia and sleepiness, some euphoria and fatigue. Higher doses caused ataxia and dysarthria. Clinically the drugs were used for psychomotor agitation and anxiety, nervousness, apprehension, and fear.

They were also found to be effective as preanesthetic medications and to reduce anxiety and fear in patients with cancer, stroke, and cardiovascular diseases. They were effective in psychosomatic disorders and those organic diseases with a heavy psychological overlay such as asthma, angina pectoris, irritable colon, gastric ulcers, and skin diseases. The benzodiazepines were used to treat neuromuscular disorders associated with cerebral palsy, multiple sclerosis, hemiplegia, paraplegia, and bone fractures. They were found to be useful in managing different forms of epilepsy, acute alcohol withdrawal symptoms, and neurotic sleep disorders (Zbinden and Randall, 1967).

A comprehensive review of all the literature dealing with these subjects would require many volumes, but we shall later describe a few representative studies and refer the reader to the cited references for further details.

Mechanisms of Action of the Benzodiazepines

As we have seen, the biochemists and pharmacologists have discovered and then improved psychopharmacological agents, but it must be admitted that in many cases the seminal discoveries have been serendipitous. For example, the barbiturates appeared when the acid from apples (malonic acid) was combined for no particular reason with urea; the propanediols were developed while searching for a bactericide and an improved muscle-relaxant; the phenothiazines were discovered while modifying a molecule having an antihistaminic action; and the benzodiazepines were developed from a compound that seemed at one time to be not even worth bothering about. This suggests that for the most part, there is no rational basis for selecting a given compound for a particular psychotherapeutic effect. Of course, once a given molecule is found that provides at least a hint of biological action, changes on the molecule can then be undertaken toward directing the action or improving the effectiveness of the compound. Following the development of an adequate compound, there then begins the search for the physiological mechanisms underlying the drug's effects. These efforts are also coupled with the obvious search for metabolic routes and drug-induced physiological pathologies or side effects.

Three areas of study are rather prominent in the search for the mechanisms of action of psychotropic agents: neurophysiology (study of EEG changes, effects on seizure activity, single cell responses, spinal reflexes, regional effects, i.e., which parts of the brain are affected); biochemical (which neurotransmitter systems are affected and how); and pharmacological (the distribution and metabolic fate of the compounds and actions of metabolites). The early work for the benzodiazepines was very intensive and is reviewed by Sternbach et al. (1964), by Randall et al. (1974), and more recently by Sepinwall and Cook (1978). We shall review only a small portion of this work, believing that our principal purpose here is to present some comparisons between the physiological effects of benzodiazepines and the other anxiolytic agents that we have discussed.

Electrophysiological Studies

The benzodiazepines have significant effects on limbic structures of the CNS. Chlordiazepoxide (CDP) inhibited after-discharges induced by electrical stimulation of the septum, hippocampus, and amygdala. In these experiments the brain structures were electrically stimulated for a few seconds; when the stimulus was shut off, the neurons of these structures continued to fire in unison by themselves. CNS-depressant drugs may prevent the occurrence of the after-discharges or their duration may be shortened. Suppressant effects with CDP occurred at a dose of 10 mg/kg, but the effective dose for meprobamate and phenobarbital was twice as great.

Electrode-implanted, unanesthetized cats were used for simultaneous observations of behavior and electrical activity of the brain. CDP at the low dose of 1.0 mg/kg slowed the frequency of spontaneous electrical activity in the hippocampus and amygdala but not in the septum or cortex. At 5.0 mg/kg, activity in the septum was also depressed but still not in the cortex; there was also some sedation. At 10 mg/kg, there was slowing in all areas, accompanied by sleep. The effects of diazepam were similar to those for chlordiazepoxide, but diazepam was more potent. There was evidence that CDP (10 mg/kg) and diazepam (2.0 mg/kg) exerted depressant effects on the amygdala but stimulant effects on the hippocampus. In contrast, meprobamate and pentobarbital depressed the amygdala, hippocampus, and septum. In studies of the reticular activating system, it was found that low doses of chlordiazepoxide (1.5 to 3.0 mg/kg) produced an activation pattern of the EEG similar to that caused by electrical stimulation of the RAS.

Chlordiazepoxide blocked convulsions induced by pentylenetetrazol and electroshock. After 3.0 mg/kg of chlordiazepoxide, the dose of the convulsant drug had to be increased by sixfold to elicit convulsant patterns in the EEG. Chlordiazepoxide at the same dose blocked the induction and spread of convulsant activity (induced by flashing lights) in the brains of cats sensitized by pentylenetetrazol. We have already discussed the study by Haefely et al., (1975), who showed that flunitrazepam and diazepam were much more potent than phenobarbital and other antiepileptic drugs in blocking seizures induced by the GABA synthesis-blocking drug theosemicarbazide (see Chapter 9).

Investigators used single-cell studies to examine the idea that GABA was the transmitter that was involved in the action of benzodiazepines in the spinal cord, brain stem, cerebellum, substantia nigra, and cortex (Haefely et al., 1975; Haefely, 1977; 1978) (Figure 14). Data indicated that diazepam enhanced GABA-mediated presynaptic inhibition in the spinal cord and that it enhanced GABA-mediated pre- and postsynaptic inhibition in the cuneate nucleus of the brain stem.

The effects of diazepam are the opposite of the depressant effects of picrotoxin and bicuculline, both GABA antagonists (see Chapter 9). Furthermore, enhanced inhibition with benzodiazepines occurred without depression of synaptic excitation, in contrast to the action of barbiturates.

Diazepam depressed spontaneous firing rates of Purkinje cells of the cerebellum, presumably by enhancing the GABA-mediated inhibition of these cells by the basket and stellate cells of the cerebellum. In contrast, convulsant drugs such as thiosemicarbazide (a GABA synthesis blocker) and picrotoxin and pentylenetetrazol (which impede GABA activity) increase the firing rate of Purkinje cells, effects that can be prevented by diazepam.

GABAergic fibers run from the caudate nucleus to the substantia nigra and act as a monosynaptic negative feedback mechanism to depress the firing of the

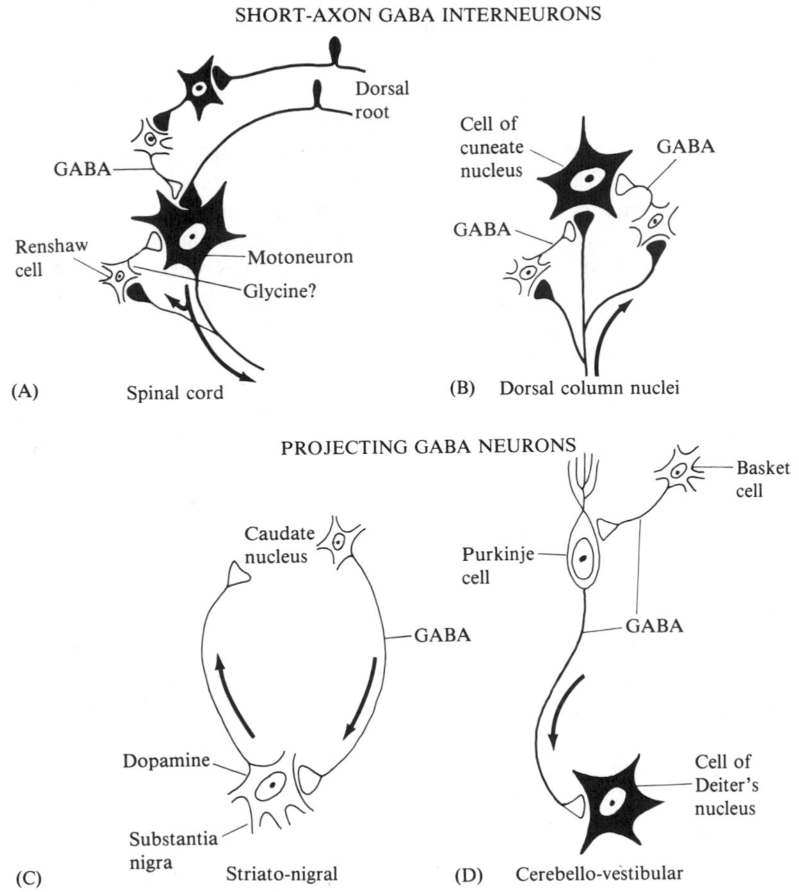

FIGURE 14 BENZODIAZEPINES FACILITATE GABA-MEDIATED SYNAPTIC INHIBITION. (A) GABA exerts a presynaptic inhibitory effect upon primary sensory neurons for touch or proprioception in a dorsal root fiber participating in a spinal reflex. The reciprocal inhibition exerted by the Renshaw cell is mediated by glycine and is not affected by benzodiazepines. (B) GABAergic interneurons exert presynaptic and postsynaptic inhibitory influences on cells of the cuneate nucleus (CN) to modify sensory impulses for touch and proprioception that project to the thalamus. (C) GABAergic fibers project from the caudate nucleus to the substantia nigra to inhibit the dopaminergic cells whose fibers project back to the caudate nucleus. (D) GABAergic fibers from the basket cells of the cerebellum inhibit the Purkinje cells, and the Purkinje cells exert effects upon cells of Deiter's nucleus associated with the vestibular system. These latter effects are depressed by the GABA antagonist picrotoxin, an effect that is reversed by the benzodiazepines. (After Haefely, 1978.)

dopaminergic fibers that run in the opposite direction. Picrotoxin causes an increase in the turnover and *in vivo* release of dopamine in the caudate nucleus as a result of the blockade of the inhibitory GABA-mediated feedback pathway; this effect is also blocked by diazepam. However, the effect might be due to the hypothermic effects of diazepam. In another study, Haefely et al. (1975) found that the peak-to-peak amplitude of evoked potentials in the substantia nigra induced by electrical stimulation of the caudate nucleus was depressed by bicuculline but not by diazepam alone. However, the diazepam dose (3.0 mg/kg) did weaken the effect of the doses of bicuculline given 2 hours later. Neuroleptics such as phenothiazines and haloperidol cause an increase in dopamine turnover in the substantia nigra. This effect occurs because the neuroleptics block dopamine receptors, and by some kind of feedback system (possibly involving presynaptic autoreceptors) the dopamine neurons produce more neurotransmitter to overcome the block. Benzodiazepines antagonize this process, presumably by enhancing the GABAergic feedback system that inhibits dopamine neuron activity. Similar effects occur in the hippocampus—GABA-mediated recurrent inhibition of hippocampal pyramidal cells is enhanced by benzodiazepines; and in functionally isolated cortex, diazepam enhances GABAergic inhibition. All of these studies explain many of the clinical effects of benzodiazepines and point to the important role played by GABA in these processes.

Benzodiazepine Effects on Neuromuscular Functions

To understand the muscle relaxant effects of the benzodiazepines, the drugs' effects on reflex activity and muscular spasticity were studied (Randall and Kappell, 1973). It was found that benzodiazepines were more potent in blocking spinal reflexes in anesthetized cats than were meprobamate and phenobarbital. The benzodiazepines were also more potent than meprobamate in blocking decerebrate rigidity, the type of spasticity of the antigravity muscles seen after damage to the cerebral cortex.

In rotarod tests of motor coordination, the effective dose (ED50) of benzodiazepines (the dose that caused 50 percent of the mice to fall off a rotating rod) was the same for an oral dose of chlordiazepoxide and phenobarbital (31 mg/kg); but eight other benzodiazepines were from 5 times (for diazepam and flurazepam) to 310 times (for flunitrazepam) more po-

tent than phenobarbital (31 mg/kg). Moreover, the lethal dose for 50 percent of the mice (LD50) ranged from 17 times (for chlordiazepoxide) to 20,000 times (for flunitrazepam) greater than the ED50 dose for either drug, whereas the ratio was only 7.8 to 1 for phenobarbital. Also, in tests of muscle-relaxant activity in cats, the potency of benzodiazepines was from 12.5 times (medazepam) to 2500 times (flunitrazepam) more potent than that of phenobarbital; and the lethal dose ranged from 100 times (chlordiazepoxide) to 20,000 times (clonazepam) the effective dose for muscle relaxation, whereas the ratio for phenobarbital was only 2 to 1 (Randall and Kappell, 1973). This illustrates the greater safety factor of the benzodiazepines compared to that of a drug even as safe as phenobarbital.

In the 1960s, the understanding of the mechanism of action of the benzodiazepines on these phenomena was impeded by the physiological complexity of spinal reflexes (Zbinden and Randall, 1967). More recently the effects of benzodiazepines on amino acid transmitters has been better understood, and these interactions now provide a basis for understanding the drug effects on neuromuscular systems.

As we have seen, the fact that benzodiazepines were potent blockers of convulsant drugs that act by blocking GABA synthesis seems to have provided clues to the many researchers who established the relationship between benzodiazepine and GABA effects. It now appears that the diazepam-induced enhancement of GABA-mediated presynaptic inhibition in the spinal cord and the brain stem and the enhanced GABA-mediated effects in the striatonigral pathway, the cerebellum, and the cerebral cortex are directly related to the antispastic and anticonvulsant effects of the benzodiazepines and thus explain the muscle relaxant effects of these drugs.

Benzodiazepine–GABA Interactions

Much is known about the precise way that benzodiazepines interact with GABA synapses, but there are still unanswered questions. First of all, benzodiazepines do not seem to act directly upon GABAergic receptors because the drugs neither produce the same effects nor compete with GABA receptors in the same way as does the GABA-mimetic muscimol; neither do they interfere with high affinity binding of [^{3}H]bicuculline at GABA-receptors. Benzodiazepines do not inhibit neuronal or glial uptake of GABA, but they may increase the sensitivity of neuronal membranes to the effects of GABA or increase the amount of GABA release by an action potential. There is evidence to show that calcium-induced, but not potassium-induced, release of GABA was enhanced by a high concentration of diazepam. In any case, the benzodiazepines exert their effects only in the presence of endogenous GABA during the activity of GABA-ergic neurons. This is borne out by the finding that presynaptic inhibition induced by diazepam is abolished when GABA synthesis is blocked by thiosemicarbazide or isoniazid. Also, diazepam does not mimic the action of GABA when added *in vitro* to isolated cerebellar Purkinje cells (Haefely, 1977).

The enhancing effect of benzodiazepines is most prominent when the GABA effect on postsynaptic receptors is submaximal, for example, in the presence of pentylenetetrazol or picrotoxin (Hafely, 1977). To account for the effect of benzodiazepines in counteracting the convulsant effect of drugs that block GABA synthesis such as thiosemicarbazide it has been proposed that diazepam may release GABA from stores that are not immediately available for release by nerve impulses (Costa et al. 1975). However, as already mentioned, thiosemicarbazide has many effects, and it will induce convulsions even when GABA levels are maintained at normal levels. It is possible, on the other hand, that measurement of brain levels of GABA may reflect glial stores that are not available for neuronal action, thus accounting for convulsions in the presence of seemingly adequate supplies of GABA. Whether benzodiazepines are capable of releasing glial GABA to block convulsions has not been established.

Brain-Specific Benzodiazepine Receptors

The ultimate elucidation of the mechanism of action of most drugs depends upon the knowledge of where a drug binds to a specific receptor and of whether it activates or blocks the receptor to induce or prevent changes in subcellular components such as enzymes or ionophores of the cell. Recent studies have shown that benzodiazepines bind with high affinity to receptors that appear to be exclusively found within the central nervous system.

Binding Properties of Benzodiazepines

The central binding of [^{3}H]diazepam was found to be highly specific, with low nonspecific binding (7 to 9 percent). The specific binding was saturable, indicating a finite number of receptor sites. Maximal binding occurred at 50 nM of [^{3}H]diazepam, with no additional effect with higher concentrations (Squires

and Braestrup, 1977). Inhibition of central [^{3}H]diazepam binding occurs only with other benzodiazepines, whose potencies in this regard correlate well with their clinically important and other pharmacological properties. Moreover, there was no IC50 (inhibition by 50 percent) for [^{3}H]diazepam binding at 3.4 nM by 19 amino acids at 0.1 mM concentration, nor, at the same concentration, by any neurotransmitter or any of their many agonists and antagonists; nor by endogenous compounds, for example, ATP, cAMP, prostaglandins, peptides such as enkephalins, and riboflavin (vitamin B$_2$); nor by numerous centrally active drugs such as phenothiazine and butyrophenone antipsychotics, antidepressants, convulsants and anticonvulsants, ethanol, phosphodiesterase inhibitors, barbiturates, propanediols, opiates and their antagonists, reserpine, and cholinergics (Table 3). Also, tests of stereospecificity of benzodiazepine binding showed that the *d* (+) enantiomers of two benzodiazepines had a 120- to 220-fold higher displacing potency than their respective pharmacologically weak *l* (−) enantiomers. Thus, binding and pharmacological potency showed parallel stereospecificity (Mohler and Okada, 1977b; Mackerer et al., 1978; Braestrup and Squires, 1978).

There was no diazepam binding in skeletal muscle or intestine, but kidney, liver, and lung showed some specific binding that differed from brain binding by having a significantly lower affinity, which was associated with a mitochondrial rather than a membrane fraction. Displacement studies with other benzodiazepines showed no correlation with clinical potency; therefore peripheral binding was clearly pharmacologically different from central binding (Braestrup and Squires, 1977). Earlier studies have shown that benzodiazepines have only weak, if any, effects upon the peripheral autonomic nervous system; consequently, typical anticholinergic effects such as blood-pressure changes, tachycardia, dry mouth, blurred vision, difficulties of urination, and constipation are rarely observed (Zbinden and Randall, 1967). These findings are now seen as being in agreement given the absence of benzodiazepine receptors on autonomically innervated structures.

Distribution of Benzodiazepine Binding Sites

Within the CNS, binding of benzodiazepines is not evenly distributed. In humans (Braestrup et al., 1977) and rats (Braestrup and Squires, 1977; Squires and Braestrup, 1977; Mackerer et al., 1978), binding was

TABLE III Chemical Compounds That Do Not Significantly Inhibit [³H]Diazepam Binding

Amino Acids

L-α-alanine	L-glutamate	L-leucine	L-threonine
β-Alanine	Glycine	L-lysine	L-tryptophan
L-arginine	Glycylglycine	L-phenylalanine	L-tyrosine
L-aspartate	L-histidine	L-proline	L-valine
L-cysteine	L-isoleucine	L-serine	

Endogenous compounds

Acetylcholine	Dopamine	Melatonin	Serotonin
ADP	Epinephrine	Met-enkephalin	Taurine
ATP	GABA	Norepinephrine	Thiamine
Bufotenine	GDP	Prostaglandin E₂	Urea
Cyclic AMP	GTP	Riboflavin	Uric acid
L-dopa	Histamine		

Psychotropic agents

Aminopyrine	Doxepin	Methocarbamol	Phenobarbital
Amitriptyline	Ethanol	α-Methyldopa	Phenoxybenzamine
Apomorphine	Ethosuximide	Methysergide	Physostigmine
Atropine	Etorphine	Molindone	Picrotoxin
Bicuculline	Haloperidol	Morphine	Pimozide
Caffeine	Harmaline	Muscimol	Propanolol
Carbamazepine	Imipramine	Nalorphine	2-Pyrrolidone
Clozapine	Isoniazid	Naloxone	Reserpine
Carisoprodol	Meprobamate	Pentobarbital	Strychnine
Chlorpromazine		Pentylenetetrazole	Theophylline
Diphenylhydantoin			Tolbutamide
			Yohimbine

(Sources: Mohler and Okada, 1977a; Squires and Braestrup, 1977; Mackerer et al., 1978; Chang and Snyder, 1978; Braestrup and Squires, 1978)

highest in the cerebral cortex, hippocampus, and cerebellum. Binding was lowest in the spinal cord, with an intermediate distribution in the midbrain, hypothalamus, corpus striatum, and medulla-pons (Williamson et al., 1978).

Cellular fractionation studies showed that benzodiazepine binding was highest in the synaptosomal component (Mackerer et al., 1978). Mohler and Okada (1977a) reported that cell fractions enriched in synaptic membranes accounted for 70 percent of [³H]diazepam binding in intact synaptosomes and that there was no uptake into brain cells of cortical slices at low concentrations. These data all suggest a site of action of the benzodiazepines on the neuron surface and not within the cell, as was the case with peripheral binding (see earlier).

Comparisons of the Binding and Pharmacological Activity among Benzodiazepines

If the [³H]diazepam binding sites are truly involved

in the behavioral effects induced by the benzodiazepines, it would be expected that their pharmacological potency *in vivo* would parallel their *in vitro* binding affinities for these receptors. The pharmacological activity, as measured in tests described by Zbinden and Randall (1967) and Randall and Kappell (1973), was correlated for 10 to 20 1,4-benzodiazepines with their relative ability to displace [³H]diazepam binding in rat or human particulate homogenates of brain tissue (Braestrup et al., 1977; Mohler and Okada, 1977a; Squires and Braestrup, 1977; Mackerer et al., 1978). Inhibition of [³H]diazepam binding was very closely correlated with benzodiazepine potency with respect to:

1. The antagonism of pentylenetetrazol-induced convulsions in mice.
2. Antiaggressive activity in fighting mice.
3. Impairment of mouse rotorod performance (a test of coordination).

4. The performance of squirrel monkeys in a conditioned avoidance test.
5. Muscle relaxant activity in the cat.
6. Antimaximal electroshock activity in the mouse (Mackerer et al., 1978); a test for electroshock-induced convulsions).
7. The clinical potency in man.

Binding inhibition was poorly correlated with:

1. The taming action on cynomolgus monkeys.
2. Conditioned avoidance in rats.
3. The inhibition of electroshock-induced convulsions in mice (Mohler and Okada, 1977a). The difference in this finding from the finding listed in 6 above may be explained by the various ways of compensating for differences in drug concentrations.

Of utmost importance here in the interpretation of these data is the validity of these behavioral tests in the prediction and determination of clinical effectiveness in man. Perhaps the most valid assessment of the pharmacological–biochemical relationship was obtained from human brain (Braestrup et al., 1977). When the clinical effectiveness of the drugs was expressed in terms of the recommended daily dosages, a correlation with binding potency suggested that the benzodiazepine receptor action *in vitro* is involved in *in vivo* drug actions.

Benzodiazepine Receptor Actions

Various neurotransmitters have been implicated at one time or another in the mediation of benzodiazepine-induced behavioral changes. At present the preponderance of evidence supports the contention that facilitation of GABAergic transmission is the essential property of benzodiazepines that is responsible for the clinical efficacy. Other transmitters have been found to undergo changes, but in most cases the effects seem to be secondary to drug–GABA interactions.

The precise molecular mechanism of action by which benzodiazepines modify GABAergic activity may now be more clearly established. Mao et al. (1975) showed that the diazepam-induced decrease in cerebellar cyclic GMP content is dependent on the continuous presence of GABA. Cyclic GMP levels in the cerebellum increase when afferents to the cerebellum are stimulated. GABA-mediated blockade of this activity causes a drop in cGMP levels. Isoniazid-induced inhibition of glutamate decarboxylase (GAD) depletes brain GABA and increases cGMP levels in the cerebellum. Therefore, cGMP can serve as a marker for GABA activity in the cerebellum (Mao et al., 1975). When GABA levels were reduced by more than 30 percent, diazepam was unable to block the increase in cGMP, indicating that benzodiazepines by themselves have no GABA-mimetic activity. The necessary presence of GABA suggests either an enhancement of presynaptic release or an indirect activation of postsynaptic receptors by benzodiazepines. The former theory was ruled out by Olson et al. (1978) because their *in vitro* studies showed that benzodiazepines do not act upon presynaptic receptors and do not increase the amount of GABA released in response to action potentials. Also, the benzodiazepines do not increase GABA turnover (MacDonald and Barker, 1978).

Because benzodiazepines are not GABA agonists and because they do not induce presynaptic release, Costa et al. (1978) investigated the possibility of a benzodiazepine-sensitive regulatory process for the affinity of GABA for its receptors. They proposed that GABA receptors are supramolecular units comprising a chloride ionophore, the GABA molecule itself, and a GABA recognition site. The recognition site can be in one of two kinetic states, that is, with either a high or a low affinity for GABA molecules. When the recognition site is in the high-affinity state, GABA molecules are able to interact with the ionophores, the consequence being a GABAergic response with a resultant decrease in cerebellar cGMP.

Support for this model comes from the fact that two types of crude synaptic membranes could be prepared from rat cerebral or cerebellar cortex. Type B (freshly prepared) had one type of receptor having a low affinity for binding [^{3}H]GABA in a Na$^+$-free medium. (A Na$^+$-free medium is employed to avoid confounding the result with Na$^+$-dependent presynaptic uptake.) Type A was obtained by additional treatments of type B membranes: several freeze–thaw steps followed by treatment with the detergent Triton X-100. This procedure disrupts the membrane and washes away any water-soluble protein that might be adhering to the lipid membrane. After this treatment, the type A membrane had two populations of receptors: one with a high affinity and the other with a low affinity for [^{3}H]GABA binding.

To investigate the possibility that type B membranes contained an endogenous inhibitor of the high-affinity GABA-binding sites found in type A preparations, various amounts of the supernatant buffer obtained by centrifuging a suspension of type B membranes were added to type A membranes. The type B supernatant fluid inhibited in a dose-related fashion the high-affinity [³H]GABA binding to type A membranes.

The supernatant fluid of type B membranes was then purified 500-fold. Less than one unit (0.33 μg) of the purified protein, having a molecular weight of approximately 15,000, completely abolished the high-affinity Na⁺-independent binding of GABA when added to type A preparations. It also changed the low-affinity binding to a still lower level. Thus, there appears to be an endogenous inhibitor of GABA that occupies sites that regulate GABA receptors.

Costa et al. (1978) further investigated the interaction of this protein with benzodiazepines. Diazepam (7×10^{-7} M) and the pharmacologically active (+) enantiomer of RO-113128 (10^{-7} M) reversed the inhibition of the high-affinity [³H]GABA binding caused by the endogenous protein inhibitor (2.5 μg). Diazepam failed to reverse the activity of 40 units (13.2 μg) of inhibitor, and the pharmacologically inactive (−) isomer of RO-113624 was unable to antagonize the endogenous protein inhibitor. It was also found that this protein inhibitor competitively inhibited [³H]diazepam binding to type A membranes.

From these findings it was seen that diazepam competes with the endogenous protein inhibitor* isolated from type B membrane preparations for the regulatory site of GABA receptors. When the site was occupied by the endogenous inhibitor, the affinity of GABA receptors for GABA molecules was maximally reduced. When diazepam occupied the regulatory site, the affinity was enhanced. Thus, the receptor site for this endogenous protein inhibitor was probably the binding site for pharmacologically active benzodiazepines. It was not known at the time if the regulatory binding sites are located adjacent to GABA synapses or in other neuronal or glial membranes where they may regulate other brain processes (Figure 15).

Later experiments verified the foregoing developments and restated the conclusions that now say that there are two types of GABA receptors designated as GABA₁ (low affinity) and GABA₂ (high affinity), corresponding to the former type B and type A receptors, respectively. These two receptors together with an endogenous regulating protein (GABA-modulin), recognition sites, and the chloride ionophore make up a supramolecular postsynaptic membrane complex, part of which binds to benzodiazepine molecules. It is

*Now called GABA-modulin (Baraldi et al., 1979).

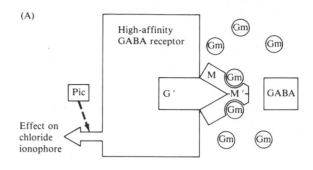

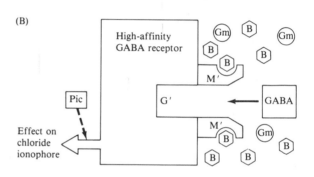

FIGURE 15 HYPOTHETICAL GABA RECEPTOR COMPLEX. The large rectangle represents a high affinity GABA receptor with G′ as its receptor site. Attached to the receptor is a satellite receptor M for GABA-modulin (Gm). When GABA-modulin binds to its receptor sites M′ the receptors (M) move to the position shown in A thereby blocking the GABA receptor site (G′). Benzodiazepine molecules (B) can compete with GABA-modulin for the receptor site M′ but they do not activate the receptor thus leaving the GABA receptor G′ open for GABA binding as shown in B. The picrotoxin molecule (Pic), unlike the benzodiazepine molecule seems to interfere directly with the action of the GABA receptors on chloride conductance channels, thereby blocking the action of benzodizepines.

believed that the benzodiazepines exert their effects by interacting with the regulating protein to effect increased GABA receptor activity and thus enhance GABAergic inhibition of postsynaptic neural elements. It is not yet known whether GABA₁ or GABA₂ receptors are separate entities or transitional states (Guidotti et al., 1979).

Physiological Significance of
Benzodiazepine Binding Sites

Skolnick et al. (1979) initiated a series of experiments in order to obtain information about the physiological significance of specific benzodiazepine receptors in the CNS. This question is similar to the question raised about the significance of opiate receptors in the CNS, which prompted research that culminated with the discovery of endogenous opiate-like substances in the body. The possibility of an endogenous benzodiazepine-like ligand serving as a neurotransmitter was considered. First it was found that rats that had electrically induced seizures showed a 21 percent increase of binding of [³H]diazepam in their brains if they were sacrificed 15 minutes after the seizure, but binding affinity was normal if the animals were sacrificed one hour after the seizure. This effect was found to be due to a rapid increase in the number of receptors rather than in a change in receptor affinity. It was also found that treating GABA receptors with pentylenetetrazol (PTZ) increased benzodiazepine binding. Subconvulsive doses of PTZ had no effect, suggesting that the seizure was necessary for the increase in benzodiazepine receptors. This enhanced binding may explain the marked potency and the rapid therapeutic effect of the benzodiazepines for the treatment of the persistent seizure condition status epilepticus. This physiological response of the receptors to seizure activity again suggests that there is an endogenous ligand that regulates GABA activity to prevent seizures.

A Possible Endogenous
Benzodiazepine-like Ligand

Extracts were made from bovine brain tissue in attempts to find substances that could serve as endogenous ligands of the benzodiazepine receptors. Ultimately inosine and hypoxanthine (which are the respective precursors of the purines adenine and guanine found in DNA and RNA) were found to be weak endogenous inhibitors of [³H]diazepam binding in vitro. When inosine and some of its derivatives were administered intraventricularly to mice challenged by PTZ, they caused a time- and dose-dependent increase in the interval between injection of PTZ and the onset of seizure activity. Thus, these substances showed at least a partial antagonism to the effects of PTZ.

Lippa et al. (1979) reported the discovery of a new, pharmacologically unique substance, CL 218,872—a drug in the class of triazolopyridazines (TPZs)—that

had much stronger inhibitory effects on benzodiazepine binding than inosine and hypoxanthine. This substance was tested on 48-hour food- and water-deprived rats in a chamber that had a spout that delivered a dextrose-water solution. After the rat located the spout, it was allowed 25-seconds of free (no shock) licking. It was then given weak (200 µA) shocks through the drinking spout (5 seconds on-5 seconds off) during the rest of the 5-minute test period. The number of shocks received were recorded. When rats were previously given CL 218,872, diazepam, or chlordiazepoxide (CDP), the number of shocks accepted was increased in a dose-related way for all three drug treatments, showing that CL 218,872 had a potency similar to that of the benzodiazepines (Figure 16).

CL 218,872 was also as potent as diazepam in antagonizing PTZ-induced seizures. But this compound was weak compared to the benzodiazepines in producing motor depression and ataxia that are common side effects of benzodiazepines especially after the early doses. CL 218,872 is quite similar in chemical structure to the purines (Figure 17), and the suggestion is that the endogenous ligand will turn out to be purine-like even though inosine or hypoxanthine may not be the actual ones.

The explanation offered for the lack of the motor depressant and ataxic effects of this and related drugs is that there are two or more brain-specific, benzodiazepine receptors (types I and II). These have been detected in the brains of codfish, rats, mice, and baboons. It seems that the benzodiazepines bind to both types of receptors with almost identical affinities. But evidence shows that the TPZs bind to type I receptors at a much higher affinity than to type II. Thus, several TPZs are active in anticonflict and anti-PTZ effects but produce little sedation or ataxia, and little potentiation of the sedative effects of ethanol or barbiturates. This suggests that anticonflict and anti-PTZ effects are mediated by type I receptors whereas the other effects are mediated by type II receptors (Squires et al., 1979). However, in a drug discrimination experiment, rats that had learned to discriminate CDP (3 mg/kg) from saline in a two-lever Skinner box paradigm for food reinforcement, responded in a dose-dependent manner to the CDP lever when CL 218,872 was substituted for CDP (Figure 18). But, when tested with CL 218,872 at a dose of 10 mg/kg, only 3 of 10 animals responded sufficiently to indicate a preference. The other 7 were mostly inactive during the 10-minute test session. Also, whereas CDP caused

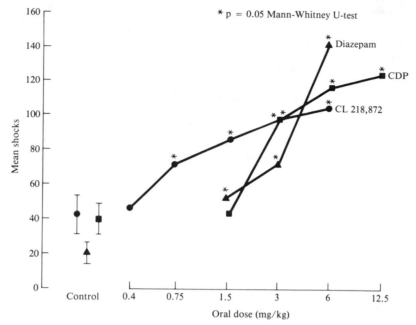

FIGURE 16   EFFECTS OF CL 218,872, DIAZEPAM, AND CHLORDIAZEPOXIDE on punished responding. Each data point represents the mean number of shocks re- ceived by hungry and thirsty rats through a drinking spout during a 5-minute test. See text for details. (From Lippa et al., 1979.)

an increase in the response rate, CL 218,872 did not, and at 10 mg/kg the rats that did respond had a response rate that was only 25 percent of the control rate (McElroy and Feldman, 1982). These doses were comparable to the antianxiety doses reported by Squires et al. (1979) and Lippa et al. (1979).

Because the 10 mg/kg dose of CL 218,872 caused sedation, another test examined the possibility that even lower doses of this drug normally cause sedation. In the tests described above, CL 218,872 was given to rats that had undergone a number of drug discrimination trials with CDP, and it is likely that these rats had developed a tolerance to the sedative effect of CDP (as shown by their increased response rates) and had possibly conferred a cross tolerance to a sedative effect of CL 218,872. Therefore a group of drug naive rats trained to bar press on the same FR-10 schedule as above, was given CL 218,872 (5 mg/kg i.p.) to observe the effect of the drug on the response rate. The result is indicated by the squared data point on the bottom half of Figure 18. It shows that the drug produced a significant decrease in response rate from the control value. Thus, it appears that CL 218,872 and the benzodiaz-

Triazolopyridazines (TPZs)

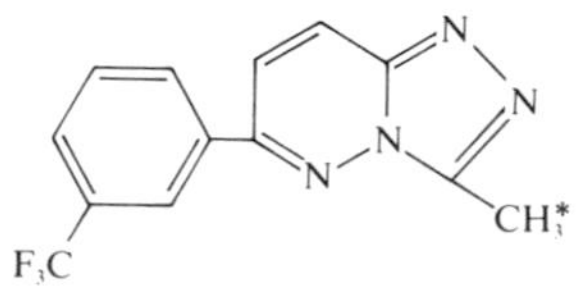

CL 218,872

3-Methyl-6-[3-(trifluoromethyl) phenyl]-1,2,4-triazolo[4,3-b] pyridazine

*Substituting H yields
  CL 218,873

*Substituting CH_2Cl yields
  CL 219,884

FIGURE 17   CHEMICAL STRUCTURE OF TRIAZOLO-PYRIDAZINES.

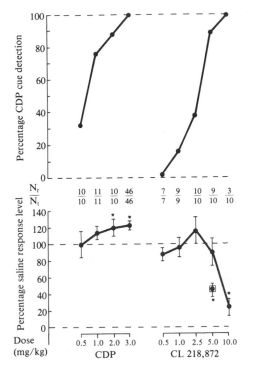

FIGURE 18 GENERALIZATION OF DISCRIMIN-ATIVE STIMULI elicited by chlordiazepoxide (CDP) and CL 218,872. Percentage cue detection refer to the mean percentage of CDP lever selection for 10 animals. The response level refers to the mean ± SEM total response output for 10 minutes expressed as a percentage of saline-control performance. Nr/Nt = number of respondents/number tested. (* = p < 0.05; Wilcoxon test). (From McElroy and Feldman, 1982.)

epines have similar sedative effects in similar dose ranges with possible cross tolerance between them. Perhaps more importantly, there is a question about whether the sedative effect is related to type II receptors, and whether the previously reported specificity of TZPs for type I receptors is significant.

The search for endogenous ligands for benzodiazepine receptors has continued, leading to the isolation of some bioactive compounds with benzodiazepine receptor binding properties from aqueous brain extracts of rats and cattle and from human urine and serum. Some have been characterized as peptides, though they have yet to be fully identified (Marangos et al., 1979; Davis and Cohen, 1980a, 1980b). Experiments have shown that injection of these sub-

stances into the ventricles of rat brains caused behavioral changes similar to those caused by the same treatment with diazepam. This was particularly evident when both diazepam and the putative endogenous ligand disinhibited punished behavior in a Geller conflict test and retarded the onset and lethality of pentylenetetrazol-induced convulsions. In both tests, the ligand and diazepam had similar potencies (Davis et al., 1981).

The demonstrated bioactivity of these compounds strengthens the hypothesis regarding the existence of endogenous benzodiazepine receptor ligands, but, as the above authors pointed out, the limited number of subjects in these experiments and the lack of complete purity of the injected material call for some reservations pending further studies.

Finally, it has been reported that there is a linkage between benzodiazepine effects and the role of calcium–calmodulin in the phosphorylation of membrane proteins. When brain membranes were incubated with diazepam, there was an inhibition of Ca^{2+}–calmodulin-stimulated phosphorylation of several, but not all, major membrane proteins. This selectivity suggested that different protein kinases were affected by the drug. Also, the drug concentrations for these effects are well within the range of plasma concentrations of diazepam that produce clinical effects in man; and the effect was shown to accompany a stereospecific membrane-binding of diazepam, indicating the involvement of a specific benzodiazepine receptor which, however, had a relatively low affinity for benzodiazepines (DeLorenzo, 1982).

Furthermore, there was a high, significant correlation between the pharmacological potencies of benzodiazepines in inhibiting electric shock-induced convulsions and their kinase inhibition potencies. However, there was no correlation between benzodiazepine kinase inhibition potency and benzodiazepine-induced muscle relaxation, inhibition of rotarod performance, inhibition of electric shock-induced fighting and conditioned avoidance, or pentylenetetrazol-induced convulsions. This suggests that other benzodiazepine receptors having higher binding affinities for benzodiazepines mediate these actions. This suggestion is supported by the finding that Ca^{2+}-calmodulin kinase activity was not affected by the GABA antagonists picrotoxin and bicuculline nor by the agnoist muscimol over a wide range of doses. In contrast, conditioned avoidance behavior and shock-induced fighting are usually affected by these drugs. Thus, the foregoing results provide additional evidence for the presence of two or more forms of benzodiazepine receptors, one of which seems to be GABA-independent and whose effects are mediated by the Ca^{2+}-calmodulin system (DeLorenzo et al., 1981).

The Site of Anxiolytic Action of the Benzodiazepines

Lippa et al. (1979) sought for the functional localization of benzodiazepine receptors in the brain. Because the highest concentration of benzodiazepine receptors is in the cerebral cortex, this area was examined first. Food- and water-deprived rats were given various doses of diazepam. Half of the animals were placed in the previously described drinking–conflict test, the other half were sacrificed and their frontal cortices examined for [³H]diazepam binding *in vitro*. As expected, there was a dose-related increase in the number of shocks taken in the conflict test, and the *in vitro* binding test showed a parallel inhibition of diazepam binding, i.e., the higher the *in vivo* dose, the more inhibition of *in vitro* binding. This means that the higher the *in vivo* dose of diazepam, the fewer receptor sites remained available for the subsequent *in vitro* test for [³H]diazepam binding. From these data it could be estimated that only 15 to 20 percent of the available receptors in the frontal cortex were necessary for a significant anticonflict effect.

Obviously these data did not by themselves establish the frontal cortex as the site for the anxiolytic effects of diazepam, but a subsequent experiment showed that rats with lesions in the frontal cortex or rats with knife cuts that isolated the frontal cortex from the rest of the brain, when tested in the drinking–conflict test, took significantly more shocks than nonoperated controls. These data supported the hypothesis of frontal cortex involvement in behavior inhibition that can be affected by the benzodiazepines.

All of these data suggested a model for the role of the frontal cortex in the anxiolytic effects of the benzodiazepines. The frontal cortex, through some unknown mechanism, is capable of behavior inhibition. Benzodiazepines can disinhibit behavior by inhibiting the cells in the frontal cortex that have benzodiazepine-binding receptors. It was also proposed that an endogenous ligand is released when an organism is subjected to anxiety-provoking stimuli, and these ligands

bind to those same sites that selectively bind benzodiazepines. This proposal is supported by the finding that there was a decrease in [³H]diazepam binding in rats subjected to inescapable shocks, which may reflect the release and occupation of the receptor sites by the endogenous ligand, leaving fewer binding sites for [₃H]diazepam (Lippa et al., 1979).

Summary

The discussion of these experiments was meant to provide a comprehensive view of the mechanisms of action of the benzodiazepines. The current view appears to be that these drugs interact with GABA receptors by way of a regulating protein that controls the activity or formation of special receptors having a high affinity for GABA, thus potentiating GABA effects. GABA is a potent inhibiting transmitter that acts upon motor systems, is involved in cortical functions, and, in addition, exerts modulating influences on other transmitter systems (Figure 19). The anticonvulsant and muscle-relaxing effects of the benzodiazepines can be traced to direct GABA effects on the motor systems of the cerebellum, the corpus striatum, and the spinal cord (and probably other systems, which are being studied), whereas the available evidence suggests that the anxiolytic effects, to be discussed later on, are

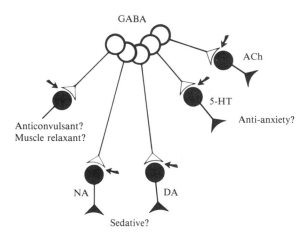

FIGURE 19 LINKS BETWEEN GABA AND OTHER NEUROTRANSMITTER SYSTEMS. Benzodiazepines potentiate the GABA system, which then exerts inhibitory effects on motor systems, the noradrenergic (NA), dopaminergic (DA), serotonergic (5-HT), and cholinergic (ACh) systems. (From Haefely, 1978.)

mediated via GABAergic inhibition of serotonergic systems. The sedative and ataxic effects may be the result of GABAergic influences upon noradrenergic or dopaminergic systems, or possibly may be mediated through different GABA receptors than those mediating anxiolytic effects.

It is also appears that the benzodiazepines represent a fortuitous discovery of substances having properties similar to those of an endogenous neurotransmitter whose function is the redress of neural balance during stress or overexcitation of the CNS. The presence of this transmitter has only been hinted at, but its identity is the object of intensive investigation at the present time. Related to this search is the recent development of drugs like the TPZs, which have the desirable antianxiety and anticonvulsive properties but may be without the sedative and ataxia-producing side effects. These compounds may have important clinical utility.

Phylogenetic and Ontogenetic Appearance of Benzodiazepine Receptors

The evolutionary appearance of benzodiazepine receptors was investigated in 18 vertebrate and 5 invertebrate species by Nielsen et al. (1978). The vertebrate classes included mammals, birds, reptiles, amphibians, bony fishes, and the more primitive jawless fishes. The invertebrates tested included annelids, molluscs, arthropods, and insects. Substantial concentrations of [^{3}H]diazepam receptors were present in the brains of all vertebrates except the hagfish, a primitive jawless agnathan. The highest levels were found in mammals, particularly in small mammals such as the rat, hamster, and mouse, with progressively less found in birds, reptiles, and amphibians. [^{3}H]Diazepam binding was not found in the invertebrates, suggesting that benzodiazepines may not elicit specific pharmacological responses in these species. Phylogenetically, then, the benzodiazepine receptors exhibit a late evolutionary appearance, first appearing in the brain of higher bony fishes, which developed from the more primitive jawless fishes.

Braestrup and Nielsen (1978) investigated the ontogenesis of the benzodiazepine receptor in the rat. Specific [^{3}H]diazepam binding was present 8 days before birth, the earliest time investigated, at 5.2 percent of the adult concentration. At birth the concentration was 35.4 percent of the adult concentration, and adult concentration was reached by the seventh day after birth. The total number of receptors increased steadily, and the maximum number was reached around the third or fourth week.

Benzodiazepine Effects upon Other Transmitter Systems

Effects on Catecholamine and Acetylcholine Systems

There is substantial evidence to indicate benzodiazepines block the turnover of dopamine (DA) in the olfactory tubercules, the nucleus accumbens, and DA in islands in the entorhinal cortex and the caudate nucleus. However, these effects seem to be due to enhanced GABA receptor activity on the dendrites and cell bodies of the DA neurons, thereby reducing the firing rate in the ascending mesolimbic DA pathway (see Figure 7 in Chapter 7). Similar inhibitory effects are found for norepinephrine; and benzodiazepine-induced enhancement of GABA-mediated inhibition of the locus caeruleus seems to be a viable explanation (Fuxe et al., 1975). This mechanism would account for the ability of chlordiazepoxide, diazepam, and nitrazepam to block the increased turnover and depletion of NE that is caused when rats are subject to stressful foot shocks and immobilization (Taylor and Laverty, 1973).

There is evidence that cholinergic systems are also affected within the CNS by benzodiazepines. At the cellular level, it was found that benzodiazepines increased ACh levels in synaptosomes in the guinea pig, mouse, and rat brain and decreased ACh turnover without affecting choline, choline acetylase, or choline esterase activity. All this suggests a blockade of ACh release. There also exists a parallelism between the increase in striatal acetylcholine levels and the duration of the muscle-relaxant action of diazepam in rats. Diazepam (17 μmoles/kg, i.v., or higher) increased ACh levels in hemispheric structures, the striatum, and hippocampus in rats, mice, and guinea pigs. These effects were also attributed to blockade of ACh release. Also the reduced turnover of ACh in the cortex and midbrain caused by diazepam was mimicked by the GABA receptor agonist muscimol. This suggests that a GABA mechanism intervenes in the effects of benzodiazepines on ACh turnover (Guidotti, 1978).

Benzodiazepine-Serotonin Interactions

We have previously mentioned that serotonin turnover was diminished by the benzodiazepines and that this is directly related to the antianxiety effects of these drugs. The question then arises as to whether benzodiazepines act directly upon serotonergic neurons or, as in other cases, is the effect mediated via GABAergic neurons.

Benzodiazepines seem to induce serotonergic effects that may not be dependent upon GABA systems. For example, Chase et al. (1970) found that diazepam had no effect upon uptake but that it did increase the retention of intracisternally injected, radioactively labeled serotonin and its metabolite 5-hydroxyindoleacetic acid (5-HIAA). This suggested that the drug interfered with 5-HT metabolism and transport of 5-HIAA from the brain. Dominic (1973) found that chlordiazepoxide, diazepam, and flurazepam depressed the serotonergic biosynthetic and metabolic pathways in the mouse brain and the effect was more evident in the teldiencephalon than in the brain stem. These effects may not be specific for benzodiazepines because Corrodi et al. (1967a) had found that anesthetic doses of pentobarbital partially blocked the depletion of serotonin in rats that had been pretreated with the 5-HT synthesis inhibitor α-propyldopacetamide. It is possible, however, that these effects may only represent a compensatory effect of GABA-mediated reduction of serotonergic activity.

Wise et al. (1972) compared the changes in NE and 5-HT turnover after a single dose or after multiple daily doses of oxazepam. Groups of rats that received either one dose or six doses of oxazepam (20 mg/kg) were matched to rats that had similar saline injections. Ten minutes before the single or the sixth dose of drug (or saline), each rat received via an indwelling cannula an intraventricular injection of [^{14}C]serotonin and [^{3}H]norepinephrine. Three hours after the injection of the radioisotopes, the animals were killed by decapitation, and the brains were removed and divided into forebrain–diencephalon and midbrain–hindbrain pieces. The radioactivity of the brain sections were ascertained. It was found that after a single dose of oxazepam the total amount of ^{14}C (from 5-HT and metabolites) and ^{3}H (from NE and metabolites) exceeded that of the saline controls in the midbrain–hindbrain regions. After six doses of oxazepam, there were increases only in the ^{14}C levels over that of the saline controls. This was interpreted as follows: There was a drug-induced blockade of 5-HT and NE turnover after one dose of oxazepam; however, after six

doses, tolerance occurred for the NE effect, and NE turnover returned to normal. On the other hand, 5-HT turnover was still depressed. There were no significant changes in monoamine turnover in the diencephalon-forebrain areas. This was consistent with earlier findings that intraventricularly injected serotonin is selectively taken up in the midbrain area containing the cell bodies of 5-HT neurons. Wise and his colleagues, on the basis of an earlier study by Margules and Stein (1968), then attributed the sedative effect of the drug, which does undergo tolerance, to the changes in NE turnover; and the anxiolytic effect of the drug, which persists after repeated dosing, to the persistent depression of 5-HT turnover. A discussion of Margules and Stein's experiment will make this point clear.

In their experiment, rats were trained to respond in a multiple schedule (VI-2 min/CRF) after the design of Geller and Seifter (1960). The rats were drug-naive in that they had never before been treated with benzodiazepines. They were run on the VI-2 min (nonpunished) schedule for milk rewards for 15 minutes, followed by 3 minutes on the CRF (punished) schedule (signaled by a continuous tone), during which each lever-press was followed by a milk reward accompanied by a mild and brief (0.25 second) foot shock. On drug-test days, oxazepam (20 mg/kg, i.p.) was given immediately before the test session, which lasted 72 minutes (four 18-minute cycles). The tests continued for 22 consecutive days. Figure 20 shows the cumulative records for a typical rat. On the control (saline) day, VI (nonpunished) responding was persistent and vigorous, but during the CRF (punished) segment, there was almost no responding. During the first oxazepam test, there was a rapid decline in the VI response rate as the drug took effect, but there was a marked appearance of ten responses during the first CRF segment. Thereafter, on that day, responding during both segments was minimal. On successive days, however, the rates for both nonpunished and punished responding markedly increased until on the fourth day nonpunished responding had almost returned to normal. By the twenty-second day, there was an above-normal rate for nonpunished responses. Meanwhile punished responses had increased from two to over a hundred for a daily session.

It was concluded that oxazepam caused a transient sedative effect marked by depressed response rates, and that oxazepam would probably have increased the rate of punished responding had the effect not been

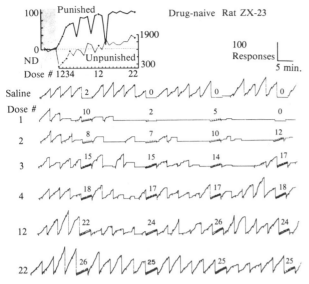

FIGURE 20 OXAZEPAM EFFECTS ON PUNISHED AND UNPUNISHED BEHAVIOR. The graph at upper left shows the daily output of punished and unpunished responses for a representative drug-naive rat during 4 no-drug (ND) days and 22 days of chronic oxazepam treatment. The scale for punished responses is on the left ordinate, that for unpunished on the right. The cumulative records are shown for the last control day and drug days as indicated. The slopes of these curves indicate the response rates. The recording pen reset after every 3 minutes. The numbers indicate the frequency of punished responses that occurred during 3-minute tone periods and the responses are indicated by short upward strokes of the pen. Downward strokes indicate rewarded responses that occurred during the unpunished periods. (From Margules and Stein, 1968.)

masked by the sedative effect of the drug. As the rat developed a tolerance for the sedative effect of the drug, the anxiolytic effect of the drug was unmasked and punished response rates increased. Nonpunished response rates also increased but proportionately less than those for punished responses. There was thus a selective effect on punished responses.

To demonstrate the tolerance effect in another way, the experimenters tested drug-sophisticated rats that had had prior injections of diazepam and chlordiazepoxide on a weekly basis for several months. When these animals were tested with oxazepam, there was an immediate and sustained increase in punished responding, but no decrease occurred for nonpunished responding.

Thus, the prior drug experiences seemed to provide the tolerance for the sedative effect in these rats.

After ten tests, oxazepam was removed for four control tests. The punished response rate fell to zero and returned to the high level only when the drug was restored. This showed that the response rate was under the control of the drug and that rate effects were not due to practice or to the cumulative effect of the drug or its metabolites (Figure 21).

We can now see how these results fit with the results of the experiment by Wise et al. on the effects of single and multiple doses of benzodiazepines on brain NE and 5-HT turnover. After a single dose, the response rates were depressed, presumably due to the temporary blockade of NE turnover; and the continuous increase in response rates, particularly that for punished responding, was presumed to be mediated by the continuous blockade of 5-HT turnover.

Cook and Sepinwall (1975) sought additional evidence about whether benzodiazepine-induced changes in NE and 5-HT turnover paralleled behavior changes as in the Wise et al. and the Margules and Stein experiments. Cook and Sepinwall used a slightly different multiple schedule that elicited punished and nonpunished responding from their rats. They then compared the effects of chlordiazepoxide on the response rates and NE and 5-HT turnover. In general their results were similar to those of the other experiments but there were some differences between the time course of the NE and 5-HT turnover and the behavioral changes. This could have been due to procedural differences. For example, they found that the depression of nonpunished responding was not correlated with the changes in NE turnover; the maximum decrease in NE turnover was observed after two drug treatments, at which time the depression of nonpunished behavior had disappeared. They also found that a weekly dose and daily doses had the same effect on behavior and amine turnover. They even found that one massive dose of chlordiazepoxide (160 mg/kg p.o.) could just as well confer a "drug sophisticated" status to rats that were tested again with a small dose 27 days later (Cook and Sepinwall, 1978). How these differences in results can be reconciled remains to be seen.

The Anxiolytic Effects of the Benzodiazepines

There are innumerable experiments that show that serotonin is involved in the anxiolytic properties of

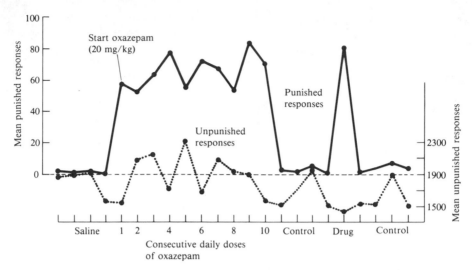

FIGURE 21 EFFECTS OF BENZODIAZEPINE PRE-TREATMENT on oxazepam effects on punished and unpunished behavior. The animals were pretreated with diazepam or chlordiazepoxide. When tested with oxazepam, there was an immediate increase in punished responding (ordinate on left) without a decrease in unpunished responding (ordinate on right). (From Margules and Stein, 1968.)

benzodiazepines. But before proceeding to a discussion of a representative group of them, the question of the involvement of GABA in the serotonergic action should again be considered.

The Role of GABA. Cook and Sepinwall (1975) tested the possibility that GABA might be involved by itself or in the serotonin-mediated effects of the benzodiazepines. We have already mentioned experiments showing that benzodiazepines and aminooxyacetic acid (AOAA), which blocks GABA metabolism and increases brain GABA levels 500-fold, can block the convulsant effects of the GABA synthesis blocker, theosemicarbazide (see Figure 5 in Chapter 9). Also Polc et al. (1974) showed that AOAA not only mimicked the presynaptic inhibitory action of diazepam in the spinal cord but also synergized the action of diazepam when both drugs were given together. Conversely, theosemicarbazide blocked the action of diazepam; and bicuculline (the GABA antagonist) competitively reduced the action of diazepam in the spinal cord. Thus, GABA agonists mimic and enhance the actions of benzodiazepines whereas GABA antagonists block them. (The interactions of the benzodiazepines with the GABA receptors have been discussed earlier in this chapter).

To assess the role of GABAergic mechanisms on antianxiety effects, Cook and Sepinwall examined the effect of AOAA on punished behavior in a modified Geller and Seifter (1960) procedure (described earlier). During drug tests, the rats were treated 40 to 50 minutes before with AOAA (2.5 to 25 mg/kg i.p.). The results showed that with 2.5 and 5 mg/kg, AOAA had no significant effect on either nonpunished or punished response rates. At doses of 10 or 25 mg/kg, both response rates were depressed about equally. Thus, AOAA did not mimic benzodiazepines in this case.

Because peak brain levels of GABA were reported to occur around 4 to 8 hours after AOAA administration, other rats were injected earlier before the tests. Similar results were found when AOAA (10 mg/kg) was given 2 hours before testing, but AOAA (25 mg/kg) given 3–4 hours before testing had insignificant effects on both punished and nonpunished response rates.

In additional tests, AOAA (10 mg/kg, i.p., 50 minutes before testing or 25 mg/kg, 3–4 hours before testing) was given along with a threshold dose of diazepam (0.62 mg/kg, p.o. 35 min before testing). The results on response rates were comparable to the effects of either dose of AOAA given alone. Thus, no synergistic anticonflict effect was found in contrast to the synergistic effects found by Polc et al. (1974) in their spinal cord experiments.

These results were regarded with caution by Cook

and Sepinwall because of the discrepancy found between the time courses of the anticonvulsant effects of AOAA and brain GABA levels. Nevertheless, the results of their experiments showed that AOAA neither had anticonflict activity nor did it synergize with diazepam in that respect. Thus, whereas GABA seems to be clearly involved in muscle relaxant, ataxic, and anticonvulsant effects of benzodiazepines, no evidence was found here for a possible role for it in antianxiety effects.

Stein et al. (1977a) addressed themselves to the same question concerning the role of GABA on benzodiazepine-induced serotonin changes. They considered the possibility that benzodiazepines increase the release of GABA at terminals that form axoaxonal synapses at serotonergic nerve endings performing presynaptic-inhibitory functions. Thus, an increase of GABA would inhibit the release of serotonin at these nerve endings. They tested this hypothesis by administering picrotoxin, a putative GABA receptor blocker, to rats receiving oxazepam (15 mg/kg) in a Geller-type conflict test. They also tested rats with the glycine antagonist strychnine.

Oxazepam, as expected, sharply increased punished responses, which leveled off after three or four doses. On subsequent days, picrotoxin (1–4 mg/kg) was given 10 minutes after the oxazepam dose. The same dose of strychnine was given in separate tests. The results were that the optimal dose of picrotoxin (2 mg/kg) significantly reduced the punishment-lessening effect of oxazepam without disturbing unpunished response rates. However, Sepinwall and Cook (1978) replicated the experiment by Stein et al. (1977) and found that 1 mg/kg of picrotoxin produced a slight, but not significant, decrease in the magnitude of the response to oxazepam, and whereas 2 mg/kg of picrotoxin significantly decreased the effect of oxazepam on punished responding, it depressed unpunished responding by about 50 percent in some rats. Given alone, this dose of picrotoxin markedly depressed both punished and unpunished responding leaving the findings of Stein et al. in doubt.

The results of the strychnine experiment by Stein et al. showed that strychnine depressed punished behavior as well as unpunished behavior. But these results are ambiguous because electrophysiological studies failed to show that benzodiazepines activate or block glycine receptors (Chapter 9). Also, strychnine has been found to exert nonspecific effects on neuronal and muscular

membranes. It was also found that benzodiazepines are weak protectors against strychnine-produced convulsions (Costa et al. 1975; Haefely, 1978). These findings diminish consideration of glycine receptors as mediating effects of the benzodiazepines.

However, with respect to the role of GABA, despite the negative findings of the GABA enhancing experiments and the questionable findings of the picrotoxin experiments, there is evidence that serotonergic neurons affected by benzodiazepines are under the influence of GABAergic systems. For example, GABAergic postsynaptic inhibition has been demonstrated for the serotonergic neurons of the midbrain raphe in that they are inhibited by iontophoretic application of GABA; and the suppression of spontaneous firing of the cells in the dorsal raphe nucleus by electrical stimulation of the ventromedial pontine reticular formation is blocked by picrotoxin but not by strychnine (Gallager and Aghajanian, 1976). The failure to obtain antianxiety effects or to enhance the antianxiety effects of diazepam by enhancing GABA levels in the brain does not rule out a role for GABA for the following reasons: First, if we grant that benzodiazepines merely make GABA receptors more sensitive to GABA molecules, it does not necessarily follow that AOAA-induced high GABA levels should cause more stimulation of saturated or only normally sensitive GABA receptors. Second, whereas the picrotoxin data is ambiguous, the precise action of picrotoxin on GABA receptors is unknown.

The Role of Serotonin. There is abundant evidence that changes in serotonin action are related to the anxiolytic action of the benzodiazepines. In an experiment utilizing the Geller conflict paradigm, rats were trained on a multiple VI-2/CRF (punishment) schedule and treated with oxazepam. The animals showed the typical increase in responding during the CRF period. In subsequent tests, oxazepam treated rats were given via indwelling cannulas intraventricular doses of NE or 5-HT, or the solvent (Locke's solution) as a control just before they were tested. The results showed that NE enhanced the effects of oxazepam, and 5-HT blocked it (Figure 22). Furthermore, stimulation via indwelling cannulas of the serotonergic dorsal nucleus of the raphe with crystalline carbachol (5 μg) caused marked suppression of punished and unpunished responses. Moreover, the carbachol effect was reversed within 10 minutes after a dose of oxazepam (10

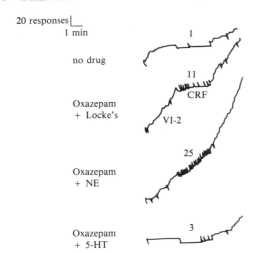

20 responses
1 min

no drug

Oxazepam + Locke's

Oxazepam + NE

Oxazepam + 5-HT

FIGURE 22 NE AND 5-HT EFFECTS ON OXAZEPAM-INDUCED DISINHIBITION. In this typical rat, systemic oxazepam and intraventricular (IVT) vehicle (Locke's solution) increase responding during the CRF (punished) period, the drug plus IVT NE increased it more, and the drug plus IVT 5-HT blocked the oxazepam effect. The numbers above the curves indicate the total of reinforcements. (From Stein et al., 1973.)

mg/kg, i.p.); the rats showed a sharp return to high levels of punished and unpunished responses (Stein et al. 1973). This demonstrated that serotonergic neurons originating in the nuclei of the raphe may play a significant role in behavior suppression.

The Effects of Serotonin Agonists and Antagonists. A number of serotonergic drugs have been found that affect responses that are suppressed by punishment. For example, methysergide, a 5-HT receptor blocker, and strangely perhaps, D-2-bromolysergic acid (BOL), which has weak central effects, both caused a marked increase in punished behavior in pigeons (Graeff and Schoenfeld, 1970). These drugs had similar effects in rats (Wise et al., 1972). The same effects were found in rats treated with PCPA, the 5-HT synthesis inhibitor; and the PCPA effect was reversed by 5-HTP, the serotonin precursor (Robichaud and Sledge, 1969). Also, additive anticonflict effects were observed with methysergide and chlordiazepoxide (Cook and Sepinwall, 1975).

Enhancing 5-HT activity with 5-HTP suppressed food rewarded behavior in the pigeon (Aprison and Ferster, 1961), and the effect was further enhanced by

the MAO inhibitor iproniazid, which had no effect by itself; the MAO inhibitor blocked 5-HT metabolism and thereby increased synaptic activity of 5-HT. Also, the serotonin receptor agonist α-methyltryptamine suppressed punished and nonpunished behavior in the rat (Stein et al., 1973) and pigeon (Graeff and Schoenfeld, 1970), and intraventricular administration of the serotonergic neurotoxin 5,6-dihydroxytryptamine yielded antipunishment activity (Stein et al., 1975).

In other experiments, Graeff (1974), using a variation of the Geller and Seifter (1960) technique, trained rats on a concurrent FI-1 (water), FR-5 (shock) schedule. In this schedule, thirsty animals were rewarded for the first lever-press that occurred after the fixed interval of 1 minute, whereas every fifth response (FR-5) caused the animals to receive a brief shock to their feet. The counter that controlled shock delivery was reset after each fixed interval. Ideally, the animal should wait 1 minute, press the lever for the water reward, then wait 1 more minute, press the lever, and so on. In this way, the animal would receive the maximum reward with least effort and no shocks. Under control (no drug) conditions, the animals made few responses and experienced few shocks. When they were injected with 5-HT receptor blockers such as methysergide, cyproheptadine, or chlordiazepoxide (Librium), there was a dose-related increase in responses over control rates (as much as 50 to 100 percent) and a sharp increase in the number of shocks. It was also found that cyproheptadine was markedly more effective in this regard than methysergide, and this correlates with the higher potency of cyproheptadine as a 5-HT receptor blocker on the isolated rat uterus, which may be related to its potency in the CNS.

Geller et al. (1974) trained rats to lever press on a liquid food multiple VI-2/CRF schedule. During CRF, each lever-press yielded food reward, but, in addition, the rats received foot shock that was aversive enough to prevent the occurrence of more than two or three responses during the CRF period. One hour before the test, the animals were given 60 mg/kg of cinanserin, a serotonin receptor blocker, followed 30 minutes later by the 5-HT agonist α-methyltryptamine (4 mg/kg) or saline; or 45 minutes later by 60 mg/kg of 5-HTP or saline. The results showed that cinanserin produced a 10- to 20-fold increase in CRF responses. Moreover, this effect was significantly diminished by combining cinanserin with 5-HTP or with the 5-HT agonist α-methyltryptamine. These experiments clearly show that serotonin antagonism is followed by an increase of responses that have been suppressed by punishment, whereas serotonin agonism causes the suppression of responses associated with punishment.

These effects are illustrated by the performance of rats in a Geller paradigm experiment (unpublished, from our laboratory) that investigated the possible interactions between CDP and the serotonin reuptake-inhibitor fluoxetine. The rats were subjected to a multiple VI-40 sec/CRF schedule of milk reinforcements, which alternated every 5 minutes. The switch to the CRF period was signaled by a light appearing over the opening for the milk dipper. All responses during the CRF period were followed by milk reward accompanied by a brief (0.5 second) foot shock. Each test session lasted one hour.

Figure 23A shows cumulative response records for one control (no drug) session and four drug sessions with increasing doses of fluoxetine (FXT). It can be seen that the response rate during the VI schedule is much higher than the CRF rate, although this lower rate is at least partly due to frequent pauses to consume the food rewards. There was little change in response rate for this rat after administering 2.5 or 5.0 mg/kg of FXT, but after 10.0 or 15.0 mg/kg there was a marked response suppression particularly of CRF (punished) responses. In Figure 23B, response records from a different rat are shown of sessions during which the rats were treated

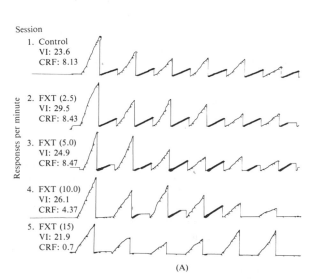

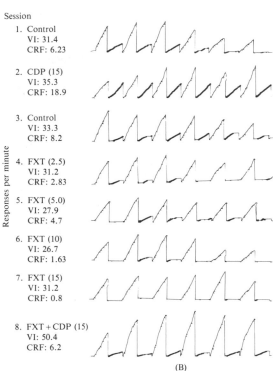

FIGURE 23 EFFECTS OF FLUOXETINE AND CHLORDIAZEPOXIDE on punished and unpunished responses. Each daily session consisted of six alternations between a VI-40 sec and a CRF schedule. Each component lasted 5 minutes, after which the recording pen reset to baseline. Reinforcements are indicated by small diagonal deflections. When reinforcements occurred close together (as in some CRF sessions) the pen marks were blurred together. The drug conditions and the response rates (responses/minute) are shown on the left of each record. (A) Typical rat on control (no drug) day and 4 additional drug tests with increasing doses of FXT. The drug selectively decreases responding during the CRF (punishment) component. (B) Records of a different rat receiving FXT and CDP alone or in combination. CDP increases VI and especially CRF responding. FXT decreases this responding, and the drugs given together mutually cancel their effects. (From Feldman, unpublished study.)

with CDP and FXT alone or in combination. In session 2, CDP (15 mg/kg) elicits only a small increase in VI responding, but a 3-fold increase in CRF responding. Giving 2.5 or 5.0 mg/kg of FXT (sessions 4 and 5) caused marked reductions in the CRF rates (65 and 47 percent, respectively), of the most recent control rate (session 3), whereas there were only small changes in the VI rates (6 and 16 percent, respectively). Sessions 6 and 7, with 10 and 15 mg/kg of FXT, showed further selective suppression of CRF rates, whereas combining CDP and FXT at 15 mg/kg caused a marked increase in the VI rate and a restoration of the CRF rate to near control levels (session 8).

The CDP–induced increase in CRF responding appears to be the result of the anxiolytic effects of the drug, since drug potency in this test correlates well with clinical potency in treating psychoneurotic disorders (see Cook and Sepinwall, 1975). CDP-induced increases in the VI component is a common feature of benzodiazepine treatment (see Figure 20), and suggests that there are aversive components in VI schedules that are also affected by the drug. With respect to the FXT-induced effect on CRF responding, the data suggest that this drug, by blocking 5-HT uptake, enhances serotonergic synaptic activity which increases the aversive consequences of CRF responses as shown by their virtual disappearance from the records. The data support the concept that blocking serotonergic activity is associated with response potentiation, whereas enhancing serotonergic activity is associated with response inhibition (Stein et al., 1977b). Furthermore, the mutual antagonism between CDP and FXT support the idea that diminished serotonin activity is involved in the anxiolytic activity of the benzodiazepines, a condition that can be blocked by drugs that enhance serotonergic activity.

Other Behavioral Effects of the Benzodiazepines

A comprehensive review of the many areas of study of benzodiazepine effects on behavior would require more space than can be accommodated in this volume. Fortunately there are many reviews, some of which have already been referenced, and a list of relevant books can be found at the end of this chapter. However, a brief overall view of some topics will indicate other areas of interest that have not been covered thus far in this chapter.

Food Consumption

Chlordiazepoxide increases food intake in food-deprived rats that are allowed to eat compared to intake in nondrugged controls, in sated rats, and even in rats that have been stomach preloaded. We have already seen that CDP-treated rats will lever-press for food (milk or food pellets) in a conflict situation when food reward was accompanied by foot shocks. Oxazepam increased eating of quinine-adulterated food (Margules and Stein, 1967); and diazepam treated pigs increased lever-pressing for food pellets on a progressive ratio schedule—a schedule calling for progressively increased responses for each reward. This procedure allows the drug-treated pig to indicate the effort it is willing to make to obtain food compared to its effort in the no-drug state (Dantzer, 1976).

It was proposed that the increase in food-related behavior was due to the anxiolytic effect of the drug, which disinhibited fear-suppressed eating in experimental situations or when offered special food rewards. But this did not explain increased eating when anxiety was at a minimum, i.e., when animals were tested in home cages with the same food for control and test conditions. An alternative hypothesis is that the benzodiazepines specifically exert their effects either by inhibiting a satiety mechanism or facilitating a hunger mechanism, but it is difficult to isolate which effect is involved if indeed they are different (Feldman and Smith, 1978).

In one study (reviewed by Dantzer, 1977), rats performed on a FR-10 or FR-15 satiation schedule, i.e., they were allowed to perform until satiated. CDP, but not diazepam or oxazepam, elicited increases in responding for more food reinforcements. This effect could not be mimicked by increasing food deprivation, presumably to make the animals more hungry. This suggested that CDP disinhibited or disrupted the mechanism regulating satiation rather than by acting directly on food motivation. Benzodiazepine-induced resistance to satiation was demonstrated in cats that had learned to consume their daily food within a 3-hour period. When benzodiazepines were given at the end of the feeding period, the animals resumed eating voraciously. Oxazepam was the most potent drug (compared to N-methyllorazepam, diazepam, and CDP) to yield this effect. Also sated rats or pigs that had learned to lever-press for food, when put into a Skinner box after diazepam treatment, started to lever-press and ate the food rewards (Dantzer, 1977).

Because serotonin systems have been implicated in the anxiolytic effects of benzodiazepines, its role in increased food intake by the drugs has been investigated.

Earlier studies showed that 5-HT depletion with PCPA induced hyperphagia in rats, whereas 5-HT infused through hepatic-portal cannulae in rabbits decreased food intake in a free-feeding test. Peripheral 5-HTP administration also decreased food intake (probably a peripheral effect, because its conversion to 5-HT limited its crossing the blood brain barrier). Also, fenfluramine is an anorectic drug that releases 5-HT and increases its turnover rate. As might be known or anticipated, the control of feeding is an enormously complicated process, with many neurotransmitter systems being involved. Also, because 90 percent of the serotonin content of the body is found in visceral tissues, changes in the peripheral role of serotonin by drugs is always a possibility (Blundell, 1977).

Feldman and Smith (1978) examined the effect of fluoxetine (FXT, a 5-HT reuptake blocker) on CDP-induced feeding enhancement. In their study, rats on an *ad libitum* diet of lab chow were injected with CDP (3.8, 7.5, and 15 mg/kg) and FXT (2.5, 5.0, and 10 mg/kg) alone or in combination just before a 4-hour test period when the amount eaten was monitored. The results showed a significant dose-dependent relationship of CDP-induced increases in food consumption and of FXT-induced decrease in food consumption, and a competitive antagonistic interaction between these two agents (Figure 24). Assuming that FXT enhanced 5-HT effects, its blocking action on the CDP effect supports the contention that 5-HT is involved in the CDP enhancement of food intake. A possible explanation for the CDP effect is that satiety is a form of food aversion that is attenuated by 5-HT blockade, thus promoting food intake.

Benzodiazepine Effects on Aggression

An earlier discussion of aggressive behavior indicated that aggression has many forms and that it is under the control of complex neurotransmitter interactions. Therefore, simple explanations for drug effects on this behavior cannot be made with confidence. Nevertheless, there is ample data that benzodiazepines have taming and antiaggressive properties if it is assumed that the experimental paradigms under which the drug is tested fall comfortably under the rubric of aggressive behavior.

Effects on muricide in rats. Muricide or mouse killing by rats is characteristic of few or many members of given rat strains. The Holtzman strain shows few and Sprague-Dawley rats show significantly more in-

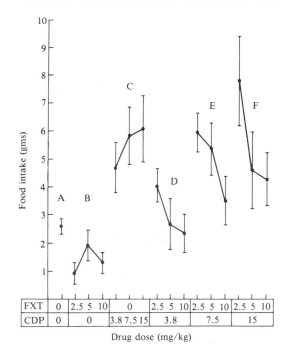

FIGURE 24 CHLORDIAZEPOXIDE AND FLUOXETINE EFFECTS ON FOOD INTAKE. Fluoxetine (FXT) decreased food intake, chlordiazepoxide (CDP) increased it; and the two drugs taken together exerted a competitive antagonism of their effects. A, control; B, FXT effects; C, CDP effects; D,E, and F, effects of CDP-FXT combinations. (From Feldman and Smith, 1978.)

dividual mouse killers. The method of identification merely involves placing a mouse in a cage with a single rat. If the rat attacks and kills the mouse within 15 minutes, usually by biting it in the back of the neck, it is designated as muricidal. Tests with low-base-rate Holtzman rats show that low doses of CDP increase muricide activity, whereas higher doses with high-base-rate (100 percent) Sprague-Dawley rats decreases muricide activity (Leaf et al., 1975).

Are the antimuricidal effects of CDP specific or secondary, that is, due to the sedative effects of the benzodiazepines? Some investigators found that mouse-killing was diminished by benzodiazepines only at doses that produce motor impairment, whereas others found that the drug was effective at doses that had no observable motor effects.

Quenzer and Feldman (1975) examined the possibility that repeated administration of CDP would cause a loss of the muricide-depressant effect. This hypothesis was based on previous observations by Margules and Stein (1968) that the sedative effect of the benzodiazepines shows tolerance and disappears after repeated dosing (see Figure 20). Support for the hypothesis was found when CDP at 50 mg/kg lost its antimuricidal effect with repeated testing (Figure 25). Results of tests with the drug at 25 mg/kg were less clear, presumably because of poorer tolerance induction and weaker muricide-depressant effects. With the drug at 75 mg/kg, the depressant effect of the drug was still evident after repeated testing, and drug toxicity was also evident because 5 of 13 rats died in this group.

Because it could be argued that the tolerance shown with repeated dosing was a behavioral tolerance (i.e., the rats learned to perform mouse-killing while under the affect of the drug), a second experiment was done on muricidal rats that received CDP for 7 days (25, 50, and 75 mg/kg) without being tested for muricide. On day 8, they were given the drug before a muricide test.

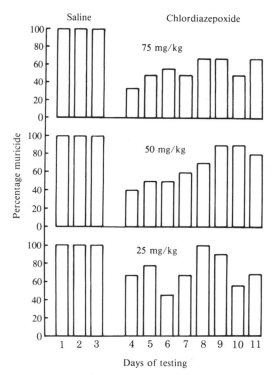

FIGURE 25 CHLORDIAZEPOXIDE EFFECTS ON MURICIDAL RATS. Comparisons of percentages of muricidal rats under no-drug (saline) and drug (CDP) conditions. Rats had to kill a mouse within 15 minutes to be considered muricidal. (From Quenzer and Feldman, 1975.)

The results showed that on day 8 all rats killed mice; but control rats that received saline injections on the first 7 days failed to kill mice on day 8 after receiving CDP at 50 mg/kg. These results clearly demonstrated that repeated dosing led to a tolerance of the antimuricide effects of CDP, and because of the experimenter's observations of the listless, indecisive, and sometimes defensive rat behaviors seen in early drug tests in the first experiment, it was concluded that the sedative effects of the drug were responsible for the antimuricidal results.

This result was buttressed by the results of a third experiment that used caffeine to antagonize the sedative effect of CDP. It showed that muricidal rats with an initial combined dose of CDP (50 mg/kg) and caffeine (75 mg/kg) killed mice, even though the latency of the kill within the 15-minute test period was somewhat longer than in the tests under saline. Tests with caffeine itself showed no effect on muricide. Thus, at the dose tested, caffeine at least partially blocked the sedative effect of CDP and allowed muricidal activity to appear.

A possible explanation for CDP-induced muricide in low-base-rate rats is that for these rats the appearance of a mouse elicits fear, and CDP attenuates that fear, which allows the emergence of muricidal behavior. Alternatively, the emergence of muricide in these rats is a drug idiosyncracy or rare side effect. Parallels are seen in the human use of sedative drugs such as alcohol and barbiturates, which sometimes elicit excitement and aggression; and treatment with diazepam (Valium) has at times elicited hyperexcitement and rage (Leaf et al., 1975).

Effects on shock-induced fighting. In another experiment, CDP was tested for its effect on intraspecies aggression in a shock-induced fighting paradigm. Pairs of rats were placed in a chamber and subjected to inescapable foot shocks daily for 10 consecutive days (0.5-second duration, 2.0 mA, every 2 seconds for 10 minutes for a total of 300 shocks). This procedure caused the rats to rear and strike each other. The number of such attacks was recorded for each pair. Before the shock sessions, one group was given CDP (15 mg/kg), one group was given saline; one CDP group was not shocked; and a fourth group was given CDP immediately after the daily shock session. After one day of rest, all animals were given 10 additional days of shock sessions with no drug.

The results showed that CDP given before the shock

sessions significantly suppressed the shock-induced fighting (Figure 26). The reduction in fighting compared to the no-drug group was 69 percent. In other tests with CDP doses of 5 mg/kg and 30 mg/kg, it was found that the lower dose resulted in an 11 percent decrease and the higher dose in a 67 percent decrease. In these animals, the drug caused the animals to respond more by jumping about randomly in response to the shock. The data also showed that there was no tolerance to the drug effects in that there were no changes over the days of testing. The group that received CDP *after* each shock session showed similar degrees of fighting behavior as the no-drug group, showing there was no cumulative drug effect that might have antagonized a tolerance effect. When shock sessions were resumed for another 10 days with no drug, the fighting responses were the same for all groups (Quenzer et al., 1974).

These experiments show that some forms of what might be called aggressive behavior, such as muricide, can be attenuated by the nonspecific sedative effects of the benzodiazepines, whereas other forms, such as shock-induced fighting, seem to be suppressed by some other specific drug-induced process. It is yet to be determined what benzodiazepine property is responsible for these effects.

Clinical Use of the Benzodiazepines

As we mentioned earlier, the benzodiazepines are enormously popular from a clinical standpoint, as indicated by the fact that they are among the most prescribed drugs of all kinds, with 100 million prescriptions being filled annually in the United States. This fact raises important questions about the clinical effectiveness and safety of these drugs compared to other anxiolytic agents, the extent to which they are justifiably prescribed, and whether or not they are associated with dependency and addiction.

Clinical Efficacy

In evaluating antianxiety agents—even in well-designed clinical trials—there are complications in demonstrating benefits when placebo effects range from 20 percent to as much as 60 percent in some kinds of patients. Moreover, it is difficult to demonstrate effectiveness for these drugs in short-lived anxiety syndromes that frequently improve without chemical intervention. Also, a favorable response from these drugs is more frequently associated with those patients from lower socioeconomic classes, those having a lack of psychological sophistication and being unable to express unhappiness verbally in terms of intrapsychic and interpersonal difficulties, and those who have

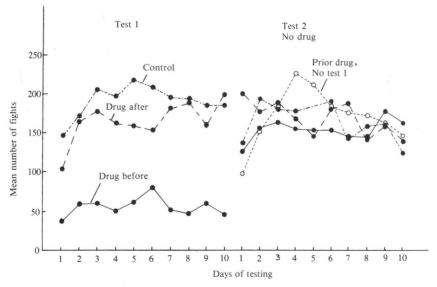

FIGURE 26 CHLORDIAZEPOXIDE EFFECTS ON SHOCK-INDUCED FIGHTING. Comparisons of the number of fighting responses among control and CDP-treated rats. Only when CDP was given *before* shock sessions was fighting response suppressed, and there was no tolerance for the effect. No drug was given during the Test 2 sessions. (From Quenzer et al., 1974.)

passive, almost magical, expectations from physicians who enthusiastically prescribe such medication (Baldessarini, 1977).

Nevertheless, a survey showed that of 25 experimental trials of short-term treatment of neurotic anxiety, 18 showed a strong benzodiazepine-placebo difference, 4 showed a trend toward a difference, and 3 showed no difference. When benzodiazepines are compared among themselves with respect to effectiveness and unwanted side effects such as sedation, the evidence was not altogether convincing in any direction. When compared to various barbiturates, there was evidence that benzodiazepines had a reasonably constant clinical superiority in efficacy with fewer side effects. Also, despite a 5- to 20-fold increase in cost of benzodiazepines over barbiturates, they are recommended because of the substantial increment of safety afforded by benzodiazepines when accidental or intentional overdosing occurs (Greenblatt and Shader, 1978).

The efficacy of the benzodiazepines for inducing muscle relaxation and the potency of their anticonvulsive characteristics have already been discussed. Chlordiazepoxide is used to control the behavior of hyperactive children, but is regarded as being somewhat less effective than amphetamines. Paradoxically, benzodiazepines sometimes elicit excitement and rage in brain-damaged children and in those individuals with a history of aggressive and impulsive behavior. Again, one may speculate that these antisocial behaviors are under aversive control (i.e., they are inhibited by the threat of punishment) and they may be disinhibited by the benzodiazepines.

The benzodiazepines that are used as sedative-hypnotics such as flurazepam (Dalmane) and nitrazepam (Mogodon, not marketed in the United States) are also immensely popular (Oswald et al., 1973). In the United States Dalmane accounts for 53 percent of the 25 million sleeping pill prescriptions filled annually for the 8 million persons who use the pills (Smith, 1979). Flurazepam is preferred by physicians over barbiturates, again for its relative safety, even though in some persons it elicits, as do the barbiturates, excessive sedation, intoxication and paradoxical excitation.

Researchers at the Sleep Research and Treatment Center of the Pennsylvania State University Medical School extensively examined the effects of flurazepam on normal and insomniac adults (Kales and Scharf, 1973). The insomniac subjects' sleep was electrically monitored (electroencephalogram, electromyogram and electroocculogram) during a placebo-baseline period; and during short (1 week), intermediate (2 weeks) and long term (8 weeks) drug treatment periods. The drug periods were followed by placebo-withdrawal periods. The general findings were that the usually prescribed dose (15 mg) was quite effective in shortening the sleep induction period, decreasing wake time and the number of awakenings. When the dose was 30 mg, a dose frequently given in obstinate cases, similar effects were observed with the addition of carryover effects; that is, when the drug was withdrawn there was a continued benefit with regard to induction time and the duration of sleep for at least a few withdrawal nights. This finding raised the question of how the drug given before retiring affected performance during the subsequent daytime hours, a question that is important for all hypnotics. However, the subjects did not complain of any difficulty during the daytime hours, and subsequently estimated that they were sleeping better than usual. The EEG data revealed no marked disturbances in the patterns of sleep, although at 30 mg there was a slight decrease in REM sleep without any evidence for REM rebound during periods of drug withdrawal.

A report from the Institute of Medicine of the National Academy of Sciences on the subject of sleeping pill use pointed out that some individuals can develop tolerance and become addicted to flurazepam, although not as rapidly nor as severely as to barbiturates (Smith, 1979). Moreover, it has been ascertained that an active metabolite of flurazepam remains in the body for more than a whole day, thus causing a buildup of this metabolite when flurazepam is routinely taken at bedtime. By the seventh night a patient may have 4 to 6 times the amount present after the first night, thus causing diminished alertness and hand-eye coordination during the day and possibly contributing to auto accidents. In contrast, barbiturates produce metabolites that leave the body at a rate that does not allow a buildup. Flurazepam is frequently given to elderly patients who exhibit insomnia as a natural consequence of aging. In nursing homes, frequently as a convenience to the nursing staff who believe that sleeping patients are good patients, the prescription rate may be as high as 94 percent. The resulting diminished alertness may be confused with irreversible senility or dementia and lead to other inappropriate medication.

A later study by Kales et al. (1978) investigated two experimental benzodiazepines, triazolam and flunitrazepam, as to their effects on sleep. They also investigated nitrazepam (Mogodon). The results showed that triazolam and nitrazepam decreased sleep latency (the time to fall asleep), the time awake after sleep onset, and the total time awake. After drug withdrawal, the time awake after sleep onset and total time awake increased significantly over baseline levels. In short-term tests with flunitrazepam there was no improvement in inducing or maintaining sleep, but sleep again worsened significantly after drug withdrawal. The results also showed that triazolam lost its effectiveness after two weeks of continuous use.

To account for the rebound phenomenon, it was proposed that the production of endogenous benzodiazepine-like molecules would be decreased by exogenous benzodiazepines or metabolites and that after drug withdrawal there would be a lag in the production and replacement of the endogenous substances. For those benzodiazepines having long-lasting metabolites, the effect might be less abrupt because the endogenous compounds would be partially restored before the active metabolites would be totally eliminated. It was also proposed that the abrupt withdrawal of anxiolytic benzodiazepines could lead to "rebound anxiety."

In conclusion, it should be noted that insomnia can be caused by many factors, and even those who complain of insomnia frequently are found during objective observations to sleep for normal durations and have a normal distribution of the various sleep patterns (see the section on sleep in Chapter 7). Furthermore it is argued that the mechanism of action of the sedative-hypnotic benzodiazepines is not related to what is now known about the physiology of sleep. Until these relationships are known, there is no rational basis for the use of these drugs. Consequently, if used at all they should be used sparingly.

Appropriate and Inappropriate Use of Benzodiazepines

The immense popularity of the benzodiazepines has raised questions about whether these drugs are always being used in the best interests of their users. One can point to the vast sums spent on advertisements and other forms of promotion—in 1973 estimated at 1.2 billion dollars per year for all drug promotions, or about 4000 dollars annually per physician (Goddard, 1973). We can then ask to what extent these influences are responsible for the millions of prescriptions of anxiolytic drugs that are being written. It was reported

that among Valium users, women outnumbered male users by 2½ to 1. This has been interpreted as showing that our society relegates women to low paying, unfulfilling jobs, family and child care, and never-ending housework. These frustrations often bring women to their physicians with vague complaints of fatigue, pressure, and anxiety. The drug industry capitalizes on this state of affairs by showing, for example, in an ad in a medical journal a picture of a woman dressed to do housework but behind prison bars with her broom and an assortment of mops. This picture is above a caption that reads, ostensibly to the physician, "You can't set her free but you can help her feel less anxious—Serax (oxazepam)." Or imagine an ad showing a well-dressed but depressed-looking woman sitting at a table in a gymnasium near a sign reading "Register Today For The Bazaar." Alongside the picture a statement reads, "MA—Fine Arts . . . PTA (President elect) . . . representations of a life currently centered around home and children, with too little time to pursue a vocation for which she has spent many years in training . . . a situation that may bespeak continuous frustration and stress: a perfect framework for her to translate the functional symptoms of psychic tension into major problems. For this kind of patient—with no demonstrable pathology yet with repeated complaints—consider the distinctive properties of Valium (diazepam)." Consider another example: an ad reads that Librium is the appropriate response to the "excessive anxiety" felt by a young college woman whose "exposure to new friends and other influences may force her to reevaluate herself and her goals."

One could certainly argue that physicians are acting out of sincere well-intentioned efforts to deal with individuals that come to them with vague complaints lacking organic causes, but because up to half of their patients are people feeling lonely, tired, anxious, unhappy, depressed, dissatisfied, or without purpose and because the physicians may lack the training for appropriate counseling or the time to practice it, they treat the complaints symptomatically rather than addressing themselves to the sources of their patients' malaise.

Benzodiazepine Toxicity and Dependency

Benzodiazepines in some respects share with most sedative drugs the possibility of daytime sedation, drowsiness, decreased mental acuity, incoordination, and increased risk of accidents. However, they are regarded as being significantly less toxic in high doses than barbiturates and the propanediols (e.g., meprobamate). They have been regarded as being "virtually suicide-proof" and that persons that have taken massive doses can be managed with far less difficulty than those with life-threatening overdoses of barbiturates and propanediols. The explanation of the relative safety of the benzodiazepines may rest upon the lack of effect of these drugs on visceral functions, particularly the mechanisms controlling respiration.

Whereas some writers report that tolerance to the anxiolytic effects of diazepam can occur, leading to self-medication of increasing doses and subsequently causing intoxication and euphoria, others say that it is probably minimal with the benzodiazepines. The explanation for the relative lack of tolerance development for these drugs is their prolonged duration of action correlated with plasma half-lives in man of 24 to 48 hours, whereas that of meprobamate is around 12 hours. Thus, doses of benzodiazepines may be less frequent because the clinical effect is more sustained. In this respect, the benzodiazepines are like phenobarbital, which also has a sustained action, and even though this barbiturate may be continually used to control epilepsy, there is little tolerance and the drug is rarely abused.

There have been reports of physical dependence on benzodiazepines, but these cases have been associated with extreme doses and duration of treatment, 10 to 20 times the usual daily doses of chlordiazepoxide and diazepam for several months. Also, there have been reports of severe withdrawal symptoms, even including convulsions, and these reports have been emphasized and exploited by detractors of the drugs, who frequently fail to point out that these effects are rare, that they occur in unstable individuals who get prescriptions simultaneously from a number of physicians, and that there was a high probability of the concurrent use of other drugs. The more usual withdrawal picture following benzodiazepine abuse is one that starts from 4 to 8 days, or as long as 2 weeks after withdrawal, and is usually moderate in intensity and rarely associated with seizures (Hollister, 1980). Such is not the case with meprobamate, which was found to be so highly addicting that it is rarely prescribed for more than a few days; consequently, it has virtually disappeared from pharmacists' shelves because of its abuse potential and life-threatening withdrawal effects.

In conclusion, it should be emphasized that fatalities associated with sedative drugs in most cases probably do not occur solely by the action of the sedative drug, but rather when it is combined with other sedatives such as alcohol. In these instances, the benzodiazepines have had their share of involvements. The recommended course of action to prevent these occurrences is for the physician to prescribe these drugs to those patients with less potential for drug abuse and addiction, where there are clear indications for potential benefits, and for a short period of time. Patients with previous histories of sedative or alcohol abuse and antisocial or impulsive traits should be given these substances with extreme caution.

With more favored patients, anxieties may be dealt with more efficaciously with psychotherapy or changes in environment and the use of these drugs should be regarded as no more than symptomatic treatment. It should be remembered, however, that activities that can cause an individual to be free of tension and to feel good have strong reinforcing effects, tendencies that are virtually built into anxiolytic drug-taking. Thus, the desire for the continuous use of these drugs is always present. To counter these tendencies, the drugs should be used only intermittently. Because anxiety states usually follow an irregular course, drugs should be used only when the symptoms are discomforting and disabling. Even the fact of knowing that relief is available may frequently help an individual over minor crises. Thus, the chance of tolerance developing and loss of efficacy is minimized and the risk of drug dependency or addiction is avoided (Hollister, 1973, 1980; Baldessarini, 1977).

So, on the one hand, there are drugs that can relieve the tension and the symptoms of anxiety, and in acute situations the anxious person can be treated quickly and effectively with low risk of untoward effects. But, on the other hand, the drugs may be misapplied by the physician who treats every personal problem or disappointment as a clinical syndrome or who offers these drugs to those with character disorders or those having histories of drug or alcohol abuse. In fairness, however, it seems that as experience has grown and the limits of chemotherapy are established, whatever abuse there has been in the past, there is now an increasing improvement in the perceptions of physicians and drug manufacturers of the proper place of these drugs in medical practice.

Conclusion

This chapter examined the area of psychopharmacology that deals with drugs that are used to allay anxiety. We have shown that anxiety is a constant presence that can at times be severe and overwhelming. Many individuals cannot deal with anxiety by adjusting their behavior either because they cannot avoid the conflicts with which they are confronted or because they do not have the stamina, skill, or intelligence that is necessary. Consequently, many anodynes have been utilized to tide people over, so to speak, during the numerous crises that arise.

Until very recently there were no drugs that were specifically formulated for this purpose. Even the benzodiazepines share many of the disadvantages of the earlier drugs: adverse side effects, a tendency to induce dependence and addiction, and their use as a device for avoiding the responsibility for direct action upon the sources of conflict. Parenthetically, it is of interest to note that although the mechanism of action of the benzodiazepines is unique, there is a cross tolerance to other sedative and anxiolytic agents, suggesting that there are some basic physiological features that are common to all of them.

Among the anxiolytic drugs that are currently in use, the benzodiazepines claim to be minimally dangerous and have thus gained a popularity that is unprecedented. Moreover, there are good rational bases for benzodiazepine use: the physiological mechanism of action is becoming well understood, and behavioral studies in animals predict their clinical usefulness. There is evidence that the drugs have an endogenous counterpart, suggesting that they merely augment natural processes. This has led to the design of agents such as the triazolopyridazines, which may improve on the anxiolytic specificity of the benzodiazepines.

The popularity of the benzodiazepines has also become a source of concern and their widespread use is controversial. This concern is partly sparked by the substantial financial rewards that accrue to the marketers of these substances. However, the consensus seems to be that the need for anxiolytic drugs is real and that the benzodiazepines are superior to most other drugs when compared on the basis of therapeutic index (indicating their low proportion of side effects and toxicity), and range of applicability. Compared to alcohol use, which is an alternative drug for many, the benefits of the benzodiazepines are even more pronounced.

A certain amount of abuse potential seems to be inherent in such medication, and alertness is required by prescription writers and dispensers of the substances to keep them out of the hands of those who would abuse them or of those who are substituting a new persistent drug habit for an old one.

Drugs by themselves do not solve personal problems, but they can interrupt the production of anxiety or suppress its symptoms so that problems can be viewed in more objective ways. Unfortunately, these drugs have been used as a panacea and unforeseen complications have emerged, but a keener appreciation of their limitations is now putting them in their appropriate place.

Recommended Readings

Blum, R.H. and Associates. (1969). *Society and Drugs, Vol. 1, Drugs.* Jossey-Bass, San Francisco. Articles on the origins of use of alcohol, opium, cannabis, tobacco, and other substances.

Blundell, J.E. (1977). Is there a role for serotonin (5-hydroxytryptamine) in feeding? *International Journal of Obesity*, 1, 15–42. An evaluation of the literature on serotonergic effects on feeding.

Boissier, J.-R. (Ed.) (1978). *Differential Psychopharmacology of Anxiolytics and Sedatives.* S. Karger, New York. A discussion of possible differences between these two classes of drugs.

Costa, E., Di Chiara, G. and Gessa, G.L. (Eds.) (1981). *GABA and Benzodiazepine Receptors, Advances in Biochemical Psychopharmacology, Vol. 26.* Raven Press, New York. A collection of papers that describe the mechanism of action of the benzodiazepines.

Dantzer, R. (1977). Behavioral effects of benzodiazepines: a review. *Behavioral Reviews*, 1, 71–86. A comprehensive evaluation of benzodiazepine effects on punishment, conditioned suppression, avoidance and escape behavior, learning and memory, food and water consumption, exploratory behavior and aggression and social dominance.

Garattini, S., Mussini, E. and Randall, L.O. (Eds.) (1973). *The Benzodiazepines*, Raven Press, New York. A collection of 47 review papers on all aspects of benzodiazepine research.

Greenblatt, D. and Shader, R.I. (1974). *Benzodiazepines in Clinical Practice.* Raven Press, New

York. Reviews and commentaries on the clinical use of benzodiazepines.

Guidotti, A. (1978). Synaptic mechanisms in the action of benzodiazepines. In *Psychopharmacology: A Generation of Progress* (M.A. Lipton, A. DiMascio and K.F. Killam, Eds.), pp. 1349–1357. Raven Press, New York. Recent developments on how benzodiazepines exert their effects.

Schallek, W., Horst, W.D. and Schlosser, W. (1979). Mechanism of action of benzodiazepines. In *Advances in Pharmacology and Chemotherapy, Vol. 16* (S. Garattini, A. Goldin, F. Hawking and I.J. Kopin, Eds.), pp. 45–87. Academic Press, New York. An evaluation of research that attempts to clarify the action of benzodiazepines.

Tallman, J.F., Paul, S.M., Skolnik, P. and Gallager, D.W. (1980). Receptors for the age of anxiety: pharmacology of the benzodiazepines. *Science*, 207, 174–281. An excellent review of current research and theory about benzodiazepines.

Valzelli, L. (Ed.) (1978). *Psychopharmacology of Aggression*. S. Karger, New York. This review evaluates the effects of benzodiazepines in the control of aggression.

CHAPTER TWELVE

Pharmacological Treatment of Schizophrenia and the Affective Disorders

Despite enormous strides in the advancement of our knowledge of the neurochemical basis of behavior and emotion, our understanding of neural mechanisms mediating behavior is still in its infancy. Many answers to our questions will not be forthcoming until more sophisticated biochemical, physiological, and behavioral measurement techniques develop. The greatest problem is the inaccessibility of the CNS to experimental manipulation and measurement. In general, we must rely on animals to study drug effects on the CNS, and a variety of animal models have been developed to study psychiatric illness. An alternate approach is to sample the accessible biological fluids (e.g., blood, urine) of patients with mental disorders. However, it is unlikely that the variety of mental illnesses stem from a common neurochemical entity. Therefore, research results will be highly dependent on the test populations chosen. Thus, increased validity and reliability in diagnosis of psychiatric conditions is critical in determining the biological correlates.

Although a genetic factor has been identified in the etiology of psychosis, psychological, biological, and sociological factors combine in a unique manner to contribute significantly to the development of mental disorders in a particular individual. For instance, it is well recognized that increased emotional stress is related to the appearance of psychotic symptoms (Paul, 1977). In addition, stress has widespread physiological effects on circulating hormone levels, as well as on CNS neurochemistry. Thus, neurochemistry, which we now assume regulates behavioral responses to environmental stimuli, is in turn regulated by external influences. The dynamic state of the intact organism in part explains why evaluating steady-state neurochemistry may not reflect the conditions in the intact organism.

This chapter describes several hypotheses regarding the etiology and pathogenesis of mental illness. For convenience, it is divided into two large sections, corresponding to major classes of psychoses as originally identified by Kraepelin in the late 1800s (Kraepelin, 1913): schizophrenia and affective disorders. Much subsequent evidence, including genetic and drug response data, supports this dichotomy (Haier, 1980). The hypotheses presented here are constantly changing as new data accumulate and old ideas are modified. In this chapter perhaps more than any other, critical evaluation of the ideas presented is urged. Only through diligent questioning and carefully controlled experiments will the frontiers of neuropsychopharmacology be extended.

The psychoses are characterized by marked distortions of reality and disturbances in perception, intellectual functioning, affect (mood), motivation, and motor behavior. The psychotic individual's incapacity is often so complete that voluntary or involuntary hospitalization is required. One class of psychoses comprise the affective psychoses (depression, mania, manic-depressive), to be discussed later in the chapter. A second class is schizophrenia, which poses a very great social problem and is responsible for filling a majority of mental hospital beds.

Schizophrenia

Schizophrenia is characterized by disturbed form and content of thought. Bizarre delusions having no basis in fact are common. Particularly prevalent are persecutory delusions involving the belief that others are spying on or planning harm to the individual. Also quite common is the delusion that one's thoughts are broadcast from one's head to the world or that thoughts and feelings are not one's own but imposed by an external source. The form of thought is disturbed, leading to confused and illogical communication patterns that frequently do not follow conventional rules of semantics. Speech may be vague or repetitive and characterized by loosening of associations such that ideas shift from one subject to another completely unrelated subject.

Disturbances in perception are also a frequent occurrence in schizophrenia. The major disturbance is hallucination, most often auditory in nature. Generally the hallucinations consist of voices, which are insulting or commanding. Tactile hallucinations also occur: usually electrical, tingling, or burning sensations.

In many schizophrenics, emotions are either absent or inappropriate to the situation. Individuals with blunted emotions show no sign of expression, speak in a monotone, and frequently report a lack of feeling. Inappropriate emotion is demonstrated by the individual who smiles or laughs while describing electrical tortures. Sudden and unpredictable changes of emotion are also common.

Schizophrenics are frequently withdrawn, preoccupied with their own thoughts and delusions. They are often withdrawn both physically and emotionally. Motor activity is generally reduced and characterized by inappropriate and bizarre postures, by rigidity that resists efforts to be moved, or by purposeless and stereotyped movements, for example, rocking or pacing.

The combination of symptoms varies significantly in schizophrenia, and the disorder has been divided into finer categories, including hebephrenic, catatonic, and paranoid. For a further account of clinical symptoms, see Snyder (1980a) or the Diagnostic and Statistical Manual of Mental Disorders (1980; DSM-III).

Diagnosis and Management

Estimates of the incidence of schizophrenia are handicapped by differences in diagnostic criteria, which depend to a large extent on the training of the clinicians making the diagnosis as well as their experience, theoretical beliefs, types of practice, and other biases (Haier, 1980; Babigian, 1975). Because diagnosis is a summary of subjectively evaluated symptoms at a given time, it is easy to see that diagnostic criteria may vary from society to society, institution to institution, or clinician to clinician. Diagnosis also may vary because psychiatric patients inevitably exhibit symptoms of more than one diagnostic category. Furthermore within even a short time span, some symptoms tend to become more prominent, while others recede. It is apparently not uncommon to find that a patient admitted with catatonic manifestations of schizophrenia may be diagnosed as a paranoid schizophrenic several years later (Weiner, 1975). Within the United States, diagnosis has two principal problems: (1) Not everyone uses the same criteria in making diagnoses. (2) Many criteria are unreliable (Haier, 1980). The most recent attempt to provide standard criteria for each category of mental illness and to test them for reliability is represented by the DSM-III, prepared by the American Psychiatric Association. However, critics of the modified criteria exist, and many of the DSM-III revisions have been controversial. Estimates of incidence also vary with the methods of quantification used, for example, records of admissions to public and/or private hospitals, field-survey data, or psychiatric case registers in urban communities. Studies in Europe and Asia, using a relatively narrow concept of schizophrenia, have found a lifetime prevalence rate of from 0.2 to 1 percent. Studies that were done in the United States and that used broader criteria suggest higher rates, at least for urban populations (DSM-III, p. 186).

Figure 1 shows a steady increase in the number of hospitalized psychiatric patients from 1900 to 1956, when the number of patients began a gradual decline. This reduction in the number of hospitalized mental patients has been attributed to a large increase in hospital discharges despite the steady increase in new cases admitted yearly. The increased discharge rate correlates temporally with the initiation of psychotropic drug therapy.

It is significant to remember that patients released from the hospital are not "cured" but are in some stage of remission. Relapse rates for psychiatric disorders are high, but drug treatment has greatly im-

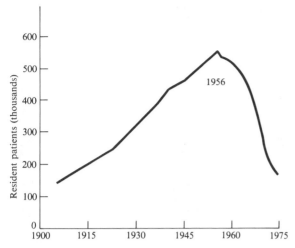

FIGURE 1   PATIENT POPULATION in public mental institutions, 1900–1975. (From Bassuk and Gerson, 1978.)

proved the condition of a large number of patients and enabled them to reenter the community, where they may avoid the general deterioration that occurs with prolonged institutionalization. A secondary benefit of community living may be that the mentally ill are now more visible to the community, thus dramatizing the need for greater social concern for mental health and removing a small portion of the social stigma connected with the disorder.

Although a return to the community is generally believed to provide mental patients with the opportunity to reestablish family ties, social responsibility, and useful employment, many patients live with poor or marginal adjustment to their environment. In addition, because many discharged patients are atypical in their dress, inept in social functioning, and marginal in their economic productivity, there is frequent community resistance to the establishment of community residences for the mentally ill (Klerman, 1977). The establishment of such residences usually occurs in areas populated by the poor, where there is less resistance. The outcome is increased social segregation of the patients. Arnhoff (1975) and others have suggested that the impact on the families of psychiatric patients may be very great. Among potential problems are increased stress on family members and exposure of children to a distorted model (parental or sibling) and increased emotional turmoil. Concern has also

been expressed for the increase in reproduction rate among severely mentally ill individuals who reside in the commuity as compared to hospitalized patients. Because a genetic factor has been identified for both schizophrenia and affective disorders, the increased reproduction rate foreshadows an increase in incidence of mental disorders in the future.

The onset of schizophrenia is most often between the ages of 15 and 54; therefore, the disease disrupts the individual's most productive years. On that basis, the direct (e.g., hospitalization costs, medication) and indirect (loss of productive employment and participation in society) costs of schizophrenia have been estimated at $40 billion a year in the United States (Strauss and Carpenter, 1981).

Epidemiology

Although the question of who is likely to develop schizophrenia has been examined repeatedly, few answers have been found uniformly. One of the strongest epidemiological findings is the inverse relationship between social class status and the incidence of schizophrenia (Dohrenwend and Dohrenwend, 1974b). Despite the fact that the relationship has been found repeatedly, it has not held true in all cases. For instance, the relationship is apparently quite strong in metropolitan centers but weak or absent in smaller cities. In addition, if one excludes the lowest social class, the differential between the remainder is not so great. Two traditional hypotheses have been suggested to explain the phenomenon (Mishler and Scotch, 1963). The first suggests that the social and economic stresses experienced by the lower class are a possible basis for the higher incidence of schizophrenia. The second hypothesis suggests that low social class is secondary to schizophrenia because schizophrenic patients, who frequently maintain bizarre behavior and are unemployed, are downwardly mobile on the socioeconomic scale.

More recently, a third hypothesis has evolved, which suggests that the reduced social network and social communication typical of the lowest class may be an explanation for the elevated numbers of schizophrenics (Hammer et al., 1978). These investigators suggest that the lower socioeconomic class has a higher risk of severed connections among individuals because of death, forced change of residence, or migration. Such disruption in the social network of an individual and its associated loss of social reinforcement and feedback may be the link to the prevalence of schizophrenia. Such disruption occurs most often in the "disorganized" parts of society, that is, where people experience excessive mobility, ethnic conflict, overcrowding, and social isolation. The advantage in identifying such factors is the possibility of developing preventive action for those individuals with the highest risk.

Although remaining controversial, the concept of schizophrenia as a unitary disease is diminishing. Heterogeneity is becoming a focus of study. Different subgroups may be identified in the future, based on biological homogeneity following a recent surge in efforts to uncover a biochemical basis for mental disorders, including schizophrenia and manic-depressive psychosis. In the past, researchers sought an abnormal toxic substance unique to schizophrenia. Current research is focused on possible abnormalities in normal biological functioning, particularly in neuronal metabolism.

The Hereditary Nature of Schizophrenia

The search for a neurochemical pathology responsible for the disease state or for a vulnerability to the disease has been encouraged by genetic studies that demonstrate the importance of heredity to the etiology of this disorder. Systematic family and adoption studies have been conducted by American–Danish teams of investigators, who have taken advantage of the excellent record-keeping system of Denmark to explore the relative contribution of heredity and environment to the development of schizophrenia (Kessler, 1980; Kety et al., 1975; Rosenthal et al., 1971; Wender et al., 1974). These studies demonstrated that relatives of schizophrenics were afflicted with the disease much more frequently than members of the general population. Indeed, the closer the relationship, the greater the probability of schizophrenia in the relative. Furthermore, monozygotic twins, even when reared apart (i.e., in different environments), have a several-fold higher probability of concordance for schizophrenia than dizygotic twins. The operation of genetic factors is strongly suggested by the finding that the offspring of a schizophrenic parent have essentially the same risk for the disorder whether or not they are raised by that parent. All of the studies suffer from relatively small sample sizes, diagnostic uncertainty, and difficulty in data collection characteristic of longitudinal studies. Never-

theless, a substantial case for the hereditary nature of schizophrenia or the propensity for schizophrenia has been accumulated (Kessler, 1980; Heston, 1970).

Pathology

Although no gross or cellular pathology has been found in the brain of schizophrenics, a number of biochemical differences between schizophrenic and normal populations have been identified. However, many of the differences may be effects of the disorder rather than causes. Biochemical differences have been attributed to long-term and multiple drug use by psychiatric patients, institutional diet and vitamin deficiency, differences in physical activity, or other effects of chronic hospitalization. Clearly, the lack of objective diagnostic criteria makes it more difficult to identify the neurochemical correlates of behavior, as it is not unlikely that the multiple types of schizophrenia are paralleled by variations in neurochemistry. Errors involved in sampling from a heterogeneous population explain the lack of confirmation of results by different research groups. Furthermore, in post mortem examination of CNS neurochemistry, experimental results must take into account a variety of enzymatic changes following death. Both death-to-morgue time and morgue-to-autopsy time have been shown to be significant variables in neurochemical studies.

Models of Schizophrenia

Neurochemical research has been further hindered by the difficulty in establishing an animal model for schizophrenia. Because one of the primary symptoms of schizophrenia is thought disorder—an obviously cortical process—we would not expect to find an identical function in animals. During the 1950s, LSD-induced hallucinations were compared to schizophrenic episodes and extensive research was initiated into the mechanism of the drug's action. However, the differences between the drug state and endogenous schizophrenia were found to be more pronounced than were the few similarities (Hollister, 1967). Of the greatest significance is the fact that the LSD-induced state is rarely confused with an endogenous schizophrenic episode by trained clinicians. In addition, drug-induced hallucinations are visual and usually pleasant, whereas in endogenous schizophrenia, hallucinations are usually auditory and threatening. Furthermore, LSD-induced hallucinations are perceived by schizophrenic patients as different from their existing disorder. Also, it has been noted that schizophrenics are highly resistant to suggestion and withdraw from interpersonal contacts. Withdrawal from personal interaction is much less frequent during drug-induced psychoses, and subjects administered LSD are highly suggestable.

In contrast with other drug-induced behaviors, the toxic psychosis following frequent high doses of amphetamine consists of well-formed paranoid delusions, various forms of stereotyped, compulsive behavior, and either visual or auditory hallucinations (Angrist and Gershon, 1970). These effects of high doses of amphetamine are apparently not due to lack of sleep, overexcitement, or precipitation of an underlying disorder (Snyder et al., 1974). The psychotic symptoms can be alleviated by the agents that are most effective in treating endogenous psychosis (Angrist and Gershon, 1970). Also, amphetamine exacerbates the existing symptoms of schizophrenia rather than superimposing new symptoms on the old (Janowsky and Davis, 1976). Furthermore, low doses of amphetamine do not affect the symptoms of manic, depressed, or neurotic patients. These similarities have led to the conclusion that the toxic reaction after high doses of amphetamine is almost indistinguishable from schizophrenia (Ellinwood and Sudilovsky, 1973).

In animals, high doses of amphetamine produce a characteristic stereotyped sniffing, licking, and gnawing that was first identified by Randrup and Munkvad (1967). Because this behavior occurs in response to high doses of amphetamine in man and is similar to the compulsive, repetitious behavior seen in schizophrenia, the amphetamine-induced stereotypy is used in the laboratory as an animal model for schizophrenia.

Dopamine Hypothesis

The finding that the sympathomimetic drug amphetamine can produce a psychotic reaction has prompted a catecholamine hypothesis of schizophrenia. Several lines of evidence suggest that a relative or absolute increase in dopamine may be involved in the development of schizophrenia (for reviews, see Snyder et al., 1974; Iversen, 1975a; Matthysse, 1977).

It is well known that amphetamine potentiates the activity of the catecholamines at the synapse by causing release of the transmitters, preventing reuptake into the presynaptic terminal, and exerting a direct action at the postsynaptic receptor. The relative impor-

tance of norepinephrine (NE) and dopamine (DA) to the various pharmacological effects of amphetamine is now established. Garver et al. (1975) found that the hyperactivity and stereotypies occurring after administration of amphetamine to rats were blocked by pretreatment with α-methyltyrosine, which inhibits synthesis of both NE and DA. Blocking DA receptors with pimozide or haloperidol before administering amphetamine also prevented the appearance of stereotypy and hyperactivity, suggesting that DA may be the significant neurotransmitter in these behaviors. Support for this conclusion comes from lesion experiments in which destruction of the DA-containing pathways reduces or abolishes amphetamine-induced stereotypy (Creese and Iversen, 1974; Costall and Naylor, 1974; Asher and Aghajanian, 1974). In addition, stereotyped behavior can be elicited by intracerebral injection of amphetamine into forebrain DA areas, including striatum and globus pallidus (Costall et al., 1972). This effect can be blocked by systemic (Costall et al., 1972) or intracerebral (Pijnenburg et al., 1975) administration of DA blockers, such as haloperidol. Thus, the DA-induced psychotomimetic effects of amphetamine prompted further investigation into the possibility that excessive DA neurotransmission is responsible for schizophrenic symptoms.

Phenothiazines and Butyrophenones. Further pharmacological support for the DA hypothesis comes from the observation that the drugs designated as neuroleptics* (the phenothiazines and butyrophenones) are effective in alleviating the primary symptoms of schizophrenia and are central DA receptor blockers. The phenothiazines are currently the largest and most commonly used class of antipsychotic drugs. They were originally synthesized in 1883 in the course of investigating two chemically related dyes but were not used until much later (1940s). The phenothiazine nucleus (Figure 2) is a three-ring structure: two benzene rings joined by sulfur and nitrogen atoms. Various substituents at R_1 and R_2 change the potency, pharmacological activity, and side effects of the different phenothiazines. Figure 2 also shows the structural relationships of several phenothiazines. The structural substituent at R_1 determines the three major subgroups of the phenothiazines: the aliphatic (e.g.,

---

*A neuroleptic drug is defined as one that selectively reduces emotionality and psychomotor activity.

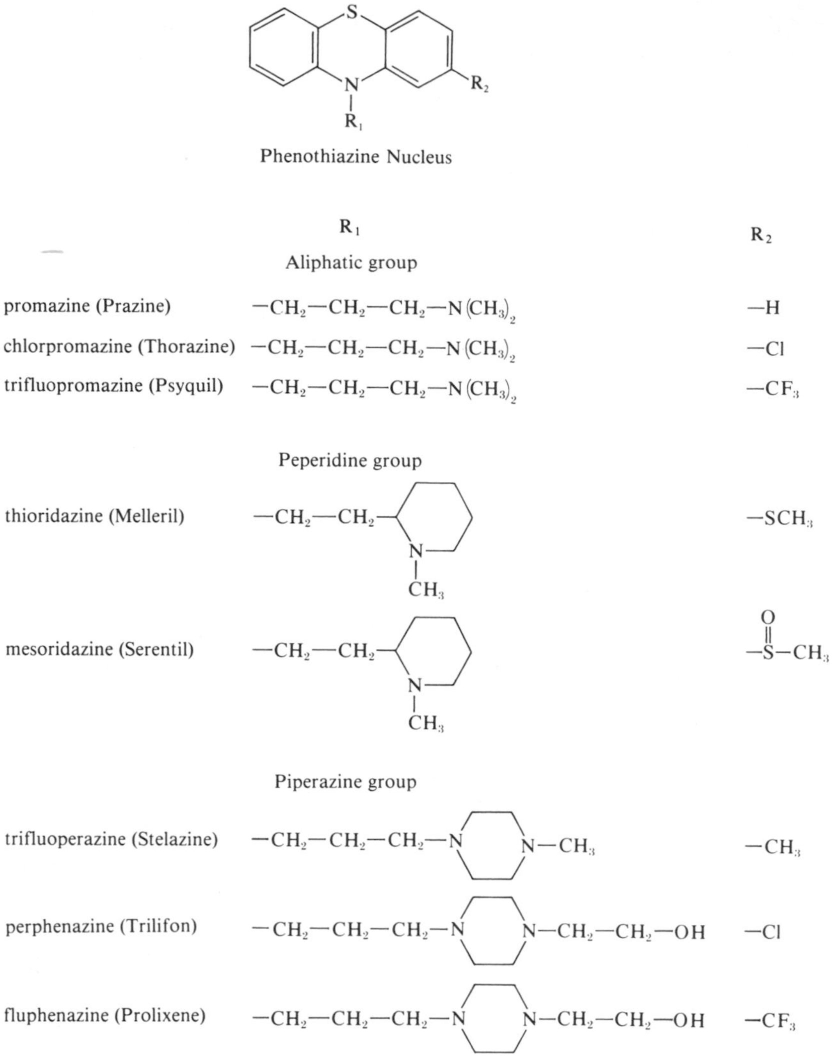

Phenothiazine Nucleus

	R_1	R_2
	Aliphatic group	
promazine (Prazine)	$-CH_2-CH_2-CH_2-N(CH_3)_2$	$-H$
chlorpromazine (Thorazine)	$-CH_2-CH_2-CH_2-N(CH_3)_2$	$-Cl$
trifluopromazine (Psyquil)	$-CH_2-CH_2-CH_2-N(CH_3)_2$	$-CF_3$

Peperidine group

thioridazine (Melleril) — $-CH_2-CH_2-$ piperidine ring with $N-CH_3$ — R_2: $-SCH_3$

mesoridazine (Serentil) — $-CH_2-CH_2-$ piperidine ring with $N-CH_3$ — R_2: $-\overset{O}{\underset{\|}{S}}-CH_3$

Piperazine group

trifluoperazine (Stelazine) — $-CH_2-CH_2-CH_2-N$ piperazine $N-CH_3$ — R_2: $-CH_3$

perphenazine (Trilifon) — $-CH_2-CH_2-CH_2-N$ piperazine $N-CH_2-CH_2-OH$ — R_2: $-Cl$

fluphenazine (Prolixene) — $-CH_2-CH_2-CH_2-N$ piperazine $N-CH_2-CH_2-OH$ — R_2: $-CF_3$

FIGURE 2   PHENOTHIAZINE NUCLEUS and related compounds.

chlorpromazine), piperidine (e.g., thioridazine), and piperazine (e.g., trifluoperazine) groups. Additional substitution at R_2 further alters potency. For example, within the aliphatic group, chlorpromazine (which has a chlorine at R_2) is much more potent pharmacologically than is promazine (which has no R_2 substituent). A —CF_3 radical at R_2 (trifluopromazine) further increases potency for depressing motor activity as well as alleviating psychotic symptoms.

The second group contains a piperidine moiety in the side chain and includes thioridazine and mesoridazine. This substitution is apparently responsible for a lower incidence of extrapyramidal side effects.

In the third group, the replacement of the propyldimethylamino side chain of the aliphatic group by a propylpiperazine side chain (e.g., the change from trifluopromazine to trifluoperazine) greatly augments the potency of the neuroleptic drugs. Within this third group, the replacement of the terminal—CH_3 on the piperazine ring (as on trifluoperazine) with—

CH_2CH_2OH (e.g., fluphenazine) further increases antipsychotic potency as well as antiemetic effects and extrapyramidal side effects.

The three-dimensional configurations of the phenothiazines, as determined by X-ray crystallography, can be superimposed on the three-dimensional structure of dopamine (Feinberg and Snyder, 1975). From that work it is apparent that a change in substituents, such as the lack of a substituent at R_2, alters the ability of the phenothiazine to conform to the structure of dopamine and thus reduces the pharmacological activity.

The phenothiazines have many biological effects, but few can be shown to correlate with clinical potency as antipsychotic agents. The best correlation is between the effect on dopamine neurons in the brain and antipsychotic efficacy. Carlsson and Lindqvist (1963) originally speculated that phenothiazines block DA receptor sites and by a feedback mechanism increase the synthesis and release (i.e., the turnover) of DA. In support of this idea, they found a large increase in O-methylated metabolites after administration of phenothiazines, indicating increased extraneuronal metabolism. They also found that the neuroleptic drugs increased the formation and disappearance of [^{14}C]DA from its precursor [^{14}C]tyrosine, demonstrating more rapid DA turnover. In addition, the antipsychotic drugs block the effects of iontophoretic DA on the firing of striatal neurons (Siggins et al., 1974) and block the effects of amphetamine on DA neurons in midbrain (Bunney and Aghajanian, 1975b).

A second major class of neuroleptic drugs comprises the butyrophenones (e.g., haloperidol and spiroperidol). These drugs are structurally unrelated to the phenothiazines, but their pharmacological effects are very similar and most resemble the piperazine phenothiazines in their actions.

Dopamine-Stimulated Adenylate Cyclase. Further evidence for the inhibition of DA systems by the phenothiazines includes their effect on the second messenger, cyclic AMP (cAMP). The formation of cAMP by adenylate cyclase in the caudate is probably regulated by two distinct catecholamine receptors: stimulated by DA and by β-adrenergic compounds (Forn et al., 1974). However, only the DA-stimulated adenylate cyclase is effectively inhibited in a competitive manner by the addition of low concentrations of neuroleptic drugs (Clement-Cormier et al., 1974). Since destroying the presynaptic cell does not prevent the effect, it is likely that the drug-induced inhibition is a postsynaptic phenomenon (Iversen, 1975a). The neuroleptic drugs also inhibit DA stimulation of adenylate cyclase in other areas of the brain that contain DA terminals, including nucleus accumbens, olfactory tubercle, amygdala, and median eminence (Clement-Cormier et al., 1974; Clement-Cormier and Robison, 1977); this inhibition may account for other effects of the drugs, such as endocrinological changes.

When various phenothiazine drugs are compared, the individual potencies as inhibitors of DA-sensitive adenylate cyclase correlate to some degree with their *in vivo* potencies as antipsychotics (Karobath and Leitich, 1974; Iversen, 1975a). There is one exception to this finding: drugs in the butyrophenone class (e.g., haloperidol), which are among the most potent antipsychotic drugs, do not demonstrate a similar efficacy in the *in vitro* test of adenylate cyclase inhibition. This discrepancy may be explained by the drugs' ability to presynaptically block stimulation-induced release of DA (Seeman and Lee, 1975). Alternatively, the discrepancy may be explained by the fact that in *in vivo* systems, the butyrophenones may accumulate more readily in the DA system than do other neuroleptic drugs, so that at a given dose, a higher concentration of drug reaches the receptor site. The importance of pharmacological factors such as rate of absorption, binding to lipid depots, and rate of excretion should be emphasized when comparing *in vivo* and *in vitro* potency, as all those factors significantly alter effective drug concentrations of *in vivo* preparations but have no effect on *in vitro* measures.

Dopamine receptor binding. The phenothiazines and butyrophenones have also been shown to inhibit the binding of [^{3}H]dopamine and [^{3}H]haloperidol to the dopamine receptor in the caudate (Creese et al., 1976). Ability to displace the labeled ligand is closely correlated with both clinical efficacy of the various drugs tested and with the drug's inhibition of DA-sensitive adenylate cyclase. Furthermore, an excellent correlation exists between the neuroleptics' inhibition of [^{3}H]haloperidol binding and their ability to inhibit amphetamine-induced stereotypy.

Although it is tempting to speculate that the mesolimbic DA system may be responsible for the drug's antipsychotic action and the nigrostriatal DA system may be responsible for the pronounced Parkinsonian side effects, there is little direct evidence for such a distinction. Most of the neurochemical effects of the neuroleptic drugs are about equipotent in the two major tracts. However, Crow et al. (1978) tested the effects of three neuroleptic drugs (chlorpromazine, fluphenazine, and thioridazine), which produce different amounts of extrapyramidal side effects, on DA turnover in the striatum and the nucleus accumbens. Their results demonstrated that the drugs' potencies were quite different in striatal DA turnover but were very similar in nucleus accumbens. Hence, they suggested that the neuroleptic effect on striatal DA is more likely to be responsible for the side effects than the DA turnover in the nucleus accumbens.

Clozapine has a strong action on DA turnover in the limbic system and a relatively weak one in the striatum. Coincidentally, clozapine has antipsychotic efficacy but very few extrapyramidal side effects. Furthermore, Bunney and Aghajanian (1975b) demonstrated that clozapine is capable of reversing amphetamine-induced depression of neuronal firing in the DA cell bodies in the ventral tegmentum (the origin of DA fibers of the mesolimbic system). Clozapine was not effective in blocking amphetamine-induced depression of neuronal cell bodies in substantia nigra (the origin of the nigrostriatal DA system). Because antipsychotic drugs that also have extrapyramidal effects inhibit amphetamine's effects on both cell groups, it is more likely that the antipsychotic effects of the neuroleptic drugs are due to action on the mesolimbic DA system. These findings demonstrate one potential problem in screening methods; correlations must be examined to determine whether they are related to the desired pharmacological effect or to one of the many side effects. Without such care, a screening test developed to identify potent antipsychotic drugs may in reality select compounds with strong extrapyramidal side effects that have some antipsychotic action.

Neuroleptic action on DA neurons has been complicated by the discovery of a second class of receptors—dopaminergic autoreceptors. Dopamine neurons apparently have receptors that are sensitive to DA, are located on their cell bodies, dendrites, and nerve terminals, and are responsible for controlling the synthesis and release of neurotransmitter. Since the idea was first suggested by Kehr et al. (1972), both biochemical and behavioral evidence for existence of the receptors has accumulated (Meltzer, 1980). Thus, application of DA or a DA agonist (apomorphine) to the DA cell bodies in the substantia nigra or ventral

tegmentum decreases the rate of firing of the DA neurons (Aghajanian and Bunney, 1977). The DA-induced inhibition can be antagonized by systemic administration of a neuroleptic drug such as chlorpromazine. In fact, the DA autoreceptors are 6–10 times more sensitive to the application of DA than are the postsynaptic receptors in the caudate (Skirboll et al., 1979). The biphasic effect of dopamine agonists on motor behavior in rats is also consistent with the notion of two types of receptors. Low doses of L-dopa, apomorphine, and other agonists inhibit motor activity and exploratory behavior, whereas higher doses increase motor activity; finally, at still higher doses, apomorphine produces stereotyped sniffing, licking, and gnawing and subsequent decrease in locomotion (Strömbom, 1977). The identification of two types of receptors means that pharmacological treatment of psychiatric and motor disorders will become more specific. It is reasonable to expect that by modifying either the dose administered or by changing the molecular structure of the drug, differential activity at the receptors will be possible.

Although pharmacological evidence supports the DA hypothesis, is there evidence for dopaminergic hyperactivity in schizophrenics? Thus far the evidence has not been convincing. Homovanillic acid, the major DA metabolite, is not increased in the cerebrospinal fluid of schizophrenics (Post et al., 1975), as one would expect in a more active DA system. Dopamine-sensitive adenylate cyclase activity was also found to be the same in postmortem brains from schizophrenics and normal controls (Carenzi et al., 1975). There has been one report of a decrease in dopamine-β-hydroxylase in schizophrenic brains postmortem (Wise et al., 1974). This enzyme would increase the levels of DA in the brain while reducing NE. However, the report was not confirmed by another group (Wyatt et al., 1975). Such discrepancies reemphasize the problems associated with neurochemical investigations after death: (1) heterogeneous populations resulting from diagnostic discrepancies, (2) previous history of chronic drug use, (3) postmortem deterioration of enzyme activity that is reflected in both death-to-morgue time and morgue-to-autopsy time. In all these cases, groups have been small and variability high. It may also be worthwhile to remember that not all schizophrenics are improved by treatment with neuroleptic drugs, and these unresponsive patients may reflect a subpopulation with distinct neurochemical pathology.

Furthermore, schizophrenia can occur in patients with Parkinson's disease—patients who, it is assumed, have depleted DA stores in the brain (Crow et al., 1978). Such should not be the case if schizophrenia is related to excessive dopamine activity.

Central Nervous System Effects
of the Neuroleptic Drugs

As with all pharmacological agents, the neuroleptic drugs have many effects on an organism in addition to the principal therapeutic effects. Acute administration of the neuroleptic drugs produces reduced motor activity and indifference to environmental stimuli. The indifference to environmental stimuli is demonstrated in conditioned avoidance experiments with animals. In one such experiment, a rat may be trained to escape electric foot shock by climbing a pole. If the shock onset is signaled by a buzzer, the rat will learn in a few trials to climb the pole whenever it hears the buzzer. After small doses of chlorpromazine, the rat ignores the buzzer even though it is able to climb the pole when the shock is applied. The ability of chlorpromazine to block the conditioned avoidance response (CAR) is characteristic for antipsychotic drugs and has been used as a screening device to identify new efficacious agents. A good correlation between antipsychotic potency and suppression of CAR has been demonstrated (Niemegeers et al., 1969; Cook and Catania, 1964).

However, to evaluate the effect of a drug on CAR, the contribution of nonspecific sedation to the suppression of the CAR must be considered. That is, the animal may merely be responding more slowly to the warning signal because of sedation. By lengthening the interval between signal and shock, the two effects can usually be separated. Under these conditions, neuroleptic drugs still produce a decrement in CAR (Lipper and Kornetsky, 1971). A second method to avoid the contaminating contribution of general sedation is to use passive avoidance procedures such as the step-down platform. In this test, the animal is placed on a platform suspended above an electrified grid floor. After several trials, a normal animal avoids the shock by remaining on the platform. Animals treated with neuroleptic drugs continue to make the step-down response, indicating that the drugs produce an indifference to environmental stimuli without significant sedation.

Clinically, tolerance to the sedative effect develops gradually although the antipsychotic effect may take weeks to develop. The difference in the time course of the pharmacological effects may thus be useful in identifying adequate screening methods, as any behavioral or neurochemical effect of the phenothiazines that undergoes tolerance is probably related to the sedative rather than to the antipsychotic action of the drug.

The phenothiazines do not produce euphoria and are often considered to have unpleasant effects, particularly in individuals who are not psychotic. For these reasons, the neuroleptic drugs are a class of drugs that are rarely, if ever, abused. Other CNS effects of the phenothiazines include inhibition of nausea and vomiting, as a result of their actions on the medullary chemical trigger zone. In addition, the neuroleptic drugs inhibit release of growth hormone and cause release of prolactin. The neuroendocrine dysfunction and the drug-induced defects in temperature regulation are most likely attributable to DA inhibition in the hypothalamus.

Side Effects of Neuroleptics

Parkinsonism. The most troublesome side effect is the appearance of extrapyramidal (Parkinsonian) symptoms which undergo remission after drug treatment stops. The incidence of these symptoms is high, and some psychiatrists have suggested that the clinical efficacy and the appearance of Parkinson's side effects are inseparable (Mattke, 1968), although this conclusion has been questioned. Because we know that Parkinson's disease is caused by a deficiency of DA in the basal ganglia, the phenothiazine-induced tremors and rigidity is probably due to the blockade of DA receptors in the caudate (a part of the basal ganglia). However, if dopamine receptor blockade were responsible for the side effects as well as the antipsychotic effects, the two should be closely correlated; for several neuroleptic drugs this is not the case. Snyder et al. (1974) found that neuroleptic drugs also bind to muscarinic cholinergic receptors in the brain and that their affinity for the acetylcholine receptors is inversely correlated with their ability to produce extrapyramidal effects. Thus, it may be possible to produce neuroleptic drugs that have high affinity for the dopamine receptors (and therefore effective antipsychotic action) and at the same time have strong anticholinergic action to minimize parkinsonian side effects. One early example, widely used clinically, is thioridazine. A second drug may be the experimental neuroleptic drug clozapine.

It has been noted that neuroleptic drug-induced parkinsonism is the result of DA receptor blockade with a resulting release of a disinhibited excessive cholinergic activity in the striatum (see Chapter 7). When neuroleptic therapy seems to be the best course of action, the presence of concomitant parkinsonism can be substantially mitigated by combining the neuroleptic treatment with an anticholinergic drug such as benztropine mesylate (Cogentin).

Tardive Dyskinesia. A second neurological syndrome associated with the prolonged use of antipsychotic drugs is tardive dyskinesia (TD), which is characterized by stereotyped involuntary movements (particularly of the face and jaw), "flycatching" darting of the tongue, and choreiform and purposeless movements of the extremities. These spontaneous movements are increased during high vigilance and agitation; drowsiness and sleep have the opposite effect. When there is voluntary use of some muscle groups which ordinarily exhibit dyskinesis the symptoms cease, while abnormal movements are enhanced in other muscle groups. For instance, during conversation the oral manifestations of TD are diminished but the dyskinesia of the hands and pelvis become more conspicuous. On the other hand, writing or the performance of a manual task abolishes spontaneous dyskinesia of the hands but seems to release oral movements (Crane, 1978).

Usually TD appears late compared to parkinsonism and other neuroleptic side effects. Investigators have diagnosed the disorder in patients who received antipsychotic drugs for from 18 months to 5 years, and a few of these patients had received the drugs 8 or 10 years prior to the appearance of the TD symptoms—hence the term tardive (late) dyskinesia.

TD appears in about 10 percent of patients treated with neuroleptics, and it may appear in any age group. Its prevalence increases in patients over 50, especially in geriatric patients who are usually vulnerable to the toxic effects of drugs due to impaired liver and kidney function. If TD develops during the course of drug treatment it tends to persist, even if treatment is discontinued. Because most patients have been treated with a variety of neuroleptics it is not possible to single out any one agent as being more toxic than any of the others (Crane, 1978).

There have been many attempts to establish the neuropathology of TD. Autopsy material is scarce and contradictory. Christensen et al. (1970) attributed the "irreversible" nature of TD to his finding of gliosis (multiplication of microglia) in the substantia nigra and other parts of the brain, which usually denotes neuron degeneration. However, other investigators failed to confirm his findings. Animal experiments have shown that lesions in the head of the caudate nucleus in the brain of a cat will cause a vast array of abnormal movements with some features in common with human TD, thus perhaps localizing the site of TD injury to the striatum.

It was also discovered that terminating neuroleptic treatment or lowering the dose aggravated the TD symptoms, and that reinstating treatment or raising the dose alleviated the symptoms. This suggested that the neuroleptics, by blocking DA receptors, had induced a DA receptor supersensitivity, and that this state could be reversed only by returning to drug treatment or by raising the drug dose (Creese et al., 1977, 1978). Snyder et al. (1977) tested this idea by investigating the effects on DA receptor binding in rats after chronic treatment with the neuroleptics haloperidol, fluphenazine and reserpine, as well as the non-antipsychotic phenothiazine promethazine, and amphetamine. One week after 21 days of treatment with the neuroleptics there was a 20 to 30 percent increase in DA receptor binding which was due to an increase in the number of [^{3}H]haloperidol binding sites rather than a change in their affinity. Chronic treatment with the nonneurolepic drugs did not increase binding. Thus, behavioral supersensitivity and tardive dyskinesia following chronic treatment with neuroleptics may be due to an increase in DA receptors.

These findings are consistent with the results of many other studies that showed that interruption of the nigrostriatal pathway will cause hypersensitivity of dopaminergic receptors due to denervation and disuse. For example, *in vitro* studies showed that dopamine sensitive adenylate cyclases become more responsive to dopamine in striatal tissue after denervation (Iversen, 1975a), and increased reactivity of dopamine receptors occurred after denervation produced by 6-hydroxy-dopamine (Ungerstedt, 1971a, 1971c) (see Chapter 7). Also, guinea pigs treated with chlorpromazine did not show symptoms until they were challenged by dopamine receptor agonists such as amphetamine and apomorphine, which produced stereotyped movements in the mouth and elsewhere (Rubovits and Klawans, 1972). In another study, after dopamine receptor hypersensitivity had been established in rats, they were pretreated with a neuroleptic before the challenge with apomorphine. This blocked the stereotypy. Similar hypersensitivity phenomena were observed with catecholamine depletors such as α-methylparatyrosine and reserpine, as well as with chlorpromazine and haloperidol. These findings appear to give strong support to the receptor supersensitivity hypothesis to explain TD, but it must be noted that the dyskinesias elicited in animals bear little resemblance to those of humans (Crane, 1978).

There is justifiable concern about long-term exposure or indiscriminate use of neuroleptics, especially in patients weakened with age since their systems cannot adequately cope with heavy chemical burdens. Also, neuroleptic drug use for the young afflicted with psychoses—who may be faced with pharmacotherapy for many years and may ultimately react to an accumulation of toxic effects—is a cause for concern. This calls for the discriminate use of neuroleptic drugs and intensified efforts to find either alternative treatments or ways to prevent the occurrence of tardive dyskinesia.

Peripheral Effects of Neuroleptics

Like many pharmacological agents, the phenothiazines have multiple effects in the periphery. In addition to dopamine blocking effects, the drugs have anticholinergic and antiadrenergic actions, as well as antihistaminic and antitryptaminic actions. The complex interactions produce widespread effects on the autonomic nervous system, endocrine system, and on the renal–urinary system. It is not within the scope of this chapter to describe in detail the intricate effects of these drugs on peripheral physiology. For further discussion refer to any standard text in medical pharmacology.

Reserpine

Reserpine (a Rauwolfia alkaloid) should be included in our discussion of effective antipsychotic drugs that reduce catecholamine activity. Reserpine was originally used to treat hypertension but caused depression in patients receiving the drug. It was adopted in the early 1950s (at about the same time as chlorpromazine) to treat mania and excited schizophrenic states. It is no longer used extensively because it is slow in onset, produces serious side effects (including severe mental depression), and is generally not as useful as the phenothiazines. However, it has proven to be very

useful in understanding the biochemistry of depression and is a keystone of the biogenic amine hypothesis of depression (see section later in this chapter on affective disorders).

Transmethylation Hypothesis

Among the other biogenic amine hypotheses of schizophrenia is the "transmethylation hypothesis" originated by Osmond and Smythies (1952) about 30 years ago. They suggested that the neurochemical basis of schizophrenia is the aberrant metabolism of a normal amine into a methylated psychotogen. One such O-methylated catecholamine is dimethoxyphenylethylamine (DMPEA), which is structurally similar to the hallucinogen mescaline, as well as the normal transmitter DA (Figure 3). DMPEA has been found in the urine of some schizophrenic patients, but no evidence of correlation between schizophrenia and the concentration of the methylated compound in the urine has been found. Furthermore, DMPEA did not produce psychotic symptoms when administered to normal individuals (Hollister and Friedhoff, 1966).

Indoleamines (e.g., 5-HT) can also be methylated to form hallucinogenic compounds such as N,N-dimethyltryptamine (DMT), psilocybin, and bufotenine (Figure 4). Although bufotenine has been found in the urine and plasma in schizophrenics and

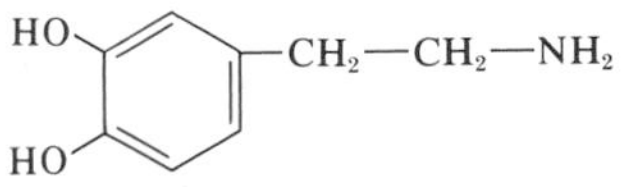

Dopamine

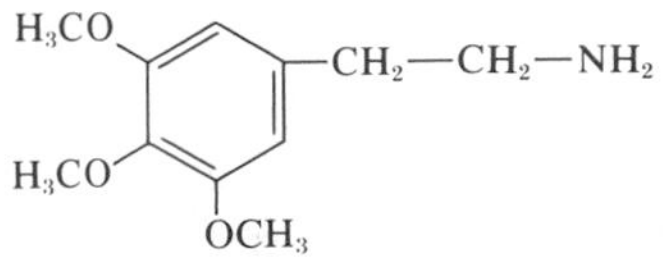

Mescaline

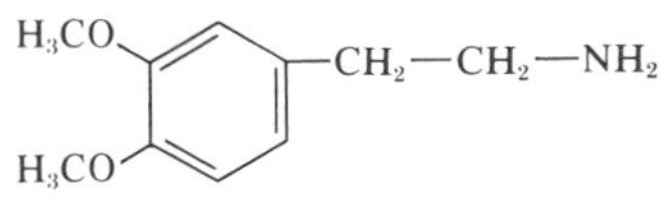

Dimethoxyphenylethylamine (DMPEA)

FIGURE 3 DOPAMINE AND RELATED O-METHYLATED CATECHOLAMINES.

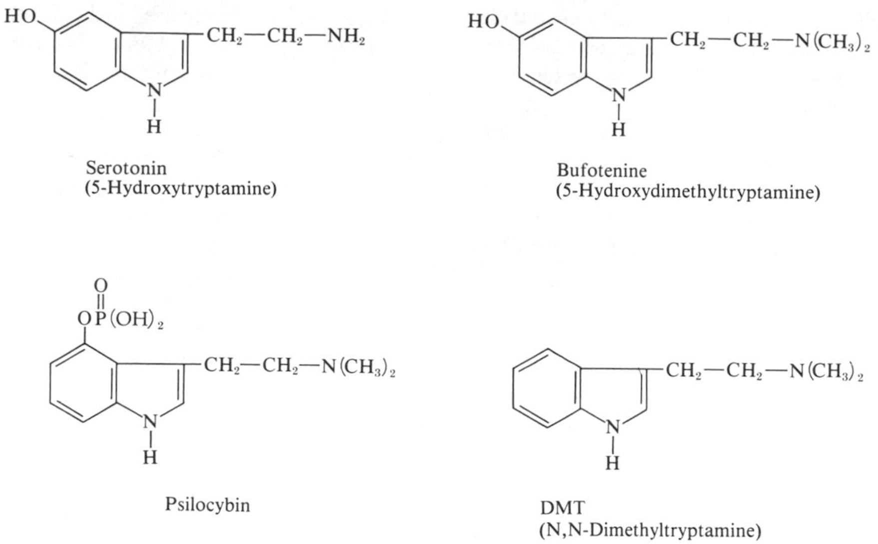

FIGURE 4 SEROTONIN AND RELATED METHYLATED COMPOUNDS.

normals, no consistent differences between the two groups have been found. The possibility must be considered that the important variable may not be absolute concentration of psychotogen but rate of accumulation or sensitivity of receptor mechanisms that would not be necessarily reflected in concentration. However, bufotenine does not induce psychosis in normal individuals, although the lack of effect may be due to an inability of bufotenine to cross the blood brain barrier.

In order for a methylated amine to be considered a psychotogen, several criteria originally proposed by Hollister (1977) must be met. Evaluation of DMT based on these criteria has been summarized by Gillin et al. (1976).

1. *The proposed schizotoxin should mimic important clinical aspects of schizophrenia.* DMT, when administered to normal volunteers, produced visual illusions, hallucinations, distortion of spatial perception and body image, speech disturbances, and euphoria (Szara, 1956). These effects are of short duration and closely follow blood levels of DMT. Although neither auditory hallucinations nor thought disorders occur, some of the psychological effects following DMT administration strongly resemble endogenous schizophrenia. Its amine precursor, tryptamine, produces effects in humans similar to the effects produced by LSD (Martin et al., 1972).

2. *The schizotoxin should be found in humans.* The data on this point are conflicting and have been summarized elsewhere (Gillin et al., 1976). There is no apparent relationship between any form of schizophrenia and the amount of DMT found in blood or urine. Also, DMT has been found in the blood and urine of normal volunteers. Thus far no conclusion has been drawn on whether DMT is an endogenously synthesized product or results from diet, bacterial infections, or other sources.

3. *The necessary precursors and synthesizing enzymes should be present in humans.* The precursor amine is probably tryptamine, which is found in the brain of many species, including humans (Martin et al., 1972), with the highest levels of tryptamine in spinal cord, hypothalamus, and basal ganglia (Saavedra, 1977). Although it has been suggested that tryptamine is formed in several neuronal systems, the amine is not considered a putative neurotransmitter because no storage mechanism has been identified, large amounts are associated with nonparticulate portions of cells, and release after nerve stimulation has not been demonstrated. However, it seems likely that tryptamine synthesis may be influenced by 5-HT content because the tryptophan hydrox-

ylase inhibitor (PCPA) decreases brain 5-HT while increasing brain tryptamine (Saavedra and Axelrod, 1973). Furthermore, levels of tryptamine can be increased by administering the amino acid L-tryptophan, inhibitors of monoamine oxidase (MAO), or drugs that prevent the conversion of tryptophan to 5-hydroxytryptophan (Koe and Weissman, 1966). Thus, an intimate relationship between 5-HT neurons and tryptamine is apparent; and the possibility that some of the behavioral effects of PCPA may be due to increases in tryptamine must also be considered.

Four indole methylating enzymes have been identified in mammalian tissues (Koslow, 1977), including brain (Mandel and Morgan, 1971; Banerjee and Snyder, 1973). These enzymes may be responsible for the formation of the methylated amine, as pictured in Figure 5. Formation of DMT *in vivo* has been found in rat brain after tryptamine administration (Saavedra, 1977). The administration of large amounts of the amino acid methionine (a methyl donor) caused an exacerbation of schizophrenic symptoms (Pollin et al., 1961), although it is not clear whether methyl donation or direct toxic action is responsible for the effect.

Of the other methylating enzymes that have been identified, at least one is capable of forming DMT in platelets (Wyatt et al., 1973b). Because MAO activity in the platelets of schizophrenics has been found to be lower than in normal subjects (Murphy

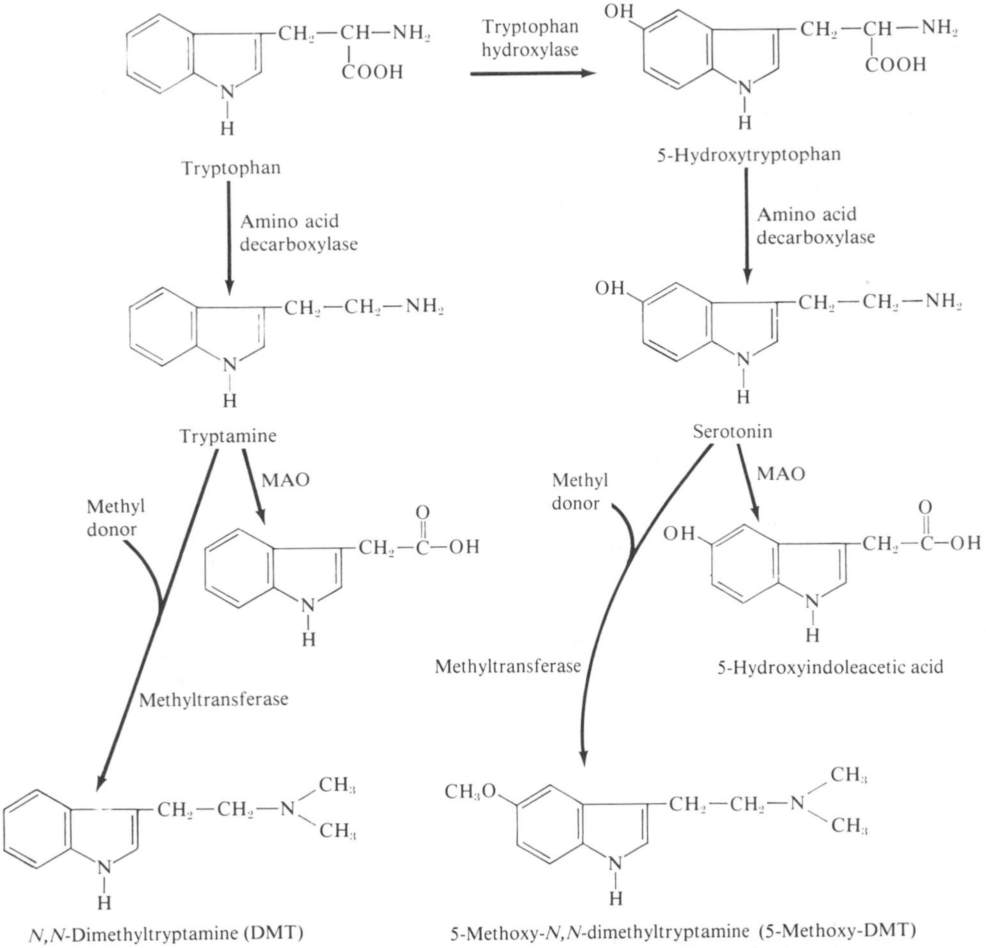

FIGURE 5 FORMATION OF DMT and 5-Methoxy-DMT by methylation.

and Wyatt, 1972) and because lower MAO activity might be expected to increase levels of tryptamine (see Figure 5), it is possible that an increase in synthesis of DMT would also occur. However, increasing the levels of the tryptamine precursor (L-tryptophan) did not change either blood levels of DMT or the patient's clinical condition (Gillin et al., 1976).

4. *The schizotoxin should be synthesized or metabolized differently in schizophrenics than in controls.* Synthesis of DMT has not been conclusively demonstrated, and there have been few studies comparing the concentration of metabolites in normals and schizophrenics. The finding that DMT is very rapidly metabolized (Kaplan et al., 1974) may explain the difficulty in comparing concentrations of DMT in the biological fluids of schizophrenics and normal volunteers. Even if the correct methylating enzyme and correct methylated amine are isolated, it is possible that the enzyme activity occurs in both normals and schizophrenics and that the major difference between the two groups is the activation or modulation of the enzyme.

5. *Tolerance to the psychotogen should not occur because schizophrenia is a disease that persists for many years and does not show a gradual diminution.* Unlike the rapid development of tolerance to LSD, psilocybin, and mescaline, tolerance to the autonomic changes or psychological effects of DMT does not seem to develop (Gillin et al., 1976). A lack of tolerance has been reported for squirrel monkeys working on an operant task after administration of DMT daily for as long as 38 days (Cole and Pieper, 1973).

6. *Neuroleptic drugs should antagonize the effects of DMT.* Once again, evidence to support the hypothesis is limited. Some results suggest that chlorpromazine or its metabolites may inhibit N-methyltransferase (Axelrod, 1962; Narasimhachari and Lin, 1974) but even less data exist on the effect of antipsychotic drugs on the metabolism of DMT or on the behavioral effects of the compound.

The transmethylation hypothesis has received limited experimental support because DMT does produce profound psychological changes that do not appear to undergo tolerance to any appreciable extent. Furthermore, the enzymatic capability to produce DMT in brain exists. However, many important criteria for establishing a methylated amine as a schizotoxin have not been met.

A family of methylated amines exists because the methylating enzymes are not specific for one substrate. Thus, we might further consider the compounds 5-methoxytryptamine, 5-methoxy-N-methyltryptamine, N-methylserotonin, N,N-dimethylserotonin, 5-methoxy-N-methyltryptamine, and so forth. Some of these have behavioral effects when administered peripherally; others produce electrophysiological changes in the CNS or alter serotonergic activity (Koslow, 1977). Each may be considered according to our criteria for putative psychotogens. Thus, we must wait for further research into the physiological significance of the methylated amines and their possible role in abnormal behavior.

Phenylethylamine Hypothesis

The model psychosis induced by doses of amphetamine closely resembles paranoid schizophrenia. Phenylethylamine (PEA) is a sympathomimetic amine that has many of the same pharmacological properties as amphetamine. PEA is a naturally occurring product of phenylalanine and is normally metabolized by MAO of the B type to phenylacetic acid. It may also be hydroxylated to form phenethanolamine (Figure 6). However, until recently the quantification techniques have not been sufficiently sensitive to make accurate measurements, so results on the concentration of PEA in brain and biological fluids vary. The PEA hypothesis suggests that biochemical abnormalities that result in increased levels of PEA might be responsible for an amphetamine-like psychotic reaction (Wyatt et al., 1977). Thus, inhibition of MAO might be expected to increase PEA. Because PEA is relatively nonpolar, it can readily cross the blood brain barrier. Therefore, low peripheral MAO activity could have a significant effect on central PEA levels. However, patients treated for a variety of disorders with MAO inhibitors rarely become psychotic. Thus, low MAO activity cannot in itself be responsible for the schizophrenic reaction.

PEA administered systemically with an MAO inhibitor produces stereotyped behavior and increased motor activity in rats (Moja et al., 1976). Repeated administration over 7 days did not reduce the behavioral effects of the agents. Thus, tolerance to the central effects of PEA apparently does not occur. The neuroleptic drugs blocked the behavioral effects of PEA and pargyline, and the order of potency roughly reflects clinical efficacy of the same compounds (Wyatt, 1976). Thus, a number of the criteria for an endogenous

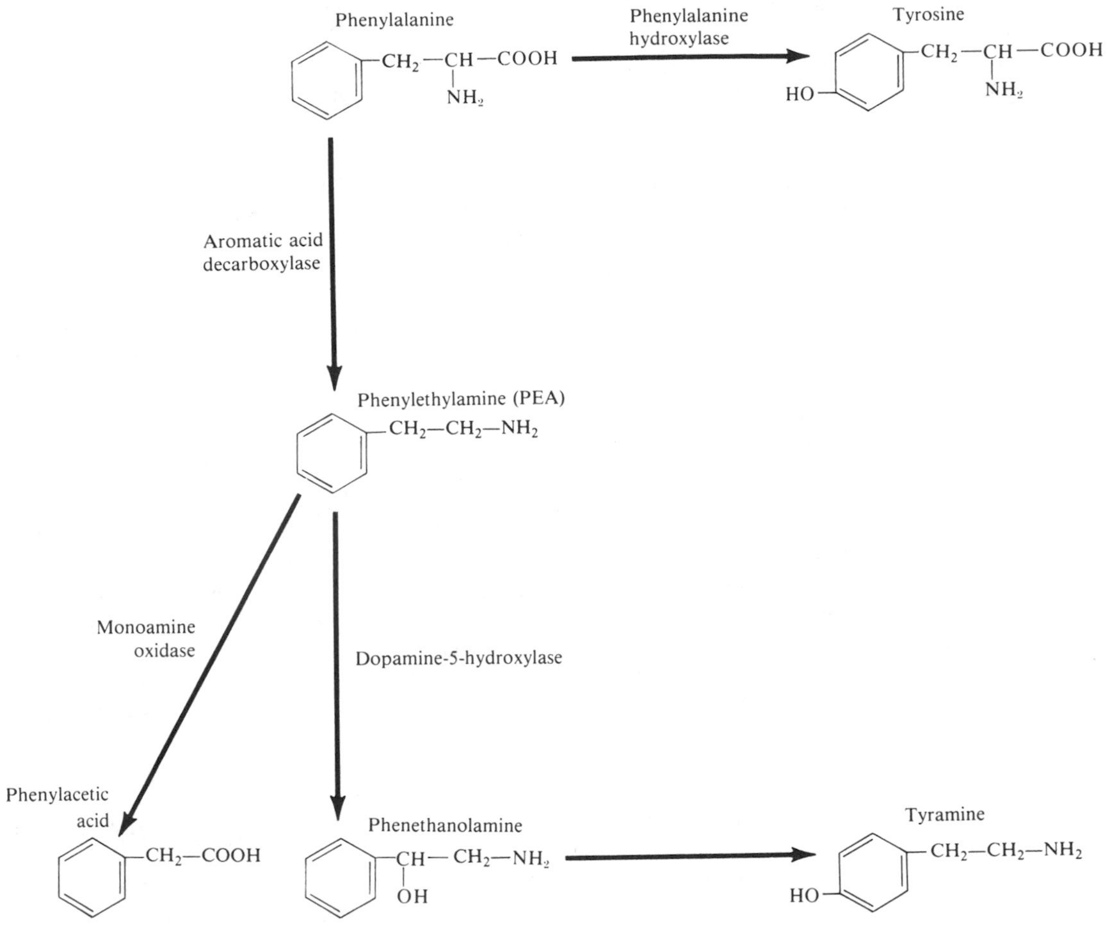

Phenylalanine

$CH_2-CH-COOH$
NH_2

Phenylalanine hydroxylase →

Tyrosine

$HO-$ $CH_2-CH-COOH$
NH_2

Aromatic acid decarboxylase

Phenylethylamine (PEA)
$CH_2-CH_2-NH_2$

Monoamine oxidase

Dopamine-5-hydroxylase

Phenylacetic acid

$-CH_2-COOH$

Phenethanolamine

$CH-CH_2-NH_2$
OH

Tyramine

$HO-$ $CH_2-CH_2-NH_2$

FIGURE 6   METABOLISM OF PHENYELTHYLAMINE (PEA) from phenylalanine.

psychotogen have been met. However, there is little evidence that PEA is found in greater concentrations in schizophrenics than normals, although until recently sensitive techniques for measurement were not available. L-Phenylalanine plus iproniazid (an MAO inhibitor) were not found to produce a mood or behavioral change in chronic schizophrenics (Pollin et al., 1961), although iproniazid is a poor inhibitor of B type MAO, which is responsible for metabolism of PEA.

Role of Monoamine Oxidase

Differences in monoamine oxidase activity have been considered in the biochemical studies investigating the etiology of schizophrenia. MAO is an en-zyme that is found in most tissues in vertebrates. The greatest enzyme activity is found in liver. In brain, different regions vary significantly in the amount of activity and in the proportions of the two major subtypes, MAO-A and MAO-B. Within the nervous system, MAO is a significant metabolic enzyme that degrades many monoamines, including NE, DA, and 5-HT. Studies of families with mono- and dizygotic twins have shown that MAO is under genetic control (Nies et al., 1973). Furthermore, abnormal amine metabolism caused by irregular MAO activity may be consistent with either the dopamine hypothesis, the transmethylation hypothesis, or the phenylethylamine hypothesis.

Most studies have used blood platelets as a ready source of the enzyme. A significant reduction in MAO activity in platelets has been found in patients with chronic schizophrenia and manic–depressive illness (Wyatt et al., 1979; Murphy and Wyatt, 1972). No difference exists between controls and acute schizophrenics or unipolar depressives. Contradictory conclusions from other laboratories again emphasize the difficulties in this type of research (Meltzer et al., 1980). A report by Schildkraut et al. (1980) suggests that reduced platelet MAO activity may only occur in a subpopulation of chronic (as compared to acute) schizophrenics and that MAO activity is increased in schizophrenia-related depressions characterized by chronic asocial or bizarre behavior. These authors (Schildkraut et al., 1976) found low MAO activity in 16 chronic schizophrenics who reported auditory hallucinations or delusions.

To avoid the necessity to control for the effects of diet, drugs, and chronic hospitalization, Wyatt and co-workers (1973a) examined platelet MAO activity in monozygotic twins discordant for schizophrenia. They found that the MAO activity of both schizophrenic and nonschizophrenic co-twins was significantly lower than for normals and that the enzyme activity was highly correlated between twins. This suggests that low platelet MAO activity is not due to drug treatment or factors related to hospitalization. It also demonstrates that low MAO activity is not a secondary result of the disease and thus is not a biochemical marker for the disease itself. However, low MAO activity may represent a genetic marker for increased vulnerability for schizophrenia.

The difficulties in interpreting the MAO data stem from the lack of proper control groups. For instance, individuals other than those who have a psychiatric disorder demonstrate altered MAO activity. Among these are individuals with Down's syndrome, essential hypertension, migraine, toxemia of pregnancy, and juvenile diabetes mellitus (Sullivan et al., 1980). The chronic use of certain drugs, for example, antidepressants, lithium carbonate, and reserpine, also alters MAO function. Both alcoholics (Major and Murphy, 1978) and heavy marijuana users (Stillman et al., 1978) have lowered MAO activity in platelets. Certain dietary deficiencies have also been correlated with altered MAO activity: iron, riboflavin, and B_{12} have been implicated (Sullivan et al., 1980). In addition, it has been demonstrated that matching age and sex of subjects is important, particularly as platelet MAO activity in the adult human female is highest just before ovulation and lowest in the postovulatory period (Belmaker et al., 1974). Additional difficulties in providing accurate evaluations of MAO involves the variables in the assay procedure itself, in the heterogeneity of platelet size, density, and age, and in the choice of substrates to be oxidized (Wise et al., 1980; Jackman and Meltzer, 1980; Robinson and Nies, 1980).

However, no difference in MAO activity has been found in the brains of schizophrenics as compared to controls in postmortem analyses, nor does inhibition of MAO activity by MAO inhibitors produce psychosis (Wyatt and Murphy, 1975). Furthermore, almost complete inhibition of brain MAO activity is necessary before it has an effect on behavior. Thus, some investigators doubt that there is a relationship between reduced brain MAO activity and pathogenesis of psychosis (Meltzer et al., 1980). However, partial MAO inhibition, especially after chronic MAO inhibitor administration, produces a change in the sensitivity of an individual to a variety of agents such as caffeine, insulin, narcotic analgesics, and amphetamine (Murphy and Kalin, 1980). Partial inhibition may also produce neuroendocrine changes, altered blood pressure, and modified sleep patterns. Thus, it is possible that MAO inhibition produces deficits in an individual's response to the environment, both external and internal, and hence may be linked to the development of abnormal behavior.

Even if MAO activity is not directly related to the development of schizophrenia, platelet MAO activity may have predictive value in identifying "high risk" groups within a given population. For example, 375 college students were screened for platelet MAO activity; the lowest 10 percent were found to have had more psychiatric or psychological counseling and to have had more frequent problems with the police (Buchbaum et al., 1976). Furthermore, families of the low MAO group had an 8-fold higher incidence of suicide or suicide attempts. However, there was no reported difference in the incidence of childhood adjustment problems, family stress, or neurological illness between the high MAO group and the low MAO group.

Thus, although MAO activity in platelets may indicate vulnerability to psychiatric illness, additional long-term longitudinal studies must be performed before predictive value can be assessed. In addition, as the enzyme has been further characterized, multiple forms that vary with both organ and species as well as with substrate and inhibitor specificities have been identified. Perhaps finer discriminations in the exact role of each of the isoenzymes in physiological and pathological states will be uncovered by future research.

Affective Disorders

The second major class of psychoses comprises the affective disorders, which are characterized by extreme and inappropriate exaggerations of mood. Disturbances of thinking and motor behavior are consistent with the mood, although the mood does not reflect a realistic appraisal of the environment at the time.

DEPRESSION refers to the affective state of sadness that occurs in response to a variety of human situations such as loss of a loved one, failure to achieve goals, or disappointment in love. Pathological depression differs only in intensity and duration or quality of the emotional state. Most depressed patients express feelings of hopelessness, worthlessness, sadness, guilt and desperation. Frequently patients exhibit loss of appetite, insomnia, crying, diminished sexual desire, loss of ambition, fatigue, and motor retardation or agitation. Physical symptoms may include localized pain, severe digestive disturbances, and difficult breathing. Self-devaluation and loss of self esteem are very common and are combined with a complete sense of hopelessness about the future, which may end in suicide.

MANIA involves symptoms that are almost the exact opposite of those of depression; elation is the primary symptom. Manics feel faultless, full of fun, bursting with energy. They tend to make impulsive decisions of the grandiose sort and have unlimited confidence in themselves. Those individuals who alternate between periods of mania and depression are MANIC-DEPRESSIVE, and are suffering from bipolar affective disorders.

Because the symptoms and consequences of depression are so severe, it is the subject of much clinical and pharmacological treatment. The patterns of symptoms vary significantly from individual to individual. This heterogeneity of the population of depressed patients adds to the variability of results in experiments attempting to correlate mental state with changes in neurochemistry. Numerous attempts have been made to identify subgroups of depressed individuals and they have been classed on the basis of several factors, including age (senile-involutional), motor activity (agitated-retarded depression), stimulus preceding onset (endogenous-exogenous), or clinical features (neurotic-psychotic). Although such classification has been useful for determining therapeutic protocol, it has been of only limited value in most biological studies.

Biogenic Amine Hypothesis

The search for a physiological factor underlying affective disorders was encouraged by the discovery of a genetic link in the disorder. The concordance of affective disorders for dizygotic twins is much higher than the general population but is significantly lower than that for monozygotic twins. In one study using birth registers cross-matched with registers of mental illness, concordance for affective disorders was 50 percent for 10 pairs of monozygotic twins and 2.6 percent for 39 pairs of male dizygotic twins (Harvald and Hauge, 1956). More recent studies of family histories have suggested that bipolar affective disorder (manic-depressive) is transmitted by an X-linked dominant gene, like color blindness (Reich et al., 1969). Furthermore, we have already mentioned that platelet MAO activity may serve as a genetic marker for vulnerability to affective disorders (Murphy and Wyatt, 1975), even if deficiencies in MAO are not causally related.

The biological hypothesis is also supported by several features of affective disorders including the accompanying somatic symptoms (e.g., sleep disturbances, loss of appetite), the circadian cycle of depression, and the incidence of endocrine and metabolic disorders (Baldessarini, 1975). In addition, during the 1950s several drugs that altered mood and behavior were tested. Many of the original observations of the neurochemical control of behavior came from the clinical literature. For instance, reserpine, which is an effective agent in treating hypertension because it reduces sympathetic (adrenergic) control of blood vessels, was found to induce depression in a significant number of patients. The prolonged central depressant properties of reserpine are due to the drug-induced inhibition of vesicular storage of the neurotransmitters, which are subsequently metabolized intraneurally by MAO. The depression in mood that follows reserpine administration is considered by clinicians to be indistinguishable from naturally occurring depression. It became evident that a number of drugs that reduced the biogenic amine levels precipitated depression, whereas those agents that elevated neurotransmitter levels were effective in alleviating depression. From this early discovery, the monoamine hypothesis of depression was formulated. It suggests that depression is related to a deficit of monoamines at critical synapses, whereas mania is associated with an excess of monoamines at critical synapses (Schildkraut, 1965).

Because reserpine is known to deplete stores of several monoamines including DA, NE, and 5-HT, the importance of each to the development of depression is not immediately clear. In this country the catecholamines have received the greatest attention, whereas in Europe serotonin has generated the most research interest. Thus far no definitive answer has been found, and because of numerous contradictions, it has been suggested that the biogenic amine neurotransmitters may act synergistically to modulate complex behaviors.

A number of years ago, Brodie and Shore (1957) suggested a synergistic action of NE and 5-HT. They hypothesized that serotonin is a transmitter in the "trophotropic" system that is involved with normal conservation and relaxation and that functions much like the parasympathetic division of the autonomic nervous system. Norepinephrine was proposed to act in the "ergotropic" system that functions during times of stress, aggression, and adaptation to environmental change and that is similar to the sympathetic division of the autonomic nervous sytem. Thus, depression may be related to a reduced adrenergic function in combination with an increase in 5-HT activity. Alternatively, it is possible that changes in 5-HT are responsible for part of the depression syndrome whereas changes in NE or DA may be related to other symptoms. In addition, it is important to remember that other neurochemical modulators (e.g., GABA, substance P) are presently being identified. Thus, historical emphasis on catecholamines, ACh, and 5-HT will need modification.

Although the question of the relative importance of the catecholamines and 5-HT to reserpine-induced depression has not been resolved, researchers have employed classic pharmacological techniques in approaching the problem. For instance, to distinguish between the possible role of two amines, heroic amounts of transmitter precursors were administered to reserpinized animals in an attempt to reverse reserpine's sedative effect. When L-dopa was administered in nonphysiological doses, the reserpine-induced depression was attenuated whereas the serotonin precursor, 5-HTP, apparently enhanced the sedation

(Carlsson et al., 1957). These results suggest that the catecholamines are particularly important to the effect of reserpine. However, we must remember in evaluating this evidence that the distribution of amines formed from exogenously administered precursors may not be identical to the distribution (and thus the function) of endogenously formed amines.

Another approach to the biogenic amine hypothesis was based on the assumption that if the level of catecholamines is the significant modulator of depression, one would expect L-dopa (the precursor of the catecholamines) to increase CA levels and elevate mood. Although this method has been used frequently, interpretation of the results of precursor experiments depends on a number of assumptions that frequently are not met. These include the following: (1) The precursor must be absorbed readily and pass through the blood brain barrier. (2) It must distribute physiologically in the brain and reach a pharmacological concentration. (3) The necessary enzymatic systems must be functioning to convert precursor to transmitter. (4) The increase in precursor or transmitter must not alter other transmitter systems. (5) The newly formed transmitter must be released normally (Burns and Mendels, 1977). Experiments performed on the basis of these assumptions, have shown that L-dopa has no effective antidepressant activity, although it occasionally produces hyperactivity (Murphy et al., 1971; Burns and Mendels, 1977). On the other hand, additional support for the role of catecholamines is found in the α-methyltyrosine (α-MT)-induced depletion of catecholamines and the subsequent appearance of sedation (Spector et al., 1965). Because α-MT reduces CA stores by inhibiting tyrosine hydroxylase, it does not deplete 5-HT. Also α-MT-induced sedation is reversed by L-dopa.

In contrast, L-tryptophan (the precursor of 5-HT) has been found by some to have a limited antidepressant action in a small number of clinical trials, as compared to imipramine (Coopen et al., 1972b). Others report no significant benefit from L-tryptophan either alone or with L-dopa, although tryptophan administered with an MAO inhibitor produced antidepressant action superior to either drug alone. Also, 5-HT can be depleted with p-chlorophenylalanine (PCPA) to 10 percent of normal levels without inducing depression. In fact, some evidence suggests that animals depleted of 5-HT may be hyperactive and more sensitive to external stimuli. If reserpine administration follows PCPA, the typical depression appears (Koe and Weissman, 1966). Thus, evidence for a role for catecholamines has accumulated.

One problem that arose in reserpine experiments was that the time course of reserpine's sedative effect did not match the time course of brain amine depletion. Reserpine-induced behavioral effects recover long before the amine stores return to their normal levels. Although initially perplexing, this difference in time course is possible because much of the transmitter may be stored in nonfunctional pools. Thus, even significant depletion of the total store may not disrupt the functional pool. Evidence for this was reported by Haggendal and Lindqvist (1964), who showed that by using a small amount of reserpine over a long period of time they could deplete most of the amines without behavioral symptoms. After reducing brain levels to about 10 percent of normal, they found an excellent temporal correlation between the behavioral effects and changes in the residual amines. Even though studies of turnover (i.e., utilization) more reliably reflect the activity within the cell, it is clear that turnover of large storage pools (which is relatively easy to measure) may mask turnover in the smaller functional pool that is essential for synaptic activity. Thus, attempting to correlate brain levels or turnover of a specific amine with behavioral changes is undoubtedly an oversimplification of the dynamic state of the organism. It is much more likely that relative changes of various amines are the critical regulators of behavior.

Metabolic Studies in Depressed Patients

One method of studying the relationship of biogenic amines to mental disorders is by examining enzyme activity or amine metabolites in accessible body fluids, including blood, urine, or cerebrospinal fluid (CSF) of depressed patients. Interpretation of such data must be cautious because in most cases no relationship has been established between enzyme activity in blood and enzyme activity in the CNS. In addition, measurements of biogenic amine metabolites in urine and other fluids represents a summation of the total metabolic processes in the body and may not reflect closely what occurs in the brain. Because CNS metabolism represents only a small proportion of total metabolism, small but significant changes in the CNS pool can easily be masked by the large concentration of peripheral metabolites. Variations in metabolite levels are so great between individuals that differences between groups

are very difficult to find. To avoid these problems, recent studies have employed postmortem brain tissue from depressed psychiatric patients. However, as discussed earlier, the potential pitfalls of postmortem measurements are not easily avoided.

If depressed synaptic activity is responsible for depression, we might expect to find lower levels of amines and metabolites in blood, urine, or CSF, reflecting the reduced utilization of the neurotransmitter amines. Unfortunately, the results of studies of amine metabolites in depressed patients have been inconsistent, and although a role for biogenic amines is suggested, no strong supportive evidence for a role of a particular amine can be presented. For instance, both low (Shaw et al., 1967) and normal (Bourne et al., 1968) concentrations of 5-HT have been found in brains from suicide victims. These differences in results may be due to differences in the ages of the victims, their diet, or time of death in relation to the natural circadian rhythm of biogenic amine levels. Additionally, the length of time between death and assay may be a significant variable (Dowson, 1969).

The major metabolite of 5-HT is 5-hydroxyindole-acetic acid (5-HIAA), both centrally and peripherally. It is generally assumed that urine levels of 5-HIAA are not a good indicator of brain activity because of the large peripheral contribution to urinary 5-HIAA (Goodwin and Potter, 1978). Thus, CSF levels are considered more reliable. Frequently, probenecid is administered before CSF sampling because probenecid inhibits the transport of 5-HIAA and homovanillic acid (HVA) out of the CSF, thus making the metabolite accumulation in the lumbar CSF greater and probably more representative of brain CSF. CSF levels of 5-HIAA have been reported to be lower (Dencker et al., 1966; Coopen et al., 1972a) or essentially normal (Goodwin et al., 1973) in depressed patients. Of those reporting lower 5-HIAA levels, Dencker et al. (1966) found a return to normal after recovery, whereas others found a persistence of low 5-HIAA for some time after recovery (Coopen et al., 1972a). The latter results suggest that low levels reflect a constitutional deviation that identifies vulnerability to the disorder rather than the degree of disorder once it has appeared. Furthermore, in patients with mania, 5-HIAA was also found to be low (Dencker et al., 1966), normal, or elevated (Goodwin et al., 1973).

One explanation for the many apparent discrepancies was provided by Asberg et al. (1976), who found that the distribution of 5-HIAA in CSF was bimodal. Thus, two biochemically distinct subpopulations could be identified. These investigators also found that in the subgroup with lower 5-HIAA levels, a significant negative correlation existed between severity of depression and concentration of 5-HIAA. For these patients having higher 5-HIAA levels, no relationship between severity of depression and 5-HIAA levels could be found. Thus, many of the discrepancies in reported results may be due to selection of subpopulations of patients. Furthermore, contaminating factors have not always been controlled. For example, exercise has been shown to significantly alter 5-HIAA levels in CSF. In addition, a commonly used antidepressant, imipramine, is also known to depress CSF levels of serotonin metabolites. Thus, the results of these studies have been difficult to interpret and have not resolved our many questions.

The question of what proportion of DA metabolites in urine originate in brain is unclear. However, for norepinephrine metabolites, the picture is much better. The major metabolites of NE are 3-methoxy-4-hydroxymandelic acid (VMA) and 3-methoxy-4-hydroxyphenylglycol (MHPG). In animals, aldehyde reductase (forming MHPG) predominates over aldehyde dehydrogenase (forming VMA) in brain, whereas the opposite is true in the periphery (Erwin, 1973). Ebert and Kopin (1975) have found that in humans the majority of urinary MHPG comes from brain metabolism of NE whereas almost all of the urinary VMA comes from metabolism of peripheral NE. Thus, most studies examine MHPG in depressed patients. However, as with the conflicting results for 5-HIAA levels, no general conclusion is possible because MHPG levels have been found to be lower in some cases and unchanged in others (Goodwin and Potter, 1978).

The summarized results cannot be taken to support the biogenic amine hypothesis of depression. However, it is possible that thus far the right questions have not been asked. For instance, it has recently been shown that there are differences in urinary MHPG between hospitalized depressed patients and normal controls when their metabolite response to changes in diet or exercise are considered (Goodwin and Potter, 1978). In the patients, the discontinuation of a low monoamine diet increased MHPG levels by 70 percent, whereas the same dietary modification did not modify control MHPG. Moderate exercise increased MHPG in depressed patients but had no effect on controls.

Results such as these suggest that changes in metabolite levels may be more important than absolute levels. Although the questions being asked are crucial to understanding the biochemistry of affective disorders, much more research with more refined methods and better controls will be needed to provide the answers.

Pharmacological Methods in Animal Models

An alternate approach to the problems of the neurochemical basis of affective disorders is a pharmacological approach using animal models. As is true for most human behavioral disorders, the establishment of an appropriate model for depression has been difficult. The manifestations of depression are described in uniquely human terms and inferences about the subjective state of an animal can be misleading. Nevertheless, sedation in animals is considered to be an analog of depression in man. However, drug-induced states of hyperactivity in animals do not necessarily indicate an antidepressant action of a drug. For instance, amphetamine, which can produce increased motor activity, is not generally considered an effective antidepressant. Thus, the results of animal experiments must be evaluated cautiously. Following tests of motor activity, the drug may be used in a battery of more elaborate behavioral tests from which a profile of drug action can be summarized and compared to other drugs that are known to be effective antidepressants.

Pharmacological Therapy in Humans with Affective Disorders

In addition to pharmacological manipulations in animals and measurement of amine metabolism in depressed patients, a third approach to understanding the relationship of amine metabolism and mood is to investigate the mechanism of action of effective antidepressant agents. Among those pharmacological treatments that are used to improve affective disorders are administration of monoamine oxidase inhibitors, tricyclic antidepressants, electroconvulsive therapy (ECT), and lithium chloride (LiCl). It is reasonable to point out that estimates of improvement in depressed patients are often difficult to substantiate because of their subjective nature and because of a high rate of spontaneous remission, that is, loss of symptoms without medical care. Furthermore, because none of the pharmacological treatments is effective for all patients, it is reasonable to assume that subpopulations of patients exist. Thus, care is required in evaluating reports of biochemical correlates of improved psychiatric condition.

Monoamine oxidase inhibitors. Earlier we said that the principal mode of terminating the action of the catecholamines is by reuptake into the presynaptic terminal, with subsequent storage in vesicles and reuse. Despite that fact, inhibition of MAO (the enzyme that intraneuronally deaminates the biogenic amines) has significant effects on behavior.

The discovery of the antidepressant action of the MAO inhibitors was serendipitous. As mentioned earlier, MAO inhibitors were developed in the early 1950s to treat tuberculosis, a property apparently unrelated to the inhibition of MAO. Clinical reports cited cases of drug-induced euphoria that prompted the clinical trials of the drugs as mood elevators. Only after the discovery of the antidepressant action was the drugs' ability to inhibit MAO discovered.

A single dose of MAO inhibitor increases norepinephrine, epinephrine, dopamine, and serotonin in brain, heart, intestine, and blood, and thus presumably prolongs and increases the action of the transmitters at their receptors. Clearly, MAO inhibitors (like all other therapeutic agents) have multiple effects that are not restricted to brain amines but occur at peripheral sites as well, producing "side effects." For example, MAO inhibitors generally cause dry mouth, blurred vision, and difficulty in urination. Although a single dose increases amine levels, several weeks of administration are usually required to produce effective antidepressant action clinically. Thus, the acute actions of the drugs are quite often different from those following chronic administration. In some cases, repeated drug treatment leads to reduced pharmacological effects (see the discussion of tolerance in Chapter 1), whereas in other instances several weeks of drug administration are required before the desired pharmacological effect occurs.

The drugs in this class often have very little effect on animal behavior and in general do not produce significant increases in motor activity. However, pretreatment with an MAO inhibitor does prevent reserpine-induced depression and may also produce behavioral excitation (Chessin et al., 1957; Spector et al., 1960). Such an effect may occur because the nonstored amine that cannot be broken down by MAO accumulates presynaptically and leaks from the terminal. It is in-

teresting to note that MAO inhibitors do not have a euphoric or stimulating effect on normal human subjects but may be dysphoric and unpleasant. However, in the depressed patient, MAO inhibitors are often effective in improving mood.

Once again the evidence on the relative importance of NE and 5-HT is inconsistent. Spector and co-workers (1960) showed that in those species (rabbits) where both catecholamines and 5-HT are increased by MAO-inhibition, the increase in motor activity was best correlated with increased levels of NE. In species (cat) where there was only an increase in 5-HT without change in NE, no behavioral excitation was observed. On the other hand, at least one study has demonstrated that the antidepressant effect of tranylcypromine (a frequently used MAO inhibitor) was reversed by depletion of 5-HT with the synthesis inhibitor *p*-chlorophenylalanine (Shopsin et al., 1976).

Clinical use of the MAO inhibitors has decreased because of the high incidence of side effects. MAO inhibitors are nonspecific and inhibit the metabolic degradation of many other drugs and biogenic amines. For instance, they drastically alter an organism's ability to metabolize barbiturates, alcohol, and opiates. In addition, it may be recalled that MAO inhibitors potentiate the action of amphetamine-like compounds and may precipitate a hypertensive crisis due to the well-known "tyramine-cheese reaction." Tyramine is a naturally occurring amine formed as a byproduct of fermentation in many foods, including cheeses, certain beers, pickled products, and others. Tyramine is normally metabolized by MAO but when the enzyme is inhibited, high levels of tyramine produce dramatic increases in blood pressure.

As mentioned earlier, several types of MAO have been identified on the basis of substrate preference and pharmacological inhibition (Johnston, 1968; McCauley, 1981). Type A MAO acts more efficiently to deaminate 5-HT and NE and is inhibited by clorgyline. Type B MAO deaminates DA and phenylethylamine (PEA) and is blocked by deprenyl. Intravenous injection of clorgyline inhibits Type A MAO in brain (and elsewhere) and increases the endogenous level of 5-HT and NE (Yang and Neff, 1974). In contrast, deprenyl significantly raised the levels of exogenously administered PEA but not NE or 5-HT. The ability to separate the effects of MAO suggests that a drug may someday be developed to selectively inhibit the metabolism of an amine in a specific area of the brain whose deficiency is related to a disease state. At the same time, the action of the other amines that are related to side effects would not increase.

Finally, just as in the case of schizophrenia, there were attempts to correlate levels of MAO activity with depressive disorders. The evidence for altered MAO activity in depressed patients is contradictory. Platelet MAO activity has been found to be higher in depressed patients than in a control group (Nies et al., 1974). Such a finding could be considered to support the amine hypothesis of depression because elevated MAO activity suggests lowered amine levels. However, others have found no significant difference in total MAO activity unless the group of depressed patients was divided into uni- and bipolar groups. In this case, bipolar patients (manic–depressive) had significantly reduced platelet MAO activity compared to either controls or unipolar depressed patients (Murphy and Wyatt, 1975). The same group noted, however, that changes in MAO activity do not seem to be correlated with clinical improvement or deterioration of condition. Although research is continuing in this area, at this time no strong case can be made for an altered MAO activity in patients with affective disorders.

Tricyclic antidepressants. Tricyclic antidepressants are the drugs most often used to treat depression and have largely replaced MAO inhibitors. Their name is derived from their characteristic structure (Figure 7) which is clearly similar to the phenothiazine nucleus (Figure 2). In fact, the prototypic tricyclic compound, imipramine, was originally tested for antipsychotic activity because of its similarity in structure to the phenothiazines. Contrary to all expectations, clinical trials showed that imipramine was ineffective in quieting agitated psychotic patients but did appear to elevate the mood of some depressed patients. Thus, further trials for its use as an antidepressant followed. Several commonly used tricyclic compounds are shown in Figure 7. Their pharmacological effects are essentially

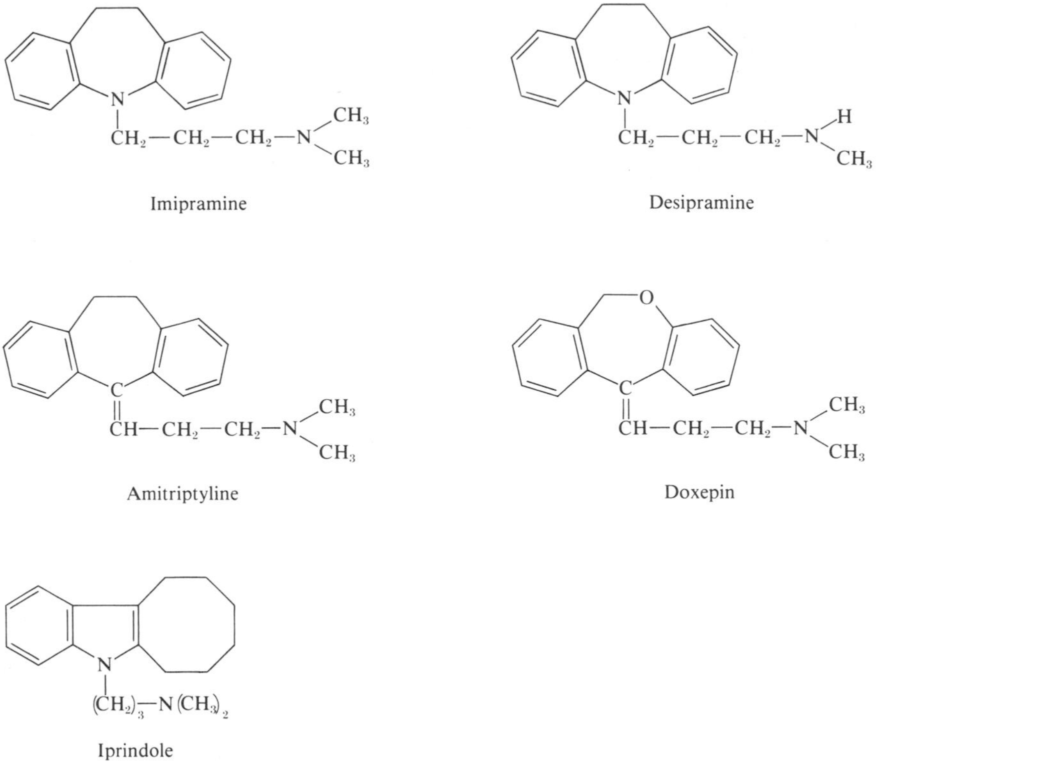

Imipramine

Desipramine

Amitriptyline

Doxepin

Iprindole

FIGURE 7   TRICYCLIC ANTIDEPRESSANT DRUGS. The tricyclic antidepressant drug iprindole is structurally and pharmacologically different from the other tricyclic antidepressant drugs shown.

the same and differ primarily in their relative potency.

An antidepressant action is generally attributed to inhibition of the neuronal uptake mechanism that normally terminates the action of the neurotransmitter. Thus, the duration of transmitter action at the synapse is prolonged. The tricyclics do not inhibit the uptake of amines into storage granules but seem to inhibit only the uptake from the extraneuronal space into the adrenergic terminal (Carlsson and Waldeck, 1965). Following intracisternal administration of ^{3}H-norepinephrine, treatment with tricyclic antidepressants has been shown to inhibit the uptake of labeled NE (Dengler et al., 1961; Glowinski and Axelrod, 1964) and increase the concentration of O-methylated metabolites without changing the amount of deaminated metabolites (Schanberg et al., 1967). The increase in O-methylated metabolites is a consequence of reuptake inhibition and the subsequent exposure to extraneuronal metabolism by COMT. Uptake inhibition by the tricyclic compounds has also been found for 5-HT but not for DA (Carlsson et al., 1969a). Carlsson found that the tertiary amine tricyclic compounds inhibit serotonin uptake much more effectively than NE uptake. These drugs, including imipramine and amitriptyline, are potent mood elevators, whereas the secondary amines (e.g., desimipramine) are more potent in increasing motor activity. The secondary amines inhibit NE uptake more effectively than 5-HT, suggesting that NE levels may be related to psychomotor depression whereas 5-HT modulates mood (Frazer, 1981).

The tricyclic compounds, like the MAO inhibitors, are dysphoric for normal individuals. When tricyclic compounds are given to a normal individual, he feels sleepy and tends to be quieter, light-headed, and ataxic. These effects, in combination with a variety of somatic side effects (e.g., dry mouth, blurred vision) make the use of these drugs unpleasant and anxiety provoking for the normal individual. In contrast, when given to a depressed patient (over a 2- to 3-week period), a definite elevation in mood occurs. The same phenomena may be seen in animals.

When given to rats, imipramine depresses spontaneous activity, causes ataxia, and prolongs hexobarbital sleeping time. However, if given before reserpine, imipramine induces excitation and exploratory behavior that is presumed to result from the spillover of free catecholamines onto receptors (Sulser et al., 1964). If imipramine is given after the effects of reser-

pine have developed or if catecholamine stores are first depleted by administration of α-methyltryosine, only partial reversal occurs. These data suggest that imipramine's antidepressant action is produced by increasing the action of catecholamines.

In addition, imipramine potentiates the action of amphetamine, a sympathomimetic that releases catecholamines from the presynaptic terminal, that is, imipramine potentiates amphetamine-induced hyperactivity (Halliwell et al., 1964). Although tricyclic compounds reduce the rate of electrical self-stimulation in positive hypothalamic sites, imipramine and amphetamine administered together produce self-stimulation at a rate much higher than amphetamine alone (Stein and Seifter, 1961). In a similar manner, imipramine intensifies and increases the duration of amphetamine-induced hyperthermia, although alone, imipramine does not increase body temperature and may in some cases lower it (Jori and Garattini, 1965).

Much of the data summarized thus far supports the hypothesis that the tricyclic compounds act by inhibiting catecholamine uptake, but a number of discrepancies exist (Barchas et al., 1977). Cocaine, which is not a tricyclic compound but is an excellent amine uptake inhibitor, has little clinically recorded antidepressant action (Post et al., 1974). In addition, the atypical tricyclic compound, iprindole, which is reported to have significant antidepressant action, does not block neuronal uptake of NE (Rosloff and Davis, 1974), alter the metabolism of NE (Freeman and Sulser, 1972), or change the turnover of NE (Rosloff and Davis, 1974). Iprindole has low potency in reversing reserpine-induced sedation (Gluckman and Baum, 1969). Others have shown that iprindole, unlike other effective tricyclic antidepressants, did not inhibit spontaneous firing of NE cells in the locus caeruleus (Nyback et al., 1975).

An additional discrepancy is that uptake inhibition occurs after a single administration of the tricyclic antidepressants, but clinical effectiveness occurs only after 2–3 weeks of daily treatment. Although somewhat puzzling, it has been shown that the effect of the drugs on the level of neurotransmitter varies, depending on the duration of drug treatment. After acute administration, NE levels are increased (Sulser et al., 1964), whereas chronic treatment produces lowered NE levels (Schildkraut et al., 1972). Changes in neurotransmitter concentration after chronic drug treatment may represent an adaptive change in neuronal activity and may explain the variability in drug effectiveness with repeated treatment.

Other investigators have examined the acute and chronic effects of antidepressants on the NE-sensitive adenylate cyclase (the enzyme that catalyzes the formation of cAMP) in limbic forebrain. It is known that reserpine both produces sedation in animals and leads to supersensitivity of the cAMP generating system (Williams and Pirch, 1974), presumably because the postsynaptic receptor responds to a reduction in impulse traffic with an increased sensitivity to a neurotransmitter applied exogenously. It has been suggested that antidepressant agents may prevent the development of reserpine-induced supersensitivity or induce subsensitivity of the receptors. In fact, chronic administration of imipramine or related tricyclics for 3–6 weeks produces a subsensitivity to NE in brain slices (Vetulani et al., 1976a; Schultz, 1976). That is, the formation of cAMP after the addition of NE to the rat cortex slices is significantly less in animals pretreated for several weeks with imipramine or another tricyclic antidepressant than in nontreated animals or in those receiving only an acute injection. Similar results were reported in an *in vivo* experiment in which pineal cAMP was measured following i.p. injection of NE (Moyer et al., 1979). Norepinephrine was found to have no effect on pineal cAMP levels when injected alone. Acute pretreatment with desmethylimipramine (which blocks catecholamine reuptake) followed by NE, increased cAMP significantly. With repeated exposure to desmethylimipramine, the ability of NE to increase cAMP was abolished. These results are reasonable when changes in receptor density are considered. Long-term, but not short-term, antidepressant treatment has been shown to reduce the number of β-adrenergic receptors in rat frontal cortex without altering the affinity of the receptor for transmitter (Wolfe et al., 1978; Peroutka and Snyder, 1980). The antidepressants tested in these experiments included several tricyclics, including iprindole and the MAO inhibitor pargyline. These results suggest that the effectiveness of the tricyclic antidepressants may be related to long-term adaptive changes (subsensitivity) in the postsynaptic cells that follow the changes in presynaptic uptake that occurs acutely.

Because similar changes were found after chronic MAO inhibitor administration (Vetulani et al., 1976b) and after electroconvulsive shock (Vetulani et al., 1976a), a revised model of antidepressant action has been proposed (Sulser et al., 1978), suggesting that depression may be a state characterized by hypersensitive catecholamine receptors and that effective antidepressant treatment desensitizes the receptor mechanism. It must be mentioned, however, that chlorpromazine, an antipsychotic agent structurally similar to imipramine but causing sedation, also produces a subsensitivity to NE (Schultz, 1976). Thus, it is possible that the change in receptor function may be unrelated to therapeutic action. Although additional evidence must be accumulated to document the hypothesis, the model is appealing and should redirect pharmacological research into the molecular mechanism of antidepressant action.

After antidepressant treatment, changes in several neurotransmitter receptors in addition to the β-adrenergic receptor have been reported. The antidepressants are potent antagonists at brain muscarinic receptors; a property that correlates well with the clinically observed anticholinergic side effects, such as difficulty in urination and exacerbation of glaucoma (Snyder and Yamamura, 1977). The relative potencies of tricyclic antidepressants at α-adrenergic receptors are similar to those at muscarinic receptors. The α-adrenergic binding of the drugs may be related to the production of sedation, hypotension, and relief of psychomotor agitation (U'Prichard et al., 1978). Peroutka and Snyder (1980) have found that chronic treatment (but not short-term treatment) with several types of antidepressants reduced the number (but not the affinity) of serotonin binding sites labeled with [^{3}H]spiroperidol (receptors called serotonin-2). Serotonin-1 receptors, which bind [^{3}H]5-HT were not altered by long-term antidepressant treatment in these experiments, although an earlier report showed that in short-term experiments tricyclic drugs displaced [^{3}H]LSD* binding (Bennett and Snyder, 1975).

The behavioral effects of these changes on receptor binding are not known. However, deMontigny and Aghajanian (1978) examined the electrophysiological response of single cells in rat forebrain to microiontophoretic application of 5-HT. They found that following 2 days of antidepressant treatment, the sensitivity of the neurons to 5-HT was not changed. After

---

*Binding of LSD is considered to occur at both serotonin-1 and serotonin-2 receptors.

4–7 days of pretreatment, the response of the cells to exogenously applied 5-HT was moderately increased. Following 15 days of antidepressant administration, there was a large increase in sensitivity to 5-HT. The time course of the physiological effect is related to the clinical antidepressant effect, that is, the antidepressant action generally requires 2 weeks of drug administration. In addition, they found that several drugs (FG-4963 and chlorpromazine) with a similar structure, but without antidepressant activity, did not increase sensitivity of the cells to 5-HT. Furthermore, iprindole, which is clinically effective but does not work by amine uptake blockade, significantly increased 5-HT sensitivity in forebrain cells. Thus, serotonin may play an important role in modulating depression, and neuronal receptor sensitivity may underlie the pathophysiology of affective disorders.

Antidepressants also act at histamine receptors of the H_1 type (Peroutka and Snyder, 1980). This action, however, does not seem to correlate with clinical effectiveness. Kanof and Greengard (1978) and Green and Maayani (1977) have found that the drugs are very effective competitive inhibitors of histamine-stimulated adenylate cyclase in hippocampus and neocortex. In these brain areas, the histamine receptor coupled to adenylate cyclase is of the H_2 type. All the antidepressants tested were capable of shifting the dose-response curve for histamine-induced cAMP production to the right, suggesting that more histamine was required to produce a given amount of cAMP. The low concentration of antidepressant required for this effect suggests that the histamine-sensitive adenylate cyclase may be antagonized *in vivo* at pharmacologically effective doses. It is unlikely that every drug that inhibits histamine stimulation of adenylate cyclase is an effective antidepressant agent. Both LSD and the phenothiazine fluphenazine are capable of such action at high concentrations, but neither has clinically demonstrated antidepressant action.

Although the physiological function of histamine neurons in brain is not known, the investigators suggest that acute blockade of histamine receptors may reduce cAMP in postsynaptic cells and hence modify the function of other neural networks. With prolonged drug administration, protein synthesis may be affected in these cells and subsequently modify the number or sensitivity of receptors to other neurotransmitters, as discussed in the preceding section. The modification of so many neurotransmitter systems by antidepressants makes the elucidation of the mechanism of action of these drugs very difficult and hence requires much more intensive investigation in the future.

Electroconvulsive therapy. In the early 1900s a Hungarian psychiatrist noted that several of his patients showed improvement in their psychiatric state after having spontaneous seizures. This observation prompted others to produce convulsions in schizophrenic patients by administering either camphor and oil or, later, a synthetic camphor derivative (pentylenetetrazol = Metrazol) or insulin. Such treatment was the predecessor of electroconvulsive therapy (ECT), which was introduced in 1938 and is used today to treat affective disorders. Although ECT has been used for about 40 years, we do not yet understand the neurochemical basis for its effectiveness. Clinical evaluations have shown ECT to be as good or better than antidepressant drugs in treating depression for certain types of patients (Klein and Davis, 1969). Although ECT produces no pain or awareness of the seizure and has a relatively low incidence of side effects, a great deal of controversy exists over its use and public concern has limited the use of this form of therapy over the last few years. However, one can view seizure therapy as a complex process to elicit persistent biochemical changes in the brain similar to those produced by the antidepressant drugs.

Fink (1977) summarizes the characteristics of ECT effectiveness. First, the behavioral changes following ECT are due to the cerebral seizure and not to convulsions, hypoxia, or other peripheral events. Curare or succinylcholine (which block cholinergic action at the muscles) prevent the convulsion (i.e., the motor effect at muscles), but not the brain seizure, and do not reduce the clinical effectivenes of the therapy. Hyperoxygenation also has no effect on the effectiveness of ECT. The physiological manifestation best correlated with antidepressant action is the appearance of EEG slow wave activity.

It is also clear that the method of producing the seizure, by either electricity, or various drugs (e.g., pentylenetetrazol, flurothyl) does not alter the effectiveness of the treatment. Electroshock is most often used because it does not produce the fear reaction that pentylenetetrazol frequently does, and ECT produces seizure more reliably than flurothyl. Furthermore,

ECT is easier and safer to administer and apparently produces the least discomfort and side effects to the patient. The type of current does not modify outcome nor does the placement of electrodes, although electrode placement does influence some of the side effects such as poor orientation, confusion, and loss of memory. This suggests that memory loss is not the basis for the therapeutic effect, as had been suggested earlier.

Also correlated with therapeutic effects on mood are improvements in sleep, appetite, menstrual cycle, and sex drive, functions normally considered under hypothalamic control. It is possible that these functions may be important to the therapeutic process. Of particular interest to neurochemists is the demonstration that the effects of ECT can be modified by psychotropic drugs. For instance, barbiturates may enhance the effectiveness of ECT in some patients. Those individuals demonstrating the enhancement by barbiturates are also those who show the best outcome after the series of shock treatments. Drugs that impede the therapeutic effectiveness of ECT are anticholinergic drugs, such as atropine, and the hallucinogens, such as LSD. Results of this type suggest that modifications in the cholinergic nervous system may be the neurochemical basis of ECT effectiveness.

Essman (1973) discusses in some detail the central neurochemical changes that accompany ECT. Clearly, there is no simple relationship to be found between widespread neurochemical changes and therapeutic effectiveness of electroshock. It has proved difficult to evaluate the neurochemical changes in animals after electroshock because there are many parameters of ECT administration that vary from laboratory to laboratory. These factors include differences in stimulating electrode properties, placement of electrodes on the skull, direction and amount of current passed through the tissue, the nature of the seizure discharge following ECT, and the acute or chronic nature of the treatment. Despite the many experimental variables, there have been a large number of reports of ECT effects on brain chemistry. A correlation between some of these biochemical changes and antidepressant action may soon be identified.

Among the possibly significant effects of ECT is a change in electrolyte concentration. Most often sodium, potassium, and calcium have been studied because changes in the concentration of these ions across cell membranes link the electrical excitation of a cell with intracellular metabolic events. Changes in cellular energy metabolism following ECT are also significant, as it is obvious that seizures and intense neuronal excitability must require large increases in energy utilization. Finally, changes in neuronal biogenic amines have been studied both in animals and in human blood, urine, and cerebrospinal fluid.

Although changes in cholinergic activity after ECT have been reported, as with the other antidepressant treatments, NE and 5-HT have received the greatest attention. In general, brain 5-HT is increased after either single or after multiple ECT treatments. An increase in 5-HT has been found even when the convulsion is pharmacologically blocked, indicating that the increase in 5-HT is dependent on current passing through the brain and is not an artifact of seizure (Garattini et al., 1960). Others have found that the ECT-induced changes in brain 5-HT may be dependent on several factors, including time after treatment, species, region of brain measured, age of the animals, and type of housing (isolated versus aggregated) (Essman, 1973).

Serotonin metabolism is apparently altered after ECT in humans. In depressed patients treated only with ECT, a significant fall occurred in CSF levels of 5-HIAA (a metabolite of 5-HT) within the first 4 hours after treatment. This decrease in 5-HIAA was followed by a significant increase, reaching a 2-fold increase 24 hr after ECT. This increase persisted for as long as 7 days after the single treatment. In contrast, repeated exposures to ECT did not produce the same changes in 5-HT and its metabolite (Nordin et al., 1971).

The preceding discussion makes clear that the many variables contributing to changes in 5-HT, its precursor, and its metabolites have been difficult to control. Although it is tempting to speculate on the importance of the ECT-induced increase in 5-HT and its metabolite, no conclusions can be drawn at this time.

The effect of ECT on catecholamines has proved to be at least equally interesting, particularly in relation to the catecholamine hypothesis of depression. Repeated electroconvulsive shocks have been shown to raise NE levels in the pons–medulla region of brain and to lower NE levels in the midbrain–hypothalamus (Feighner et al., 1972). Others have reported reduced NE levels after chronic ECT in conjunction with increases in NE metabolites, normetanephrine, or homovanillic acid (Schildkraut et al., 1967; Essman, 1973), and increases in NE synthesis by tyrosine hydroxylase

(Musacchio et al., 1969). These results support the idea that ECT produces an increase in NE turnover in discrete areas of the brain.

In addition, Hendley and Welch (1975) have found that acute ECT produces a decrease in NE uptake in chronically reserpinized rats; this decrease would prolong the neurotransmitter action in the synapse. However, after daily electroconvulsive shocks for 9 days, they found that the uptake affinity (K_m) remained low but the V_{max} of the kinetic reaction increased. These results suggest that the number of uptake sites increased (as reflected by an increased V_{max}), perhaps as an adaptive response to the decreased affinity of the uptake system that is characteristic of the acute ECT treatment.

Further support for increased NE turnover is provided by Vetulani et al. (1976a), who showed that administration of ECT for 8 days significantly reduced the sensitivity of limbic forebrain adenylate cyclase to stimulation by NE. Similar subsensitivity of the enzyme did not occur acutely (after 4 administrations), suggesting that chronic overexposure to NE is responsible for the change in enzyme sensitivity. ECT also prevented the development of hypersensitivity of the limbic forebrain system after reserpine administration (Vetulani and Sulser, 1975). Thus, the therapeutic effects of antidepressant drugs and ECT may be related to the development of subsensitivity of the postsynaptic adenylate cyclase that is responsive to NE (Sulser et al., 1978).

In addition, Bergstrom and Kellar (1979) and Pandey et al. (1979a) have each shown that chronic treatment with electroconvulsive shock reduces the number of β-adrenergic receptors in rat cerebral cortex. It is tempting to speculate that the reuptake block by the tricyclic compounds produces longer exposure of adenylate cyclase-coupled β-receptors to NE and subsequently produces subsensitivity. However, iprindole, which does not block reuptake, also alters the number of β-receptors. Thus, a mechanism other than reuptake blockade must be assumed. These results have encouraged the speculation that depression might be associated with increased sensitivity of central NE receptors.

Other laboratories have investigated the effect of ECT on dopamine systems. Chronic administration of several antidepressants counteracted the hypomotility elicited by small doses of apomorphine, prevented the apomorphine-induced reduction in DA metabolism,

and potentiated the stimulant effects of apomorphine at higher doses (Serra et al., 1979). These authors suggest that tricyclic drugs decrease the sensitivity of DA receptors normally stimulated by apomorphine. Using more direct measures, Chiodo and Antelman (1980a,b) have found that both typical (amitriptyline and imipramine) and atypical (iprindole) antidepressants reduce the sensitivity of dopaminergic autoreceptors (DA receptors on the soma and dendrites of DA-containing neurons in the substantia nigra). In their experiments, the responses of single DA cells were recorded following administration of apomorphine, a DA agonist known to inhibit the spontaneous electrical activity of the autoreceptors. After either 2 or 10 days of antidepressant treatment, the inhibitory effect of apomorphine was attenuated. When ECT was examined, the same investigators found that ECT also gradually reduces DA autoreceptor sensitivity and that the effect depends more on the passage of time than on repeated shock treatment. That is, a single shock treatment decreased receptor sensitivity 7 days later as effectively as one shock treatment a day for 6 days. Therefore, we can conclude that the action of ECT on the receptors is a time-dependent phenomenon. The delay is consistent with the slow onset of clinical therapeutic effects. Possibly depression is caused by supersensitive DA autoreceptors, which would reduce dopaminergic transmission and hence reduce response to the environment. The use of tricyclic antidepressants or ECT may gradually reverse the supersensitivity, thus attenuating depression. Although this hypothesis, as well as the others presented in this chapter, are highly speculative, they provide a basis for testing and will stimulate research into this field.

Lithium. Thus far we have discussed pharmacological agents effective in treating depression with the hope that understanding the neurochemical effects of the therapeutic agents may elucidate a neurochemical mechanism underlying depression. The second major class within affective disorders is the bipolar depression (manic–depressive) syndrome, which is characterized by extreme mood swings varying from mania to severe depression. Manic episodes may be characterized by euphoria, extreme hyperactivity, increased sexual activity, extreme financial irresponsibility, hostility, and violence. The most effective pharmacological agent to improve mania is lithium. Although lithium has no psychotropic effect when given to a normal individual, it has acute anti-manic effects. It is also useful for preventing the recurrence of both mania and depression, although it has no acute antidepressant action (Davis, 1976). It may be interesting to compare the acute and chronic biochemical effects of lithium with the drug's acute effectiveness against mania and its prophylactic action for mania and depression (Schildkraut, 1973).

In humans, the effective therapeutic range of lithium concentration in blood is 0.7–1.2 mM (depending on body weight), whereas toxic effects occur at blood levels of 2.0 mM (Shaw, 1975). This means that the therapeutic index is quite low and patient's blood level of lithium must be monitored closely. Acute toxic effects include vomiting, diarrhea, polydipsia, ataxia, tremor, fatigue, coma, and seizures (Baldessarini and Lipinski, 1975). The low therapeutic index also means that in animal experiments it is difficult to determine whether the effects of lithium on neurochemistry or neurophysiology are related to the therapeutic or the toxic effects of the drug.

Electrolytes are essential for neuronal function, for carrying the current and also for the maintenance of neurotransmitter and its release. Because lithium belongs to the same group of elements as sodium and potassium and has a monovalent charge when ionized, it is reasonable to suspect that lithium, which has no known biological function, may exert its therapeutic effect by modifying the neuronal ionic mechanism. Lithium also has an ionic radius similar to those of magnesium and calcium; thus its action may also be related to interaction with these divalent cations. In some biological systems (e.g., isolated nerve preparation), lithium can partially substitute for sodium in carrying the current. However, the substitution is not complete because lithium is not extruded by the active, energy-requiring sodium pump (Peach, 1975). Hence, its antimanic action may be related to its ability to alter membrane excitability.

Several investigators have found that in red blood cells the ratio of intracellular to extracellular lithium ion (Li$^+$) is higher in bipolar patients than in normal controls when both have been administered lithium (Ramsey, 1981). Li$^+$ is moved across the membrane by a Li$^+$–Na$^+$ countertransport system that does not require energy but is driven by the electrochemical gradient for Na$^+$ across the membrane. Because the system appears to be under genetic control (Pandey et al., 1979b), it is possible that the altered Li$^+$ concen-

tration in red blood cells of manic–depressive individuals represents a genetic deficiency in cell membrane transport. Although the blood cell may not be directly related to the psychotropic action of Li$^+$, it acts as a model and suggests an important potential site for the drug action within the CNS.

On the whole, results of studies that examined Li$^+$ interaction with or substitution for K$^+$, Na$^+$, and Mg^{2+} have been quite inconsistent. A relationship between lithium's therapeutic effect in the treatment of mania and its effect on these ions has not been found (Ramsey, 1981). The best evidence for an ionic mechanism of action for Li$^+$ involves calcium. Abnormal Ca^{2+} metabolism is known to frequently produce emotional symptoms that disappear when normal function is restored. Carman et al. (1977, 1979) have found a correlation between CSF levels of Ca^{2+} and the severity of depression. They have also reported a change in plasma Ca^{2+} with the onset of mania. Finally, they show consistent decreases in total calcium in CSF and serum following successful electroconvulsive shock treatment. The decrease does not occur initially but develops after 3–4 treatments, in close relation with clinical improvement. Unfortunately, although Li$^+$ has been found to antagonize Ca^{2+} in some patients treated with the antimanic drug, results once again are not consistent. Furthermore, administration of parathyroid hormone (which acutely increases serum Ca^{2+} levels) to manic–depressive individuals has not been found to alter their mood (Gerner et al., 1977).

In addition to acting on neuronal ionic mechanisms, lithium has a wide range of biological effects on a variety of systems such as carbohydrate metabolism, antidiuretic hormone secretion, and thyroid function. Furthermore, Li$^+$ has an action on biogenic amine metabolism.

The ability of lithium to decrease catecholamine activity has been cited in support of the catecholamine hypothesis of affective disorders. Lithium apparently enhances the uptake of NE and 5-HT into synaptosomes from rat brain (Colburn et al., 1967) and thus reduces the action of the neurotransmitters in the synapse. Lithium also reduces the release of [^{3}H]NE from electrically stimulated brain slices but does not change the spontaneous release of the amine (Katz et al., 1968). It is likely that this action of lithium is related to its competitive interference with the role of calcium in the excitation–secretion coupling mechanism (Katz and Kopin, 1969). The inhibition of release by lithium can be reversed by adding excess calcium.

The effect of lithium on turnover of NE is not so clear. Corrodi et al. (1967a, 1967b) found that acute administration of LiCl increased the rate of disappearance of NE after treatment with the synthesis inhibitor α-methyltyrosine. Schildkraut et al. (1966) found a similar decrease in [^{3}H]NE after intracisternal injection of the labeled amine. An increase in ^{3}H-labeled deaminated metabolite and decrease in [^{3}H]normetanephrine suggests that lithium increases intracellular deamination by MAO, a result in accord with the enhanced uptake by lithium. Others have reported, however, that prolonged lithium administration produces no change in NE or DA turnover (Corrodi et al., 1969; Ho et al., 1970; Bliss and Ailion, 1970). Thus, it is difficult to see a relationship between long-term clinical efficacy of lithium and its ability to alter NE turnover.

Lithium also inhibits the production of cAMP by adenylate cyclase in many brain regions, including cerebral cortex, caudate, and hippocampus but not in brain stem or cerebellum (Walker, 1974). In addition, lithium reduces the ability of NE to stimulate further adenylate cyclase activity (Walker, 1974; Forn and Valdecasas, 1971), suggesting that the postsynaptic action of NE is also reduced in addition to its reduced release and enhanced uptake. The inhibition of cAMP formation is particularly interesting because at the onset of mania, one patient population showed increased urinary excretion of cAMP (Abdulla and Hamadah, 1970; Paul et al., 1970). Unfortunately, no difference in CSF levels of cAMP have been found in either manic or depressed stages of the disorder (Robison et al., 1970), so the urinary levels probably do not reflect changes in brain chemistry but rather in a peripheral source. In addition, Eccleston et al. (1970) showed that exercise increases the 24-hour excretion of cAMP in normal individuals. Thus, the increased cAMP excretion in manic patients probably reflects their increased motor activity rather than the essential psychopathology.

In addition to its effects on brain NE and NE-sensitive adenylate cyclase, lithium also alters the metabolism of other neurotransmitters, including 5-HT, acetylcholine, and GABA. However, the results of experiments investigating their role in lithium's therapeutic action have not produced a cohesive model of drug action. An excellent series of reviews can be found in Johnson (1975).

From this discussion of drug treatment for affective disorders, it should be clear that the mechanism of action of the most effective agents is not always known. Even clinically the course of therapy for individual patients is most often empirically derived. However, subpopulations of patients responding to a particular pharmacological treatment will be identified and this information will provide an essential step in the understanding of pharmacological treatment, CNS biochemistry, and its relationship to the affective disorders.

Conclusion

This chapter has discussed the most recent hypotheses regarding the neurochemical bases for the major mental illnesses, schizophrenia and affective psychoses. The dopamine hypothesis of schizophrenia has received the greatest attention and also has the most empirical support. However, as with the transmethylation and phenylethylamine hypotheses, it suffers from numerous discrepancies and lacks sufficient, rigorously controlled testing. Despite these weaknesses, the models have generated a great deal of information about CNS neurochemistry and provide a direction for future research.

The biogenic amine hypothesis of depression and mania has received greatest support from pharmacological research involving reserpine-induced depression. Although the therapeutic effectiveness of the tricyclic antidepressants and the MAO inhibitors gives further support to the importance of the amine neurotransmitters, there is still much to be learned about the drugs' mechanisms of action. Clinical correlations between amine levels in biological fluids and the status of mental health in patient populations remain difficult to interpret.

Quite clearly the research described has produced as many questions as answers. We hope that the critical assessment of the various hypotheses will not discourage, but rather will inspire, greater efforts in all the neuroscience fields toward more refined quantitative methods, better controlled experimental designs, and novel approaches to a most significant problem.

Recommended Readings

Crane, G.E. (1978). Tardive dyskinesia and related neurologic disorders. In *Handbook of Psychopharmacology, Volume 10* (L.L. Iversen, S.D. Iversen and

S.H. Snyder, Eds.), pp. 165–196, Plenum Press, New York. A thorough discussion of one of the most serious and most common side effects of antipsychotic drug treatments.

Iversen, L.L., Iversen, S.D. and Snyder, S.H. (1978). *Handbook of Psychopharmacology, Volume 14, Affective Disorders: Drug Actions in Animals and Man.* Plenum Press, New York. This volume of eight papers is a rich source of experimental findings on the mode of action and use of antidepressant and antimanic drugs.

Palmer, G.C. (Ed.) (1981). *Neuropharmacology of the Central Nervous System and Behavioral Disorders.* Academic Press, New York. This book contains several excellent chapters on tricyclic antidepressants, monoamine oxidase inhibitors, and lithium.

Roberts, P.J., Woodruff, G.N. and Iversen, L.L. (Eds.) (1978). *Advances in Biochemical Psychopharmacology, Volume 19, Dopamine.* Raven Press, New York. This entire volume is devoted to dopamine—its receptors, its relationship to adenylate cyclase, and

the syndromes associated with the disfunction of dopamine systems.

Snyder, S.H. (1980). *Biological Aspects of Mental Disorders.* Oxford University Press, New York. An up-to-date discussion of the major psychiatric syndromes, hypotheses of their biological bases, and usual modes of treatment.

Usdin, E., Hamburg, D.A. and Barchas, J.D. (Eds.) (1977). *Neuroregulators and Psychiatric Disorders.* Oxford University Press, New York. A collection of sixty-four papers summarizing information about the role of neurotransmitters in mental illness, chemical substances that may be of diagnostic and therapeutic use, and the mechanisms of action of psychotropic substances.

Wyatt, R.J., Potkin, S.G., Bridge, T.P., Phelps, B.H. and Wise, C.D. (1980). Monoamine oxidase in schizophrenia: An overview. *Schizophrenia Bulletin,* 6, 199–207. This article discusses the behavioral, biochemical, and pharmacological aspects of monoamine oxidase activity.

CHAPTER THIRTEEN

The Opiates

The opiates comprise a class of drugs known as the narcotic analgesics. Their principal effect is pain reduction, and for acute pain the opiates and their synthetic analogs are vastly superior to all other analgesics. Opiates have a distinctive chemical structure, although slight or substantial modifications of the natural substances can cause pronounced changes in their pharmacological effects.

In addition to inducing analgesia, opiates not only have a spectrum of annoying side effects but also produce a sense of well-being and euphoria that leads to increased opiate use. In itself, this may not be undesirable, but coupled with the development of tolerance and of physiological addiction, the possibility of fatal overdosing, and the social strictures against drug dependence, serious medical, social, and legal problems surround the use of these substances. One consequence of these problems has been a search for compounds that will maximize desired therapeutic effects and minimize undesired side effects.

The opiates were once considered unique because their efficacy was coupled with a great need for substances for obtunding pain. Indeed, in 1680, Syndenham wrote, "Among the remedies which it has pleased Almighty God to give to man to relieve his suffering, none is so universal and so efficacious as opium." However, this uniqueness rested primarily upon ignorance about the mechanism and site of action, and as this ignorance has given way before contemporary research, the opiates are seen as no more unique than other pharmacologically valuable drugs. From another standpoint, however, the opiates are unique in that they contribute to a more complete understanding of the mechanisms of pain, tolerance, and physical dependence, and on the molecular level, to the mechanism of drug-receptor interactions.

History, Use, and Identity

The opiates, being unsurpassed in reducing pain, have been used as analgesics and for other purposes for centuries and are still widely used in all branches of medicine despite their undesirable side effects and their addiction potential. Reference to the use of opiates is found in the writings of Theophrastus as early as the third century B.C. For a long time opium was administered as a vapor or given through punctures in the skin. Because of the extreme variability of the opium content and the variable rate of absorption, the opiate's effects varied from inadequate analgesia to respiratory depression and death. Fatalities were not uncommon because, lacking our modern narcotic antagonists, futile attempts were made to revive patients from opium-induced unconsciousness by placing a sponge dipped in vinegar under the nose or by dripping the juice of rue (a plant with evergreen leaves that produce an acrid, volatile oil) into the ears (May and Sargent, 1924).

The administration of opium was greatly improved after 1803 when the German chemist Sertürner isolated the active ingredient in opium, which he called morphine after the god of dreams, Morpheus. The effects of morphine were more potent and significantly more predictable than those of the parent compound opium, although the problem of accurate administration persisted until 1853, when Pravaz invented the syringe and Alexander Wood developed the hollow needle (Foldes et al., 1964).

Opium is prepared by drying and powdering the milky juice taken from the seed capsules of the opium poppy, *Papaver somniferum*, just prior to ripening. Experimental cultivation of the opium poppy has been successful in the temperate zone as far north as England and Denmark, but the majority of the world's supply comes from Southeast Asia, India, China, Iran, Turkey, USSR, and Southeast Europe.

The active ingredients in opium include over 25 alkaloids, which make up 25 percent of its content by weight. Although the content varies with different specimens of opium, the percentage by weight of the most important alkaloids are approximately 10 percent morphine, 0.5 percent codeine, 0.3 percent thebaine, 1 percent papaverine, 6 percent narcotine, and 0.2 percent narceine (Reynolds and Randall, 1957). Of these alkaloids, morphine and codeine have the widest clinical use.

In addition to their analgesic effects, the opiates, acting on the CNS, have hypnotic effects and produce drowsiness, mood changes, and mental clouding. Act-

ing on the GI tract, opiates produce decreased gastric motility and reduced gastric and intestinal secretion, causing constipation. Another autonomic effect is the telltale pupil constriction.

Structure-Activity Relationships

Although morphine was separated from opium in the early 1800s, the structure of morphine was not identified until 1925 by Gulland and Robinson. The structures of morphine and related compounds are shown in Figure 1. The naturally occurring opiate alkaloid codeine is identical in structure to morphine except for the substitution of a methoxy ($-OCH_3$) for a hydroxyl moiety ($-OH$), producing a compound that tends to have less pharmacological activity. Although codeine's analgesic effects are much weaker than those of morphine, its analgesic potency is adequate for the relief of moderate pain. Its advantage over morphine is that its hypnotic property is also less and is not increased significantly by increased dosage. Thus, ordinarily, codeine alleviates moderate pain with fewer side effects.

Of great interest to synthetic chemists and pharmacologists was the discovery that simple modifica-

FIGURE 1 STRUCTURES OF OPIOIDS AND NARCOTIC ANTAGONISTS chemically related to morphine.

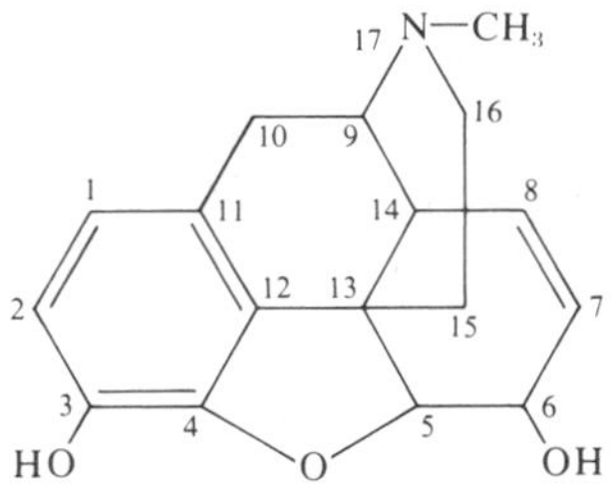

Opiate	3*	6*	17*	Other Changes
Morphine	$-OH$	$-OH$	$-CH_3$	none
Heroin	$-OCOCH_3$	$-OCOCH_3$	$-CH_3$	none
Codeine	$-OCH_3$	$-OH$	$-CH_3$	none
Nalorphine	$-OH$	$-OH$	$-CH_2CH=CH_2$	none
Naloxone	$-OH$	$=O$	$-CH_2CH=CH_2$	Single instead of double bond between C7 and C8
Naltrexone	$-OH$	$=O$	$-CH_2CH-CH_2$ (with CH_2 bridge)	Single instead of double bond between C7 and C8

*The numbers 3, 6, and 17 refer to positions in the morphine molecule, as shown above

tions of the morphine molecule produce great variations in pharmacological potency. In 1874, a minor chemical modification of the morphine molecule (i.e., the addition of two acetyl groups, CH_3-COO^-), produced the compound diacetylmorphine or heroin. At the time, the new compound was promoted as a more potent, nonaddicting substitute for morphine. Today we know that the pharmacological effects of morphine and heroin are identical because heroin is converted to monoacetylmorphine (MAM) and then to morphine in the brain. Heroin is, however, faster acting because the diacetylation makes the drug less polar and thus more lipid soluble. Great lipid solubility renders the drug more readily accessible to the brain, where it can act at brain receptors.

In more recent years, synthetic narcotics have been developed with the hope of producing more potent analgesic activity accompanied by reduced physical and psychological dependence. Some synthetic compounds, such as etorphine, are potent analgesics and have many of the same pharmacological effects as morphine, but all of them still possess some potential for addiction.

Four chemical classes of drugs show pharmacological activity in humans similar to that of morphine. They are the 4-phenylpiperidines (e.g., pethidine), the diphenylpropylamines (e.g., methadone), the morphinans (e.g., levorphanol), and the 6,7-benzomorphans (e.g., metazocine) (Figure 2). The compounds in these groups share the capacity to produce analgesia, respiratory depression, gastrointestinal spasm, and morphine-like physical dependence. Upon examination, the flat two-dimensional representations of these structurally diverse compounds appear to be quite different and one may question whether there is indeed a common mechanism of action for these drugs. Three-

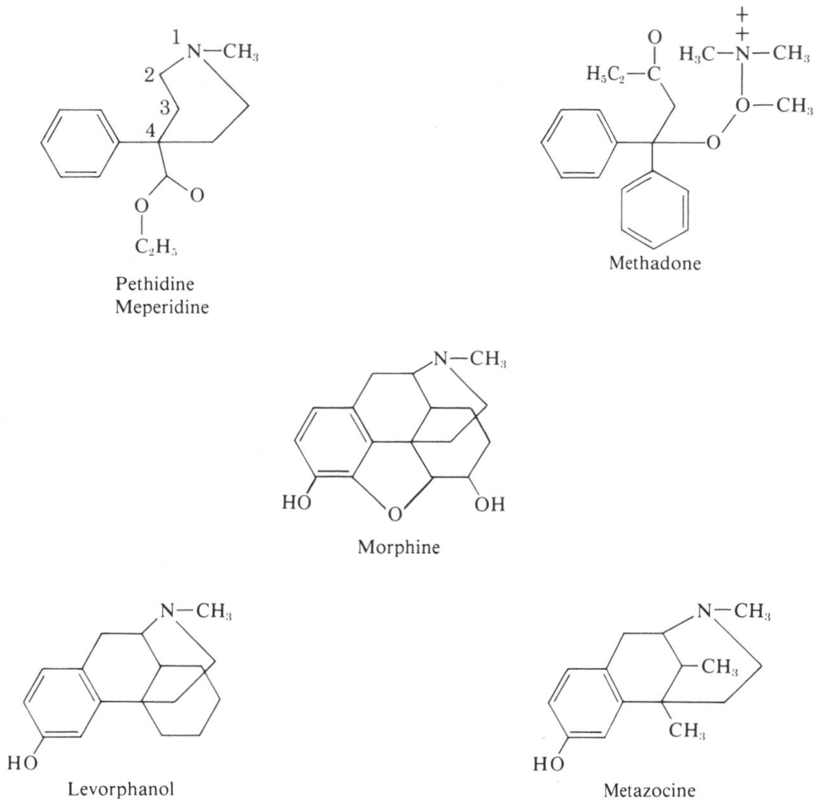

Pethidine
Meperidine

Methadone

Morphine

Levorphanol

Metazocine

FIGURE 2 FOUR CHEMICAL CLASSES OF NARCOTIC ANALGESICS. The similarities in their structures to one another and to morphine explain in part their common pharmacological effects and mechanisms of action.

dimensional molecular models, however, show that the drugs of these different classes can all simulate a piperidine ring. In addition, most have a nitrogen and a methyl group attached to the ring as well as a variety of other bulky groups.

Other chemical modifications, such as the substitution of an allyl group ($-CH_2CH = CH$) for the methyl group on the nitrogen atom of morphine produce the narcotic antagonists naloxone and nalorphine (Figure 1). Opiate antagonists are drugs that have structures similar to those of the opiates but produce no pharmacological activity of their own. These drugs can prevent or reverse the effect of administered opiates because of their ability to occupy opiate receptor sites. As receptor occupation is not an all-or-none phenomenon, we can consider most opiates to be mixed agonists–antagonists even though naloxone, for example, has an antagonist–agonist potency ratio that is so large that naloxone is considered to be a "pure" antagonist.

Pharmacodynamics: Administration and Excretion

Morphine is readily absorbed through most mucous membranes and is administered most commonly by subcutaneous injection. Oral administration, however, is not uncommon; neither is absorption from the nasal mucosa (as when heroin is used as snuff); nor from the lung (as when opium is smoked). Once absorbed, morphine's distribution is fairly uniform in most tissues. Despite the fact that morphine has its greatest effects on the CNS, the drug does not seem to concentrate there. In fact, only small quantities are capable of passing the blood brain barrier. It is worthwhile to mention that opiates apparently are capable of passing the placental barrier. Consequently, newborns of opiate-addicted mothers suffer withdrawal symptoms within several hours of birth. Although opiate withdrawal is not considered life-threatening in the adult addict, the syndrome may have severe consequences for the newborn, particularly if his nutritional state is poor as a result of inadequate prenatal care.

The kidney is the principal route of excretion. Most of the administered drug is found in the urine within 24 hours of treatment, whereas only 7–10 percent eventually appears in the feces. Some of the morphine is excreted unchanged, but the largest portion is combined with glucuronic acid. The conjugate has an increased filtration rate in the kidney because of the altered ionic charge of the molecule.

Physiological Effects

Central Nervous System

In terms of both pharmacodynamics and physiological effects, the prototypic opiate is morphine. The related opiates have qualitatively similar effects that vary primarily in potency and duration. Morphine has its most pronounced effects on the CNS, and, as we might expect, these drug-induced effects are dose related. At small to moderate doses (5–10 mg), the principal subjective effects are drowsiness, decreased sensitivity to external and internal stimuli, and loss of anxiety and inhibition. At this dose, muscle relaxation occurs, pain is relieved, respiration is somewhat depressed, and pupils are constricted. The ability to concentrate is impaired and this effect is often followed by a dreamy sleep.

At slightly higher doses, an abnormal state of elation or euphoria may develop that is quite different from the usual sense of well-being. The literature frequently refers to the "kick," "bang," or "rush" that the addict feels immediately after injecting morphine or heroin into a vein. This rush is likened to an "abdominal orgasm." Nonaddicts describe it as a sudden flush of warmth, localized in the pit of the stomach. Individuals who take opiates orally or who smoke, sniff, or inject them subcutaneously or intramuscularly do not experience the rush. Because these latter individuals can be just as dependent on opiates as the "mainliners" (i.e., those who inject i.v.), it is clear that the rush is not the basis for addiction. It is interesting to note that the euphoric effect of morphine does not always accompany analgesia. In fact, in well-adjusted, stable individuals who are free of pain, the administration of morphine may produce a dysphoria (restlessness and anxiety). The elation occurs most often in those who are either abnormally depressed or highly excited (Reynolds and Randall, 1957).

The nausea that often accompanies even small therapeutic doses of morphine is increased with the higher doses. The nausea is also a CNS effect of the drug and involves the action of morphine on the chemical trigger zone in the medulla, which ultimately contributes to vagal input to the gut. For the addict, the nauseous episode may become a "good sick" because it has attained secondary reinforcing properties by signaling the onset of euphoria.

At the highest doses of morphine, depression deepens to unconsciousness. Pupils are now quite constricted and respiratory rate is further depressed. At this dose, the respiratory center in the brain stem, which normally responds to high CO_2 levels in the blood by triggering increased rate and depth of respiration, is severely depressed and may be the ultimate cause of death. Of great significance is the fact that even at the highest doses, morphine does not cause slurred speech, significant motor incoordination, or severe mental clouding, unlike other agents (such as nitrous oxide) that cause analgesia only when accompanied by mental confusion or unconsciousness.

Gastrointestinal Effects

Apart from the CNS, effects of morphine are greatest on the gastrointestinal tract. Opium was used for relief of diarrhea and dysentery even before it was used for analgesia. The digestive processes, on the whole, are slowed in most species, and in humans constipation is a common and disturbing side effect of morphine use, even in the addicted person. Morphine also alters the tonus and motility of the stomach and intestines, thereby slowing the passage of the contents and permitting greater absorption of water and increase in fecal viscosity. However, with repeated administration of morphine, most of the pharmacological effects are diminished in magnitude. Demonstrating the phenomena of "rebound," frequent and copious diarrhea is a prominent part of the syndrome following abrupt withdrawal of morphine after prolonged drug usage.

Analgesia

Of the many pharmacological properties of the opiates, their analgesic effects have received the most attention; a voluminous literature exists on this topic. However, despite great efforts, the mechanism by which morphine produces analgesia is just beginning to be understood. Basic to this problem is the difficulty in identifying and measuring pain.

Pain may be considered to be a sensation resulting from any tissue-damaging stimulus; therefore, it is essential for survival. However, pain is not a single modality. Pain receptors, unlike the more specialized receptors of the other senses, can be activated by a variety of stimuli, including radiant heat, extreme cold, electrical impulses, pressure or stretching, cuts or tears, and chemical irritants. The quality of pain also varies and may be described as pricking, stabbing,

burning, throbbing, aching, and so on. Cutaneous pain may be considered to be "bright" or "dull" but usually involves little emotional reaction (Winter, 1965). On the other hand, pain that is deeper is accompanied by autonomic responses, such as sweating, fall in blood pressure, or nausea, and a strong emotional component. This emotional response to pain is one that is not usually found in conjunction with other sensory systems such as audition or taste. The separation of the two components is particularly clear in the patient who, after receiving morphine for protracted pain, maintains that the pain is present and as intense as ever but is no longer aversive. The ability of morphine to modify the emotional component of pain may explain why it is more effective in alleviating chronic or pathological pain than acute pain. Presumably the sensory component of pain is the same for all persons given the identical stimulus, but the reaction process to the initial sensation may be quite different for different subjects. Furthermore, it is never certain that all subjects in an experiment on pain are describing the same experience.

In a lengthy review of the subject, Beecher (1957) suggested that the reaction process is influenced by the patient's concept of the sensation, by its significance based on past experience, and by its degree of seriousness. For instance, Beecher suggests that a strong emotional reaction may be generated in the patient with a characteristic ache beneath the sternum suggesting heart failure and possibly death, whereas a pain of the same intensity and duration in the arm is considered trivial and is disregarded. Further evidence of the influence of emotion on pain is the often cited example of the soldier who, during the heat of the battle, is unaware of his mortal wounds. Sexual arousal is also known to block pain. Furthermore, hypnosis, which under some conditions can effectively block the response to pain, must be considered to reduce the reaction component rather than the sensory component of pain. The effectiveness of analgesics may then be due to (1) reduced sensation, (2) reduced process of recognition, or (3) altered processes of discrimination, memory, or judgment that follow recognition (Winter, 1965).

Quantification of Pain

Although we can get subjective verbal reports of the sensation of pain, quantification is difficult, particularly in the clinical setting. There are a number of response-biasing factors that must be considered when evaluating clinical reports of analgesic effects generated by the patient self-reporting technique. Anxiety may be related to the anticipation of more pain or to the lack of knowledge of the cause of pain and plays an important part in how a patient responds to drug treatment. This fact is emphasized by the finding that opiates, under certain experimental test situations (such as responding to heat stimuli), do not reliably raise pain thresholds in humans, although they are very effective in the treatment of pathological pain. The tests of analgesia using animal models compare more closely with the tests of human pathological pain than with tests of human experimental pain. The differences that exist may be due to the fact that the human subject exposed to experimental pain realizes that the stimulus poses no real threat, whereas for the animal subject, all pain is serious and may represent a stimulus that is life threatening.

Although we know that morphine significantly reduces the reactive component of pain, we must keep in mind that drugs that reduce anxiety (e.g., chlordiazepoxide) do not have significant analgesic properties. Furthermore, depressant or anxiolytic drugs such as the barbiturates and meprobamate do not have analgesic effects except at doses that produce gross intoxication.

The Placebo Effect

A second important response-biasing factor is the placebo effect. A PLACEBO is a pharmacologically inert compound administered to the subject as part of the ritual of drug administration. For a substantial number of patients, the placebo provides striking therapeutic effects as well as a variety of side effects. It has been reported that when surgical patients suffering from steady, severe wound pain are injected subcutaneously with saline, three or four out of ten report satisfactory relief of pain (Lasagna et al., 1954). It is important to remember that the placebo effect may be either psychological or physical; it may make the patient feel better for psychological reasons or it may produce actual physiological changes, such as changes in gastric secretion for an ulcer patient (Beecher, 1957).

In investigations of drug effects, the placebo is an essential part of the experimental design because it enables the elimination of bias on the part of the patient and also the separation of the effect of the drug from suggestion. Every therapeutic treatment must be considered to contribute to placebo effects. One might consider an active drug as a placebo overlaid by active drug effects. Morphine's effectiveness, then, is the sum of a placebo effect and its pharmacological drug effect. If 70 percent of a group tested for pain relief were satisfactorily improved by morphine, 30–40 percent of the total number experiencing pain relief must be subtracted as placebo responders in order to determine the true effectiveness of the drug.

There seems to be no simple, reliable way to eliminate those subjects in the group who will be placebo responders because neither superficial observations nor classic measures of intelligence are correlated with the response. With more elaborate psychological testing, placebo reactors have been found to be generally less mature, somewhat self-centered, and more preoccupied with bodily processes (Lasagna et al., 1954). The group also tends to be more anxious than those who do not respond to the placebo and to be more emotionally labile.

Because of the large contribution of emotional factors and the high incidence of placebo responders, the DOUBLE-BLIND EXPERIMENT is highly desirable. In these experiments, neither the patient nor the observer knows what treatment the patient has received. Such precautions ensure that the results of any given treatment will not be colored by overt or covert prejudices either on the part of the patient or the observer. Obviously, the ability to maintain the blind is reduced if the drug has noticeable side effects. Unfortunately, appropriate design and controls are not often readily applicable in the clinical setting. For instance, the patient is not likely to appreciate suffering for a long period of time in order to provide information on the drug's time course of action.

Experimental Procedures

The laboratory, on the other hand, provides a more controlled setting for the measurement of the analgesic properties of the opiates, but the experimental paradigms available to the laboratory scientist do not lend themselves well to the study of chronic or pathological pain. We have already mentioned that the human laboratory subject is aware that the pain is of only minor and temporary significance, so analgesic properties of drugs are poorly defined. The methods used to induce pain at threshold, such as the application of sudden pressure, pinpricks, or stabs, show ineffective or inconsistent analgesic effects even with opiates. The experimental methods that show more consistent results with the analgesics are those techniques that produce slowly developing or sustained pain. One such technique is the occlusion of blood flow with a tourniquet on an exercising muscle (Lewis et al., 1931). Using this method, the pain is slow in onset and is directly related to the amount of exercise. Cutaneous pain in man can be produced by the intradermal injection of various chemicals. In order to avoid undependable results, however, the outer layer of epidermis is removed after the formation of a blister with canthardin (Armstrong et al., 1951). The blister base is used for testing with the application of small quantities of various agents. Bathing the area with isotonic solutions enables repeated testing within 10–15 minutes without changing the sensitivity of the nerve endings. Techniques that have been designed to produce more intense or more persistent pain are infrequently used as finding subjects willing to participate in the experiments is more difficult.

An alternative and common method to measure analgesic properties uses animal models. For a detailed description of the most commonly used animal tests for analgesia, see Chapter 2.

Mechanism of Action of Opiates

Although the opiates have been used for centuries, the cellular mechanism of action for each of morphine's many effects is not known. Many attempts have been made, but no clear relationship has been found between the neurochemical changes following morphine administration and morphine-induced analgesia. It is now generally assumed that specific membrane-bound receptors for the opiates exist, and extensive work to identify, characterize, and isolate these receptors is currently underway. In addition, there is an intense interest in the endogenous opiate-like substances, which may represent a class of neurotransmitters involved in modulation of pain transmission. The discussion of morphine's mechanism of action will center on the opiate receptor and the endogenous opiates because of the great interest in this new topic in neurobiology and because the research techniques used to study the opiate receptors provide a model for studying neurotransmitter receptors in general.

In addition to the literature on the search for the endogenous opiate, a large body of literature exists on the interaction of the opiates with each of the known neurotransmitters, including the catecholamines, acetylcholine, and 5-hydroxytryptamine. Within this latter body of literature, there are many apparent inconsistencies in reported results. The frequently contradictory results have been attributed to several factors, including variability in available analgesic testing methods, marked differences in drug effects among species, and the interfering peripheral pharmacological effects of morphine that may alter central neurotransmitter metabolism (Calcutt et al., 1973).

The opiates are known to have multiple effects on catecholamine metabolism. Moderate doses of morphine decrease norepinephrine (NE) levels in various areas of the brain of cats and mice (Vogt, 1954; Reis et al., 1971; Fennessy and Lee, 1972), although the synthesis rate is accelerated (Smith et al., 1972; Clouet and Ratner, 1970). In contrast, in the rat much higher doses of morphine are required to produce an effect, which may be either an increase (Gunne, 1963) or a decrease (Maynert and Klingman, 1962) in NE levels. In addition, it has been found that NE turnover in whole brain is unchanged after treatment with morphine (Clouet and Ratner, 1970), but both increased (Sugrue, 1973) and decreased (Clouet and Ratner, 1970) turnover have been reported for selected areas of the brain.

Changes in dopaminergic activity have been found after both acute and chronic morphine administration. An acute morphine-induced increase in dopamine (DA) turnover has been suggested by (1) an increased conversion of tyrosine to DA, (2) an increase in DA metabolism, and (3) an increase in depletion of brain DA after DA synthesis inhibition (reviewed in Lal, 1975). It is not known whether any of the morphine-induced changes in neurotransmitter metabolism are direct effects of the opiate. For instance, morphine does not directly change the affinity of tyrosine hydroxylase (the rate-limiting enzyme in the biosynthesis of NE and DA) for its substrate (tyrosine) or its cofactor, nor does it change the feedback inhibition of the enzyme by the catecholamines (CA) (Cicero et al., 1973). Yet morphine under some conditions significantly increases CA synthesis.

The relationship of NE to analgesia is also complex. Whether NE increases or reduces morphine-induced analgesia may depend on both the species tested and the particular test of analgesia used. In rats and mice, intraventricular NE significantly attenuates the analgesia produced by morphine when measured with the tail-flick test (Calcutt et al., 1973). However, the same laboratory, along with many others, has shown that in mice intraventricular NE has a significant analgesic property when measured with the hot plate test. Clearly, in the mouse, different tests produce different results.

The picture is not much clearer for the role of 5-hydroxytryptamine (5-HT) in analgesia. Using the tail-flick test or the hot plate test, several investigators found an antagonism between 5-HT- and morphine-induced analgesia, whereas others have reported that increases in brain 5-HT potentiate the analgesic effects of morphine (Calcutt et al., 1973). In addition, electrical stimulation of the 5-HT cell bodies in the raphe nucleus produces analgesia (Liebeskind et al., 1973), and Vogt (1974) has described a loss of morphine-induced analgesia after destruction of 5-HT-containing fibers. In an attempt to reconcile the discrepancies, several investigators have proposed dual control of analgesia by several neurotransmitters (Calcutt et al., 1973; Harris and Dewey, 1973; Akil and Liebeskind, 1975).

The opiates have also been found to act on cholinergic neurotransmission. In the guinea pig ileum bioassay, a concentration of morphine as low as 100 nM depresses the electrically induced contraction of the longitudinal muscle by reducing the release of acetylcholine (ACh) (Lees et al., 1973). A good correlation has been found between the potency for guinea pig ileum twitch inhibition and clinical potency for analgesia. In the CNS, a significant inhibition of ACh release as well as an elevation of brain ACh levels has been found, but the effects of the narcotic antagonists on ACh levels and their effectiveness in blocking the opiate-induced increase in ACh level differs from laboratory to laboratory. In addition, no simple correlation exists between brain ACh level and analgesia.

Clearly, the effects of the opiates on neurotransmitters are diverse and complex. It is also quite likely that in the brain the activity of any single neurotransmitter cannot be altered without resultant changes in other neurotransmitters. In addition, the endogenous opiates have a potential role as neurotransmitters in the pain pathways, although their function is not yet clear.

The Opiate Receptor

In-depth analysis of the molecular structures of the opioid drugs provides sufficient information to hypothesize definite structural features of the opiate receptor. Very early it became clear that the piperidine ring was essential for the pharmacological activity of opiates (Figure 1). The nitrogen atom of this ring is normally positively charged, so it is likely that one important element of the drug–receptor interaction is the attraction of the drug molecule to a negatively charged site on the receptor surface. It is also evident from the three-dimensional model of morphine that the receptor must have the shape of an irregular pouch into which the morphine molecule can fit, allowing the essential contacts to be made on different walls of the pouch.

The importance of "fit" of the molecule to the receptor is demonstrated by the D-isomers of the morphine series. The D-isomers are identical to the active L-isomers in structure but are mirror images; thus, they are excluded from the receptor site by their "wrong" geometry and have neither agonist nor antagonist activity. The structural requirements of the opiate receptor provide an excellent means to demonstrate the specificity of any opiate pharmacological effect. Thus, if it is suspected that a compound has an opiate effect, that effect must be blocked by a specific opiate receptor antagonist such as naloxone and not be produced by D-isomers of the test compound.

Opiates' actions in the CNS may tell us something about normal brain functions, particularly those involving pain transmission. Several lines of evidence suggest that opiate actions must involve highly specific receptors in the brain. The fairly stringent molecular requirements for opiate activity, the great potency of these compounds, and the stereospecificity of the drugs (i.e., the optical isomers of the analgesic compounds are inactive) all support the hypothesis of a specific opiate receptor.

OPIATE RECEPTORS are hypothetical, stereospecific tissue constituents to which morphine and other opiate agonists bind to initiate their pharmacological effects. The methods used for the identification and characterization of the opiate receptors are similar to those used to identify other membrane-localized receptors (such as those for insulin, prolactin, and angiotensin), as well as the receptors for the putative neurotransmitters acetylcholine, β-catecholamines, serotonin, and glycine.

Receptor Binding Studies

The general approach is to study the physiochemical interaction between a radioactive ligand and the plasma membrane, either in the intact cell or in an isolated membrane preparation. Under optimum conditions, the initial binding studies should be done on a very simple system so that tissue preparative procedures that may disrupt the cellular organization and membrane integrity are avoided (Cuatrecasas, 1974b). A simple intact system is also necessary to compare the receptor binding capacity and the biological activity of the hormone in the same preparation. But intact tissue is not necessarily the best preparation, because one must also be concerned with the homogeneity of the cell population as well as with the presence of connective tissue or other elements that may hamper the diffusion of test agents.

Opiates, apparently, will bind to almost any biological or nonbiological membrane. Thus, one cannot add radioactively labeled opiate to the tissue homogenate and assume that if the labeled drug molecules are associated with some subcellular fraction that it represents drug "binding" to a specific recognition site. In addition to binding at specific recognition sites (i.e., receptors), the labeled ligand can also be dissolved nonspecifically in the lipid membrane, or it may nonspecifically bind to anionic groups in the membrane because of the positively charged atoms in the opiate molecule.

Goldstein et al. (1971) developed a method for detecting specific opiate receptors in mouse brain. In this method one sample (A) of membranes known to bind opiates is incubated with a radioactive opiate, levorphanol. The result is radioactive tissue that includes (1) a nonsaturable solution of opiate molecules in the lipid membranes, (2) a nonspecific saturable binding due to electrostatic attraction, and (3) stereospecific saturable binding on opiate receptors. A second sample (B) is first incubated with an excess of nonradioactive dextrorphan, an opiate in the wrong (+) configuration. This also dissolves in the lipid membranes and fills up nonspecific electrostatic sites. But this opiate ligand cannot bind to specific opiate receptors. When sample B is then treated with radioactive levorphanol, the labeled drug will be excluded from nonspecific sites but will bind to the specific sites. The difference in radioactivity (A minus B) measures the nonspecific saturable binding. A third sample (C) is first incubated with excess nonradioactive levorphanol and then with radioactive levorphanol. Now the labeled opiate is excluded from both specific and nonspecific sites. The difference in radioactivity (B minus C) yields a measure of stereospecific receptor binding. The residual radioactivity in sample C indicates

the nonspecific nonsaturable interaction (Goldstein, 1976).

Although our discussion described only opiate binding, the principle of receptor binding with radioactive ligands has been used successfully to identify many other receptors in the CNS. Some of these include the β-adrenergic receptors (Lefkowitz et al., 1974), serotonin receptors (Bennett and Aghajanian, 1974), and glycine receptors (Young and Snyder, 1974).

The separation of specific binding from nonspecific binding is of great importance because physiological membrane receptors are, as a rule, present in small numbers. There are many more nonspecific binding sites, which may show quite high affinity for the ligand. Goldstein's initial attempt to identify the opiate receptor in brain homogenates found only 2 percent stereospecific binding (Goldstein et al., 1971). The technique was greatly improved and used more successfully when radioactive opiates with higher specific radioactivity (e.g., 40 Ci/nmol for [³H]naloxone) were developed. Use of the "hotter" ligand means that even a small number of receptors with high affinity can be measured over and above background values.

Biochemical Characterization of Opiate Binding

In addition to steric specificity, several other criteria should be met to confirm the specificity (Cuatrecasas, 1974b).

Using [³H]naloxone as the primary ligand, Pert and Snyder (1973) found [³H]naloxone binding to be saturable, with half saturation occurring at about 1.6×10^{-8} M with 18 mg tissue. Figure 3 shows that with increasing amounts of [³H]naloxone, stereospecific binding increases and gradually reaches a plateau. The asymptotic curve indicates saturation of the binding sites, which suggests that a finite number of receptors exists. In this case, the concentration of the opiate needed to saturate the receptors is within a concentration range that is meaningfully related to the concentration of agonist necessary to elicit a pharmacological response.

Opiate binding sites have high affinity for narcotic analgesics and their antagonists. Affinities range from very high for a potent narcotic analgesic (etorphine) to very low or undetectable for drugs that do not have analgesic effects (Simon, 1976). It is also of interest to examine both the rate of association of the opiate and receptor and the dissociation of the complex, as a ratio of dissociation to association gives an independent

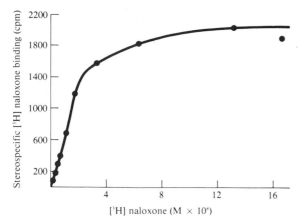

FIGURE 3   STEREOSPECIFIC BINDING OF [³H]NAL-OXONE to rat brain homogenate. By increasing the concentration of the opiate, saturation of the opiate receptors occurs. (From Pert and Snyder, 1973.)

estimate of affinity. That is, if a substance dissociates from tissue about as rapidly as it associates with it, then that substance is not as likely to be as physiologically active as a substance that dissociates significantly more slowly than it associates. Moreover, the rate of dissociation of the ligand–receptor complex is consistent with the loss of pharmacological effect observed in a bioassay when the drug is removed from the medium.

Further biochemical studies have shown that stereospecific opiate binding is greatly impaired by proteolytic enzymes such as trypsin and pronase (Pasternak and Snyder, 1974; Simon et al., 1973) and by sulfhydryl reagents (Pasternak and Snyder, 1974). This observation strongly supports the idea of a protein receptor with a sulfhydryl group occupying a position at or near the binding site. Pasternak and Snyder (1974) also showed that stereospecific opiate binding is very sensitive to phospholipase A, which alters the lipid constituents in the membrane or in the receptor itself and thus retards binding. The finding that phospholipase C is less effective than phospholipase A suggests that the more polar moieties of the phospholipids that are attacked by phospholipase C are less important to opiate binding.

Ionic Requirements

Simon et al. (1973) reported that the addition of sodium to the binding assay produced a dose-depen-dent decrease in etorphine binding. Pert and Snyder (1974) found that sodium, but not other alkali metal ions (except lithium to a limited extent), enhanced the binding of opiate antagonists and greatly reduced the binding of agonists. For example, the binding of the virtually pure antagonist, [³H]naloxone, is increased by 60 percent by the addition of 1 mM sodium, and this antagonist binding continues to increase as the sodium ion concentration is raised to 40–50 mM. Conversely, binding of the agonists levorphanol, oxymorphone, or dihydromorphine is depressed by the addition of Na$^+$. The ability of Na$^+$ to alter the degree to which opiates bind correlates well with the agonist–antagonist properties of these drugs.

The fact that the effect of Na$^+$ is highly specific and can only be elicited by Na$^+$ and Li$^+$, but not by Rb$^+$, Cs$^+$, K$^+$, or other mono- or divalent cations (Pert and Snyder, 1974, Snyder and Pert, 1975) suggests that the ions interact with sites on the membrane that can transform the receptors so that they are less likely to bind agonists and more likely to bind antagonists. Despite the fact that Na$^+$ alters agonist–antagonist binding, it is not yet clear whether Na$^+$ alters the number of opiate receptors or the affinity of the receptors for the ligand. However, both Simon (1975) and Snyder (1975b) have proposed models in which the opiate receptor shifts conformation and binds either agonists or antagonists, depending on its molecular state. Figure 4 shows that, according to their model, the addition of Na$^+$ shifts the receptor to the an-

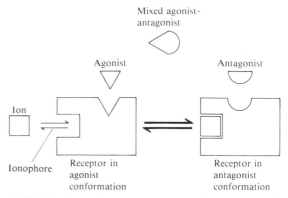

FIGURE 4   MODEL OF OPIATE RECEPTOR to explain the sodium effect by postulating that the receptor can exist in two different conformations: a no-sodium binding form with a high affinity for agonists and a sodium form with a high affinity for antagonists. Sodium effect is selective; of the other positively charged ions, only lithium has a similar effect. (From Snyder, 1975b.)

tagonist state, so antagonists bind effectively whereas agonists show less ability to bind. Removal of Na$^+$ shifts the receptor back to the agonist form, and antagonists bind less effectively.

Subcellular Localization

Opiate receptor binding seems to be confined to nervous tissue, primarily within the CNS and the myenteric plexus of the guinea pig intestine. It is of interest to determine where in the neuron binding takes place. We might expect, for instance, that if the opiates act by altering synaptic activity, then opiate binding should occur in the area of synaptic membrane rather than in the nuclear portion of the cell or within the cytosol (cell plasma). Using the combined methods of differential centrifugation and sucrose gradients, Pert et al. (1974) recovered the subcellular fractions shown in Figure 5. When the various fractions were assayed for opiate binding, they found that the greatest amount of binding occurred in the synaptic membrane fraction, with much less in the mitochondrial or nuclear fractions. A similar result was reported by Terenius (1973). The localization of opiate binding to the synaptic membrane fraction suggests that opiates exert their primary pharmacological effects by altering synaptic function.

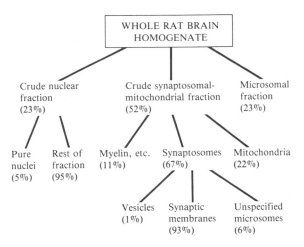

FIGURE 5 SUBCELLULAR DISTRIBUTION of stereospecific opiate receptor binding. The proportion of opiate binding in each fraction is indicated as a percentage of the binding of the parent fraction. (From Snyder and Pert, 1975.)

Localization within the Central Nervous System

Opiate receptor binding varied quite dramatically when localization within the brain was measured. Using monkey brain, Kuhar et al. (1973a) found a 30-fold difference in binding between the anterior portion of the amygdala, which had the greatest binding per milligram protein, when compared to very low or nondetectable binding in the corpus callosum, corona radiata, fornix, optic chiasma, cortex and dentate nucleus of the cerebellum, and in lower brain stem and spinal cord. Binding in posterior amygdala was about 0.5 times that in the anterior portion and equaled that in the periaqueductal area of the midbrain. The hypothalamus and medial thalamus showed about 0.4 times the binding found in anterior amygdala. Although there were no regional differences within the hypothalamus, the medial thalamus had 3 times as much binding as did the lateral thalamus. In the head of the caudate receptor binding was 0.8 times that in the hypothalamus, 2 times that in the body and tail of the caudate, and 1.7 times that in putamen. Binding in the putamen was approximately equal to that in the hippocampus, superior colliculi, interpeduncular nucleus, and the frontal pole and superior temporal gyrus of the cerebral cortex.

Within the cortex, the precentral gyrus and occipital pole had less than 0.25 times that in frontal cortex. A grossly similar distribution is reported for human brain after autopsy (Heller et al., 1973). In addition, two laboratories have measured specific opiate binding *in vivo* using autoradiography (Pert et al., 1975; Schubert et al., 1975). In both rats and mice, the specific binding of the radioactive opiate was high in caudate–putamen, substantia nigra, locus caeruleus, amygdala, thalamus, periventricular substance, hypothalamus, and habenula; sites in good agreement with earlier *in vitro* studies.

Pain Pathways. Distribution of opiate receptor binding is of interest in terms of its correlation with the neuroanatomical centers normally associated with pain transmission. The principal ascending fiber bundle mediating pain and temperature is the lateral spinothalamic tract. The collaterals and ramifications of this tract, as described by Nauta (1975), may be responsible for the various components of the sensation we call pain.

The lateral spinothalamic tract projects from dorsal horn neurons to the thalamus. It has been mapped by injecting horseradish peroxidase (HP) into the thalamic cells of adult cats. Several days after the injection, the brains were removed, fixed, sliced and stained, showing that the HP underwent retrograde transport to the cells of lamina V at the base of the dorsal horn. These cells react to noxious (as well as to nonnoxious) stimuli. The cells containing the retrograde HP were also processed for enkephalin binding using immunocytochemical staining. The results revealed that enkephalin immunoreactive axonal endings synapse on the same cells identified by HP in lamina V, suggesting that enkephalin modulates the pain information carried from the periphery to higher centers (Ruda, 1982). Thus, it appears that enkephalins modulate the release of substance P at the first order synapses in laminae I and II of the dorsal horn (see Chapter 10) as well as modulating second order synapses in lamina /V of the pain pathway to higher centers.

In addition to modifying the pain signal the opiates modify the awareness of or emotional response to pain. A great many of the lateral spinothalamic fibers synapse at brain stem levels below the thalamus, such as the tegmental reticular formation (which may have an alerting function). Furthermore, a number of fibers synapse in the central gray of the midbrain, and pathways originating here go to the hypothalamus and in turn connect this center with limbic structures that may be responsible for the emotional component of pain. Functionally, then, morphine may act by blocking a flow from the nociceptive pathway to higher sensory areas as well as to limbic structures. The mapping of opiate receptors (Kuhar et al., 1973a; Heller et al., 1973) suggests that significant binding occurs in limbic structures as well as in the hypothalamus and medial thalamus (neural centers receiving nociceptive input).

The medial thalamus has been further implicated in morphine's effect because Wei et al. (1972) showed that applying naloxone crystals to the medial thalamic area in morphine-dependent rats precipitated dramatic withdrawal symptoms that were not seen after treatment in other areas such as the neocortex, hippocampus, or lateral thalamus. They found a similar effect by applying naloxone to a medial area at the junction of the diencephalon and mesencephalon, an area Kuhar et al. (1973) found to bind labeled opiates selectively. Interpretation of these findings is complicated by the fact that naloxone had little effect when applied to the hypothalamus or striatum, although these areas did show significant opiate receptor binding.

Electrically Induced Analgesia. The central gray areas around the aqueduct have been found not only to bind opiates strongly but also to produce analgesia when stimulated electrically. In fact, both focal electrical stimulation-induced analgesia and analgesia produced by microinjection of opiates appear to exert their effects at sites surrounding the third ventricle, the cerebral aqueduct, and rostral portions of the fourth ventricle (Mayer and Liebeskind, 1974; Herz et al., 1970; Jacquet and Lajtha, 1974; Sharpe et al., 1974). In addition, some cross tolerance occurs between the analgesic effects of electrical stimulation in the mesencephalic central gray area and subcutaneous administration of morphine (Mayer and Hayes, 1975). Akil et al. (1976) also showed that naloxone could partially antagonize the analgesia produced by focal electrical stimulation of the periaqueductal gray area in rats without altering responsiveness to other stimuli. The fact that even large doses of naloxone were no more than 38 percent effective in blocking the analgesia might mean that the analgesia does not result from the activation of a single underlying mechanism. The authors suggest that electrical stimulation might release a morphine-like substance onto postsynaptic receptor sites that could be blocked by naloxone. The stimulation might also have a direct postsynaptic action, which Akil et al. (1976) feel might not be blocked by the opiate antagonist (Watkins and Mayer, 1982).

Evidence from the variety of sources described in the preceding paragraph suggests that the central gray surrounding the third and fourth ventricles and the aqueduct is a significant neural locus for analgesia. Neuroanatomically, the central gray core from periaqueductal to periventricular and medial thalamic area may be considered a functional unit because of reciprocal connections established between the central gray of the midbrain and the periventricular region of the diencephalon by the dorsal longitudinal fasciculus of Schütz (Nauta, 1975). In addition, Nauta describes fibers that connect the central gray substance with a large area of midbrain tegmentum and with the intralaminar nuclei of the thalamus.

Pharmacological Significance in Analgesia

As yet, we have said very little about the pharmacological significance of the opiate receptors. Without some correlation with a physiological response, the hypothetical opiate receptor is of merely heuristic value. Pert and Snyder (1974), however, have shown that there is, in general, a correlation between the effectiveness of an opiate in producing or antagonizing analgesia and its ability to bind specifically to the opiate receptors. As would be expected, the parallel is not perfect. For instance, although etorphine is about 100 times more potent than morphine *in vivo*, it has only 20 times the affinity of morphine for the receptor. Such discrepancies can often be resolved by determining the lipid solubility of the opiate and the speed at which it can reach the binding sites in brain after systemic administration. In the case of etorphine, we find that it is many times more efficient than morphine in entering the brain. Thus, its affinity for the opiate receptor is not the sole factor in determining *in vivo* potency. In all studies in which an *in vivo* pharmacological effect or the clinical efficacy of a compound is compared to its activity in an *in vitro* system, one must be aware of the physiological and pharmacological factors altering absorption, binding, solubility, and metabolism. Better correlations are found between the ability of an opiate to bind to receptors and its effect on an isolated preparation *in vitro*.

Opiate Bioassay

The bioassay considered to measure opioid activity most accurately uses the guinea pig ileum longitudinal muscle–myenteric plexus preparation developed by Kosterlitz and co-workers (Kosterlitz et al., 1970). After dissection, the tissue is maintained in a physiological solution that is aerated with a 95% O_2:5% CO_2 mixture and kept at 37°C. The muscle preparation is fastened at each end to maintain a fixed tension so that when the postganglionic cholinergic neurons are electrically stimulated, the release of ACh induces a twitch of the longitudinal smooth muscle that can be recorded on a polygraph. The release of ACh and the resulting twitch is inhibited by opiate drugs. Although a variety of compounds inhibit the twitch response, the specificity of this effect for the opiates is demonstrated by naloxone reversal. Kosterlitz and co-workers (Kosterlitz et al., 1973b; Kosterlitz and Waterfield, 1975) showed that the naloxone-reversible twitch inhibition is almost perfectly correlated with the ability of the opiates to relieve pain in man.

Creese and Snyder (1975) found a very good correlation between the extent of muscle-twitch inhibition by the opiates tested and their affinity for stereospecific binding sites in the guinea pig intestine. Furthermore,

they found that the relative affinities of opiates and the degree of stereospecificity for intestinal binding sites is very similar to that in brain. Thus, it is apparent that a correlation exists between analgesic effect *in vivo*, muscle-twitch inhibition in the bioassay, and ability to bind stereospecifically to opiate receptors.

The bioassay has provided the most reliable and accurate measure of opioid activity. In addition, the same muscle preparation can be used many times without a great loss in sensitivity by washing out each test agent. Discrepancies do exist between studies, probably because the procedure has several potential pitfalls, which can be avoided by maintaining the proper controls. Goldstein (1976) describes several of the possible variables. First, the lipid solubility of the different opiate compounds is of considerable significance. Second, one must also be aware of the activity of enzymes (e.g., peptidase) in the muscle preparation. Not only is it likely that opioid-like peptides will be broken down into smaller peptides, but the activity of these enzymes varies from preparation to preparation, thus increasing experimental variability. Third, sensitivity to opiates varies from muscle strip to muscle strip because of differences in dissection or preparation of the strip or differences among animals. Thus, for each experiment, the strip must be tested with a standard (such as normorphine) against which test compounds can be measured. In addition, the duration of viability of each tissue in its bathing medium is different, so frequent control tests with the standard (normorphine) is essential. The variables described are typical of any bioassay. Therefore, with these factors in mind, the assay does provide important information on opioid activity.

Endogenous Opiate-Like Peptides

Although opiate receptor binding appears to be localized in neural centers that are believed to be involved with pain transmission and although subcellular localization to the synaptic membrane portion of the cell indicates that opiates do exert their primary effect on synaptic activity, the distribution of opiate receptor binding fails to parallel the regional distribution of any previously known neurotransmitter. Although it is possible that several neurotransmitters are responsible for the opiate's analgesic effect, none of the known neurotransmitters alters opiate receptor binding. Furthermore, Kuhar et al. (1973a) found that electrolytic lesions that depleted stores of NE, 5-HT, or ACh failed to alter opiate receptor binding at terminals of these tracts. These findings suggested the possibility that an as-yet-unidentified neurotransmitter or perhaps an endogenous opiate-like compound mediates synaptic activity in the pain pathways.

In 1974, two independent laboratories identified a peptide in brain extracts that mimicked opiate activity both in its ability to inhibit electrically induced contraction in the guinea pig ileum (Kraulis et al., 1975; Hughes, 1975) and to bind to opiate receptors (Terenius and Wahlstrom, 1974). This discovery stimulated a tremendous effort toward further identification and characterization of the endogenous opiates. The family of endogenous peptides that act as agonists at opiate receptor sites are called "endorphins," from *endo* signifying endogenous and *orphin* from a common suffix in the names of opiates. Several peptides of low molecular weight having opiate agonist properties were found in pig brain (Hughes et al., 1975), beef brain (Pasternak et al., 1975), human cerebrospinal fluid (Terenius and Wahlstrom, 1975), and pituitary extracts (Teschmacher et al., 1975). Hughes et al. (1975) sequenced the amino acids of two pentapeptides, Met-enkephalin* (H-Tyr-Gly-Gly-Phe-Met-OH) and Leu-enkephalin (H-Tyr-Gly-Gly-Phe-Leu-OH), which differ only in the terminal amino acid (Figure 6A). The peptides have many of the pharmacological effects of the opiates. They can produce analgesia (Belluzzi et al., 1976; Buscher et al., 1976; Chang et al., 1976; Jacquet et al., 1976; Loh et al., 1976; Cox et al., 1976), inhibit electrical stimulation-induced muscle twitch of guinea pig ileum (Kraulis et al., 1975; Hughes, 1975; Cox et al., 1976), depress neuronal firing in various areas of the brain and spinal cord (Lamotte et al., 1976; Duggan et al., 1976; Frederickson and Norris, 1976), and produce physical dependence (Wei and Loh, 1976a; 1976b).

Within a short time, it was discovered that the amino acid sequence of Met-enkephalin is identical to a peptide sequence within β-lipotropin, a 91-amino acid peptide that was first found in the pituitary (Li and Chung, 1976) and that also has some opioid properties (Kosterlitz, 1976). Further work identified a number of other β-lipotropin fragments with varying degrees of opioid activity. For example, three fragments designated as α-, β-, and γ-endorphin consist of amino acid chains 61 to 76, 61 to 91, and 61 to

*Since these substances were found in the brain, they were named enkephalin, which is Greek for "from the head."

77, respectively (Figure 6B). Figure 6B shows the amino acid sequence of β-lipotropin and several related endogenous opiates. The figure also shows the relationship to two other psychoactive fragments: β-MSH (melanocyte stimulating hormone) and ACTH [4–10]. That a parent ACTH and lipotropin are both contained within a common precursor makes it apparent that considerable processing of this molecule must occur to give rise to the large number of peptides found in the pituitary as well as in the brain. It quickly became clear that each of the active opiate-like fragments contained the 5-amino acid chain (61–65) that constitutes Met-enkephalin. The question now being asked is whether the larger endogenous opiates serve as prohormones for the smaller peptides or whether the enkephalins are degradation products of the larger active peptides. Using specific antisera to β-lipotropin, Watson et al. (1977) have found β-lipotropin localized in the cytoplasm and axons of nerve cells in hypothalamus, periventricular nucleus of the thalamus, substantia nigra, and periaqueductal gray, as well as other areas. Because β-endorphin is only one cleavage step from β-lipotropin, the 91-amino acid peptide may be the immediate precursor and storage form for the opiate. The relationship between β-lipotropin and Met-enkephalin is still unclear because some brain areas contain both substances, whereas others contain only one or the other. Because Met-enkephalin is found in brain areas that are devoid of β-lipotropin, it is unlikely that β-lipotropin is a direct precursor for Met-enkephalin. It is known that the peptides found in the brain are not first manufactured in the pituitary because hypophysectomy (removal of the pituitary) does not reduce brain levels of the opiate peptides (Cheung and Goldstein, 1976).

Localization

The 5-amino acid enkephalins have been extensively studied. Pasternak et al. (1976) have shown that enkephalin binding to opiate receptors is selectively facilitated by manganese and inhibited by sodium to an extent similar to that of the opiate agonists. The subcellular distribution of enkephalins resembles most neurotransmitters, that is, enkephalin activity is most concentrated in the nerve terminal or synaptic fraction. Simantov et al. (1976) have examined the relative distribution of enkephalin activity (i.e., its ability to bind to opiate receptors) in 34 areas of rhesus monkey brain. Table I shows that pronounced regional varia-

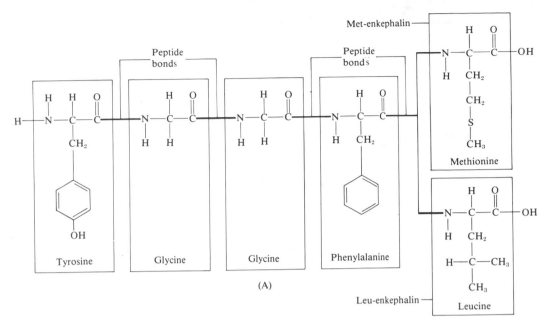

(A)

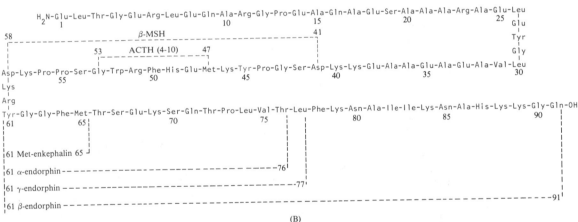

(B)

FIGURE 6 AMINO ACID STRUCTURE OF EN-
KEPHALINS AND β-LIPOTROPIN. A. Structure of Met-
enkephalin and Leu-enkephalin. The peptides have identical
amino acid sequences except for their terminal units. B.
Structure of sheep β-lipotropin (91 amino acids). The dashed
lines mark several psychoactive peptides within the larger
peptide: ACTH[4-10] (composed of amino acids 47-53 of
β-lipotropin); β-MSH (41-58); β-endorphin (61-91);
α-endorphin (61-76); and Met-enkephalin (61-65).

tions exist and that highest enkephalin activity is
associated with limbic and extrapyramidal areas of the
brain. Table I also shows the amount of opiate receptor binding in the same 34 brain areas. It is clear that
some discrepancies exist between the highest receptor
densities and the greatest concentrations of enkephalin. The amygdala, for instance, has the highest density of opiate receptor binding but only moderate to
low levels of enkephalin. Also, both the periaqueductal gray and the medial thalamus show high receptor
binding but only moderate amounts of enkephalin.
Some of these discrepancies may be explained in

TABLE I Regional Distribution of Enkephalin in Monkey Brain

Region	Enkephalin concentration (Units/mg protein)	Opiate receptor density (fmole stereospecific [³H]dihydromorphine bound/mg protein)
Cerebral cortex		
Superior temporal gyrus	0.88 ± 0.11	10.8
Inferior temporal gyrus	0.55 ± 0.07	6.0
Postcentral gyrus	0.46 ± 0.05	2.8
Precentral gyrus	0.41 ± 0.07	3.4
Temporal pole	0.36 ± 0.07	
Frontal pole	0.35 ± 0.04	11.9
Occipital pole	0.24 ± 0.04	2.3
White matter areas		
Corpus callosum posterior	0.56 ± 0.05	< 2 (Whole)
Corpus callosum anterior	0.53 ± 0.05	
Optic chiasma	0.40 ± 0.06	< 2
Corona radiata	0.34 ± 0.02	< 2
Limbic cortex		
Amygdala	1.68 ± 0.16	65.1 (Anterior) 34.1 (Posterior)
Hippocampus	0.52 ± 0.07	12.5
Hypothalamus		
Anterior hypothalamus	4.20 ± 0.47	24.3
Posterior hypothalamus	1.35 ± 0.11	24.7
Thalamus		
Medial thalamus	0.57 ± 0.04	24.6
Lateral thalamus	0.25 ± 0.02	7.8
Pulvinar	0.19 ± 0.02	
Extrapyramidal areas		
Head of caudate nucleus	5.28 ± 0.40	19.4
Globus pallidus interior	4.96 ± 0.41	7.7 (Whole globus pallidus)
Globus pallidus exterior	4.92 ± 0.34	
Body of caudate nucleus	3.04 ± 0.37	9.0
Tail of caudate nucleus	1.72 ± 0.20	8.9
Putamen	0.96 ± 0.07	11.7
Midbrain		
Periaqueductal gray	1.48 ± 0.16	31.1
Raphe area	1.08 ± 0.06	8.2
Superior colliculi	0.72 ± 0.05	10.6
Inferior colliculi	0.46 ± 0.03	6.7
Cerebellum-lower brain stem		
Floor of fourth ventricle	1.14 ± 0.08	6.3
Lower medulla oblongata	0.44 ± 0.04	5.8
Deep nucleus	0.17 ± 0.02	
Cerebellar cortex	0.16 ± 0.02	< 2
Spinal cord (cervical)		
Dorsal cord (white and gray)	0.72	3.1 (White)
Ventral cord (white and gray)	0.72	3.3 (White)

(From Simantov et al., 1976)

part by the finding that β-endorphin-containing cells and enkephalin-containing cells are not identical (Rossier et al., 1977). Using a radioimmunoassay procedure, they found that β-endorphin concentrations are highest in the hypothalamus, followed by the septum, midbrain, and brain stem. β-Endorphin was not detected with this assay in the hippocampus, cerebral cortex, cerebellum, or striatum. In contrast, enkephalin was most heavily localized in the striatum and hypothalamus. Based on results of this type, Figure 7 shows the location of the β-endorphin-rich and enkephalin-rich areas of the brain along with some of the pathways that may be involved in endogenous opiate activity. The right half of the figure shows areas containing enkephalin. The left half of the figure shows localization of β-endorphin as well as β-lipotropin (β-LPH) and ACTH. β-LPH and ACTH were included because each has sufficient similarity in structure to β-endorphin to react immunologically with the antibody to β-endorphin. It should also be mentioned that the β-endorphin antibody may react with various basic myelin proteins in the membrane, and for that reason some contamination of results is possible (North and Tonini, 1976).

The existence of distinct neurons for the two endogenous opiates suggests that receptor populations may also vary. Not only are there distinct neurons for the two endogenous opiates, but there also appear to be two unique receptors, called mu and delta (Chang and Cuatrecasas, 1979; Snyder and Goodman, 1980). Mu receptors preferentially bind morphine, delta receptors bind enkephalin derivates. Autoradiographs of mu receptors show that they are most dense in discrete layers of the cerebral cortex where they may serve a function in sensory integration. Delta receptors are found in the limbic system, suggesting a role in the emotional component of pain. Snyder (1980b) found that brain regions having more mu than delta receptors (e.g., hippocampus and thalamus) also have more Met-enkephalin than Leu-enkephalin neurons. Areas with more delta than mu receptors (e.g., amygdala) have more Leu-enkephalin than Met-enkephalin neurons. Thus, Snyder proposed that Met- and Leu-enkephalin neurons interact with mu and delta receptors, respectively.

Based on the localization studies, Barchas et al. (1978) have suggested that enkephalin may have a true neurotransmitter function in pain transmission, emo-

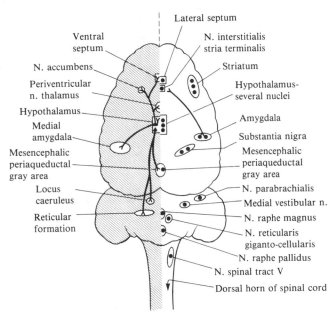

FIGURE 7 ENDOGENOUS OPIOID LOCALIZATION IN RAT BRAIN. This simplified horizontal cross section of the brain shows pathways of cells that are immunoreactive to β-LPH, β-endorphin, and ACTH (solid triangles). Cells that react to antibodies against enkephalin are identified as solid circles. (From Barchas et al., 1978.)

tional response to pain, and hormonal response to pain, whereas β-endorphin may influence other systems as a "neuromodulator" of nerve activity. The relationship with ACTH is also of interest because β-lipotropin, β-endorphin, and ACTH are found in the same cells in the anterior and intermediate portions of the pituitary. ACTH is known to be released from the pituitary into the blood in response to various forms of stress. ACTH acts on the adrenal gland and causes secretion of glucocorticoids, which in turn increase the availability of energy-rich carbohydrates. It has been found (Guillemin et al., 1977) that β-endorphin is released from the pituitary under conditions identical to those that release ACTH. A role for pituitary endorphin in modulating stress or the emotional response to stress has been suggested, and is supported by experimental findings. Mice that were defeated after being attacked by other mice demonstrate analgesia to radiant heat focused on their tails (Miczek et al., 1982). The magnitude and duration of analgesia is directly related to the number of attacks sustained by the mouse. The analgesia was blocked by pretreatment with naloxone and was attenuated by prior morphine tolerance. The demonstration of antagonism by naloxone is important, because some forms of stress-induced analgesia are apparently not mediated by endogenous opiates (Lewis et al., 1981).

More direct evidence for an interaction between pituitary β-endorphin and ACTH-regulated corticosterone release from the adrenal has been provided (MacLennan et al., 1982). Hypophysectomy completely blocked electrically-induced analgesia when measured with the tail flick test. Pretreatment with dexamethasone, which reduces stress-induced release of pituitary ACTH as well as β-endorphin, also prevented the electrically-induced analgesia. To identify the relative importance of ACTH and β-endorphin one group of animals was adrenalectomized. If ACTH is critical, adrenalectomy (which elevates plasma levels of the opioid) should decrease stress-induced analgesia. In these experiments, adrenalectomy completely blocked the analgesia—results consistent with the idea that corticosterone, rather than β-endorphin, is critical for the appearance of analgesia. Furthermore, treatment of adrenalectomized rats with corticosterone reinstated the analgesia. Thus, corticosterone has an important role in stress-induced analgesia. Since the analgesia is antagonized by naloxone, it is likely that brain endorphin regulates the pituitary-adrenal axis.

Alternatively it is possible that circulating corticosterone and brain endorphins act at higher centers, such as the midbrain serotonin system, which is believed to be involved in both opiate- and pain-induced analgesia.

Analgesic Effects of Enkephalin

Using the tail-flick test, several investigators have shown that enkephalin administered intraventricularly or injected into the periaqueductal gray produces analgesia (Belluzzi et al., 1976; Buscher et al., 1976; Chang et al., 1976; Malick and Goldstein, 1977). Jacquet et al. (1976), however, report that with other tests of analgesia, including pinpricks and thermal stimuli, β-endorphin—but not α-endorphin, Leu-enkephalin, or Met-enkephalin—has a significant analgesic effect. Cox et al. (1976) have also shown a potent analgesic effect of β-endorphin. Furthermore, tryptic digestion of β-endorphin destroyed most of its analgesic potency, indicating that the intact molecule is necessary for full activity. There is general agreement that, compared to morphine in the same analgesic test, the enkephalins reach their maximum effect much more rapidly, but that the effects are of a very short duration (Buscher et al., 1976). This difference may be due to the rapid enzymatic degradation of enkephalin (Kraulis et al., 1975; Pasternak et al., 1975).

It has been found that electrical stimulation of periventricular brain sites in humans suffering from intractable pain produces relief and also produces a significant increase in enkephalin in cerebrospinal fluid (Akil et al., 1978; Hosobuchi et al., 1979). The finding that prestimulation levels of endogenous opiate were lower in these patients than in normal controls further suggests that the brain levels of the peptide may be closely related to the report of pain.

Activity of Endogenous Opiates in Bioassay

It is interesting to compare the analgesic potency of the endogenous opiates with their potencies in the guinea pig ileum bioassay and in the stereospecific opiate binding assay. Cox et al. (1976) showed that β-endorphin was 2–3 times more potent and enkephalin was 0.2 times as potent as normorphine in the binding assay. The same group showed that in the guinea pig ileum preparation, β-endorphin and enkephalin were about equally potent but less potent than normorphine. Loh et al. (1976) found β-endorphin in vivo was 18–33 times more potent than morphine in producing analgesia whereas enkephalin was inactive. Other discrepancies of this type exist in the ever-expanding literature. The differences may be explained in terms of permeability factors in *in vitro* assays (Cox et al., 1976), of the access of the peptides to the brain, or of variability in rate of degradation of the peptides (Loh et al., 1976).

Electrophysiological Effects

The electrophysiological changes after application of enkephalin to cells are similar to those found for morphine. Using intracellular recordings from myenteric ganglia of the guinea pig ileum, North and Williams (1976) found that those cells that showed normorphine-induced hyperpolarization showed the same changes after application of Leu- or Met-enkephalin. The hyperpolarization was blocked by naloxone.

At the level of the spinal cord, opiate receptor binding has been found in substantia gelatinosa (Lamotte et al., 1976), an area where pain fibers synapse on their way to higher neural centers. Duggan et al. (1976) recorded an increase in firing rate in cells of the substantia gelatinosa in cats in response to the nonnoxious deflection of hair and the noxious application of heat. The authors found that both morphine and enkephalin inhibited the heat-induced increase in firing but not the increase in firing due to the nonnoxious stimulus of hair deflection.

Enkephalin, applied microiontophoretically, depressed spontaneous and glutamate-induced firing of selected single neurons in frontal cortex, caudate, and periaqueductal gray (Frederickson and Norris, 1976). Many, but not all, depressions were blocked by naloxone. These results support the hypothesis that enkephalin acts as a neurotransmitter that may be released upon electrical stimulation of select neurons. The first evidence of this release has been reported by Puig et al. (1977), who electrically stimulated the myenteric plexus of the guinea pig. These investigators suggested that the inhibition of the ileum twitch by electrical stimulation at 10 Hz is due to the release of endogenous opiate receptor. Specificity of the effect is shown by naloxone and naltrexone antagonism.

Release of β-endorphin from brain slices also has been demonstrated (Osborne et al., 1979). These investigators showed that by depolarizing (with elevated K^+) slices prepared from rat hypothalamus, β-endorphin was released into the bathing medium. The fact that the

release was dependent on the presence of calcium suggests that the release is similar to that of putative neurotransmitters in the CNS. Because of methodological difficulties, the *in vivo* measurement of release of the opiate peptides has not yet been possible.

Behavioral Effects

A particularly intriguing aspect of endorphin research is the effect of the peptides on behavioral measures apart from analgesia. Several laboratories have shown that intracranial injection of the identified endogenous opiates produces a loss of righting reflex, profound sedation, and prolonged muscular rigidity similar to a catatonic schizophrenic state (Bloom et al., 1976; Jacquet and Marks, 1976). Each of these behavioral effects is antagonized by naloxone. These empirical results support the report that cerebrospinal fluid levels of endorphin are correlated with the severity of symptoms in schizophrenic patients (Gunne et al., 1977). Furthermore, this group has found that naloxone reduced the auditory hallucinations of four chronic schizophrenics in a single blind test. Another laboratory, however, found no significant overall improvement in 19 schizophrenic patients treated with naloxone, although an improvement in thought content was reported (Davis et al., 1977). In addition, the improved condition of some schizophrenic patients after hemodialysis (the cleansing of the blood with an artificial kidney) has suggested that an endogenous opiate peptide may be a schizotoxic substance (Wagemaker and Cade, 1977).

There were other attempts to attenuate schizophrenic symptoms by hemodialysis and to understand the dialysis with respect to endorphins, but the results were sometimes positive, sometimes negative, with many differences in the control procedures. Another study attempted to resolve this issue with a carefully controlled double-blind study on eight patients that had been diagnosed as schizophrenic using 1978 research diagnostic criteria. The group was homogeneous with respect to age and duration of illness, and all medications were terminated 4 to 6 weeks prior to the hemodialysis series. The patients, five women and three men, each served as their own control. Each of them received 10 active and 10 sham dialysis treatments once per week for 10 weeks for 5 hours.

The patients were evaluated weekly (double-blind) by psychiatrists using one standardized scale and daily by psychiatric nurses using a different scale. The psychiatrists' and the nurses' ratings correlated highly. The patients were evaluated during the 2 weeks before dialysis, during the last 2 weeks of the active dialysis, during the first 2 weeks after the last dialysis, and during the last 2 weeks of the sham dialysis period.

According to questionnaires answered by the patients, they were unable to detect whether they were receiving active or sham dialysis treatment. With respect to the effect that dialysis had upon schizophrenic symptoms, there were no significant decreases in global psychosis ratings during any of the observation periods nor were there any significant differences in individual symptoms during any observation session (symptoms such as thought disorder, hallucinatory behavior, unusual thought content, conceptual disorganization, and suspiciousness). Individual data showed that four patients remained unchanged and four became more psychotic by the end of dialysis. The investigators concluded that hemodialysis should not be considered as a treatment for schizophrenia at the present time (Schultz et al., 1981).

A second developing area of research is the relationship of the endorphins to feeding behavior. Food deprivation in the rat results in significant analgesia, as measured with the tail-flick test (McGivern et al., 1979). The food deprivation-induced analgesia was diminished by naloxone. Because a variety of stressful conditions are known to produce analgesia that can be attenuated by opiate antagonists, it was suggested that food deprivation, by increasing stress, may trigger release of endogenous opiates, subsequently producing analgesia.

More convincing evidence of a direct action of endorphins on feeding comes from the injection of β-endorphin into the "satiety center" (ventromedial nucleus of the hypothalamus) of rats (Grandison and Guidotti, 1977). Satiated rats treated in this manner begin to eat, much as if the nucleus had been destroyed electrolytically. The apparent inhibitory action of endorphin could be blocked by either an opiate antagonist or by bicuculline, an antagonist of GABA.

Systemically administered naloxone suppressed food intake in rats fed *ad libitum* (Brands et al., 1979). Body weight declined initially, the growth rate was reduced, and the recovery of weight gain lagged behind the return of food intake. Although each of these observations has been interpreted to mean that the endorphins are involved in the modulation of feeding, it is also

possible that high doses of naloxone are in themselves aversive. Evidence for naloxone-induced vomiting and aversion have been reported (Costello and Borison, 1977).

Margules and co-workers (1978) have shown that small doses of naloxone abolished overeating in genetically obese animals without affecting the eating of lean littermates. Furthermore, the pituitaries of the obese animals contained twice as much β-endorphin as those of the lean animals, whereas plasma levels were three times higher than in normal rats. Because no differences in brain levels were found, it is possible that peripheral sites of action (e.g., opiate receptors in ileum) are involved in the production of obesity by excess levels of β-endorphin.

Others have shown that levels of β-endorphin and α-MSH are higher in the pituitaries of genetically obese mice than in controls (Rossier et al., 1979). However, because the elevation of peptides temporally follows the appearance of obesity, they are probably a consequence rather than a cause of obesity. However, Leu-enkephalin in the posterior pituitary was 200 percent of control levels in the obese mice, and the increase was correlated with increasing body weight. Thus, the relationship of the endogenous opiates to food regulation requires further investigation.

Drug Dependence

Drug Abuse

DRUG ABUSE is defined as the self-administered use of any drug in a manner that deviates from the approved medical or social patterns within a given culture (Jaffe, 1975). According to this definition, misuse of drugs can include agents with profound CNS effects, but might also include tobacco, laxatives, antibiotics, or vitamins. Exactly what constitutes drug abuse at any one time is determined by society and is variable not only from culture to culture but also within one culture from time to time. During times of rapid social change, drug abuse tends to increase within the society. Because adolescents are most vulnerable to rapidly changing mores, it is not surprising that drug abuse is highest within this age group.

Tolerance

Compulsive drug use may involve three independent components: tolerance, psychological dependence, and physical dependence. TOLERANCE produces a need to increase the dose of the drug after several administrations in order to achieve the same magnitude of effect. Tolerance to the opiates develops quite rapidly, although not all the pharmacological effects of morphine undergo tolerance to the same extent. For instance, the euphoria and analgesia show rapid tolerance, but the constipating effect persists even after prolonged opiate use. Although some of the tolerance is due to an increased rate of metabolism (drug disposition tolerance) of morphine, most of the tolerance is apparently of the pharmacodynamic type; that is, the cells become accustomed to the presence of the drug. (See Chapter 1 for a more detailed discussion of tolerance.)

Physical Dependence

Some drugs also induce PHYSICAL DEPENDENCE, which is an adaptive state produced by repeated drug administration and which manifests itself by intense physical disturbance when drug administration is halted. The WITHDRAWAL SYNDROME or ABSTINENCE SYNDROME comprises a specific array of psychic and physiological symptoms that are characteristic of each drug type. The degree of physical dependence can only be measured by the severity of withdrawal symptoms. For drugs such as alcohol, barbiturates, and the narcotic analgesics, the withdrawal symptoms are so unpleasant that they can be important factors in motivating drug-seeking behavior.

The withdrawal symptoms characteristic for the opiates can vary in intensity from quite mild to severe, depending on the extent and duration of the drug use as well as the health and personality of the addict. Opiate withdrawal is not considered to be life-threatening. Most sources say that the symptoms are flu-like and peak at 48 to 72 hours after the last administration of morphine. The symptoms include widely dilated pupils, lacrimation, weakness and depression, nausea and vomiting, intestinal spasm and diarrhea, runny nose, marked chilliness alternating with sweating, gooseflesh and piloerection, weight loss and dehydration, and abdominal cramps and muscular spasm (that may be the source for the term "kick the habit"). The observable symptoms disappear within 7 to 10 days, and readministration of the opiate at any point will dramatically suppress all the symptoms. Furthermore, cross-dependence exists among the opiates. Consequently, administration of a sufficient quantity of any opiate will stop the withdrawal symptoms after cessation of morphine. The same withdrawal syndrome will appear if a specific narcotic antagonist (e.g., naloxone) is administered to an opiate user. In fact, the rapid displacement of morphine from its receptor sites by naloxone produces more severe withdrawal than mere abstinence.

Psychological Dependence

PSYCHOLOGICAL DEPENDENCE is a condition characterized by an intense drive or craving for a drug whose effects the user feels are necessary for a sense of well-being. Psychological dependence varies both with personality characteristics of the individual and with specific drug effects. When the desire to continue taking the drug becomes a "psychic craving" or "compulsion" and the user becomes preoccupied with drug taking, there exists the basis for compulsive drug use (Jaffe, 1975).

Psychological dependence is the most poorly defined of the three factors contributing to compulsive drug use and continues to be the most difficult to identify and quantify. One approach is to examine the behavioral aspects of drug dependence within the framework of operant conditioning principles. The basis of operant conditioning is the premise that behavior that acts upon the environment is controlled by the behavioral consequences, and consequences that increase the behavior are designated as REINFORCERS. Many experiments have demonstrated that drugs act as reinforcers and have further examined the biological and environmental variables that alter the drug's reinforcing property (Schuster and Thompson, 1969).

Drug Self-Administration

Using a preference technique, the earliest studies demonstrated that physically dependent animals who are deprived of morphine will prefer a bitter-tasting morphine solution to plain water (Thompson and Schuster, 1964; Nichols, 1963). Apparently the animals associated morphine ingestion with the relief of abstinence symptoms. The strengthening of an operant response (using the morphine drinking tube) by the termination of aversive stimuli (the withdrawal symptoms) is called NEGATIVE REINFORCEMENT. Although not insurmountable with appropriate controls, several empirical problems presented themselves: (1) palatability may have altered the reinforcing properties; (2) "position habit" may have biased the probability of ingestion from one tube; (3) prior deprivation was generally required; and (4) variability in time and amount of drug absorption was great (Schuster and Thompson, 1969).

In addition, the question was asked whether the drug acts as a reinforcer because it prevented withdrawal symptoms or whether the drug itself had positive reinforcing properties. A new intravenous self-administration technique for animals provided a means to examine this question as well as the patterns of self-administration. Weeks (1964) developed the technique of implanting a cannula into the jugular vein and connecting the tube to an injection device that the animal could control by pressing a lever. With modification, the device could be operated without restraint of the animal.

Using the self-administration technique, it has been found that both rats and rhesus monkeys self-administer compounds from several major drug classes. Table II lists some of the drugs that have been self-administered by rhesus monkeys and thus act as primary reinforcers. It is highly significant that one characteristic common to all the drugs listed as reinforcers is that these drugs are all self-administered by humans and have a significant abuse potential. The drugs listed are not equally reinforcing, but Meyer (1972) has observed that the daily patterns of self-administration are quite similar to those seen in humans. In addition, chlorpromazine, an antipsychotic drug that is not abused in humans, is not self-administered by the monkeys. Furthermore, hallucinogens are rarely self-injected by animals, and it is rare to see compulsive self-administration in humans. The finding that nearly all monkeys will self-inject particular psychotropic drugs suggests that self-administration of these compounds is not abnormal but is restrained in humans by social values and customs.

Experiments with rhesus monkeys have shown that if 1 mg morphine/kg body weight is available with each injection, self-injection frequency gradually increases over time until the monkeys self-administer a stable amount of drug (30–45 mg/kg•24 hr) after 30–90 days (Woods and Schuster, 1968; Thompson and Schuster, 1968). Under these conditions, the animals do not have to be made physically dependent before they will self-administer morphine. This experiment demonstrates that morphine itself is reinforcing. However, once dependence has developed, the reinforcing effectiveness of morphine is greatly amplified by the relief of withdrawal symptoms.

It is interesting to find that the administration of

TABLE II Drugs Acting as Reinforcers in the Rhesus Monkey

Central stimulants	Narcotics	CNS depressants
Cocaine	Morphine	Pentobarbital
Amphetamine	Methadone	Amobarbital
Pipradrol	Meperidine	Phenobarbital
Methylphenidate	Codeine	Hexobarbital
Nicotine	Pentazocine	Chlordiazepoxide
Caffeine		Ethanol

naloxone increases the response rate of morphine self-administration to a rate similar to that seen during morphine abstinence (Weeks and Collins, 1964). In contrast, pretreatment with morphine, codeine, or meperidine reduces intravenous self-administration of morphine. It is evident from these studies that the animals learn to regulate with some accuracy the amount of morphine that they require.

Thompson and Pickens (1970) have described several features of self-administration of morphine (compared to self-administration of CNS stimulants) in terms of acquisition, patterning of self-infusions, and pattern of extinction (responding after reinforcement is discontinued). Not only did morphine self-infusion increase gradually over 30 days or more (Woods and Schuster, 1970; Thompson and Schuster, 1968) until a stable dose was achieved, but there was great variability in the interadministration intervals. In the case of cocaine, the initial high rate of stimulant self-infusion was maintained throughout, at a very regular rate that varied with dosage per infusion (Thompson and Pickens, 1970). However, stimulant self-infusion tended to be cyclic, with regular periods of high self-administration and abstinence, (Deneau, 1969), whereas opiate self-administration showed no such patterning. When drug reinforcement was discontinued, animals self-administering cocaine emitted a very high number of responses for a short time. During extinction, animals that had been self-administering opiates tended to persist in emitting responses at the usual rate for long periods and made responses at a lower rate for weeks or months (Thompson and Schuster, 1968). Although comparisons between drugs of this type must be made with caution, the differences may provide significant information about the nature of drug reinforcement and dependence.

The results of behavioral studies with animals suggest that compulsive drug taking is related both to an effort to reduce the pain of withdrawal and to the primary reinforcement, independent of the development of physical dependence. Results with human addicts present a more complex picture, but one that clearly has significant implications for the treatment of addictive behaviors.

Using male, opiate addicts in a research ward environment, Meyer and Mirin (1979) have attempted to answer some of the many questions surrounding drug use that involve primary reinforcement, sociological and environmental components, and avoidance of pain. For instance, what is the role of the subjective emotional state of the individual in drug-taking behavior? How important are interoceptive cues as triggers for the behavior? Are there environmental conditions associated with altered heroin use? What is the effect of narcotic antagonist administration on the drug-seeking behavior? Can psychological factors predict which individuals will continue to self-administer heroin in the presence of a narcotic antagonist?

None of the answers to the questions posed are simple, and the methodology needed to achieve the answers is fraught with difficulties. The participation of chronic opiate users in research that involves drug self-administration raises several ethical considerations: (1) How voluntary are the "volunteers" referred by social service agencies. (2) How complete should the informed consent be. (3) How adequate are the methods to maintain confidentiality. (4) How thoroughly can the risks to subjects be determined and contrasted to potential benefits. In addition, appropriate controls in the experiments are much more difficult to achieve with human subjects, whose environment and behavior cannot be as rigorously regulated as animal subjects. Nevertheless, the intriguing results produced by these types of studies should encourage more investigations of a similar nature.

Neurochemical Models of Dependence

Several comprehensive reviews on the neurochemical basis for narcotic tolerance and dependence have appeared. Researchers (Clouet and Iwatsubo, 1975; Takemori, 1975; Lal, 1975; Kuschinsky, 1977; Cochin, 1970) generally believe that tolerance to the opiates is more likely to be due to a biochemical or neuronal compensation than to a change in drug–receptor interaction. In support of this hypothesis is the finding that no significant difference in the number of receptors has been found in tolerant mice (Höllt et al., 1975; Lang et al., 1975; Gispen et al., 1975; Klee and Streaty, 1974), though some change in the affinity of the opiate receptors has been noted (Takemori, 1975).

The classical hypothesis on the mechanism of tolerance and physical dependence on opiates was formulated by Himmelsbach in 1943. His hypothesis, depicted in Figure 8, suggests that although acute administration of morphine disrupts the organism's homeostasis, repeated administration of the drug induces some undetermined adaptive mechanism that compensates for the acute effects of morphine and restores the original homeostasis. At this point, tolerance to the effects of morphine is said to have occurred, as administration of

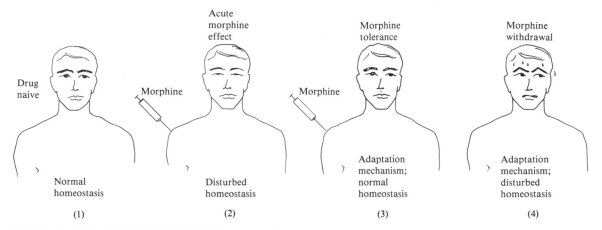

FIGURE 8   THE HOMEOSTASIS THEORY of morphine tolerance and dependence.

the same size dose of morphine no longer produces the original physiological disturbance. The abrupt cessation of morphine administration stops all drug effects but leaves the adaptive mechanism active; it then overcompensates and produces a new disturbance in homeostasis that might be equated with withdrawal.

Several other possible mechanisms to explain the organism's capacity to develop tolerance have been suggested. Collier (1968) and Jaffe and Sharpless (1968) suggested that decreased neurotransmission might lead to a "pharmacological denervation supersensitivity," that is, more receptors might develop to compensate for the reduced neural activity. Little evidence exists to support this hypothesis, at least for the effects of opiates in the CNS.

Martin (1970) suggested that morphine may selectively inhibit one neuronal pathway, permitting a normally inactive, redundant pathway to compensate for the reduced function. Such a mechanism would explain the appearance of tolerance. Upon withdrawal of the morphine, both pathways would be active, thus producing overactivity corresponding to withdrawal.

The "surfeit theory" as described by Paton (1969) is based on the assumption that opiates reduce the amount of some neurotransmitter released into the synaptic cleft. As larger amounts of transmitter are built up, more opiate is needed to block its release and tolerance has developed. When the drug is withdrawn suddenly, an exaggerated release of transmitter substance takes place, producing the withdrawal syndrome. A mechanism of this type might be useful in explaining the rapid development of acute tolerance to morphine that occurs within 6 to 8 hours of slow infusion.

Goldstein and Goldstein (1961) suggested that the acute effects of morphine are due to the inhibition of a synthesizing enzyme. However, this enzyme increases its activity with repeated exposure to morphine because by feedback regulation the low amount of product signals the need for more synthesis. Once the synthesis rate is adjusted to compensate for the inhibition produced by morphine, tolerance has developed. When the morphine is suddenly withdrawn, its inhibitory effect on enzyme activity is eliminated, the increased synthesis rate is left untouched, and significantly more product is formed than under normal conditions. The high enzyme activity is responsible for the withdrawal syndrome. Ultimately endproduct inhibition occurs and enzyme synthesizing activity slowly returns to normal.

Role of Cyclic Adenosine Monophosphate

One enzyme that may play a part in mediating opiate effects and that apparently demonstrates an initial inhibition and a fairly rapid development of tolerance is adenylate cyclase, the enzyme responsible for the synthesis of cAMP. Collier and Roy (1974) showed that morphine blocks the increased production of cAMP following the addition of prostaglandin E_1 (PGE_1) to rat brain homogenate. (PGE_1 normally stimulates cAMP production.) The morphine-induced inhibition was blocked by naloxone and was mimicked by levorphanol but not by the inactive isomer, dextrorphan (Roy and Collier, 1975). Furthermore, the rank order of potency of several opiates to inhibit PGE_1-stimulated adenylate cyclase correlated well with the drugs' analgesic potency (Traber et al., 1975). Because morphine inhibits the stimulation of adenylate cyclase by other agents (e.g., dopamine) (Miller and Iversen, 1974), inhibition of PGE_1 effects may be of little physiological significance.

Cyclic AMP has been further implicated in opioid action by the finding that intracerebral administration of cAMP or dibutyryl-cAMP significantly reduced the ability of morphine to produce analgesia in the tail-flick test (Ho et al., 1973). Collier and Francis (1975; Francis et al., 1975) found that drugs that increase cAMP enhance morphine withdrawal symptoms. They also found that administration of a phosphodiesterase inhibitor (3-isobutyl-1-methylxanthine), which increases cAMP, plus the morphine antagonist naloxone produced withdrawal-like symptoms even in morphine-naive animals.

In a much simpler system, neuroblastoma cells (cancerous cells from neural tissue) were crossed with glial cells to produce neuroblastoma × glioma hybrid cells having opiate receptors. These receptors are stereospecific for narcotic binding and have affinities that are similar to those for rat brain (Sharma et al., 1975a). As Collier and Roy (1974) found in rat brain homogenate, morphine inhibited PGE_1-stimulated adenylate cyclase in the cultured cells. The inhibition was noncompetitive (Traber et al., 1974), suggesting that morphine and PGE_1 may not act at the same site. Nevertheless, Sharma et al. (1975b) found an excellent correlation between the receptor binding affinity of various opiates and the ability of the drugs to inhibit adenylate cyclase.

Using the same cultured cell preparation, this group

(Sharma et al., 1975a) also showed that with prolonged exposure to morphine in the culture medium, the cells showed an increase in adenylate cyclase activity. After 2 days of culture with morphine present, the cells demonstrated tolerance to the acutely inhibitory effect of morphine by developing the capacity to produce cAMP to the same extent as control cells. When the opiate was abruptly removed from the cell culture medium, the concentration of cAMP rose significantly above control levels. The rebound in cAMP levels is considered to correspond to the withdrawal phenomena. The changes in cAMP levels under these conditions can be seen in Figure 9.

A related finding shows that incubation of the cells with Met-enkephalin results in a similar increase in adenylate cyclase activity that is mediated by the opiate receptor (Lampert et al., 1976). These results do not reveal the role, if any, that cAMP plays in pain transmission, but they do suggest that cAMP may be implicated in opiate-induced analgesia, tolerance, and dependence. The hypothesis of Kosterlitz and Hughes (1975),—a modification of several of the earlier models—suggests a modulatory role for enkephalin in the development of tolerance and dependence. Enkephalin can have an inhibitory effect on pain pathways in three possible ways, as shown in Figure 10.

The first model (postsynaptic inhibition) shows that enkephalin serves directly as an inhibitory transmitter. The second (presynaptic inhibition) shows that enkephalin may produce presynaptic inhibition by slightly depolarizing terminals, thereby diminishing the release of the excitatory transmitter. The third model (inhibitory modulation) shows a nerve terminal that secretes enkephalin, which then acts back upon the terminal to inhibit its release of an excitatory transmitter.

Thus far there is little evidence to support any one of the three models, although electrophysiological data from the cat spinal cord makes direct postsynaptic action least likely, as intracellular recordings showed that both morphine and enkephalin produced depressant effects on cell firing without the hyperpolarizing action of morphine on neurons in the myenteric plexus of the guinea pig ileum. In either of the other models, enkephalin has inhibitory control of the release of an excitatory neurotransmitter. It is well known that the opiates can inhibit neurotransmitter release from a variety of neurons (Lees et al., 1973; Kosterlitz and Hughes, 1975). Taube et al. (1976) found that Met-enkephalin inhibited the release of [^{3}H]norepinephrine

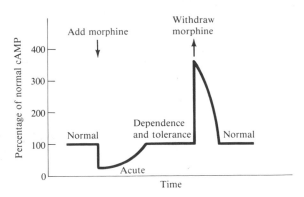

FIGURE 9 MORPHINE-INDUCED EFFECTS ON cAMP. Changes in cAMP levels in cultured cells during acute morphine administration, tolerance, and withdrawal of the drug. (Adapted from Sharma et al., 1975a.)

from rat occipital cortex slices, whereas Henderson (Henderson and Hughes, 1976) showed that the endogenous opiate inhibited evoked, but not spontaneous, release of norepinephrine from mouse vas deferens.

Jessell and Iversen (1977) have found that a stable Met-enkephalin analog suppressed the K^+-evoked release of substance P, a putative neurotransmitter, from the trigeminal nucleus in the brain stem. Enkephalin had no effect on resting efflux, suggesting that the opioid may act at the level of the stimulus–secretion coupling mechanism. The enkephalin-induced inhibition was readily reversed by naloxone.

The interaction between endogenous opiates and substance P is particularly intriguing because the latter peptide has been suggested to be a transmitter in primary sensory afferents. For instance, substance P selectively excites cells in the dorsal horn of the spinal cord that respond to noxious stimuli but not to light pressure applied to the skin (Randic and Miletic, 1977). On the basis of immunohistochemical evidence, it has been suggested that enkephalinergic interneurons may synapse axoaxonically with pain afferent terminals containing substance P (Hökfelt et al., 1977). Hökfelt has identified a striking overlap in distribution of Met-enkephalin and substance P cell bodies and nerve terminals in the periaqueductal gray, nucleus raphe magnus, the caudal trigeminal nucleus, and the marginal layer and substantia gelatinosa of the dorsal horn of the spinal cord. A proposed mechanism of action between these two peptides is that the enkephalinergic

Postsynaptic
inhibition

Presynaptic
inhibition

Inhibitory
modulation

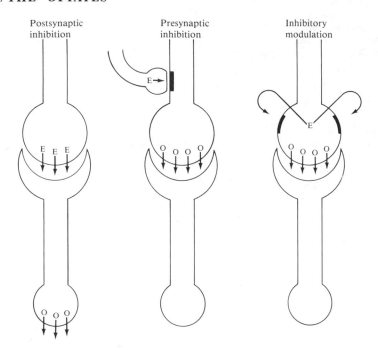

FIGURE 10   INHIBITORY ACTION OF ENKEPHALIN.
Enkephalin (E) may inhibit nerve activity either by postsynaptic inhibition, presynaptic inhibition or via inhibitory
modulation. (0 represents excitatory transmitter.) (From
Kosterlitz and Hughes, 1975.)

axoaxonic synapses serve to block the release of sub-stance P via presynaptic inhibition (see Chapter 10). It is interesting that intraventricular or systemic administration of substance P produces naloxone-reversible analgesia (Stewart et al., 1976; Starr et al., 1978).

Regardless of the molecular site of action, tolerance to administered opiates may occur because the opiates act at the enkephalin receptor sites, and by a negative feedback mechanism the synthesis of enkephalin will be reduced. Tolerance develops because more opiate is necessary to inhibit transmission in the pain pathway. Abrupt withdrawal of the opiate plus the low levels of enkephalin leave the pain fiber uninhibited, producing withdrawal symptoms. The duration of withdrawal symptoms will depend on the rate of enkephalin synthesis and the return of receptor sensitivity (which was reduced by the prolonged high concentration of opiates). The *in vivo* significance of the endogenous opiates is yet to be demonstrated. However, their interaction with administered opiates may be the basis for the appearance of opiate tolerance and dependence.

Finally, Snyder et al. (1975) proposed a model of opiate addiction that accounts for the finding that as animals or humans become progressively more dependent on opiates, the dose of an antagonist that is needed to precipitate abstinence symptoms becomes progressively smaller. These same individuals display tolerance to the agonist properties of the opiates and thus require larger doses of the drug to achieve that same pharmacological effect. Thus, it appears that the addicted state is associated with increased sensitivity to opiate antagonists and a reduced sensitivity to opiate agonists. Snyder and co-workers had previously demonstrated that an increase in sodium ion (Na^+) concentration increases the binding of opiate antagonists and decreases binding of opiate agonists *in vitro*, whereas a reduced Na^+ concentration has the opposite effects. Their results lead to the speculation that tolerance and physical dependence are due to a progressive Na^+-dependent alteration of the opiate receptor conformation, such that with repeated drug use the antagonist (high Na^+) conformation is favored. It is not yet clear whether or not opiates act directly on the Na^+-ionophore in cell membranes to bring about a change in cellular Na^+ concentrations.

Testing this model will be difficult because alterations in receptor conformation may "wash out" and be undetectable when the animal dies and its brain is homogenized and subject to the many procedures that are necessary for examining the chemical nature of the opiate receptor. An additional shortcoming of this model is that there is no proposal as to how withdrawal effects might be related to the posited drug-induced alterations in opiate receptor conformation or whether the withdrawal effect is even relevant to it.

Very little empirical evidence exists for any of the models proposed in this chapter, but each model provides a stimulus for greater research on this problem. No one model is necessarily correct, and it is likely that the answer will be a composite based on the results of intense effort in a variety of experimental fields.

Behavioral Models of Tolerance and Dependence

Despite the emphasis on the physiological basis for tolerance and dependence, many investigators have identified a conditioning component to the phenomena. The conditioning theory as described by Siegel (1975) proposes that narcotic tolerance is the result of the learning of an association between the systemic effects of the drug and those environmental cues that reliably precede the drug effects. Several experiments have shown that the anticipatory response of the animal, which occurs when he experiences the administration procedure without the active drug, is compensatory in nature. For instance, in animals repeatedly experiencing the hypoglycemic effects of injected insulin, the injection procedure alone (in the same environment) leads to an elevation of blood sugar. Thus, it is argued that tolerance to the analgesic effects of morphine results because environmental cues regularly paired with drug administration begin to elicit the compensatory response (hyperalgesia), which algebraically sums with the stable effects of morphine. With longer drug administration, the association between environment and hyperalgesia become stronger, leading to the appearance of tolerance. The importance of environment is dramatized in a series of experiments (Siegel, 1976) in which rats were made tolerant to morphine in one of two distinct environments (colony room or experimental room where white noise was a constant background). Tolerance to morphine-induced analgesia was demonstrated by those rats tested in the same environment in which they previously received morphine, but not in the alternate room.

Using the same reasoning, morphine tolerance should be retarded by the administration of the drug in the absence of environmental cues. To test the hypothesis, rats were exposed both to morphine and to an environmental cue (overhead illumination) before analgesia testing with a hot plate (Siegel et al., 1981). In the control group the light and morphine were paired. In the experimental group the cue signaled a drug-free period. Both groups were subsequently administered morphine in the presence of the cue and the amount of analgesic tolerance was measured. Although both groups demonstrated increasing analgesic tolerance over the test sessions, the rate of development of tolerance was significantly slower in the experimental (unpaired) group. Thus the animals' experiences with the drug administration environment contribute significantly to the appearance of tolerance.

Operant conditioning also plays a part in drug dependence. Although it is frequently noted that the peer group is important in understanding the initiation of drug use, it should be made clear that the drug-using subculture with its camaraderie, drug-taking rituals, and drug-acquisition procedures become a potent secondary reinforcement to the ongoing drug-taking behavior. Similar to the way in which a light previously paired with food reinforcement will significantly slow the rate of extinction when the primary reinforcer is withheld, many aspects of drug-taking behavior (the membership in a group, the peer acceptance, and new status) act like green lights and are in themselves reinforcing, apart from the primary reinforcement of the drug. Animal studies have shown that acute drug effects, withdrawal symptoms, and relief of withdrawal symptoms can each be conditioned to environmental stimuli (Roffman et al., 1972; Wikler, 1973; Goldberg, 1970). Roffman et al. (1972) found that after repeated pairing of morphine injection and the sounding of a bell during the development of physical dependence, the sounding of the bell alone was sufficient to prevent withdrawal hypothermia after the cessation of morphine injection. These results may explain why the various rituals and procedures of drug procurement and use may elicit reinforcing effects similar to the drug itself. An example of this phenomenon is the "needle freak" who by the act of injection alone or the injection of pharmacologically inert substances derives significant reinforcement.

Wikler (1973; 1965) has maintained that abstinence symptoms can likewise be classically conditioned to the environment and that the "conditioned abstinence" may be responsible for the great tendency to relapse after detoxification of the addict and return to the environment that elicits the unpleasant effects. He demonstrated that rats show an increase in withdrawal "wet dog" shakes when returned to a cage where they had undergone morphine withdrawal several months earlier.

In another experiment, Goldberg and Schuster (1967) trained morphine-dependent monkeys to respond for food reinforcement. During the food reinforcement sessions, a buzzer was presented and followed by an i.v. injection of nalorphine (an opiate antagonist), which produced withdrawal and depressed their responding for food. After several pairings, the buzzer alone elicited the signs of withdrawal (salivation, emesis, change in heart rate, and suppression of responding). The conditioned withdrawal signs could be elicited as long as 4 months after the withdrawal of morphine. A recent report demonstrated that both objective (respiration rate, skin temperature, heart rate) and subjective elements of narcotic withdrawal symptoms can be experimentally conditioned to environmental stimuli in human subjects (O'Brien et al., 1977). This empirical evidence is in direct support of the clinical reports that former addicts experience withdrawal symptoms when they visit areas of prior drug use (O'Brien, 1975). The high relapse rate may then be due to the conditioned abstinence syndrome in the old environment plus more reinforcement by the opiate because of long-term physiological changes found even after many months of abstinence (Martin, 1967).

These results suggest that one effective mode of treatment might be response extinction brought about by eliminating the reinforcement following the operant response. The use of specific narcotic antagonists that block the reinforcing properties of the opiates have been used as a pharmacological support in a number of treatment programs.

Drug Addiction

According to Jaffe (1975), drug abuse becomes an ADDICTION when the compulsive use of the drug is characterized by "overwhelming involvement with the use of the drug, the securing of its supply, and a high tendency to relapse after withdrawal." We have already discussed some of the factors that may contribute to the habitual use of a drug; however, the question of what prompts the initial drug use has never been resolved. No addictive personality type has been identified, although some psychoanalysts see drug abuse as part of a spectrum of dependency, along with thumb sucking, compulsive eating, nail biting, and compulsive masturbation (Frosch, 1970). Among those characteristics most often associated with drug abusers is intolerance of frustration and anxiety, sense of futility, expectation of failure, impulsivity, narcissism, and general depression.

Epidemiological evidence shows that addiction is greatest among male adolescents in the inner city neighborhoods that have recently undergone rapid population change, leading to breakdown in community stability and established social control (Hughes and Crawford, 1972; Chein et al., 1964). In addition, the areas of high incidence of drug use are characterized by impoverished and disrupted families, by ethnic groups most discriminated against, and by those groups that are least urbanized (Chein et al., 1964). However, as yet no one has been able to determine why many adolescents living under the same conditions do not have a history of drug abuse. Hughes and Crawford (1972) state that the pattern of heroin addiction follows the course of contagious disease, and the initial contact is most often a close friend rather than the adult pusher. Hughes and many others have stressed the role of the peer group in the spread of addiction. The adolescents who became addicts are almost inevitably related to the delinquent subculture, whose orientation consists of moods of pessimism, unhappiness, a sense of futility, mistrust, negativism, defiance, and a manipulative attitude on how to get the most out of life (Chein et al., 1964).

Modes of Treatment for Addiction

When evaluating the methods of treatment for addiction, we must remember that the addict population is a very heterogeneous one and that most addicts abuse multiple drugs. Even within the narcotics-using population, there is a diverse pattern of drug use, and the conditions for initiating drug-taking behavior and reasons for relapse vary widely. Just as there has been no way to predict which individual within a given group will become addicted, there is no reliable way to predict which types of narcotics users will respond to the various modes of treatment. On the whole, it has been found (Meyer, 1972) that older addicts do better in most treatments than do younger addicts. Also, as might be expected, addicts having some employment skills and job experience and having little criminal history do show more improvement than other groups.

The three principal treatment modalities include (1) psychological treatment, (2) pharmacological support, and (3) enforced treatment. In general, the highly idealistic goals of any treatment program are to help narcotics addicts to become emotionally mature, law-abiding, productive members of society who require no drugs or medical or social support to maintain this behavior (Jaffe, 1970). Clearly, these goals are rarely achievable with any treatment program, and we must accept improvement in these areas as a measure of success. The particular criterion emphasized will determine the method of evaluation and play a critical part in measuring the program's success. Thus, incarceration and forced abstinence are effective means of detoxifying the addict and clearly reduce criminal activities throughout the duration of "treatment." However, the method by itself does not meet the rehabilitative goals of treatment (increased employment and social responsibility, improved self-esteem, etc.), and relapse rate is extremely high.

Brill and Lieberman (1969; Lieberman and Brill, 1972), however, have emphasized the need to use "rational authority" in drug addiction programs. RATIONAL AUTHORITY is authority not intended as a punitive end in itself but as a means to ensure a durable relationship with the addict, that is, hold unmotivated addicts in a sustained treatment program. We have already said that addicts tend to be impulsive and easily frustrated and come from groups that have high delinquency rates. Thus, Brill and Lieberman proposed that a graduated series of sanctions be offered to the addict, giving him more responsibility and minimizing the addict's "acting out." Such control helps him to conform to socially acceptable standards and ultimately internalize the controls he lacks. Most often the rational authority is wielded in conjunction with parole and the threat of a return to prison. Some element of authority has been found necessary in most treatment modalities, although the control may be chemical, custodial, or autocratic, as in the case of the therapeutic community (Meyer, 1972).

Pharmacological Treatment Programs

Methadone Maintenance. Of the pharmacological support methods, the most popular is the methadone maintenance program originally developed by Dole and Nyswander (1965, 1966; Dole et al., 1966). They proposed to make addicts more amenable to rehabilitative efforts by providing pharmacological relief for narcotic craving without producing sedation or apathy. Methadone is a synthetic narcotic analgesic that has pharmacological effects qualitatively similar to morphine and that can substitute for morphine or the other opiates and prevent withdrawal (that is, there is said to be a cross-dependence between methadone and the other opiates). Although it is pharmacologically similar to morphine, oral methadone has only mild euphoric actions. In fact, in sufficient doses, methadone will prevent heroin-induced euphoria because of the cross-tolerance between heroin and methadone. The euphoria "blockade," however, can be overcome by large doses of heroin because a high concentration of heroin can effectively compete with methadone for the opiate receptors. Furthermore, methadone itself can, if administered intravenously, produce a "rush" of euphoria (Lennard et al., 1972), and in those programs where methadone is self-administered at home, a significant amount of abuse occurs.

Methadone has the advantage of being pharmacologically effective when given orally, so its use reduces the use of the needle by the addict and the ritual surrounding its use. In addition, oral administration alleviates the danger of disease due to unsterile injection techniques. Furthermore, methadone is longer lasting than most opiates, so that over a 24-hour period a more constant blood level is achieved. A more stable blood level means that the extremes of drug effect are avoided and greater stability is afforded.

One significant problem with methadone use is that it

Methadone

is addictive, and withdrawal symptoms occur with abrupt abstinence. Because the drug is long acting, however, withdrawal symptoms are comparatively mild, although longer lasting than those following morphine withdrawal. Critics of the methadone program claim that at the high doses of methadone required, abstinence can produce quite intense withdrawal symptoms (Lennard et al., 1972). The underlying philosophy of the methadone maintenance programs assumes that protracted and perhaps irreversible metabolic changes exist in opiate addicts and that the use of methadone represents a prolonged maintenance treatment (Langrod et al., 1972).

Furthermore, some authors have suggested that methadone dependence is beneficial because it provides an essential control mechanism, allowing repeated interaction with the clinical staff who can provide nonpharmacological support and encourage social rehabilitation (Bourne and Slade, 1974). The daily return to the clinic for methadone may be particularly significant for female addicts who are pregnant and who are provided with the prenatal obstetrical care that they normally do not receive. A methadone program with massive psychological support has been reported to alleviate many of the common maternal problems associated with addiction in pregnancy, such as syphilis and hepatitis. However, neither the high incidence of lowered birth weight in infants nor the infant withdrawal signs including CNS hyperactivity (tremors, irritability, twitching, seizures) and GI disturbances (vomiting, diarrhea, poor feeding) is prevented by maintenance on methadone (Harper et al., 1974).

Perhaps of greatest importance is the fact that the methadone treatment is considered far more acceptable to the addicts than the alternative therapeutic approaches (Meyer, 1972). However, we may want to pause and ask whether the prolonged administration of a potent psychotropic drug is in fact reinforcing the illusion that any drug can be "a fast, cheap, and magical answer to complex human and social problems" (Lennard et al., 1972).

Therapy with Narcotic Antagonists. An alternative pharmacological treatment modality originally proposed by Martin (Martin et al., 1966) is the use of a specific narcotic antagonist like naloxone, naltrexone, or cyclazocine. The use of the narcotic antagonists in the treatment of addiction is based on the belief that the compulsive drug abuser has acquired a complex set of operantly and classically conditioned responses that both perpetuate his drug-taking behavior and make relapse after detoxification highly probable. The antagonist, by binding to the opiate receptor site but having little or no activity, will block the reinforcing properties of the opiate. Under these conditions, extinction of the response should occur. That is, when reinforcement is stopped, the behavior should gradually stop.

Cyclazocine

Because of the nature of the extinction process, the antagonist administration is best for those addicts with a short drug reinforcement history. However, the short duration of action makes the narcotic antagonists difficult to administer on an outpatient basis. For instance, naloxone would have to be administered six times a day because it is effective for approximately 3–4 hours. It should be pointed out that the addict who stops taking the antagonist and injects heroin will suffer severe withdrawal symptoms if the antagonist is again administered. In this case, the administration of the antagonist acts as a negative reinforcer.

Cyclazocine is the most popular antagonist because its effects last up to 18 hours, but addicts are still found to inject heroin when the shielding effects of the antagonist are the lowest. Cyclazocine has significant analgesic properties and also possesses a respiratory depressant effect. In addition, large doses may produce irritability, uncontrolled thoughts, delusions, hallucinations, and motor incoordination. Despite the fact that tolerance to these unpleasant side effects develops, abuse potential is very low. Cessation after prolonged use of the drug causes withdrawal symptoms that include periods of weakness and loss of environmental contact. Because of the undesirable side effects, including a noxious taste, and because there is little motivation to substitute an unpleasant drug for one with highly reinforcing properties, the antagonist treatment modality is not a preferred method among addicts. Usually external motivation (e.g., threat of prison) is needed to initiate this type of treatment.

STEPS Program. A more recent modification of the pharmacological support technique is the "sequential treatment employing pharmacological supports" (STEPS) program outlined by Goldstein (1976a). This method employs both pharmacological and psychological support and is based on the belief that because addiction is self-inflicted and self-maintained, any addiction method must evolve from the positive motivation of the addict. Goldstein proposes a stepwise program in which the addict can progress in small steps toward two major goals: (1) elimination of heroin use and (2) change of life-style that will remove the addict from the drug-taking environment. The use of pharmacological supports allows gradual withdrawal from drug use, while social rehabilitation helps the addict to find alternative satisfactions and greater reinforcement for non-drug-taking behavior and improves the addict's self image and sense of worth. The steps shown in Figure 11 represent gradual decrements in the intensity of the drug experience.

The initial period of staff-administered intravenous morphine eliminates the dangers of illicit morphine use, such as drug overdose and disease related to unsterile equipment. It also reduces the need for criminal activities to support the drug habit. This first step also provides a limited time (1 month maximum) in which to establish a therapeutic relationship between the staff and the addict. Subcutaneous morphine (step 2) does not provide the "rush" that follows intravenous morphine, but tranquilization still occurs. In step 3, the daily oral methadone produces a still more reduced subjective euphoria than the morphine and provides the benefits described earlier for the traditional methadone program. The narcotic, levo-α-acetyl-methadol (LAAM) (step 4), provides greater freedom to the addict because it is longer lasting and can be administered orally three times a week rather than on a daily basis. At this point, a very stable state of opiate dependence exists, and it is desirable that during this period (up to 1 year) the addict has demonstrated some social development by participating in a vocational training course, maintaining a part-time job, doing volunteer work, being reunited with family, assuming some family responsibility, or participating in community affairs.

Levo-α-acetyl-methadol (LAAM)

The fifth pharmacological step is the withdrawal from LAAM and complete abstinence with or without assistance by the administration of the narcotic antagonist, naltrexone (see Figure 1). During the period of abstinence, the addicts are encouraged to work with

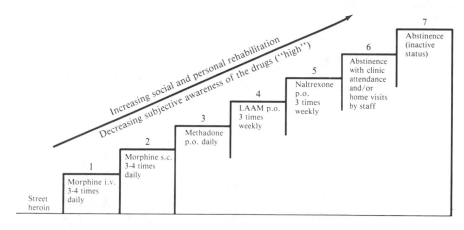

FIGURE 11   STAGES OF TREATMENT of opiate addicts in the STEPS program. (From Goldstein, 1976a.)

other addicts in the hope that providing assistance to others is in itself reinforcing and that acting as a model further encourages mature drug-free behavior.

One unusual feature of the program, as set up by Goldstein, is that it is not an all-or-none affair, and at any point in the program an addict is permitted to fall back one or several steps without being penalized. Each addict's success is measured only by gradual and continual progress upward. The rates of program completion vary from a minimum of 1–2 years up to 5 years. The clinic is always ready to help if a relapse occurs even after program completion.

Psychological Treatment Programs

Among the psychological treatment programs is traditional psychotherapy, which is considered generally unsuccessful unless teamed with other methods. A second type is the "self-help" or "communal" therapy, which includes residence programs like Synanon, Day Top, Horizon House, and others (Brill and Lieberman, 1969; Cherkas, 1965). These programs are run almost entirely by former addicts and are based on the belief that their "extended family" members are able to stay drug free because of membership in the group. Criticism by the group and banishment from the unit are the primary means of punishment and social control.

In order to enter the group, the addict must demonstrate sufficient motivation by withstanding a traumatic first interview in which he is confronted by the successful exaddicts with his own weakness. Once accepted into the group, he must stop all use of drugs "cold turkey," (i.e., without pharmacological aid) but with a large amount of emotional support. No "cure" is expected, but the program provides basic living needs, including medical care, and strives to understand the addict and help him find need-satisfying roles in a drug-free community. The addicts, who rarely leave the residence unit permanently, provide support and services for others within the group or in a similar group elsewhere.

The group is run on a strict hierarchical basis, and work projects and chores are assigned accordingly. With time and effort, the addict works his way up the hierarchy. With increasing status, daily tasks become less menial and living arrangements become less supervised and somewhat more luxurious. Intensive group self-appraisal sessions are held regularly during which highly hostile assaults may take place. Addicts in this setting find that their previous patterns of behavior, their values, and their expectations are vehemently rejected. The reward for conformity is acceptance by the group. Although there is little theoretical basis for the methods used in the self-help programs, several authors have discussed the treatment method in terms of sociological principles and therapeutic tools (Meyer, 1972; Casriel, 1963; Volkmann and Cressy, 1963).

Summary

This chapter discussed the chemical nature of opiates and their synthetic analogs, their pharmacological effects, their mechanisms of action, and their licit and illicit use. The opiates deaden pain; the effect is similar in some respects to that of anesthetics, but most anesthetics merely block nerve impulse transmission. Opiates, on the other hand, act upon specific receptors and interact with neurotransmitters such as serotonin, enkephalins, and substance P. The relationships between opiate receptors and known neural pathways for pain perception make for a robust theory about opiate action. But, how antipsychotic drugs suppress schizophrenic symptoms by blocking dopamine receptors, or how the benzodiazepines attenuate anxiety by facilitating GABAergic mechanisms and by blocking serotonergic mechanisms still elude us.

Virtually every drug has a physiological cost, and in the case of psychotropic agents there is usually a psychological cost as well. The opiates—whose remarkable properties are highly appreciated—can also cause major physical infirmity and social degradation. They serve as an object lesson of the need for the rational understanding of all drugs in use in our society.

Recommended Reading

Barchas, J.D., Akil, H., Elliott, G.R., Halman, R.B., and Watson, S.J. (1978). Behavioral neurochemistry: Neuroregulators and behavioral states. *Science*, 200, 964–973. An overview of neuropeptides and their role in behavior.

Clouet, D.H. (1971). *Narcotic Drugs: Biochemical Pharmacology*. Plenum Press, New York. A series of papers on the biochemical effects of opiates.

Goldstein, A. (1976). Opioid peptides (endorphins) in pituitary and brain. *Science*, 193, 1081–1086. The discovery of the endogenous opiates and their essential characteristics are reviewed.

Houde, R. and Wallenstein, S. (1953). A method for

evaluating analgesics in patients with chronic pain. *Drug Addiction and Narcotics Bulletin*, Appendix F, 660–682. A detailed discussion of the experimental design and methodology for evaluating clinical pain.

Kosterlitz, H.W., Collier, H.O.J. and Villarreal, J.E. (Eds.) (1973). *Agonist and Antagonist Actions of Narcotic Analgesic Drugs*. University Park Press, Baltimore. A collection of papers on the biochemical and physiological effects of narcotics.

Kuschinsky, K. (1977). Opiate dependence. *Progress in Pharmacology*, 1, 1–39. A discussion of the proposed mechanism for drug dependence.

Lal, H. (1975). Narcotic dependence, narcotic action and dopamine receptors. *Life Sciences*, 17, 483–495. A summary of evidence supporting a role for brain dopamine in the actions of opiates.

Snyder, S.H. (1977). Opiate receptors and internal opiates. *Scientific American*, 236, 3, 44–56. A well-illustrated article in this respected periodical describing the discovery and the significance of internal opiates.

Wasacz, J. (1981). Natural and synthetic narcotic drugs. *American Scientist*, 69, 318–324. A brief history of the development of narcotic drugs.

Abbreviations

AAAD Aromatic amino acid decarboxylase
AAOA Aminooxyacetic acid
ACTH Adrenocorticotrophic hormone
ADP Adenosine diphosphate
AMPT See α-MPT
ANS Autonomic nervous system
ARAS Ascending reticular activating system
AT-II Angiotensin-II
ATP Adenosine triphosphate

BOL 2-Bromo-LSD

C Carbon
Ca Calcium
CA Catecholamine, catecholaminergic
cAMP Cyclic adenosine monophosphate
CAT Choline acetyltransferase
CDP Chlordiazepoxide
cGMP Cyclic guanosine monophosphate
ChAc Choline acetylase
Cl Chlorine, chloride
CNS Central nervous system
CRF Corticotropin releasing factor
Cu Copper

d Dextrorotatory; to the right, as the in (+) isomer, *d*-amphetamine
DA Dopamine, dopaminergic
DBH Dopamine beta hydroxylase
DDC Diethyldithiocarbamate
5,6-DHT 5,6-Dihydroxytryptamine
DMPEA Dimethylphenylethylamine
DMT *N,N*-Dimethyltryptamine

DNA Deoxyribonucleic acid
DNB Dorsal noradrenergic bundle
DNP 2,4-Dinitrophenol
DOPAC Dihydroxyphenylacetic acid
DRL Differential reinforcement of low rates of responding
D-sleep Deep sleep; REM sleep
DZP Diazepam

ECT Electroconvulsive therapy
ED50 Effective dose 50
EDTA (Ethylenedinitrilo) tetraacetic acid
EEG Electroencephalograph
EGTA Ethyleneglycol-bis (β-aminoethyl ether) -N,N' tetraacetic acid
EPI Epinephrine (adrenaline)
EPSP Excitatory postsynaptic potential
ER Endoplasmic reticulum

F Fluorine, fluoride
Fe Iron
FEN Fenfluramine
FI Fixed interval
FR Fixed ratio
FXT Fluoxetine

g Gram
GABA Gamma amino butyric acid
GABA-T GABA-α-ketoglutarate transferase
GAD Glutamic acid decarboxylase
GCS Glycine cleavage system
GDEE L-Glutamic acid diethyl ester
GTP Guanosine triphosphate

HAP   1-Hydroxy-3-aminopyrrolid-2-one
HC-3   Hemicholinium
5-HIA   5-Hydroxyindole acetaldehyde
5-HIAA   5-Hydroxyindole acetic acid
HNMT   Histamine-N-methyl transferase
5-HT   5-Hydroxytryptamine
5-HTP   5-Hydroxytryptophan
5-HTP-D   5-Hydroxytryptophan decarboxylase
Hz   Hertz; waves/sec

i.c.   Intracisternal
i.m.   Intramuscular
i.p.   Intraperitoneal
IPSP   Inhibitory postsynaptic potential
i.v.   Intravenous
i.v.t.   Intraventricular

K   Kalium (potassium)
K$_m$ Michaelis constant
kg   Kilogram
α-**KGT**   Alpha ketoglutarate transaminase

l   Levorotatory; to the left, as in the isomer, L-dopa
LD50   Lethal dose 50
LH   Luteinizing hormone
LH-RH   Luteinizing hormone releasing hormone
Li   Lithium
LiCl   Lithium chloride
LVP   Lycine-8-vasopressin

M   Mole
MAO   Monoamine oxidase
MAOI   Monoamine oxidase inihibitor
MEPP   Miniature end-plate potential
MFB   Medial forebrain bundle
Mg   Magnesium
mg   Milligram
MHPG   3-methoxy-4-hydroxyphenylglycol
MHPGA   3-methoxy-4-hydroxyphenylglycoaldehyde
MIF   Melanocyte stimulating hormone inhibiting factor
MK-485   Carbidopa
mM   Millimole
α-**MNE**   Alpha methylnorepinephrine
MPB   Meprobamate
α-**MPT**   Alpha methylparatyrosine
MRF   Melanocyte stimulating hormone releasing factor
MSG   Monosodium glutamate

MSH   Melanocyte stimulating hormone
mV   Millivolt (10^{-3} volt)
μ Mu, micron (10^{-6} meter)
μ**m**   Micrometer (10^{-6} meter)
μ**l**   Microliter (10^{-6} liter)
μ**M**   Micromole (10^{-6} mole)

Na   Natrium (sodium)
nA   Nanoampere (10^{-9} ampere)
NAD   Nicotinamide adenine dinucleotide
NADP   NAD phosphate
NADPH   The reduced form of NADP
NAT N-acetyl transferase

2-OAT   2-Oxoglutarate amino transferase
6-OHDA   6-Hydroxydopamine

PCA   Parachloroamphetamine
PCPA   Parachlorophenylalanine
PEA   Phenylethylamine
PGO spikes   Nerve discharges from pons, lateral geniculate, and occipital lobe
p.o.   *per os* (orally)
PKU   Phenylketonuria

REM sleep   Rapid eye movement sleep
RNA   Ribonucleic acid

SAM S-adenosylmethionine
S.E.M.   Standard error of the mean
s.c.   Subcutaneous
SHMT   Serine hydroxymethyl transferase
SP   Substance P
SSA   Succinic semialdehyde
SSADH   Succinic semialdehyde dehydrogenase
S-sleep   Slow wave sleep (SWS)
SRIF   Somatotropin release-inhibiting factor

TAB   Trimedoxime, atropine, and benactyzine
TEC   Triethylcholine
TH   Tyrosine hydroxylase
TPH   Tryptophan hydroxylase
TRH   Thyrotropin releasing hormone
TSC   Thiosemicarbazide
TSH   Thyroid stimulating hormone, thyrotropin

VI   Variable interval
VMA   Vanillylmandelic acid
VR   Variable ratio

Glossary

absolute refractory period A brief period following an action potential during which a second action potential cannot be generated regardless of the stimulus intensity.

abstinence syndrome Physiological and behavioral symptoms that occur upon the sudden withdrawal of a drug that has been continually used. Drugs that can produce the abstinence syndrome effects include the opiates, the barbituates and alcohol.

acetylation The addition of the acetyl radical ($CH_3CO–$) into the molecular structure of an organic compound, usually by reactions with acetic acid ($CH_3–COOH$).

actin A protein that interacts with myosin, another protein, to effect muscular contractions.

action potential A regional voltage shift on part of a neuron membrane that is quickly propagated non-decrementally. It is characterized by a reversal of the neuron's internal negative polarity to positive, and then a return to negative polarity.

active transport A process by which molecules are transported across membranes by way of an hypothesized "carrier" involving an energy expenditure. It is a major vehicle for membrane transport of large molecules, and small molecules against a concentration gradient.

active zones The areas of a presynaptic membrane where the vesicle contents are ejected into the synaptic cleft.

addiction Compulsive drug use, characterized by overwhelming involvement with the use of the drug, the securing of its supply and a high probability of relapse after withdrawal.

adrenal medulla The central core of the adrenal gland which synthesizes and releases norepinephrine and epinephrine in response to sympathetic stimulation.

adrenergic A general term that refers to neural systems that secrete adrenalin or noradrenalin, drugs that are adrenalin or noradrenalin agonists or antagonists, and to the receptors that are affected by those neurotransmitters.

aerobic metabolism The stepwise oxidation of pyruvic acid, the product of anaerobic metabolism, to form acetyl coenzyme A which then enters the tricarboxylic acid cycle to yield energy.

affinity chromatography A sensitive separation technique based on the attraction of a chemical or cellular constituent for a specific ligand attached to a chromatography column.

afterpotential A brief period of depolarization or hyperpolarization of a neuron membrane following an action potential.

agonist A substance which when acting on a receptor produces a pharmacological response. Example: apomorphine has the same effects as dopamine on dopamine receptors; hence apomorphine is a dopamine agonist.

alkane A hydrocarbon having saturated carbon bonds such as methane, CH_4 or ethane, C_2H_6.

amino acids Organic compounds of the general formula $R—CH—NH_2—COOH$ (R represents hydrogen or any organic radical). They are the structural units of proteins.

amphipathic Designating molecules that have parts that are polar and soluble in water (hydrophilic), and parts that are non-polar and are not soluble in water (hydrophobic).

anaerobic glycolysis   The metabolism of glycogen in the absence of oxygen.

analeptic   A class of drugs that stimulates the nervous system; e.g., caffeine, amphetamine and metrazol.

analgesia   A reduction of pain without loss of consciousness.

angina pectoris   Paroxysmal pain in the chest accompanied by feelings of suffocation and fainting due to poor circulation and lack of oxygen to the heart muscles.

antagonist   Any substance that reduces or blocks the physiological action of a different substance. In pharmacology, an antagonist is an agent that binds to the same site as would an active compound (agonist) and blocks the action of the agonist.

antibody   A specific substance (usually a protein) produced in and by an animal as a reaction to a foreign material (an antigen). The antibody combines with great specificity to an antigen which triggers its synthesis.

antidromic   The artificially induced propagation of action potentials *toward* the cell body of a neuron. Action potentials normally propagate away from the cell body toward the axon terminals, a condition known as prodromic propagation.

antigen   A substance which when introduced into the blood or tissues incites the formation of antibodies. Antigens include toxins and foreign protein substances.

anxiolytic   Antianxiety, as in anxiolytic drugs.

Aplysia californica   A large sea snail used for experiments in neurophysiology.

area postrema   A narrow zone on the lateral wall of the fourth ventricle of the brain. It consists of neurons forming the chemical trigger zone that induces vomiting.

arrhythmia   Any irregular heart beat.

ascending reticular activating system   A cluster of small nerve cells and processes found in the central core of the mesencephalon. These cells are affected by collaterals of sensory systems and project to the intralaminar nuclei of the thalamus.

astrocyte   A star-shaped glial cell; astroglia. *See* neuroglia.

astroglia   *See* neuroglia.

autonomic nervous system   The sympathetic and parasympathetic systems which control the functions of the cardiac and smooth muscle and glandular systems.

autoradiography   A method of localizing a compound within cells and organs. Following administration of a radioactive substance to an animal, a thin slice of tissue is placed in contact with a photographic film. After some time the film is developed. The radioactivity will cause dark spots to appear on the film where the substance is concentrated.

autoreceptors   Receptors found on the somata or presynaptic axon terminals of a neuron. The receptors are sensitive to the neurotransmitter substance of the neuron and exert feedback control for the release or synthesis of the neurotransmitter.

axoaxonic synapse   A synapse formed by an axon terminal upon another axon terminal.

axodendritic synapse   A synapse formed by an axon terminal and a dendritic spine.

axolemma   A thin membrane surrounding the axon cylinder lying beneath the myelin sheath.

axon   The cell process of a neuron that transmits the nerve impulses from the soma to terminals where a neurotransmitter is released.

axon collateral   An axon branch that leads to the stimulation of a large number of recipient cells, as well as to the parent cell for feedback purposes.

axon hillock   A part of the neuron cell body that is free of Nissl granules and gives rise to the axon.

axoplasm   The axon fluid which contains organelles, sugars, proteins, fats, mitochondria, neurotransmitters in various stages of synthesis and other substances. The axoplasm serves as a vehicle for the transport of these substances.

axoplasmic flow   The flow of cellular materials from the cell body of a neuron primarily to other parts of the cell including the axon terminals.

axosomatic synapse   A synapse formed by an axon terminal upon the cell body of an adjacent neuron.

barbiturates   A class of drugs that are sedatives, hypnotics (sleep inducers) and anesthetics which produce unconsciousness. Examples are phenobarbital, pentobarbital and pentothal.

basement membrane An amorphous mucopolysaccharide matrix surrounding the capillaries.

basket cells A variety of cells found in the cerebellar cortex that exert inhibitory influences upon the Purkinje cells.

behavioral tolerance Behavioral adaptation to a drug's effects following repeated administration.

benzodiazepines A large class of drugs having muscle relaxant, anticonvulsive, anxiolytic and hypnotic characteristics. Included in this class are chlordiazepoxide, diazepam, oxazepam, flurazepam, nitrazepam, clorazepate and flunitrazepam.

biotransformation Changes in the chemical nature of a drug due to biochemical processes.

blood brain barrier Differences in the structure of the capillaries in the brain that prevent certain molecules from passing from the blood stream into brain tissue and *vice versa*. *See* tight junctions.

Bowman's capsule The sac surrounding the glomerulus of the kidney.

butyrophenones A class of drugs used to relieve the symptoms of schizophrenia. It includes the drugs haloperidol and spiroperidol. This class of drugs is also known as the phenyl butylpiperidines.

catalepsy The abnormal maintenance of distorted posture.

catecholamine A compound containing the catechol nucleus and an amine group such as NH_2.

cellular tolerance *See* pharmacodynamic tolerance.

cerebellum The division of the brain behind the cerebrum and dorsal to the pons and medulla. It receives inputs from the vestibular apparatus, the spinal cord and the cerebral cortex, and projects to the spinal cord, thalamus and midbrain for the coordination of movement.

cerebrosides A class of lipids containing a sugar and the amino alcohol molecule sphingosine.

cerebrospinal fluid The fluid in the ventricles of the brain and within the sheaths of the spinal cord. This fluid serves as a protective shock absorber for the brain, and as a "sink" function for the accumulation and clearing of molecules not needed by the brain.

chelating agent A substance that combines with metal ions to make them inert.

chemical trigger zone A cell group in the area postrema of the medulla. It is sensitive to toxic substances and controls emesis (vomiting).

cholinergic Pertaining to acetylcholine. Thus, cholinergic drugs are those that affect acetylcholine systems and cholinergic receptors are those affected by acetylcholine.

cholinomimetic A substance that mimics the action of acetylcholine.

choroid plexus Elongated, lobulated, invaginated processes having a vascular plexus which projects into the ventricles of the brain and secretes the cerebrospinal fluid.

chromaffin granules Vesicles in the adrenal medulla containing epinephrine. The vesicles are so named because they are readily stained by chromium salts.

chromatography The separation of closely related compounds by allowing a solution or mixture of them to seep through an adsorbent material such as clay or paper. Each compound becomes adsorbed in a separate, often distinctly colored layer. The appropriate layer can be "developed" with a reagent that produces a colored product which can then be analyzed for its chemical constituents.

chromatolysis The dispersion of Nissl granules in the soma of a neuron found after injury to the axon.

circadian rhythms The daily rhythms of sleeping, feeding, etc.

clonic seizures A convulsant state characterized by muscle contractions.

coenzyme A cofactor that is needed for the activation of an enzyme.

cofactor A compound or molecule that is necessary to activate an enzyme in a metabolic sequence.

competitive antagonist A substance which binds reversibly with the same site as an agonist and can be displaced by an excess of agonist.

conditioned avoidance procedure or **signalled escape procedure** A test procedure in which a noxious stimulus, previously paired with a cue, can be avoided by the subject if a correct response is made to that cue preceding the stimulus (e.g., pole climbing following a buzzer to avoid a subsequent foot shock).

conditioned emotional response procedure Following the training of any operant response, an unavoidable shock is introduced preceded by a signal. After several pairings the signal produces a suppression of responding.

conductance   The ability of a material to conduct electrons or ions; the opposite of resistance. Conductance in neurons refers to the passage of ions through membranes.

congener   A drug that belongs to a group of chemical compounds having the same parent compound.

conjugation   The chemical coupling of a drug or metabolite with an endogenous substance. The enzyme-mediated conversion forms a pharmacologically inert product, one that is more water soluble and readily excreted from the kidney.

corpus striatum or **basal ganglia**   Cell groups in the telencephalon having the principal function of integrating motor functions.

cross tolerance   The diminished pharmacological effectiveness of a drug following the repeated administration of a related drug. For example, the tolerance developed to morphine after repeated administration will be conferred upon codeine at the first dose.

crossed reflexes   Spinal reflexes that integrate the musculature on both sides of the body. For example, during walking the flexion of one leg leads to the extension of the opposite leg to support the weight of the body.

cyclic AMP (cAMP)   Cyclic adenosine $3'$, $5'$-monophosphate. A compound that is required for the phosphorylation of protein molecules resulting in a wide variety of physiological processes, such as sugar metabolism, fat metabolism, membrane depolarization, synthesis regulation, etc.

cyclic GMP (cGMP)   Cyclic guanosine $3'$, $5'$-monophosphate. A compound that phosphorylates proteins leading to succeeding physiological events.

cytoplasm   The fluid content of a cell body in which the organelles and other substances are suspended.

cytoplasmic membrane   The membrane that encloses the cell body or soma. This is in contrast to membranes that enclose the nucleus, vesicles and other organelles within a cell.

deep sleep   *See* paradoxical sleep.

Deiter's nucleus   The lateral vestibular nucleus of the brain stem.

dendrites   The finely branched processes usually found near the soma of a neuron. Their usual function is to receive excitatory or inhibitory effects via neurotransmitters.

depolarization   The decrease in the postsynaptic membrane resting potential that results from synaptic stimulation.

dibenzodiazepines   A class of antipsychotic drugs which includes clozapine. Among other actions, these drugs block dopamine receptors.

differential centrifugation   A process in which homogenized tissue is centrifuged in layers of increasing density of sucrose in order to separate the different cell constituents (membranes, nuclei, mitochondria, synaptosomes, etc.) for analysis.

differential reinforcement of low rate of responding (DRL)   A schedule of operant conditioning that encourages delay of responding by rewarding the response only after a specified waiting period.

diphenylbutylpiperidines   A class of antipsychotic drugs related to the butyrophenones, e.g. Pimozide. These drugs act by blocking dopamine receptors.

distal   The part of a cut nerve that has been separated from the cell body.

dose-response   The relationship between the size of the dose of a drug and the magnitude of the physiological or behavioral response.

double-blind   An experimental procedure in which neither the subject in the experiment nor the observer knows what treatment the subject has received.

drug disposition tolerance   The tolerance to a drug due to the induction of more metabolizing enzymes in the liver.

drug half-life or **drug half-time**   The time for a drug concentration in the blood plasma to fall to one-half of its peak or highest value.

dysphoria   Physical discomfort, accompanied by a sense of being ill at ease, feelings of impatience, restlessness, anxiety and fidgetiness.

effective dose 50 (ED 50)   The dose of a drug that produces a given pharmacological effect in 50 percent of the subjects tested.

electroencephalogram (EEG)   Recordings of the gross electrical activity of brain areas.

electrophoresis   The separation of components of a mixture in solution by applying a voltage to electrodes that are in contact with the solution. The more highly charged particles will move more readily to one of the electrodes which can then be collected and analyzed.

electrostatic attraction   The force that draws together bodies which carry opposite charges of electricity.

encephalitis lethargica   A viral inflammation of the brain characterized by increasing languor, apathy and drowsiness passing into lethargy.

endocytosis   The process whereby an extracellular substance is engulfed by a cell membrane forming a sac which incorporates the substance into the cell.

endogenous   Naturally occurring in the body.

endoplasmic reticulum, rough or **granular**   A membraneous network within the cell soma to which ribosomes are attached whose function is the synthesis of proteins.

endoplasmic reticulum, smooth or **agranular**   A membraneous network found in the cell soma and said to extend into the axon of neurons. Its functions include the transport of products synthesized in the rough endoplasmic reticulum, the synthesis of lipids, and the formation of terminal vesicles in axon terminals.

endorphins   Endogenous morphine–like compounds that can be reproduced as segments of β-lipotropin.

endothelium   A layer of contiguous thin, flat cells that line the inner surface of the heart and blood vessels, and other closed cavities.

end-plate potential   The membrane depolarization that occurs on muscle membranes leading to muscle contraction.

enkephalins   Endogenous pentapeptides perhaps derived from β-lipotropin that bind to the same brain sites as morphine and other opiates.

enterochromaffin cells   Cells containing catecholamine granules that are stained by chromium salts, found in the wall of the intestines.

epileptic focus   A circumscribed area in the brain which is presumed to be pathologic from which epileptic activity emanates.

epithelium   The coverings of the skin, mucous membranes, and the various organs of the body. The cells of the epithelium are varied depending upon the function of the organ surface.

equilibrium potential   The membrane potential that is sufficient to block the membrane transport of an ion. Example: an internal voltage of $+50$ mV will prevent the influx of Na^+ into a nerve cell.

ergot   A parasitic fungus found on wheat and rye. Derivatives of this substance are potent vasoconstrictors useful in controlling migraine headaches and hemorrhage.

ergotropic   Referring to those functions of arousal, excitement, increased muscle tone and sympathetic nervous activity. *See* trophotropic.

esterase   An enzyme that by hydrolysis cleaves esteratic groups from compounds.

esteratic site   A positively charged portion of a molecule to which negatively charged esters can be bound. *See* esters.

esters   Molecules that are derivatives of carboxylic acids (acids containing carboxyl groups, COOH, such as acetic acid CH_3COOH) in which the hydroxyl (OH) group is replaced by O-R. Acetylcholine contains an ester linkage, between the acetyl group and choline.

estrogens   Hormones that are involved in the maturation of the primary sex organs and the secondary sexual characteristics of the female. They also play a role in the female sexual cycle. Estradiol is typical of this group.

euphoria   An abnormal state of elation.

excitation-secretion coupling   The mechanism through which action potentials arriving at an axon terminal lead to the release of a neurotransmitter from the terminal.

excitatory postsynaptic potential (EPSP)   The slight and transient depolarization of a postjunctional neuron membrane following the release of a neurotransmitter from a presynaptic terminal.

exocytosis   The expulsion of material from secretory cells into the extracellular space. In neurons, neurotransmitters are expelled from synaptic vesicles or possibly from the cytoplasm itself into the synaptic cleft.

extrastriate cortex   The cerebral cortex surrounding the striate or visual cortex.

facilitated diffusion   The passage of lipid–insoluble, ionized substances from one side of a membrane to the other with the aid of a carrier protein.

Factor I An inhibitory substance found in the crayfish nervous system that consists largely of GABA.

fatty acid Any one of a group of acids such as stearic or palmitic acid that occur in natural fats, and are fat-like substances.

feedback inhibition The slowing of an activity by the end–product of the action. Example: a high concentration of norepinephrine (NE) in the axon terminals will slow NE synthesis in the cell bodies.

fenestra(e) Any small opening, such as the opening in the walls of some capillaries. They are not found in the capillaries in the central nervous system.

fibrillation A muscular tremor.

filtration The passage of water–soluble molecules through water–filled pores in membranes. The direction of flow is determined by a pressure gradient; the flow being from the high pressure side of a membrane to the low pressure side.

fixative A substance that terminates the biological activity in tissue; or that firmly attaches tissue to microscope slides for analysis.

fixed interval schedule (FI) An operant conditioning schedule which provides reinforcement at fixed times after the last reinforcement, but only if an appropriate response occurs.

fixed ratio schedule (FR) An operant conditioning schedule which requires a fixed number of responses before a reinforcer is delivered.

fluorescence photomicrography The photographing of microscopic views of fluorescing tissue components.

fluorophores Tissue granules that have been made to fluoresce.

fourth ventricle The cavity of the brain lying between the roof of the medulla and pons and the cerebellum.

freeze-fracturing technique A method by which tissue is frozen, then broken apart for preparation for microscopy. The lines of cleavage or splitting occur not between the surfaces of two adjacent cells, but between the bilayers of cell membranes allowing analysis of the particles lying within the membranes.

functional hypoglycemia A condition in which cells cannot metabolize glucose even when a sufficient amount of glucose is available.

ganglion A cluster of cell bodies lying outside the central nervous system. Examples: spinal ganglia contain the cell bodies of afferent spinal nerves; autonomic ganglia contain cell bodies of nerves innervating visceral organs.

gangliosides A class of lipids found in the cytoplasmic membranes of nerve terminals having a high affinity for calcium ions.

gap junctions Spaces between neurons or between glia and neurons that are very narrow; they may exist between dendrites as well as between axons and dendrites. Transmission across gap junctions does not depend on neurotransmitters.

Geller procedure An operant conflict task in which the subject is trained to respond to reinforcement, e.g., food. After the behavior is established the presentation of the food reward is accompanied by foot shock. Rates of responding can be regulated by varying the level of reward and shock.

glaucoma A disease of the eyes characterized by an abnormal internal ocular pressure that is destructive to the retina.

glia *See* neuroglia.

glomerulus A tuft of capillary loops in the kidney that provide the point of input for the functional cell of the kidney, the nephron.

glucocorticoids A class of substances that are secreted from the adrenal cortex in response to stress. They include hydrocortisone, cortisone and corticosterone.

glucoreceptors Specialized cells in the hypothalamus which monitor plasma glucose levels.

glycine cleavage system The process that converts glycine to its metabolite 5,10 methyline FH_4.

glycogen A form of carbohydrate formed in the liver which can be converted to glucose. Glucose can then be used as a fuel to provide energy for cellular functions.

glycogenolysis The splitting of glycogen to form dextrose (glucose).

glycolysis Glucose metabolism that ultimately leads to the production of energy in the form of ATP and water. *See* anaerobic and aerobic metabolism.

glycoproteins Protein molecules containing carbohydrate groups.

Golgi apparatus An organelle present in all cells near the nucleus but prominent in secretory cells and neurons. It appears as an array of crescentric membranes about 6.0 nm in thickness that encloses secretory material prior to transport of the material to its secretory sites.

gram equivalent Number of grams equal to the atomic weight. Example: the atomic weight of hydrogen is 1, thus the gram equivalent is 1 gm. Oxygen, O = 8; gram equivalent of O = 8 gm.

histofluorescence A method of treating tissues so that certain compounds glow in ultraviolet light thereby revealing their presence in the tissue. The treatment is useful in locating monoamine neurotransmitters.

hot plate test A test usually used to measure the potency of analgesics. An animal is placed on a metal plate that is gradually warmed. The temperatures at which animals respond to the heat are compared for the drug and no-drug condition.

Huntington's chorea An inherited disease of the central nervous system characterized by cell destruction in the corpus striatum causing uncontrolled movements and dementia. The disease usually appears during the third or fourth decade of life.

hydrocarbon A chemical unit or compound containing only carbon and hydrogen.

hydrolysis A chemical process in which water molecules are involved in the alteration of a chemical substance. Example: hydrolysis occurs when water molecules cleave ATP (adenosine triphosphate) to form ADP (adenosine diphosphate) and phosphate.

hydrophilic Designating compounds that are water soluble.

hydrophobic Designating compounds that are insoluble in water such as oils and waxes.

hyperpolarization An increase in the postsynaptic membrane potential that results from synaptic action.

hypertention High blood pressure.

hypnotic A drug that produces sleep.

hypoglycemia A deficiency of blood sugar.

hypothalamo-hypophyseal system Neurons whose cell bodies are found in the hypothalamus and whose axons are found in the hypophysis (the pituitary stalk).

These neurons exert influences upon the secretory cells of the posterior pituitary gland.

hypothalamus A cluster of cell nuclei at the base of the brain primarily serving autonomic functions.

immunoassay A method of quantification of a chemical substance based on a competition between radioactive and non-radioactive antigens for a fixed number of antibody binding sites. Also called immunocytochemical technique, or radio immunoassay.

immunologically active substance A substance that acts as an antigen and induces the formation of antibodies.

indolealkylamine A compound such as serotonin which contains an indole nucleus, an alkyl group (e.g. ethyl), and an amine (e.g. NH_2).

indoleamine A compound containing the indole nucleus and an amine group. *See* indolealkylamine.

inhibitory postsynaptic potential (IPSP) A slight and transient hyperpolarization of a neuron membrane caused by the release of transmitter from the presynaptic terminal.

initial segment A short non-myelinated section of an axon just beyond the axon hillock. In some neurons the action potential originates at that site.

intercellular clefts Small spaces between the endothelial cells of some capillaries.

interneuron A neuron with a short axon interposed between two other neurons. They frequently exert inhibitory effects on the adjacent neurons.

intersegmental reflex A spinal reflex that integrates the activities associated with two or more spinal segments such as those integrating the muscles of the trunk with those of the limbs.

intracarotid Pertaining to the injection of substances directly into the carotid artery.

intracisternal (i.c.) Referring to injection directly into the cisterns containing the cerebral spinal fluid of the brain.

intraperitoneal (i.p.) The hypodermic injection of a substance into the visceral cavity for rapid absorption into the blood stream.

intrathecal injection Injection within a sheath such as within the coverings of the spinal cord.

intravenous (i.v.)   The hypodermic injection of a substance into veins for the most rapid distribution of that substance.

intraventricular (IVT)   Usually referring to direct injection of substances into the ventricles of the brain. It is one way to administer drugs into the brain which do not normally pass the blood brain barrier.

ionic bond   A bond formed between two atoms when one or more electrons are transferred from one atom to another thereby completing a stable electron configuration for each. Example: sodium (Na$^+$) and chloride (Cl$^-$) form ionic bonds to make the stable substance NaCl.

ionization   The addition or subtraction of electrons from an atom or group of atoms resulting in a positive or negative charge.

ionophore   A molecule that facilitates the transfer of an ion across a membrane.

ionotropic   The putative character of a neurotransmitter that has the ability to directly affect the permeability of a membrane to various ions.

iontophoresis   *See* microiontophoresis.

isoenzymes   Enzymes which occur in more than one molecular form within the same species, tissues or even cells.

isomer   A compound made up of the same elements in the same proportion as those in another compound but having different chemical properties because of a difference in the arrangement of the elements.

isoquinolines   A group of compounds formed from catecholamines and indolealkylamines. When treated with formaldehyde gas the compounds formed with the amines fluoresce when viewed under ultraviolet light. The wave length of the emitted light depends upon which amine was treated making it possible to identify the presence of these neurotransmitters.

junctional folds   *See* subneural clefts.

ketone   A compound having a carbonyl group O in the keto form

$$\begin{matrix} & O \\ & \| \\ & C \\ & / \ \backslash \\ & R \quad R \end{matrix}$$

Phenylpyruvic acid contains this group and is an α-keto acid.

knife cuts   Small cuts made in animal brains by a short (1-2 mm) stiff wire that is extended from a thin hollow tube. The procedure is designed for severing specific nerve bundles.

Krebs cycle   *See* tricarboxylic acid cycle.

length constant   The distance along an axon at which a stimulus-induced voltage change falls to 37 percent of its peak value.

lethal dose 50 (LD 50)   The dose of a drug that kills 50 percent of the subjects tested.

ligand   A molecule that donates the necessary electrons to form bonds. In general, a neurotransmitter or drug molecule that is bound to a receptor molecule.

lipid   A water-insoluble organic substance largely composed of fatty acids. Lipids serve as the structural components of membranes and as storage forms of metabolic fuel.

lipid solubility   The degree to which a substance will dissolve in the lipid layers of a membrane. *See* partition coefficient.

local potential   A slight decrease or increase of the membrane potential of a neuron or muscle cell resulting from stimulation at a synaptic junction. So named because the electrical change does not extend very far from the point of stimulation. *See* excitatory or inhibitory postsynaptic potential.

locus caeruleus   A nerve cell group in the dorsal pons that gives rise to the axons that make up the ascending dorsal noradrenergic bundle. The locus caeruleus is so named because the nucleus contains a slightly bluish pigment.

lordosis   The sexual response of the female rodent to male stimulation. The animal crouches, raises its head and hind quarters, and moves its tail to the side. The lordosis quotient is a measure of sexual reactivity expressed as the ratio of lordosis responses to mounts by vigorous males.

lysis   The dissolving and disintegration of cells.

lysosomes   Microscopically small membrane-bound sacs containing digestive enzymes.

manic-depressive psychosis   A mental disorder characterized by marked changes in mood from mania to depression and back again.

marker enzymes   Enzymes that can be identified by

stains or chemical reactions. They are used to identify the specific cell components with which they are normally associated.

mast cells Cells normally found in connective tissue or plasma which contain potent vasoactive amines, e.g., histamine, that cause local inflammatory reactions.

median eminence A midline prominence in the floor of the third ventricle above the pituitary stalk. It is the point of discharge of the hypothalamic releasing and inhibiting factors of the anterior pituitary gland.

medulla or **medulla oblongata** The part of the brain stem contiguous with the most rostral part of the spinal cord.

meningitis An inflammation (infection) of the meninges, the membraneous coverings of the brain and spinal cord.

metabolizing tolerance *See* drug disposition tolerance.

metabotropic The putative characteristic of a neurotransmitter that will set metabolic changes in motion and result in permeability changes of a membrane to various ions.

methylation The addition of a methyl group (CH_3) to a compound.

Michaelis constant (K_m) The concentration of a substrate that would yield one-half of the maximum reaction for a given amount of receptor protein. This also refers to the transport of substances across membranes by protein "carriers" or drug-receptor interactions.

microglia *See* neuroglia.

microiontophoresis A method by which neurotransmitters or drugs can be applied to selected cells in measured molecular amounts. The substances are ejected from micropipettes by application of electric currents to the substances in solution. Another name for this method is iontophoresis.

micrometer (μm) 1×10^{-6} meter.

micromolar (μM) Pertaining to a solution containing 1 micromole (10^{-6} mole) of solute per liter of solvent.

microsomal enzymes Enzymes formed by the rough endoplasmic reticulum.

microsomal fraction The cell fraction obtained by differential centrifugation and which contains ribosomes and fragments of the endoplasmic reticulum.

microtubules A tubular network found in the soma and axons of neurons. They function in the rapid transport of substances necessary for the nutrition and repair of the cell, as well as the transport of the neurotransmitters or their precursors.

minor tranquilizer Any antianxiety (anxiolytic) drug. The term is becoming obsolete.

mitochondria Subcellular organelles that serve primarily to provide energy for a cell through the process of oxidative metabolism.

moiety A functional unit of a molecule; thus COOH is the carboxyl moiety of acetic acid, CH_3COOH.

mole The number of grams of a compound equal to the molecular weight of the compound. Example: a mole of sodium chloride (NaCl) is equal to the sum of atomic weights of sodium (11) and chlorine (17) or 28 grams.

molecular weight The weight of a molecule of any substance representative of the sum of the weights of its constituent atoms.

monoamines Neurotransmitters having only one amine group such as NH_2.

mucopolysaccharides Long chains of carbohydrate (sugar) units that form thin, flexible, sticky cell coatings in higher animal tissues.

muscle end-plate A specialized part of a muscle membrane where axon terminals initiate muscle contraction.

myasthenia gravis A disease characterized by progressive muscular weakness and fatigability caused by the degeneration of acetylcholine receptors in the neuromuscular junction.

myelin Fatty cells which form a sheath or covering around axons. It serves to insulate one axon from another and aids in the speed of impulse transmission along the axon.

nanometer (nm) 1×10^{-9} meter.

narcotic Any analgesic drug of the opiate class that reduces pain and induces sleep.

negative reinforcement procedure An operant conditioning technique in which the removal of aversive stimuli as a consequence of a predetermined response will increase the probability of repeated responding to avoid the aversive stimuli.

nephron The functional unit of the kidney. These filtering units consist of the glomerulus and its capsule, and the uriniferous tubule enmeshed in its capillary bed.

neurilemma   A thin membrane surrounding the myelin sheath of an axon or the axon cylinder of a nonmyelinated axon.

neuroeffector junction   The junction between axon terminals and cells of muscles or glands. Nerve impulses in the axons lead to excitation of the muscle or gland by mechanisms similar to those of synapses.

neurofilaments or **microfilaments**   Tubular structures about 10 μm in diameter in the dendrites, soma and axons of neurons. They may be involved in the translocation of organelles such as mitochondria from their site of production in the perikaryon to dendritic and axonal sites of utilization.

neuroglia   Neuroglia are a class of cells. There are three types: astroglia, microglia and oligodendroglia. Astroglia are supporting cells found between blood capillaries and nerve cells, and microglia are small cells that are migratory and act as phagocytes of the waste material and damaged parts of nerve cells. The oligodendroglia participate in the formation of the myelin sheaths of neurons within the central nervous system.

neuroleptic   A neuropharmacologic agent that has an antipsychotic action.

neuropil   A dense network of unmyelinated nerve fibers.

neurosis   Any of a variety of personality disorders of which the principal disturbance is a group of symptoms that is distressing to the individual and recognized by that individual as unacceptable. The symptoms might include general anxiety up to states of panic.

neurostenin   A protein that causes a muscle contractile action upon synaptic vesicles that results in the emptying of the neurotransmitter from the axon terminals into the synaptic space.

neurotransmitter   A chemical substance that is released from axon terminals by action potentials and stimulates or inhibits adjacent neurons or stimulates effector organs such as muscles and glands.

nicotinic   Pertaining to drugs that mimic nicotine, or receptors that are affected by nicotine.

Nissl granules   Parts of the rough endoplasmic reticulum largely composed of RNA involved in protein synthesis. Also known as chromophil substances or tigroid bodies.

nociception   The perception of pain.

nodes of Ranvier   Short sections of naked axon between longer sections of myelinated axon. It is where the action potentials occur in myelinated axons.

non-competitive antagonist   An antagonist substance whose effects cannot be overcome by increasing the concentration of the agonist.

non-synthetic reaction   The modification of a drug by oxidation, reduction or hydrolysis to form a metabolite that is inactive or more active than the parent drug.

noradrenergic   Pertaining to drugs affecting systems that utilize noradrenalin (norepinephrine) as their normal neurotransmitter. Also pertains to receptors utilizing norepinephrine.

nucleus   That part of a cell which contains the cell's chromatin (genetic material). Nucleus also refers to a group of cells in the central nervous system having well defined connections and functions. Example: the vagus nucleus of the medulla are the cell bodies that provide many of the axons making up the vagus nerve.

oligodendroglia   *See* neuroglia.

opiates   A class of drugs derived from opium. Also called narcotic analgesics, these drugs include morphine, codeine, heroin, and papaverine all of which reduce pain and induce sleep.

opiate withdrawal symptoms   The physiological reactions that occur when opiate use is terminated after prolonged use.

optic tectum   The dorsal-most layers (the roof) of the superior colliculus of the midbrain. This area receives visual as well as other sensory inputs which are integrated in higher animals for orienting and localizing responses.

organelles   The microscopic structures found within cells. Examples: mitochondria, lysosomes, endoplasmic reticulum.

organophosphorus compounds   Phosphorus containing anticholinesterase compounds. These compounds are used as insecticides and chemical warfare agents, but still have some medical utility as potent anticholinesterases.

oxidation   A chemical process in which a carbon atom increases its covalent bonds to either oxygen or nitrogen.

oxidative metabolism   *See* oxidative phosphorylation.

oxidative phosphorylation   The enzymatic conversion of ADP (adenosine diphosphate) to ATP (adenosine triphosphate), a process that requires the presence of oxygen. The process is also called oxidative metabolism.

paradoxical sleep   A deep state of sleep characterized by a paradoxical EEG denoting mental alertness, rapid eye movements, dreams, muscular relaxation, and other phenomena. Also known as deep sleep and REM sleep.

parasympatholytic   Referring to substances that block the action of the parasympathetic nervous system.

paraventricular nucleus   A cell group in the anterior part of the hypothalamus along the wall of the third ventricle. These cells secrete the hormone oxytocin which is transported to the posterior pituitary gland where it enters the blood stream. The hormone controls contractions of the uterus and ejection of milk from the breasts.

paravertebral ganglia   Twenty-one groups of cell bodies lying on each side of the vertebral column interconnected by the axons of the sympathetic trunk. The axons of the ganglia innervate the smooth muscles of the blood vessels, and eye lids, hair follicles, the sweat, tear and salivary glands, the respiratory organs, the heart, the iris, and other structures. Also known as the sympathetic ganglia or chain ganglia.

Parkinsonism   Referring to symptoms of Parkinson's disease, or drug-induced symptoms that resemble those of Parkinson's disease.

Parkinson's disease   A central nervous system disorder characterized by cellular degeneration in the substantia nigra causing tremor, muscle spacticity and an inability to initiate movement.

paroxysmal tachycardia   Acute increases in heart rate following a sudden release of epinephrine into the blood stream. *See* pheochromocytoma.

partition coefficient   The ratio of the lipid solubility of a substance in an organic solvent (n-heptane, benzene, ether) to its solubility in water.

passive diffusion   The passage of lipid soluble, unionized substances from the high concentration side of a membrane to the low concentration side by dissolving in the lipid portion of the membrane.

pentapeptide   A peptide chain containing five amino acids.

peptide   Two or more amino acids joined by peptide bonds.

peptide bond   A covalent bond between two amino acids in which the α-amino group of one is covalently bonded to the α-carboxyl group of the other through the removal of a molecule of water.

perikaryon   The cell body of a neuron. Also known as the soma.

peristalsis   The waves of contraction that pass along the alimentary canal thereby propelling its contents to adjacent sections.

PGO spikes   Bursts of phasic electrical activity seen in the EEG that originate in the pons (P) followed by activity in the lateral geniculate (G) nucleus and optic (O) cortex. These spikes are a characteristic precursor of REM sleep.

pH   The negative logarithm of the effective hydrogen ion concentration in gram equivalents per liter; used in expressing both acidity and alkalinity on a scale whose values run from 0 to 14 with 7 representing neutrality. Numbers less than 7 denote increasing acidity, and numbers greater than 7 denote increasing alkalinity. Thus $7 = 10^{-7}$ grams of H^+/liter; $1 = 10^{-1}$ or .1 gram H^+/liter.

phantasticants   Drugs such as LSD, DMT, mescaline, etc. that produce vivid visual phenomena regarded as phantasmagoria.

pharmacodynamic tolerance   An adaptation to the effects of a drug even when plasma levels of the drug are high. It is attributed to a diminished number of receptors or lower affinity of the receptors for the drug.

pharmacological denervation   A drug-induced condition resembling surgical destruction of nerves. Long term loss of neuronal activity frequently results in increased sensitivity to the missing neurotransmitter.

phenylquinine writhing test   The i.p. injection of phenylquinine causes pain and writhing in animals. It is used to test the efficacy of analgesics.

pheochromocytoma   A tumor of the adrenal gland which results in abnormal production and release of epinephrine. *See* paroxysmal tachycardia.

pheromone   A chemical substance used in communication between animals of the same species.

physical dependence   A compulsion for repeated drug use which serves to forestall the appearance of withdrawal symptoms.

picogram One trillionth (10^{-12}) gram.

pineal gland A small outgrowth of the epithalamus that rests upon the dorsal surface of the mesencephalon between the superior colliculi. Its synthesis of the hormone melatonin and 5-hydroxy-tryptophol is circadian in nature and is driven by a pacemaker in the brain.

pinocytosis A type of absorption by cells in which the cellular membrane forms a saccular structure, engulfs the extracellular substance, and closes so that the saccule becomes a vesicle within the cell.

$_p K_a$ The negative logarithm of the acid dissociation constant (K_a) which is a measure of the strength of an acid. The higher the value of K_a the greater the number of hydrogen ions liberated per mole of acid in solution, and hence the stronger the acid. The $_p K_a$ is equal to the pH of the solution in which a drug is 50 percent ionized and 50 percent unionized.

placebo A pharmacologically inert substance that is usually administered as a control substance during studies on the effectiveness of drugs.

placebo effect A physiological or behavioral reaction to a pharmacologically inert substance.

placental barrier The characteristics of the placenta that prevent the passage of some substances from the blood stream of the mother to that of the fetus.

plasma proteins Proteins (e.g. albumin) that are found in blood plasma. Some drugs are inactivated by binding to these proteins.

polypeptides Molecules consisting of a chain length of more than 10 amino acids.

polyribosomes A cellular complex consisting of a thread of messenger RNA and ribosomes which is involved in protein synthesis in the soma of cells.

poor vesicle axon terminal An axon terminal having uncharacteristically few synaptic vesicles.

positive reinforcement A reward or reinforcement that will increase the probability of the response that led to the reward.

presynaptic inhibition Inhibition of a postsynaptic cell by a prior depolarization of a presynaptic terminal via an axoaxonic synapse. The inhibition is presumably due to a diminished release of the neurotransmitter from the presynaptic terminal.

prevertebral ganglia Clusters of nerve cell bodies found in the abdominal cavity whose axons innervate the organs of the viscera sympathetically. They are named the coeliac, the superior mesenteric and inferior mesenteric ganglia.

progesterone A hormone that is synthesized in the ovary. It prepares the lining of the uterus for the implantation of the fertilized ovum, and increases the secretion of milk from the breasts. It also inhibits the contractions of the uterus.

proteolipid A macromolecule containing protein and lipid elements.

proteolytic enzymes Enzymes that degrade the bonds between the amino acids that make up protein, for example, trypsin.

proximal The part of a cut nerve that is still attached to the cell body.

psychological dependence An intense craving or drive to take a drug; a feeling that drug use is necessary to perform at optimum levels.

psychomotor epilepsy A form of epilepsy characterized by motor activity of which the patient is unaware.

psychoses A classification of serious psychiatric disorders usually requiring hospitalization, and characterized by marked distorts of reality and disturbances in perception, intellectual functioning, affect (mood), motivation, and motor behavior.

pulvinar A nucleus of nerve cells at the posterior pole of the dorsal thalamus serving to integrate visual inputs between other thalamic centers and the associative cortex.

Purkinje cells Giant nerve cells of the cerebellar cortex providing the output from the cortex of the cerebellum.

pyramidal cells Large, pyramid-shaped nerve cells in the motor cortex whose function is fine motor control of the upper extremities.

quaternary amine A compound containing a quaternary nitrogen, a positively charged nitrogen atom to which are attached four organic groups such as CH_3. Choline is a quaternary amine.

quantum A given quantity, or a sufficient quantity for a given effect.

radioimmunoassay *See* immunoassay.

raphe (ruh-PHAY) A region in the midbrain situated along the midline just dorsal to the Aqueduct of Sylvius.

receptor site   A locus on the surface of a cell probably occupied by a specific molecule that interacts with an endogenous hormone or neurotransmitter, or with exogenous drugs that alter functions of those cells.

reciprocal reflex or **reciprocal innervation**   A reflex that integrates the muscles of the body or of a limb to permit purposive action. For example, to permit the arm to be flexed by contracting the biceps, the triceps are reciprocally inhibited. Thus the action of a muscle leads to the inhibition of the antagonist muscle.

reduction   A chemical process in which a carbon atom reduces its number of bonds to oxygen or nitrogen.

reinforcement   Any event that follows a behavioral response and increases the probability of recurrence of the response.

relative refractory period   A brief period following an action potential when a second action potential can be generated only if the stimulus is somewhat greater than usual. These periods occur during afterpotentials.

REM sleep   Rapid eye movement sleep. *See* paradoxical sleep.

Renshaw cells   Small internuncial cells found in the ventral horn of the spinal cord. They form connections between axon recurrent collaterals and the cell bodies of motoneurons thus providing inhibitory feedback to motoneurons.

resting potential   The voltage difference between the inside and outside surfaces of a cell membrane when the membrane is at rest. In nerve cell membranes the resting potential is approximately -70 mV with the inside surface being negative, the outside positive.

ribosome   Small cellular organelles involved in protein synthesis.

Ringer's solution   A solution that contains sodium chloride, potassium chloride, sodium bicarbonate, monosodium phosphate, magnesium chloride, and dextrose. Resembling normal body fluids, it is used as a vehicle for injecting drugs and to maintain cells and tissue *in vitro* in an isosmotic state.

saturation   A state in which all available drug receptors have been bound to drug molecules. Saturation can refer to an organic compound in which hydrogen atoms are linked to every carbon bond.

Schwann cells   Cells which are associated with neuraxons in the peripheral nervous system. The function of Schwann cells is the formation of myelin sheaths around the axons.

septal lesions   Experimental brain lesions involving the septum, a nuclear structure in the brain of animals.

shuttle-box avoidance procedure   A conditioned avoidance procedure in which animals are given a warning signal to cross to an opposite compartment. Failure to do so within a short period (10 sec) leads to foot shocks until the animal escapes to the opposite compartment.

side effects   Secondary effects of a drug that are usually undesirable and different from its therapeutic effect. Example: constipation is a side effect when morphine or codeine is administered to relieve severe pain.

Sidman avoidance procedure or **continuous avoidance procedure**   The operant procedure involving the delivery of brief periods of shock or other aversive stimuli at fixed intervals. The aversive stimulus presentation can be delayed by a fixed interval if the subject makes the appropriate response.

silent receptors   Receptors or accumulation sites at which a drug will bind producing no observable physiological response.

sleep factor delta   A proposed peptide in the cerebral spinal fluid of a sleep-deprived dog that will induce sleep in a normal recipient dog.

slow wave sleep   A stage of sleep that is associated with an EEG showing 1-4 Hz electrical fluctuations with peak voltages of 30 to 150 uV. Also known as S-sleep.

sodium dependent   Physiological reactions that depend upon the presence of sodium.

sodium pump or **sodium potassium pump**   The hypothesized mechanism that maintains the proper balance between cytoplasmic sodium and potassium ions by expelling excess sodium and replacing potassium deficiencies.

soma   The cell body of a neuron.

somatostatin or **somatotropin release inhibiting factor (SRIF)**   A peptide released from the hypothalamus that controls the release of somatotropin from the pituitary gland. Somatostatin is also found in other sites of the CNS and in other tissues, and probably has a neurotransmitter role.

somatotropin   The pituitary hormone that controls body growth.

spatial summation The additive effect of post-synaptic potentials when two or more occur in close spatial proximity on a neuron membrane.

species-specific behavior A type of behavior that is regarded as specific for a particular species. For example, the building of a unique nest structure by birds of the same species.

splanchnic nerves The nerves that have their origin in the lateral horns of the spinal cord and terminate in the prevertebral ganglia from whence postganglionic fibers proceed to the visceral organs for sympathetic innervation.

S-sleep *See* slow wave sleep.

state dependent learning Learning that takes place during a drug-induced state or a no-drug state which then fails to generalize to the opposite state.

stereospecific A characteristic of receptors that permits them to bind to a chemical compound but not to its optical isomer.

stereotaxic apparatus A device which holds the head of an animal or person, permitting accurate placement into the brain of electrodes, cannulas, or cutting instruments.

subcellular fractionation A process by which the parts of cells can be separated for microscopic and chemical analysis. Usually the cells are broken and centrifuged in sucrose layers of different densities to separate the lighter from the heavier cellular fragments.

subcutaneous injection The hypodermic injection of a substance between the layers of the skin for slow diffusion into the blood stream.

subneural clefts or **junctional folds** A series of invaginations underlying the synaptic gutter of a neuromyal junction. They apparently serve to maximize the surface contact between a nerve ending and a somatic muscle membrane.

substrate A substance upon which an enzyme acts.

sucrose gradient centrifugation The centrifugation of cellular particles through layers of increasing densities of sucrose. In this way cell constituents of different weights can be separated.

suprachiasmatic nucleus A nucleus lying dorsal to the optic chiasma in the diencephalon, that plays a role in circadian rhythms. Sometimes, perhaps erroneously referred to as the biological clock.

supra-optic nucleus A cell group of the hypothalamus located directly above the optic chiasma. Its stimulation leads to a release of vasopressin [also known as the anti-diuretic hormone (ADH)], from the posterior pituitary gland.

sympatholytic That which inhibits the sympathetic branch of the autonomic nervous system. Example: a sympatholytic drug would block adrenergic receptors.

sympathomimetic That which mimics the sympathetic branch of the autonomic nervous system. Example: a drug that enhances catecholamine synaptic transmission.

synapse The junction usually between the axon terminals of one neuron and the dendrites or soma of an adjacent neuron. Nerve impulses in the axon cause a release of neurotransmitters at the synapse that act upon the adjacent neuron either to excite or inhibit it.

synaptic cleft or **synaptic gap** The narrow space that separates the presynaptic membrane from the postsynaptic membrane.

synaptic gap substance A mucilagenous protein material that is found in the synaptic gap. It is suggested that these materials contribute to the proper adherence of the presynaptic to the postsynaptic membranes.

synaptic knob The axon terminal, swelling or bouton that makes up the presynaptic part of the synapse.

synaptic varicosities Synaptic swellings that occur at frequent intervals along axons, especially those found in axons of the autonomic nervous system. This arrangement assures wide distribution of a neuron's effect upon a gland or muscle. Within the CNS such neurons may form contacts with thousands of other neurons.

synaptopores Putative openings or pores in the presynaptic membrane through which the neurotransmitter molecules pass to the synaptic cleft.

synaptosomes Nerve cell material obtained by subcellular fractionation that contains the membrane-enclosed synaptic terminals containing vesicles and neurotransmitters. Frequently parts of the postsynaptic membrane adhere to the terminals.

synthetic reaction *See* conjugation.

tachyphylaxis The rapid adaptation (tolerance) to the pharmacological effect of a drug.

teldiencephalon A transitional zone between the hypothalamic nuclei of the diencephalon and the medial limbic structures of the telencephalon. The zone includes the preoptic area and the suprachiasmatic nucleus.

temporal summation The additive effect of postsynaptic potentials when two or more occur close together in time. (See spatial summation.)

thalamus Cell groups in the diencephalon having the principal functions of integration and projection of sensory nerve impulses to the cerebral hemispheres.

therapeutic index The ratio of the median lethal dose (LD 50) to the median effective dose (ED 50). The higher the ratio, the safer the drug for therapeutic purposes. *See* effective dose 50 and lethal dose 50.

theta activity Electrical waves of 4-7 Hz that are recorded from the hippocampus. These waves correlate with desynchronized low voltage waves from the cerebral cortex signifying a state of arousal.

tight junctions The junctions formed by the endothelial cells of capillaries in the central nervous system. The cells are tightly pressed against each other preventing most substances from passing between them.

tolerance The reduction in potency of a given drug following repeated use of that drug or a related drug.

torpedo or **ray** One of a group of cartilagenous fishes, that have the ability to administer electric shocks into their prey or enemies.

toxic dose 50 (TD 50) The dose of a drug that produces a given toxic effect in 50 percent of the subjects tested.

tricarboxylic acid cycle (the Krebs cycle) A series of metabolic actions that occur in mitochondria that result in the oxidation of fuels obtained from food to release energy.

tricyclic anti-depressants Compounds used to relieve symptoms of depression. Derived from phenothiazines, they block the reuptake of monoamines.

trophotropic Descriptive of decreased responsiveness, decreased muscle tone, and increased activity of the parasympathetic nervous system.

troponin-myosin system A mechanism which inhibits the reaction between actin and myosin in muscle tissue and thus blocks muscle contractions.

tuberoinfundibular DA neurons Neurons originating in the arcuate nucleus of the hypothalamus and projecting to the median eminence and the pituitary gland.

tubulin A soluble protein found abundantly in the brain. The protein is composed of two different polypeptides that form microtubules in neurons. It is a major protein that is found in axoplasmic transport.

turnover time With respect to neurotransmitters, this refers to the rate of enzyme synthesis, release and metabolism.

unipolar depression Depressed states that do not alternate with periods of excitement or mania.

vagus nerve The 10th cranial nerve, part of which arises from the medulla and distributes its axons to the parasympathetically innervated structures of the viscera except those in the pelvic region.

variable interval schedule (VI) An operant schedule which encourages high rates of responding. Reinforcement is dependent upon a response following a variable time after the previous reinforcement.

vasoconstrictor A drug or hormone that constricts blood vessels thereby limiting blood flow and raising blood pressure.

vesicles Small (20-120 nm) membrane-enclosed spherical units containing neurotransmitter molecules found in large numbers in the synaptic terminals of axons. They are referred to as storage, terminal, or synaptic vesicles.

vigilance task A behavioral test requiring high arousal and close attention in order to detect weak stimuli that are randomly presented.

withdrawal symptoms *See* abstinence syndrome.

X-ray diffraction An analytical method of determining the molecular structure of a substance. A thin section or drop of a substance is irradiated by a narrow X-ray beam and its molecular structure is interpreted from the dispersal pattern that the X-ray particles deposit on a film.

Bibliography

Abdulla, Y.H. and Hamadah, K. (1970), 3', 5'-Cyclic adenosine monophosphate in depression and mania. *Lancet,* 1, 378–381.

Adams, E. (1958). Barbiturates. *Sci Am.,* 198, 1, 60–64.

Agarwal, R.A., Rastogi, R.B. and Singhal, R.L. (1977). Enhancement of locomotor activity and catecholamine and 5-hydroxytryptamine metabolism by thyrotropin-releasing hormone. *Neuroendocrinol.,* 23, 236–247.

Aghajanian, G.K. and Bunney, B.S. (1973). Central dopaminergic neurons: neurophysiological identification and responses to drugs. In *Frontiers in Catecholamine Research* (E. Usdin and S. Snyder, Eds.), pp. 643–648. Pergamon Press, Elmsford, New York.

Aghajanian, G.K. and Bunney, B.S. (1977). Dopamine "autoreceptors": pharmocological characterization by microiontophoretic single cell recording studies. *Arch. Pharmacol.,* 297, 1–7.

Aghajanian, G.K., Cedarbaum, J.M. and Wang, R.Y. (1977). Evidence for norepinephrine-mediated collateral inhibitions of locus ceruleus neurons. *Brain Res.,* 136, 570–577.

Aghajanian, G.K., Graham, A.W. and Sheard, M.H. (1970). Serotonin-containing neurons in brain: depression of firing by monoamine oxidase inhibitors. *Science,* 169, 1100–1102.

Aghajanian, G.K. and Haigler, H.J. (1974). Mode of action of LSD on serotonergic neurons. In *Advances in Biochemical Psychopharmacology, Vol. 10* (E. Costa, G.L. Gessa, M. Sandler, Eds.), pp. 167–178. Raven Press, New York.

Aghajanian, G.K. Haigler, H.J. and Bennett, J.L. (1975). Amine receptors in CNS. III, 5-hydroxytryptamine in brain. In *Handbook of Psychopharmacology, Vol. 6* (L.L. Iversen, S.D. Iversen and S.H. Snyder, Eds.), pp. 63–96. Plenum Press, New York.

Aghajanian, G.K., Rosecrans, J.A. and Sheard, M.H. (1967). Serotonin: release in the forebrain by stimulation of midbrain raphe. *Science,* 156, 402–403.

Aghajanian, G.K. and Wang, R.Y. (1977). Habenular and other midbrain raphe afferents demonstrated by a modified retrograde tracing technique. *Brain Res.,* 122, 229–242.

Aghajanian, G.K. and Wang, R.Y. (1978). Physiology and pharmacology of central serotonergic neurons. In *Psychopharmacology: A Generation of Progress* (M.A. Lipton, A. DiMascio and K.F. Killam, Eds.), pp. 171–183. Raven Press, New York.

Agranoff, B.W., Burrell, H.R., Dokas, L.A. and Springer, A.D. (1978). Progress in biochemical approaches to learning and memory. In *Psychopharmacology: A Generation of Progress* (M.A. Lipton, A. DiMascio and K.F. Killam, Eds.), pp. 623–635. Raven Press, New York.

Ahlquist, R.P. (1948). A study of adrenotropic receptors. *Am. J. Physiol.,* 153, 586–600.

Ahlquist, R.P. (1979). Adrenoreceptors. *Trends in Pharmacological Sciences,* 1, 16–17.

Ahlskog, J.E. and Hoebel, B.G. (1973). Overeating and obesity from damage to a noradrenergic system in the brain. *Science,* 182, 166–169.

Ajmone Marsan, C. and Traczyk, W.Z. (Eds.) (1980). Neuropeptides and neural transmission. In *International Brain Research Organization Monograph Series, Vol. 7.* Raven Press, New York.

Akert, K., Moore, K., Pfenninger, K. and Sandri, C. (1969). Contributions of new impregnation methods and freeze etching to the problems of synaptic fine structure. In *Progress in Brain Research, Vol. 31* (K. Akert and P.G. Waser, Eds.), pp. 223–240. Elsevier, Amsterdam.

Akert, K., Peper, K. and Sandri, C. (1975). Structural organization of motor end plate and central synapses. In *Cholinergic Mechanisms* (P.G. Waser, Ed.), pp. 43–57. Raven Press, New York.

451

Akil, H. and Liebeskind, J.C. (1975). Monoaminergic mechanisms of stimulation-produced analgesia. *Brain Res.*, 94, 279-296.

Akil, H., Mayer, D.J. and Liebeskind, J.C. (1976). Antagonism of stimulation-produced analgesia by naloxone, a narcotic antagonist. *Science*, 191, 961-962.

Akil, H., Richardson, D.E., Hughes, J. and Barchas, J.D. (1978). Enkephalin-like material elevated in ventricular cerebrospinal fluid of pain patients after analgesic focal stimulation. *Science*, 201, 463-465.

Anden, N.E. (1974). Effect of acute axotomy (spinal cord transection) on the turnover of 5-hydroxytryptamine. In *Advances in Biochemical Psychopharmacology, Vol. 10* (E. Costa, G.L. Gessa and M. Sandler, Eds.), pp. 35-43. Raven Press, New York.

Andersson, K. (1975). Effects of cigarette smoking on learning and retention. *Psychopharmacologia*, 41, 1-5.

Angrist, B. and Sudilovsky, A. (1978). Central nervous system stimulants: historical aspects and clinical effects. In *Handbook of Psychopharmacology, Vol. 11* (L.L. Iversen, S.D. Iversen and S.H. Snyder, Eds.), pp. 99-165. Plenum Press, New York.

Angrist, B. and Gershon, S. (1970). The phenomenology of experimentally induced amphetamine psychosis. Preliminary observations. *Biol. Psychiatry*, 2, 95-107.

Anlezark, G.M., Crow, T.J. and Greenway, A.P. (1973). Impaired learning and decreased cortical norepinephrine after bilateral locus caeruleus lesions. *Science*, 181, 682-684.

Antelman, S.M. and Caggiula, A.R. (1977). Norepinephrine-dopamine interactions and behavior. *Science*, 195, 646-653.

Appel, J.B. (1968). The effects of "psychotomimetic" drugs on animal behavior. In *Psychopharmacology-A Review of Progress* (D.H. Efron, Ed.), Public Health Service Publication No. 1836. U.S. Gov't Printing Office, Washington, D.C.

Appel, S.H. and Day, E.D. (1976). Cellular and subcellular fractionation. In *Basic Neurochemistry* (G.J. Siegel, R.W. Alberts, R. Katzman and B.W. Agranoff, Eds.), pp. 34-59. Little, Brown, Boston.

Aprison, M.H. (1978). Glycine as a neurotransmitter. In *Psychopharmacology: A Generation of Progress* (M.A. Lipton, A. DiMascio and K.F. Killam, Eds.), pp. 333-346. Raven Press, New York.

Aprison, M.H. and Daly, E.C. (1975). Biochemical aspects of transmission at inhibitory synapses: the role of glycine. In *Advances in Neurochemistry, Vol. 3* (B.W. Agranoff and M.H. Aprison, Eds.), pp. 203-294. Plenum Press, New York.

Aprison, M.H., Daly, E.C., Shank, R.P. and McBride, W.J. (1975). Neurochemical evidence for glycine as a transmitter and a model for its intrasynaptosomal compartmentation. In *Metabolic Compartmentation and Neurotransmission* (S. Berl, D.D. Clarke and D. Schneider, Eds.), pp. 37-63. Plenum Press, New York.

Aprison, M.H. and Ferster, C.B. (1961). Neurochemical correlates of behavior. II. Correlation of brain monoamine oxidase activity with behavioral changes after iproniazid and 5-hydroxytryptophan. *J. Neurochem.*, 6, 350-357.

Aprison, M.H., Shank, R.P., Davidoff, R.A. and Werman, R. (1968). The distribution of glycine, a neurotransmitter suspect in the central nervous system of several vertebrate species. *Life Sci.*, 7, Part 1, 583-590.

Aprison, M.H. and Werman, R. (1965). The distribution of glycine in cat spinal cord and roots. *Life Sci.*, 4, 2075-2083.

Armstrong, C.M. and Hille, B. (1972). The inner *quaternary* ammonium ion receptor in potassium channels of the node of Ranvier. *J. Gen. Physiol.*, 59, 388-400.

Armstrong, D., Dry, R.M., Keele, C.A. and Markham, J.W. (1951). Method for studying chemical excitants of cutaneous pain in man. *J. Physiol.*, 115, 59P-61P.

Arnhoff, F.N. (1975). Social consequences of policy toward mental illness. *Science*, 188, 1277-1281.

Aronson, B. and Osmond, H. (1970). *Psychedelics*. Doubleday, Garden City, New York.

Arvanitaki, A. and Chalazonitis, N. (1961). Excitatory and inhibitory processes. In *Nervous Inhibition* (E. Florey, Ed.), pp. 194-231. Pergamon Press, London.

Asberg, M., Thoren, P., Traskman, L., Bertilsson, L. and Ringberger, V. (1976). "Serotonin Depression" - a biochemical subgroup within the affective disorders? *Science*, 191, 478-480.

Asher, I.M. and Aghajanian, G.K. (1974). 6-Hydroxydopamine lesions of olfactory tubercles and caudate nuclei: effect on amphetamine-induced sterotyped behavior in rats. *Brain Res.*, 82, 1-12.

Axelrod, J. (1957). *O*-Methylation of epinephrine and other catechols in vitro and in vivo. *Science*, 126, 1657-1660.

Axelrod, J. (1962). The enzymatic *N*-methylation of serotonin and other amines. *J. Pharmacol. Exp. Ther.*, 138, 28-33.

Axelrod, J. (1971). Noradrenaline: fate and control of its biosynthesis. *Science*, 173, 598-606.

Axelrod, J. (1974a). Regulation of the neurotransmitter norepinephrine. In *The Neurosciences, Third Study Program* (F.O. Schmitt and F.G. Worden, Eds.), pp. 863-876. MIT Press, Cambridge, Massachusetts.

Axelrod, J. (1974b). The pineal gland: a neurochemical transducer. *Science*, 184, 1341-1348.

Ayd, F.J., Jr. (1977). Ethical and legal dilemmas posed by tardive dyskinesia. *Int. Drug Ther. Newsl.* 12, 29-36.

Azmitia, E.C. (1978). The serotonin-producing neurons of the midbrain median and dorsal nuclei. In *Handbook of Psychopharmacology, Vol. 9* (L.L. Iversen, S.D. Iversen, and S.H. Snyder, Eds.), pp. 233-314. Plenum Press, New York.

Babigian, H.M. (1975). Schizophrenia: epidemiology. In *Comprehensive Textbook of Psychiatry, Vol. 11* (A.M. Freedman, H.I. Kaplan and B.J. Sadock, Eds.), pp. 860–866. Williams and Wilkins, Baltimore.

Balasz, R., Machiyama, Y., Hammond, B.J., Julian, T. and Richter, D. (1970). The operation of γ-aminobutyrate bypath of the tricarboxylic acid cycle in brain tissue in vitro. *Biochem. J.,* 116, 445–461.

Baldessarini, R.J. (1975). The basis for amine hypotheses in affective disorders. *Arch. Gen. Psychiat.,* 32, 1087–1093.

Baldessarini, R.J. (1977). *Chemotherapy in Psychiatry,* Harvard Univ. Press, Cambridge, Massachusetts.

Baldessarini, R.J. and Lipinski, J.F. (1975). Lithium salts: 1970–1975. *Ann. Intern. Med.,* 83, 527–533.

Banerjee, S.P. and Snyder, S.H. (1973). Methyl tetrahydrofolic acid mediates *N*- and *O*-methylation of biogenic amines. *Science,* 182, 74–75.

Baraldi, M., Guidotti, A., Schwarz, J.P. and Costa, E. (1979). GABA receptors in clonal cell lines: a model for study of benzodiazepine action at molecular level. *Science,* 205, 821–823.

Barbeau, A. (1978). The last ten years of progress in the clinical pharmacology of extrapyramidal symptoms. In *Psychopharmacology: A General of Progress* (M.A. Lipton, A. DiMascio, and K.F. Killam, Eds.), pp. 771–776. Raven, New York.

Barchas, J.D., Akil, H., Elliott, G.R., Holman, R.B. and Watson, S.J. (1978). Behavioral neurochemistry: neuroregulators and behavioral states. *Science,* 200, 964–973.

Barchas, J.D., Berger, P.A., Mathysse, S. and Wyatt, R.J. (1977). The biochemistry of affective disorders and schizophrenia. In *Principles of Psychopharmacology* (W.G. Clark and J. del Giudice, Eds.). Academic Press, New York.

Barker, J.L. and Gainer, H. (1973). Pentobarbital: selective depression of excitatory postsynaptic potentials. *Science,* 182, 720–722.

Barker, J.L. and Smith, T.G. (Eds.) (1980). *The Role of Peptides in Neuronal Function.* Marcel Dekker, New York.

Barnea, A. (1978). Demonstration of a temperature-dependent association of thyrotropin releasing hormone, α-melanocyte stimulating hormone and α-leutinizing hormone-releasing hormone with subneural particles in hypothalamic synaptosomes. *J. Neurochem.,* 31, 1125–1130.

Barnea, A., Neaves, W.B., Cho, G. and Porter, J.C. (1978). A subcellular pool of hyposmotically resistant particles containing thyrotropin releasing hormone, a malanocyte stimulating hormone, and leutenizing hormone-releasing hormone in the rat hypothalamus. *J. Neurochem.,* 30, 937–948.

Bassuk, E.L. and Gerson, S. (1978). Deinstitutionalization and mental health services. *Sci. Am.,* 238, 2, 46–53.

Bazemore, A.W., Elliott, K.A.C. and Florey, E. (1957). Isolation of Factor I. *J. Neurochem.,* 1, 334–339.

Beecher, H.K. (1957). The measurement of pain. *Pharmacol. Rev.,* 9, 59–209.

Belin, M., Kauyoumdjian, J.C., Bardakdjian, J., Duhault, J. and Gonnard, P. (1976). Effect of fenfluramine on accumulation of 5-hydroxytryptamine and other transmitters into synaptosomes of rat brain. *Neuropharmacol.,* 15, 613–617.

Belluzzi, J.D., Grant, D., Gorsky, V., Sarantakis, D., Wise, C.D. and Stein, L. (1976). Analgesia induced in vivo by central administration of enkephalin in rat. *Nature,* 260, 625–626.

Belmaker, R., Murphy, D., Wyatt, R.J. and Lorieux, D.L. (1974). Human platelet monoamine oxidase changes during the menstrual cycle. *Arch. Gen. Psychiatry, 31, 557–560.*

Benjamin, A.M. and Quastel, J.H. (1981). Acetylcholine synthesis in synaptosomes: mode of transfer of mitochondrial acetyl coenzyme A. *Science,* 213, 1495–1497.

Bennett, J.L. and Aghajanian, G.K. (1974). D-LSD binding to brain homogenates: possible relationship to serotonin receptors. *Life Sci.,* 15, 1935–1944.

Bennett, J.P. and Snyder, S.H. (1975). Stereospecific binding of *d*-lysergic acid diethylamide (LSD) to brain membranes: relationship to serotonin receptors. *Brain Res.,* 94, 523–544.

Bennett, M.V.L. (Ed.) (1974). *Synaptic Transmission and Neuronal Interaction.* Raven Press, New York.

Benuck, M. and Marks, N. (1975). Enzymatic inactivation of substance P by a partially purified enzyme from rat brain. *Biochem. Biophys. Res. Commun.,* 65, 153–160.

Berger, B., Thierry, A.M., Tassin, J.P. and Moyne, M.A. (1976). Dopaminergic innervation of the rat prefrontal cortex: a fluorescence histochemical study. *Brain Res.,* 106, 133–145.

Berger, F.M. (1962). Pharmacodynamics of meprobamate: differences between meprobamate and barbiturates. In *Psychosomatic Medicine* (J.A. Nodine and J.H. Moyer, Eds.), pp. 495–501. Lea and Febiger, Philadelphia.

Berger, F.M. and Ludwig, B.J. (1964). Meprobamate and related compounds. In *Medicinal Chemistry, Vol. 1, Psychopharmacological Agents* (M. Gordon, Ed.), pp. 103–135. Academic Press, New York.

Berger, P.A. (1977). Antidepressant medications in the treatment of depression. In *Psychopharmacology: From Theory to Practice* (J.D. Barchas, P.A. Berger, R.D. Ciaranello and G.R. Elliott, Eds.), pp. 174–207. Oxford Univ. Press, New York.

Berger, P.A. and Tinklenberg, J.R. (1977). Treatment of abusers of alcohol and other addictive drugs. In *Psychopharmacology: From Theory to Practice* (J.D. Barchas, P.A. Berger, R.D. Ciaranello and G.R. Elliott, Eds.), pp. 355–382. Oxford Univ. Press, New York.

Bergstrom, D.A. and Kellar, K.J. (1979). Effect of electro-convulsive shock on monoaminergic receptor binding sites in rat brain. *Nature*, 278, 464–466.

Berl, S. (1975). The actomyosin-like system in nervous tissue. In *The Nervous System, Vol. 1, The Basic Neurosciences* (D.B. Tower, Ed.) pp. 565–573. Raven Press, New York.

Berl, S., Puszkin S. and Nicklas, W.J. (1973). Actomyosin-like protein in brain. *Science*, 179, 441–446.

Berman, J. and Yi-Yung Hsia, D. (1970). Nutritional psycho-pharmacology: inherited metabolic disorders and mental retardation. In *Principles of Psychopharmacology* (W.G. Clark and J. del Guidice, Eds.), pp. 355–371. Academic Press, New York.

Bickerton, R.K. and Buckley, J.P. (1961). Evidence for a central mechanism of angiotensin induced hypertension. *Proc. Soc. Exp. Biol. Med.*, 106, 834.

Biel, J.H. and Bopp, B.A. (1978). Amphetamine: structure-activity relationships. In *Handbook of Psychopharmacology, Vol. 11* (L.L. Iversen, S.D. Iversen and S.H. Snyder, Eds.), pp. 1–39. Plenum Press, New York.

Bignami, G. (1978). Effects of neuroleptics, ethanol, hypnotic-sedatives, tranquilizers, narcotics, and minor stimulants in aversive paradigms. In *Psychopharmacology of Aversively Motivated Behavior* (H. Anisman and G. Bignami, Eds.), pp. 385–453. Plenum Press, New York.

Bignami, G. and Michalek, H. (1978). Cholinergic mechanisms and aversely motivated behaviors. In *Psychopharmacology and Aversely Motivated Behavior* (H. Anisman and G. Bignami, Eds.), pp. 173–255. Plenum Press, New York.

Bird, E.D., Spokes, E.G. and Iversen, L.L. (1979). Brain norepinephrine and dopamine in schizophrenia. *Science*, 204, 93–94.

Bird, S.J. and Aghajanian, G.K. (1975). Denervation super-sensitivity in the cholinergic septohippocampal pathway: a microiontophoretic study. *Brain Res.*, 100, 355–370.

Birks, R. and MacIntosh, F.C. (1961). Actylcholine metabolism of a sympathetic ganglion. *Can. J. Biochem. Physiol.*, 39, 787–827.

Biscoe, T.J. and Straughan, D.W. (1966). Micro-electro-phoretic studies of neurons in the cat hippocampus. *J. Physiol. (London)*, 201, 341–359.

Björklund, A. Baumgarten, H-G. and Nobin, A. (1974). Chemical lesioning of central monoamine axons by means of 5,6-dihydroxytryptamine and 5,7-dihydroxytryptamine. In *Advances in Biochemical Pharmacology, Vol. 10* (E. Costa, G.L. Gessa and M. Sandler, Eds.), pp. 13–33. Raven Press, New York.

Björklund, A. and Lindvall, O. (1975). Dopamine in dendrites of substantia nigra neurons: suggestions for a role in dendritic terminals. *Brain Res.*, 83, 531–553.

Björklund, A. Lindvall, O. and Nobin, A. (1975). Evidence of an incertohypothalamic dopamine neurone system in the rat. *Brain Res.*, 89, 29–42.

Blackshear, P.J. (1979). Implantable drug-delivery systems. *Sci. Am.*, 241, 6, 66–73.

Blackwell, B. (1973). Psychotropic drugs in use today. The role of diazepam in medical practice. *J. Am. Med. Assoc.*, 225, 1637–1641.

Blaschko, H. (1939). The specific action of L-dopa decarboxylase. *J. Physiol.*, 96, 50–51.

Bliss, E.L. and Ailion, J. (1970). The effect of lithium upon brain neuroamines. *Brain Res.*, 24, 305–310.

Bloch, R.G., Dooneief, A.S., Buchberg, A.S. and Spellman, S. (1954). The clinical effect of isoniazid and iproniazid in the treatment of pulmonary tuberculosis. *Ann. Intern. Med.*, 40, 881–900.

Bloom, F.E. (1981). Neuropeptides. *Sci. Am.*, 245, 4, 148–168.

Bloom, F.E., Hoffer, B.J. and Siggins, G.R. (1973). Central noradrenergic receptors: localization, function, and molecular mechanisms. In *New Concepts in Neurotransmitter Regulation* (A.J. Mandell, Ed.), pp. 223–238. Plenum Press, New York.

Bloom, F.E. and Iversen, L.L. (1971). Localizing ^{3}H-GABA in nerve terminals of rat cerebral cortex by electron microscopic autoradiography. *Nature*, 229, 629–630.

Bloom, F.E., Segal, D., Ling, N. and Guillemin, R. (1976). Endorphins: profound behaviorial effects in rats suggest new etiological factors in mental illness. *Science*, 194, 630–632.

Bloom, W. and Fawcett, D.W. (1968). *A Textbook of Histology*. Saunders, Philadelphia.

Blum, R.H. and Associates (1969). *Society and Drugs, Vol. 1, Drugs*. Jossey-Bass, San Francisco.

Blundell, J.E. (1977). Is there a role for serotonin (5-hydroxy-tryptamine) in feeding? *Int. J. Obesity*, 1, 15–42.

Bodian, D. (1962). The generalized vertebrate neuron. *Science*, 137, 323–326.

Bodian, D. (1972). Neuron junctions: a revolutionary decade. *Anat. Rec.*, 174, 73–82.

Bohus, B., Van Wimersma Greidanus, T.B. and de Wied, D. (1975). Behavioral and endocrine responses of rats with hereditary hypothalamic diabetes insipidus (Brattleboro strain). *Physiol. Behav.*, 14, 609–615.

Boissier, J.-R. (Ed.) (1978). *Differential Psychopharmacology of Anxiolytics and Sedatives*. S. Karger, New York.

Bourne, H.R., Bunney, W.E. and Colburn, R.W. (1968). Noradrenalin, 5-hydroxytryptamine, and 5-hydroxyindoleacetic acid in the hindbrains of suicidal patients. *Lancet*, 2, 805–808.

Bourne, P.G. and Slade, J.D. (1974). Methadone: the mechanism of its success. *J. Nerv. Ment. Dis.*, 159, 371–375.

Bradley, K., Easton, D.M. and Eccles, J.C. (1953). An investigation of primary or direct inhibition. *J. Physiol.*, 122, 474–488.

Brady, J.P. (1968). Drugs in behavior therapy. In *Psychopharmacology: A Review of Progress 1957-1967* (D.H.

Efron, Ed.), pp. 271–280. PHS Publ. 1836 U.S. Gov't. Printing Office, Washington, D.C.

Brady, J.V. (1956). Assessment of drug effects on emotional behavior. *Science,* 123, 1033–1034.

Braestrup, C., Albrechtsen, R. and Squires, R.F. (1977). High densities of benzodiazepine receptors in human cortical areas. *Nature,* 269, 702–704.

Braestrup, C. and Nielsen, H. (1978). Ontogenetic development of benzodiazepine receptors in the rat brain. *Brain Res.,* 147, 170–173.

Braestrup, C. and Squires, R.F. (1977). Specific benzodiazepine receptors in rat brain characterized by high affinity ^{3}H-diazepam binding. *Proc. Natl. Acad. Sci. U.S.A.,* 74, 3805–3809.

Braestrup, C. and Squires, R.F. (1978). Pharmacological characterization of benzodiazepine receptors in the brain. *Eur. J. Pharmacol.,* 48, 263–270.

Brands, B., Thornhill, J.A., Hirst, M. and Gowdey, C.W. (1979). Suppression of food intake and body weight gain by naloxone in rats. *Life Sci.,* 24, 1773–1778.

Brazier, M.A.B. (1961). *A History of the Electrical Activity of the Brain.* Pitman Medical Publ. Co., Ltd., London.

Brecher, E.M. (1972). *Licit and Illicit Drugs.* Little, Brown, Boston.

Breese, G.R. and Cooper, B.R. (1975). Behavioral and biochemical interactions of 5,7-DHT with various drugs when administered intracisternally to adult and developing rats. *Brain Res.,* 98, 517–528.

Breese, G.R., Cott, J.M., Cooper, B.R., Prange, A.J., Lipton, M.A. and Plotnikoff, N.P. (1975). Effects of thyrotropin-releasing hormone (TRH) on the actions of pentobarbital and other centrally acting drugs. *J. Pharmacol. Exp. Ther.,* 193, 11–22.

Bretscher, M.S. (1973). Membrane structure: some general principles. *Science,* 181, 622–629.

Brill, L. and Lieberman, L. (1969). *Authority and Addiction.* Little, Brown, Boston.

Brinley, F.J. (1974). Excitation and conduction in nerve fibers. In *Medical Physiology, Vol. 1* (V.B. Mountcastle, Ed.), pp. 34–76. The C.V. Mosby Co., St. Louis.

Brodie, B.B. and Shore, P.A. (1957). A concept for the role of serotonin and norepinephrine as chemical mediators in the brain. *Ann. N.Y. Acad. Sci.,* 66, 631–642.

Brown, D.A., Caulfield, M.P. and Kirby, P.J. (1979). Relation between catecholamine-induced cyclic AMP changes and hyperpolarization in isolated rat sympathetic ganglia. *J. Physiol.,* 290, 441–451.

Brownstein, M.J. (1978). Peptides in mammalian nervous tissue. In *Psychopharmacology: A Generation of Progress* (M.A. Lipton, A. DiMascio and K.F. Killam, Eds.), pp. 397–401. Raven Press, New York.

Brownstein, M.J., Saavedra, J.M., Palkovitz, M. and Axelrod, J. (1974). Histamine content of hypothalamic nuclei of the rat. *Brain Res.,* 77, 151–156.

Buchbaum, M.S., Coursey, R.D. and Murphy, D.L. (1976). The biochemical high-risk paradigm: behavioral and familial correlates of low platelet monoamine oxidase activity. *Science,* 194, 339–341.

Buckley, J.P., Smookler, H.H., Severs, W.B. and Deuben, R.R. (1977). A central site of action of angiotensin II. In *Central Actions of Angiotensin and Related Hormones* (J.P. Buckley and A. Ferrario, Eds.), pp. 149–155. Pergamon Press, New York.

Bunney, B.S. and Aghajanian, G.K. (1975a). Evidence for drug action on both pre- and postsynaptic catecholamine receptors in the CNS. In *Pre- and Postsynaptic Receptors* (E. Usdin and W.E. Bunney, Eds.), pp. 89–122. Marcel Dekker, New York.

Bunney, B.S. and Aghajanian, G.K. (1975b). Antipsychotic drugs and central dopaminergic neurons: a model for predicting therapeutic efficacy and incidence of extrapyramidal side effects. In *Predictability in Psychopharmacology: Preclinical and Clinical Correlations* (A. Sudilovsky, S. Gershon and B. Beer, Eds.), pp. 225–245. Raven Press, New York.

Bunney, B.S. and Aghajanian, G.K. (1978). Mesolimbic and mesocortical dopaminergic systems: physiology and pharmacology. In *Psychopharmacology: A Generation of Progress* (M.A. Lipton, A. DiMascio and K.F. Killam, Eds.), pp. 159–169. Raven Press, New York.

Burgen, A.S.V. and Iversen, L.L. (1965). The inhibition of norepinephrine uptake by sympathomimetic amines in the rat isolated heart. *Br. J. Phamacol.,* 25, 34–49.

Burns, D. and Mendels, J. (1977). Biogenic amine precursors and affective illness. In *Phenomenology and Treatment of Depression* (W.E. Fann, I. Karacan, A.D. Pokorny and R.L. Williams, Eds.), pp. 33–67. Spectrum Publications, New York.

Burnstock, G. (1970). Structure of smooth muscle and its innervation. In *Smooth Muscle* (E. Bülbring, A.F. Brading, A.W. Jones and T. Tomita, Eds.), pp. 1–69. Edward Arnold, London.

Burt, D.R. and Snyder, S.H. (1975). Thyrotropin-releasing hormone: apparent receptor binding in rat brain membranes. *Brain Res.,* 93, 309–328.

Buscher, H.H., Hill, R.C., Romer, D., Cardinaux, F., Closse, A., Hauser, D. and Pless, J. (1976). Evidence for analgesic activity of enkephalin in the mouse. *Nature,* 261, 423–425.

Calcutt, C.R., Handley, S.L., Sparkes, C.G. and Spencer, P.S.J. (1973). Roles on noradrenaline and 5-hydroxytryptamine in the antinociceptive effects of morphine. In *Agonist and Antagonist Actions of Narcotic Analgesic Drugs* (H.W. Kosterlitz, H.O.J. Collier and J.E. Villarreal, Eds.), pp. 176–191. University Park Press, Baltimore.

Caldwell, A.E. (1970). History of psychopharmacology. In *Principles of Psychopharmacology* (W.G. Clarke and J. del

Guidice, Eds.), pp. 9–30. Academic Press, New York.

Capaldi, R.A. (1974). A dynamic model of cell membranes. *Sci. Am.,* 230, 3, 26–28.

Caporael, L.R. (1976). Ergotism: the satan loosed in Salem? *Science,* 192, 21–26.

Carenzi, A., Gillin, J.C., Guidotti, A., Schwartz, M.A., Trabucchi, M. and Wyatt, R.J. (1975). Dopamine-sensitive adenylyl cyclase in human caudate nucleus. *Arch. Gen. Psychiatry,* 32, 1056–1059.

Carlson, N.R. (1981). *Physiology of Behavior,* Allyn and Bacon, Boston.

Carlsson, A. (1974). Measurements of monoamine synthesis and turnover with special reference to 5-hydroxytryptamine. In *Advances in Biochemical Psychopharmacology, Vol. 10,* (E. Costa, G.L. Gessa, and M. Sandler, Eds.), pp. 75–81. Raven Press, New York.

Carlsson, A. (1978). Mechanism of action of neuroleptic drugs. In *Psychopharmacology: A Generation of Progress* (M.A. Lipton, A. DiMascio and K.F. Killam, Eds.), pp. 1057–1070. Raven Press, New York.

Carlsson, A., Corrodi, H., Fuxe, K. and Hökfelt, T. (1969). Effect of antidepressant drugs on the depletion of intraneuronal brain 5-hydroxytryptamine stores caused by 4-methyl-1-ethyl-meta-tyramine. *Eur. J. Pharmacol.,* 5, 357–366.

Carlsson, A., Falck, B. Fuxe, K. and Hillarp, N.A. (1964), Cellular localization of monoamines in the spinal cord. *Acta Physiol. Scand.,* 60, 112–119.

Carlsson, A., Jonason, J. and Lindqvist, M. (1969). On the mechanism of 5-hydroxytryptamine release by thymoleptics. *J. Pharm. Pharmacol.,* 21, 769–773.

Carlsson, A. and Lindqvist, M. (1963). Effect of chlorpromazine or haloperidol on the formation of 3-methoxytyramine and normetanephrine in mouse brain. *Acta Pharmacol. Toxicol.,* 20, 140–144.

Carlsson, A., Lindqvist, M. and Magnusson, T. (1957). 3, 5-dihydroxyphenylalanine and 5-hydroxytryptophan as reserpine antagonists. *Nature,* 180, 1200–1202.

Carlsson, A. and Waldeck, B. (1965). Inhibition of ^{3}H-metaraminol uptake of antidepressive and related agents. *J. Pharm. Pharmacol.,* 17, 243–244.

Carman, J.S., Post, R.M., Goodwin, G.K. and Bunney, W.E. (1977). Calcium and electroconvulsive therapy of severe depressive illness. *Biol. Psychiat.,* 12, 5–17.

Carman, J.S., Post, R.M., Runkle, D.C., Bunney, W.E. and Wyatt, R.J. (1979). Increased serum calcium and phosphorous states. *Br. J. Psychiat.,* 135, 55–61.

Carpenter, M.B. (1976). *Human Neuroanatomy, 7th Ed.* Williams and Wilkins, Baltimore.

Carter, C.S., Bahr, J.M. and Ramirez, V.D. (1978). Monoamines, estrogen and female sexual behavior in the golden hamster. *Brain Res.,* 144, 109–121.

Carter, C.S. and Davis, J.M. (1977). Biogenic amines, reproductive hormones and female sexual behavior: a review. *Behav. Rev.,* 1, 213–224.

Casriel, D. (1963). *So Fair a House: Story of Synanon.* Prentice Hall, Englewood Cliffs, New Jersey.

Ceccarelli, B., Hurlbut, W.P. and Mauro, A. (1972). Depletion of vesicles from frog neuromuscular junctions by prolonged tetanic stimulation. *J. Cell Biol.,* 54, 30–38.

Cedarbaum, J.M. and Aghajanian, G.K. (1976). Noradrenergic neurons of the locus ceruleus: inhibition by epinephrine and activation by the α–antagonist piperoxane. *Brain Res.,* 112, 413–419.

Cedarbaum, J.M. and Aghajanian, G.K. (1977). Catecholamine receptors on locus ceruleus neurons: pharmacological characterization. *Eur. J. Pharmacol.,* 44, 375–385.

Chang, J.K., Fong, B.T.W., Pert, C.B. and Pert, A. (1976). Opiate receptor affinities and behavioral effects of enkephalin: structure-activity relationship of ten synthetic peptide analogues. *Life Sci.,* 18, 1473–1482.

Chang, K-J. and Cuatrecasas, P. (1979). Multiple opiate receptors. *J. Biol. Chem.,* 254, 2610–2618.

Chang, R.S.L. and Snyder, S.H. (1978). Benzodiazepine receptors: labelling in intact animals with ^{3}H flunitrazepam. *Eur. J. Pharmacol.,* 48, 213–218.

Changeux, J.P. (1975). The cholinergic receptor protein from fish electric organ. In *Handbook of Psychopharmacology, Vol. 6* (L.L. Iversen, S.D. Iversen and S.H. Snyder, Eds.), pp. 235–301. Plenum Press, New York.

Chan-Palay, V. (1977). Morphological correlates for transmitter synthesis, transport, release, uptake and catabolism: a study of serotonin neurons in the nucleus paragigantocellularis lateralis. In *Amino Acids as Chemical Transmitters* (F. Fonnum, Ed.), pp. 1–30. Plenum Press, New York.

Chase, T.N. (1974). Serotonergic-dopaminergic interactions and extrapyramidal function. In *Advances in Biochemical Psychopharmacology, Vol. 11* (E. Costa, G.L. Gessa and M. Sandler, Eds.), pp. 377–386. Raven Press, New York.

Chase, T.N., Breese, G.R. and Kopin, I.J. (1967). Serotonin release from brain slices by electrical stimulation: regional differences and effects of LSD. *Science,* 157, 1461–1463.

Chase, T.N., Katz, R.I. and Kopin, I.J. (1970). Effects of diazepam on fate of intracisternally injected serotonin-C^{14} *Neuropharmacol.,* 9, 103–108.

Chase, T.N., Woods, A.C. and Glaubiger, G.A. (1974). Parkinson's disease treated with a suspected dopamine receptor agonist. *Arch. Neurol.,* 30, 383–386.

Chein, I., Gerard, D.L., Lee, R.S. and Rosenfeld, E. (1964). *The Road to H.* Basic Books, New York.

Cheney, D.L. and Costa, E. (1978). Biochemical pharmacology of cholinergic neurons. In *Psychopharmacology: A Generation of Progress* (M.A. Lipton, A. DiMascio and K.F. Killam, Eds.), pp. 283–292. Raven Press, New York.

Cherkas, M.S. (1965). Synanon foundation—a radical approach to the problem of addiction. *Am. J. Psychiatry,* 121, 1065–1068.

Chessin, M., Kramer, E.R. and Scott, C.C. (1957). Modifications of the pharmacology of reserpine and serotonin by iproniazid. *J. Pharamacol. Exp. Ther.,* 119, 453–460.

Cheung, A.L. and Goldstein, A. (1976). Failure of hypophysectomy to alter brain content of opioid peptides (endorphins). *Life Sci.,* 19, 1005–1008.

Cheung, W.Y. (1980). Calmodulin plays a pivotal role in cellular regulation. *Science,* 207, 19–27.

Chiodo, L.A. and Antelman, S.M. (1980a). Electroconvulsive shock: progressive dopamine autoreceptor subsensitivity independent of repeated treatment. *Science,* 210, 799–801.

Chiodo, L.A. and Antelman, S.M. (1980b). Tricyclic antidepressants induce subsensitivity of presynaptic dopamine autoreceptors. *Eur. J. Pharmacol.,* 64, 203–204.

Chiueh, C.C. and Moore, K.E. (1975). Blockade by reserpine of methylphenidate-induced release of brain dopamine. *J. Pharmacol. Exp. Ther.,* 193, 559–563.

Christensen, E., Moller, J.E. and Faurbye, A. (1970). Neuropathological investigation of 28 brains from patients with dyskinesia. *Acta Psychiat. Scand.,* 46, 14.

Cicero, T.J., Wilcox, C.E., Smithloff, B.R., Meyer, E.R. and Lawrence, C.S. (1973). Effects of morphine in vitro and in vivo on tyrosine hydroxylase activity in rat brain. *Biochem. Pharmacol.,* 22, 3237–3246.

Clark, A.W., Hurlbut, W.P. and Mauro, A. (1972). Changes in the fine structure of the neuromuscular functioning of the frog caused by black widow spider venom. *J. Cell Biol.,* 42, 1–14.

Clark, B.J. (1976). Pharmacology of β-adrenergic blocking drugs. In *β-Adrenoceptor Blocking Agents* (P.R. Saxena and R.P. Forsythe, Eds.), pp. 45–60. North Holland, Amsterdam.

Clark, F.C. and Steele, B.J. (1966). Effects of *d*-amphetamine on performance under a multiple schedule in the rat. *Psychopharmacologia,* 9, 157–169.

Clavier, R.M. and Fibiger, D.A. (1977). On the role of ascending catecholaminergic projections in intracranial self-stimulation of the substantia nigra. *Brain Res.,* 131, 271–286.

Clement-Cormier, Y.C., Kebabian, J.W., Petzold, G.L. and Greengard, P. (1974). Dopamine-sensitive adenylate cyclase in mammalian brain: a possible site of action of antipsychotic drugs. *Proc. Nat. Acad. Sci.,* 71, 1113–1117.

Clement-Cormier, Y.C. and Robison, G.A. (1977). Adenylate cyclase from various dopaminergic areas of the brain and the action of antipsychotic drugs. *Biochem. Pharmacol.,* 26, 1719–1722.

Clouet, D.H. (Ed.) (1971). *Narcotic Drugs: Biochemical Pharmacology.* Plenum Press, New York.

Clouet, D.H. and Iwatsubo, K. (1975). Mechanisms of tolerance to and dependence on narcotic analgesic drugs. *Annu. Rev. Pharmacol.,* 15, 49–71.

Clouet, D.H. and Ratner, M. (1970). Catecholamine biosynthesis in brains of rats treated with morphine. *Science,* 168, 854–856.

Cochin, J. (1970). Possible mechanisms in development of tolerance. *Fed. Proc.,* 1, 19–27.

Cohn, S. (1969). *Hearings before the Subcommittee to Investigate Juvenile Delinquency of the Committee on the Judiciary, U.S. Senate, 91st Cong. 1st Session, Sept. 17, 1969,* p. 293. U.S. Govt. Printing Office, Washington, D.C.

Cohen, S. (1970). The hallucinogens. In *Principles of Psychopharmacology.* (W.G. Clarke and J. del Guidice, Eds.), pp. 489–503. Academic Press, New York.

Colburn, R.W., Goodwin, F.K., Bunney, W.E. and Davis, J.M. (1967). Effect of lithium on the uptake of noradrenaline by synaptosomes. *Nature,* 215, 1395–1397.

Cole, J.M. and Pieper, W.A. (1973). The effects of *N, N*-dimethyltryptamine on operant behavior in squirrel monkeys. *Psychopharmacologia,* 29, 107–112.

Collier, B. (1979). Synaptic vesicles and acetylcholine quanta. *Trends in Neuroscience,* Nov., 285–287.

Collier, H.O.J. (1968). Supersensitivity and dependence. *Nature,* 220, 228–231.

Collier, H.O.J. and Francis, D.L. (1975). Morphine abstinence is associated with increased brain cyclic AMP. *Nature,* 255, 159–162.

Collier, H.O.J. and Roy, A.C. (1974). Morphine-like drugs inhibit the stimulation by E prostaglandins of cyclic AMP formation by rat brain homogenate. *Nature,* 248, 24–27.

Constantinidis, J., Geissbuhler, F., Gaillard, J.M., Hovaguimian, T. and Tissot, R. (1974). Enhancement of cerebral noradrenalin turnover by thyrotropin releasing hormone: evidence by fluorescent histochemistry *Experientia,* 30, 1182–1183.

Cook, L. and Catania, A.C. (1964). Effects of drugs on avoidance and escape behavior. *Fed. Proc.,* 23, 818–835.

Cook, L. and Davidson, A.B. (1973). Effects of behaviorally active drugs in a conflict-punishment procedure in rats. In *The Benzodiazepines* (S. Garattini, E. Mussini and L.O. Randall, Eds.), pp. 327–345, Raven Press, New York.

Cook, L. and Sepinwall, J. (1975). Behavoral analysis of the effects and mechanisms of action of benzodiazepines. In *Advances in Biochemical Psychopharmacology, Vol. 14* (E. Costa and P. Greengard, Eds.), pp. 1–28. Raven Press, New York.

Cools, A.R. and van Rossum, J.M. (1976). Excitation-mediating and inhibition-mediating dopamine-receptors: a new concept towards a better understanding of electrophysiological, biochemical, pharmacological, functional and clinical data. *Psychopharmacologia,* 45, 243–254.

Coopen, A., Prange, A.J., Whybrow, P.C. and Noguera, R. (1972a). Abnormalities of the indoleamines in affective disorders. *Arch. Gen. Psychiat.,* 26, 474–478.

Coopen, A., Whybrow, P.C., Noguera, R., Maggs, R. and Prange, A.J. (1972b). The comparative antidepressent value of L-tryptophan and imipramine with and without attempted potentiation by biothyronine. *Arch. Gen. Psychiat.* 26, 234–241.

Cooper, J.R., Bloom, F.E. and Roth, R.H. (1978). *The Biochemical Basis of Neuropharmacology.* Oxford Univ. Press, New York.

458   BIBLIOGRAPHY

Corrodi, H., Fuxe, K. and Hökfelt, T. (1967a). The effect of some psychoactive drugs on central monoamine neurons. *Pharmacol.,* 1, 363–368.

Corrodi, H., Fuxe, K., Hökfelt, T. and Schou, M. (1967b). The effect of lithium on cerebral monoamine neurons. *Psychopharmacologia,* 11, 345–353.

Corrodi, H., Fuxe, K. and Schou, M. (1969). The effect of prolonged lithium administration on cerebral monoamine neurons in the rat. *Life Sci.,* 8, 643–651, Part 1.

Costa, E., Di Chiara, G. and Gessa, G.L. (Eds.) (1981). *Advances in Biochemical Psychopharmacology, Vol. 26 GABA and Benzodiazepine Receptors.* Raven Press, New York.

Costa, E., Gessa, G.L. and Sandler, M. (Eds.) (1974). *Advances in Biochemical Psychopharmacology, Vol. 10 Serotonin: New Vistas, Histochemistry and Pharmacology.* Raven Press, New York.

Costa, E., Gessa, G.L. and Sandler, M. (Eds.) (1974a). *Advances in Biochemical Psychopharmacology, Vol. 11 Serotonin—New Vistas, Biochemical and Clinical Studies.* Raven Press, New York.

Costa, E., Giacobini, E. and Paoletti, R. (Eds.) (1976). *Advances in Biochemical Psychoparmacology, Vol. 15, First and Second Messengers—New Vistas.* Raven Press, New York.

Costa, E., Guidotti, A., Mao, C.C. and Suria, A. (1975). New concepts on the mechanism of action of benzodiazepines. *Life Sci.,* 17, 167–186.

Costa, E., Guidotti, A. and Toffano, G. (1978). Molecular mechanisms mediating the action of diazepam on GABA receptors. *Br. J. Psychiatry,* 133, 239–248.

Costa, E. and Trabucchi, M. (1975). Regulations of brain dopamine turnover rate: pharmacological implications. In *Catecholamines and Behavior, Vol. 1* (A.J. Friedhoff, Ed.), pp. 201–227. Plenum Press, New York.

Costall, B. and Naylor, R.J. (1974). Extrapyramidal and mesolimbic involvement with the stereotypic activity of d-and l-amphetamine. *Eur. J. Pharmacol.,* 25, 121–129.

Costall, B., Naylor, R.J. and Olley, J.E. (1972). Stereotypic and anti-cataleptic activities of amphetamine after intracerebral injections. *Eur. J. Pharmacol.,* 18, 83–94.

Costello, D.J. and Borison, H.L. (1977). Naloxone antagonizes narcotic self-blockade of emesis in the cat. *J. Pharmacol. Exp. Ther.,* 203, 222–230.

Cotman, C.W. and Hamberger, A. (1978). Glutamate as a CNS neurotransmitter: properties of release, inactivation and biosynthesis. In *Amino Acids as Chemical Transmitters* (F. Fonnum, Ed.), pp. 379–412. Plenum Press, New York.

Cotman, C.W., Poste, G. and Nicolson, G.L. (Eds.) (1980) *The Cell Surface and Neuronal Function.* Elsevier, New York.

Cott, J.M., Breese, G.R., Cooper, B.R., Barlow, T.S. and Prange, A.J. Jr. (1976). Investigation into the mechanism of reduction of ethanol sleep by thyrotropin releasing hormones (TRH). *J. Pharmacol. Exp. Ther.,* 196, 594–604.

Cotzias, G.C., Papavasiliou, P.S. and Gellene, R. (1969). Modification of Parkinsonism—chronic treatment with L-dopa. *N. Engl. J. Med.,* 280, 337–345.

Cotzias, G.C., Papavasiliou, P.S., Ginos, J.Z. and Tolosa, E.S. (1975). Treatment of Parkinson's disease and allied conditions. In *The Nervous System, Vol. 2, The Clinical Neurosciences* (D.B. Tower, Ed.), pp. 323–329. Raven Press, New York.

Cotzias, G.C., Van Woert, M.H. and Schiffer, L.M. (1967). Aromatic amino acids and modification of Parkinsonism. *N. Engl. J. Med.,* 276, 374–379.

Couch, J.R. (1970). Responses of neurons in the raphe nucleus to serotonin, norepinephrine and acetylcholine and their correlations with an excitatory synaptic input. *Brain Res.,* 19, 137–150.

Couteaux, R. (1958). Neurophysiological and cytochemical observations on the postsynaptic membrane at motor end-plates and ganglionic synapses. *Exp. Cell Res., Suppl. 5,* 294–322.

Cox, B.M., Goldstein, A. and Li, C.H. (1976). Opioid activity of a peptide, β-lipotropin-(61-91) derived from β-lipotropin. *Proc. Nat. Acad. Sci.,* 73, 1821-1823.

Cramer, H., Johnson, D.G., Hanbauer, I., Silberstein, N.D. and Kopin, I.J. (1973). Accumulation of adenosine 3', 5'-monophosphate induced by catecholamines in the rat superior cervical ganglion in vitro. *Brain Res.,* 53, 97–104.

Crane, G.E. (1978). Tardive diskinesia and related neurologic disorders. In *Handbook of Psychopharmacology, Vol. 10* (L.L. Iversen, S.D. Iversen and S.H. Snyder, Eds.), pp. 165–196. Plenum Press, New York.

Creese, I., Burt, D.R. and Snyder, S. (1976). Dopamine receptor binding predicts clinical and pharmacological potencies of anti-schizophrenic drugs. *Science,* 194, 481–483.

Creese, I., Burt, D.R. and Snyder, S.H. (1977). Dopamine receptor binding enhancement accompanies lesion-induced behavioral supersensitivity. *Science,* 197, 596–598.

Creese, I, Burt, D.R. and Snyder, S.H. (1978). Biochemical actions of neuroleptic drugs: focus on the dopamine receptor. In *Handbook of Psychopharmacology, Vol. 10* (L.L. Iversen, S.D. Iversen and S.H. Snyder, Eds.), pp. 38–89. Plenum Press, New York.

Creese, I. and Iversen, S.D. (1974). The role of forebrain dopamine systems in amphetamine-induced stereotyped behavior in the rat. *Psychopharmacologia,* 39, 345–357.

Creese, I. and Snyder, S.H. (1975). Receptor binding and pharamacological activity of opiates in the guinea-pig intestine. *J. Pharmacol. Exp. Ther.,* 194, 205–219.

Creese, I. and Snyder, S.H. (1978). Behavioral and biochemical properties of the dopamine receptor. In *Psychopharmacology: A Generation of Progress* (M.A. Lipton, A. DiMascio and K.F. Killam, Eds.), pp. 377–388. Raven Press, New York.

Crosby, E.C., Humphrey, T. and Lauer, E.W. (1962). *Correlative Anatomy of the Nervous System*. Macmillan, New York.

Crow, T.J., Johnston, E.C., Longden, A. and Owen, F. (1978). Dopamine and schizophrenia. *Adv. Biochem. Psychopharmacol.,* 19, 301–309.

Crowley, W.R., Ward, I.L. and Margules, D.L. (1975). Female lordotic behavior mediated by monoamines in male rats. *J. Comp. Physiol. Psychol.,* 88, 62–68.

Cuatrecasas, P. (1974a). Insulin receptors, cell membranes and hormone action. *Biochem. Pharmacol.,* 23, 2353–2361.

Cuatrecasas, P. (1974b). Membrane receptors. *Annu. Rev. Biochem.,* 43, 169–214.

Curtis, B.A., Jacobson, S. and Marcus, E.M. (1972). *An Introduction to the Neurosciences*. Saunders, Philadelphia.

Curtis, D.R., Duggan, A.W. and Johnston, G.A.R. (1971). The specificity of strychnine in the mammalian spinal cord. *Exp. Brain Res.,* 12, 544–565.

Curtis, D.R. and Eccles, R.M. (1958). The excitation of Renshaw cells by pharmacological agents applied electrophoretically. *J. Physiol.,* 141, 435–445.

Dahlström, A. (1965). Observations on the accumulation of noradrenaline in the proximal and distal parts of peripheral adrenergic nerves after compression. *J. Anat.,* 99, 677–689.

Dahlström, A. (1970). The effects of drugs on axonal transport of amine storage granules. In *New Aspects of Storage and Release Mechanisms of Catecholamines* (H.J. Schulmann and G. Kroneberg, Eds.), pp. 20–38. Springer-Verlag, New York.

Dahlström, A. and Fuxe, K. (1964). Evidence for the existence of monoamine-containing neurons in the central nervous system. I. Demonstration of monoamines in the cell bodies of brainstem neurons. *Acta Physiol. Scand., (Suppl. 232),* 62, 1–55.

Dahlström, A. and Fuxe, K. (1965). Evidence for the existence of monoamine neurons in the central nervous system. II. Experimentally induced changes in the interneuronal amine levels of the bulbospinal neuron systems. *Acta Physiol. Scand., (Suppl. 247),* 1–36.

Dahlström, A., Fuxe, K. and Hillarp, N.A. (1965a). Site of action of reserpine. *Acta Pharm. Toxicol., (Copenhagen),* 22, 277–292.

Dahlström, A., Fuxe, K., Kernell, D. and Sedvall, G. (1965b). Reduction of the monoamine stores in the terminals of the bulbospinal neurons following stimulation in the medulla oblongata. *Life Sci.,* 4, 1207–1212.

Dairman, W. and Udenfriend, S. (1971). Decrease in adrenal tyrosine hydroxylase and increase in norepinephrine synthesis in rats given L-dopa. *Science,* 171, 1022–1024.

Dale, H.H. (1914). The action of certain esters and ethers of choline and their relation to muscarine. *J. Pharmacol.,* 6, 147–190.

Dale, H.H., Feldberg, W. and Vogt, M. (1936). Release of acetylcholine at voluntary motor nerve endings. *J. Physiol.,* 86, 353–380.

D'Amour, F.E. and Smith, D.L. (1941). A method for determining loss of pain sensation. *J. Pharmacol., Exp. Ther.,* 72, 74–79.

Dantzer, R. (1976). Effects of diazepam on performance of pigs in a progressive ratio schedule. *Physiol. Behav.,* 17, 161–163.

Dantzer, R. (1977). Behavioral effects of benzodiazepines: a review. *Biobehav. Rev.,* 1, 71–86.

Davidoff, R.A., Graham, L.T., Shank, R.P., Werman, R. and Aprison, M.H. (1967). Changes in amino acid concentrations associated with the loss of spinal interneurons. *J. Neurochem.,* 14, 1025–1031.

Davis, G.C., Bunney, W.E., DeFraites, E.G., Kleinman, J.E., van Kammen, D.P., Post, R.M. and Wyatt, R.J. (1977). Intravenous naloxone administration in schizophrenia and affective illness. *Science,* 197, 74–77.

Davis, J.M. (1976). Maintenance therapy in psychiatry 1. Affective disorders. *Am. J. Psychiatry,* 133, 1–13.

Davis, J.M., Klerman, G.L. and Schildkraut, J.J. (1968). Drugs used in the treatment of depression. In *Psychopharmacology, A Review of Progress* (D.H. Efron, Ed.), pp. 719–747. Public Health Service Publ. No. 1836, U.S. Gov't Printing Office, Washington, D.C.

Davis, K.L. (1977). Psychological effects of nonpsychiatric drugs. In *Psychopharmacology: From Theory to Practice* (J.D. Barchas, P.A. Berger, R.D. Ciaranello, G.R. Elliott, Eds.), pp. 469–480. Oxford Univ. Press, New York.

Davis, L.G. and Cohen, R.K. (1980a). Inhibition of ³H-diazepam binding by an endogenous fraction from rat brain synaptosomes. *J. Pharmacol.,* 32, 218–219.

Davis, L.G. and Cohen, R.K. (1980b). Characterization of an endogenous peptide for the benzodiazepine receptor. *Biochem. Biophys. Res. Commun.,* 92, 141–148.

Davis, L.G., McIntosh, H. and Reker, D. (1981). An endogenous ligand to the benzodiazepine receptor: preliminary evaluation of its bioactivity. *Pharmacol. Biochem. Beh.,* 14, 839–844.

Davison, G.C. and Neale, J.M. (1978). *Abnormal Psychology: An Experimental Clinical Approach*. Wiley, New York.

Davson, H. (1972). The blood brain barrier. In *The Structure and Function of Nervous Tissue, Vol. IV* (G.H. Bourne, Ed.), pp. 321–345. Academic Press, New York.

DeFeudis, F.V. (1974). *Central Cholinergic Systems and Behavior*. Academic Press, New York.

Del Castillo, J. and Katz, B. (1955). On the location of the acetylcholine receptors. *J. Physiol. (London),* 128, 157–181.

DeLorenzo, R.J. (1980a). Role of calmodulin in neurotransmitter release and synaptic function. In *Calmodulin and Cell Function* (D.M. Watterson and F.F. Vincenzi, Eds.), Vol. 356, pp. 92–109, N.Y. Acad. Sci. Publ., New York.

DeLorenzo, R.J. (1980b). Phenytoin: calcium- and calmodulin-dependent protein phosphorylation and neurotransmitter release. In *Advances in Neurology: Antiepileptic Drugs Mechanism of Action, Vol. 27* (G.H. Glaser, J.K. Penry and D.M. Woodbury, Eds.), pp. 399–414. Raven Press, New York.

DeLorenzo, R.J. (1981). The calmodulin hypothesis of neurotransmission. *Cell Calcium,* 2, 365–385.

DeLorenzo, R.J. (1982). Calmodulin in neurotransmitter release and synaptic function. *Fed. Proc.* 41, 2265–2272.

DeLorenzo, R.J., Burdette, S., and Holderness, J. (1981). Benzodiazepine inhibition of the calcium-calmodulin system in brain membrane. *Science,* 213, 546–549.

De Montigny, C. and Aghajanian, G.K. (1978). Tricyclic antidepressants: long term treatment increases responsivity of rat forebrain neurons to serotonin. *Science,* 202, 1303–1306.

Dencker, S.J., Malm, U., Roos, B.E. and Werdinius, B. (1966). Acid monoamine metabolites of cerebrospinal fluid in mental depression and mania. *J. Neurochem.,* 13, 1545–1548.

Deneau, G.A. (1969). Psychogenic dependence in monkeys. In *Scientific Basis of Drug Dependence* (H. Steinberg, Ed.), pp. 199–207. Churchill, London.

Dengler, H.G., Speigel, H.E. and Titus, E.O. (1961). Effect of drugs on uptake of isotopic norepinephrine by cat tissues. *Nature,* 191, 816–817.

De Robertis, E. (1967). Ultrastructure and cytochemistry of the synaptic region. *Science,* 156, 907–914.

De Robertis, E. (1971). Molecular biology of synaptic receptors. *Science* 171, 963–971.

De Robertis, E. and Bennett, H.S. (1954). Submicroscopic vesicular component in the synapse. *Fed. Proc.,* 13, 53.

De Robertis, E. and Bennett, H.S. (1955). Some features of the submicroscopic morphology of synapses in frog and earthworm. *J. Biophys. Biochem. Cytol.,* 1, 47–58.

De Robertis, E., Fiszer de Plazas, S., Llorente de Carlin, C., Aquilar, J.S. and Schlieper, P. (1978). Synaptic receptor proteolipids: isolation and molecular biology. In *Advances in Pharmacology and Therapeutics, Vol. 1* (J. Jacob, Ed.), pp. 235–255. Pergamon Press, Elmsford, New York.

De Robertis, E., Rodrigues de Lores Arnaiz, G. and Pallegrino de Iraldi, A. (1962). Isolation of synaptic vesicles from nerve endings of rat brain. *Nature,* 194, 794–795.

Dews, P.B. (1955). Studies on behavior. I. Differential sensitivity to pentobarbital of pecking performance in pigeons depending on the schedule of reward. *J. Pharmacol. Exp. Ther.,* 113, 393–401.

Dews, P.B. (1958). Studies on behavior. IV. Stimulant actions of methamphetamine. *J. Pharm. Exp. Ther.,* 122, 137–147.

Dixon, W.E. (1906). Vagus inhibition. *Br. Med. J.,* ii, 1807.

Dohrenwend, B.S. and Dohrenwend, B.P. (Eds.) (1974a) *Stressful Life Events: Their Nature and Effects.* Wiley, New York.

Dohrenwend, B.S. and Dohrenwend, B.P. (1974b) Social and cultural influences in psychopathology. *Annu. Rev. Psychol.,* 25, 417–452.

Dole, V.P. and Nyswander, M.E. (1965). A medical treatment for diacetylmorphine (heroin) addiction. *J. Am. Med. Assoc.,* 193, 646–650.

Dole, V.P. and Nyswander, M.E. (1966). Rehabilitation of heroin addicts after blockade with methadone. *N.Y. State J. Med.,* 55, 2011–2017.

Dole, V.P., Nyswander, M.E. and Kreek, M.J. (1966). Narcotic blockade. *Arch. Intern Med.,* 118, 304–309.

Dominguez, M. and Longo, V.G. (1970). Effects of *p*-chlorophenylalanine, α-methylparatyrosine and other indole- and catechol-amine depletors on the hyperirritability syndrome of septal rats. *Physiol. Behav.,* 5, 607–610.

Dominic, J.A. (1973). Suppression of brain serotonin synthesis and metabolism by benzodiazepine minor tranquilizers. In *Serotonin and Behavior* (J. Barchas and E. Usdin, Eds.), pp. 149–155. Academic Press, New York.

Donahoe, J.W. and Wessells, M.G. (1980). *Learning, Language, and Memory.* Harper & Row, New York.

Douglas, W.W. (1975). Histamine and antihistamines. In *The Pharmacological Basis of Therapeutics, 5th Edition,* (L.S. Goodman and A. Gilman, Eds.), pp. 590–629. Macmillan, New York.

Dowson, J.H. (1969). The significance of brain amine concentrations. *Lancet,* 2, 596–597.

Drachman, D.A. (1978). Central cholinergic system and memory. In *Psychopharmacology: A Generation of Progress* (M.A. Lipton, A. DiMascio, and K.F. Killam, Eds.), pp. 651–662. Raven Press, New York.

Droz, B. (1975). Synthetic machinery and axoplasmic transport: maintenance of neural connectivity. In *The Nervous System, Vol. 1, The Basic Neurosciences* (D.B. Tower, Ed.), pp. 111–127. Raven Press, New York.

Du Bois-Reymond, E. (1877). Gesammelte Abhandl. d. allgem. *Muskel-und Nervenphysik,* 2, 700.

Dudar, J.D. (1975). The effect of septal nuclei stimulation on the release of acetylcholine from the rabbit hippocampus. *Brain Res.,* 83, 123–133.

Duggan, A.W., Hall, J.G. and Headly P.M. (1976). Morphine, enkephalin and the substantia gelatinosa, *Nature,* 264, 456–458.

Dun, N.J., Nishi, S. and Karczmar, A.G. (1978). An analysis of angiotensin II on mammalian ganglion cells. *J. Pharm. Exp. Ther.,* 204, 669–675.

Dunant, Y. and Israël, M. (1979). When the vesicular hypothesis is no longer the vesicular hypothesis. *Trends in Neuroscience,* May, 130–132.

Dunn, A.J. and Bondy, S.C. (1974). *Functional Chemistry of the Brain.* Spectrum, Flushing, New York.

Dyson, R.D. (1978). *Cell Biology, A Molecular Approach.* Allyn and Bacon, Boston.

Ebert, M.H. and Kopin, I.J. (1975). Differential labelling of origins of urinary catecholamine metabolites by dopamine C^{14}. *Trans. Assoc. Am. Physicians,* 88, 256-264.

Eccles, J.C. (1964a). Ionic mechanisms of postsynaptic inhibition. *Science,* 145, 1140-1147.

Eccles, J.C. (1964b). *The Physiology of Synapses.* Academic Press, New York.

Eccles, J.C. (1967). Postsynaptic inhibition in the central nervous system. In *The Neurosciences, A Study Program* (G.C. Quarton, T. Melnechuk, and F.O. Schmitt, Eds.), pp. 408-426. Rockefeller Univ. Press, New York.

Eccles, J.C. (1977). *Understanding the Brain, 2nd Edition.* McGraw-Hill, New York.

Eccles, J.C., Schmidt, R. and Willis, W.D. (1963). Pharmacological studies on presynaptic inhibition. *J. Physiol.,* 168, 500-530.

Eccleston, D., Loose, R., Pullar, I.A. and Sugden, R.F. (1970). Exercise and urinary excretion of cyclic AMP. *Lancet,* 2, 612-613.

Efron, D.H. (Ed.) (1968). *Psychopharmacology: A Review of Progress, 1957-1967.* Public Health Service Publ. No. 1836, U.S. Gov't Printing Office, Washington, D.C.

Ellinwood, E.H., Jr. (1974). Assault and homocide associated with amphetamine abuse. In *Amphetamines: Medical and Psychological Studies* (Whitlock, et al., Eds.), pp. 138-151. MSS Information Corp., New York.

Ellinwood, E.H., Jr. and Sudilovsky, A. (1973). The relationship of the amphetamine model psychosis to schizophrenia. In *Psychopharmacology, Sexual Disorders and Drug Abuse* (T.A. Bau, et al. Eds.), pp. 189-203. North-Holland, Amsterdam.

Elliott, G.R., Edelman, A.M., Renson, J.F. and Berger, P.A. (1977). Indoleamines and other neuroregulators. In *Psychopharmacology: From Theory to Practice* (J.D. Barchas, P.A. Berger, R.D. Cicaranello and G.R. Elliott, Eds.), pp. 33-50. Oxford Univ. Press, New York.

Elliott, T.R. (1904). On the action of adrenalin. *J. Physiol. (London),* 31, XX-XXI.

Elliott, T.R. (1905). The action of adrenaline. *J. Physiol.,* 32, 401-467.

Epelbaum, J., Brazeau, P., Tsang, D. and Brawer, J. (1977a). Subcellular distribution of radioimmunoassayable somatostatin in rat brain. *Brain Res.,* 126, 309-323.

Epelbaum, J., Willoughby, J.O., Brazeau, P. and Martin, J.B. (1977b). Effects of brain lesions and hypothalamic deafferentation on somatostatin distribution in the rat brain. *Endocrinol.,* 101, 1495-1502.

Eränkö, O. (1955). Histochemistry of noradrenaline in the adrenal medulla of rats and mice. *Endocrinol.,* 57, 363-367.

Eränkö, O. (Ed.) (1976). *Structure and Function of the Small Intensely Fluorescent Sympathetic Cells. Fogarty International Center Proceedings, No. 30 DHEW Publication No. (NIH) 76-942,* Supt. of Documents, Washington, D.C.

Erspamer, V. and Boretti, G. (1951). Identification and characterization by paper chromatography, of enteramine, octopamine, tyramine, histamine, and allied substances, in extracts of posterior salivary glands of octopoda and in other tissue extracts of vertebrates and invertebrates. *Arch. Int. Pharmacodyn. Ther.,* 88, 296-332.

Erwin, G.V. (1973). Oxidative-reductive pathways for metabolism of biogenic aldehydes. In *Frontiers of Catecholamine Research* (E. Usdin, Ed.), pp. 161-166. Pergamon Press, New York.

Esplin, D.W. and Zablocka, B. (1965). Central nervous system stimulants. In *The Pharmacological Basis of Therapeutics* (L.S. Goodman and A. Gilman, Eds.), pp. 345-353. Macmillan, New York.

Essig, C. (1970). Barbiturate dependence. In *Drug Dependence* (R.T. Harris, W.M. McIsaac and C.R. Schuster, Jr., Eds.), pp. 219-140. Univ. of Texas Press, Austin, Texas.

Essman, W.B. (1973). *Neurochemistry of Cerebral Electroshock.* Spectrum, New York.

Estes, W.K. and Skinner, B.F. (1941). Some quantitative properties of anxiety. *J. Exp. Psychol.,* 29, 390-400.

Eterović, V.A. and Bennet E.L. (1974). Nicotinic cholinergic receptor in brain detected by binding of ^3H-α-bungaratoxin. *Biochim. Biophys. Acta,* 362, 246-355.

Evans, W.O. (1961). A new technique for the investigation of some analgesic drugs on a reflexive behavior in the rat. *Psychopharmacologia,* 2, 318-325.

Everett, G.M. (1974). Effect of 5-hydroxytryptophan on brain levels of dopamine, norepinephrine, and serotonin in mice. In *Advances in Biochemical Psychopharmacology, Vol. 10* (E. Costa, G.L. Gessa and M. Sandler, Eds.), pp. 261-262. Raven Press, New York.

Fahn, S. and Coté, L.J. (1968). Regional distribution of γ-aminobutyric acid in brain of the Rhesus monkey. *J. Neurochem.,* 15, 209-213.

Falck, B., Hillarp, N.A., Thieme, G. and Thorp, A. (1962). Fluorescence of catecholamines and related compounds condensed with formaldehyde. *J. Histochem. Cytochem.,* 10, 348-354.

Fatt, P. and Katz, B. (1952). Spontaneous subthreshold activity of motor nerve endings. *J. Physiol.,* 117, 109-128.

Feighner, J.P., Lao, L., King, L.J. and Ross, W.J. (1972). Brain serotonin and norepinephrine after convulsions and resperpine. *J. Neurochem.,* 19, 905-907.

Feinberg, A.P. and Snyder, S.H. (1975). Phenothiazine drugs: structure-activity relationships explained by a conformation that mimics dopamine. *Proc. Nat. Acad. Sci.,* 72, 1899-1903.

Feldman, R.S. (1962). The prevention of fixations with chlordiazepoxide. *J. Neuropsychiatry,* 3, 254-259.

Feldman, R.S. (1968). The mechanism of fixation prevention and "dissociation" learning with chlordiazepoxide. *Psychopharmacologia,* 12, 384-399.

Feldman, R.S. and Smith, W.C. (1978). Chlordiazepoxide-fluoxetine interactions on food-intake in free-feeding rats. *Pharmacol. Biochem. Behav.,* 8, 749–752.

Fennessy, M.R. and Lee, J.R. (1972). Comparison of the dose-response effects of morphine on brain amines, analgesia and activity in mice. *Br. J. Pharmacol.,* 45, 240–248.

Ferguson, J., Henriksen, S., Cohen, H., Mitchell, G., Barchas, J. and Dement, W. (1970). Hypersexuality and changes in aggressive and perceptual behavior caused by chronic administration of parachlorophenylalanine in cats. *Science,* 168, 499–501.

Fernstrom, J.D. and Wurtman, F.J. (1974). Control of brain serotonin levels by the diet. In *Advances in Biochemical Psychopharmacology, Vol. 11* (E. Costa, G.L. Gessa and M. Sandler, Eds.), pp. 133–142. Raven Press, New York.

Fibiger, H.C. (1978). Drugs and reinforcement mechanisms: a critical review of the catecholamine theory. *Annu. Rev. Pharmacol. Toxicol.,* 18, 37–56.

Fibiger, H.C., Carter, D.A. and Phillips, A.G. (1976). Decreased intracranial self-stimulation after neuroleptics or 6-hydroxydopamine: evidence for mediation by motor deficits rather than by reduced rewards. *Psychopharmacology,* 47, 21–27.

Fink, M. (1977). EST: a special case of pharmacotherapy. In *Phenomenology and Treatment of Depression* (W.E. Fann, Ed.), pp. 285–294. Spectrum, New York.

Fiszer, S. and De Robertis, E. (1969). Subcellular distribution and chemical nature of the receptor of 5-hydroxy-tryptamine in the central nervous system. *Neurochem.,* 16, 1201–1209.

Fitzsimons, J.T. (1975). The renin-angiotensin system and drinking behavior. *Prog. Brain Res.,* 42, 215–233.

Florey, E. (1954). An inhibitory and an excitatory factor of mammalian central nervous system, and their action on a single sensory neuron. *Arch. Int. Physiol.,* 62, 33–53.

Foldes, F.F., Swerdlow, M. and Siker, C.S. (1964). *Narcotics and Narcotic Antagonists.* Thomas, Springfield, Illinois.

Fonnum, F. (Ed.) (1978). *Amino Acids as Chemical Transmitters.* Plenum Press, New York.

Fonnum, F. and Storm-Mathisen, J. (1978). Localization of GABA-ergic neurons in the CNS. In *Handbook of Psychopharmacology, Vol. 9* (L.L. Iversen, S.D. Iversen and S.H. Snyder, Eds.), pp. 357–401. Plenum Press, New York.

Forn, J., Krueger, B.K. and Greengard, P. (1974). Adenosine 3',5'-monophosphate content in rat caudate nucleus: demonstration of dopaminergic and adrenergic receptors. *Science,* 186, 1118–1120.

Forn, J. and Valdecasas, F.G. (1971). Effects of lithium on brain adenyl cyclase activity. *Biochem. Pharmacol.,* 20, 2773–2779.

Fort, J. (1970). A world view of drugs. In *Society and Drugs* (R.H. Blum and Associates, Eds.), pp. 229–243. Jossey-Bass, San Francisco.

Fox, C.F. (1972). The structure of cell membranes. *Sci. Am.,* 226, 2, 30–38.

Francis, D.L., Roy, A.C. and Collier, H.O.J. (1975). Morphine abstinence and quasi-abstinence effects after phosphodiesterase inhibitors and naloxone. *Life Sci.,* 16, 1901–1906.

Fraser, H.F., Wikler, A., Essig, C. and Isbell, H. (1958). Degree of physical dependence induced by secobarbital or pentorbarbital. *J. Am. Med. Assoc.,* 166, 126.

Frazer, A. (1981). Tricyclic antidepressants: basic considerations. In *Neuropharmacology of the CNS and Behavioral Disorders* (G.C. Palmer, Ed.), pp. 73–91. Academic Press, New York.

Frederickson, R.C.A., Burgis, V., Harrell, C.E. and Edwards, J.D. (1978). Dual actions of substance P on nociception: possible role of endogenous opioids. *Science,* 199, 1359–1361.

Frederickson, R.C.A. and Norris, F.H. (1976). Enkephalin-induced depression of single neurons in brain areas with opiate receptors—antagonism by naloxone. *Science,* 194, 440–442.

Freeman, J.J. and Sulser, F. (1972). Imprindoleamphetamine interactions in the rat: the role of aromatic hydroxylation of amphetamine in its mode of action. *J. Pharmacol. Exp. Ther.,* 183, 307–315.

Freud, S. (1936). *The Problem of Anxiety.* Norton, New York.

Fried, P.A. (1972). Septum and behavior: a review. *Psychol. Bull.* 78, 292–310.

Fried, P.A. (1973). The septum and hyperactivity: a review. *Br. J. Psychol.,* 64, 267–275.

Friedman, M.I. and Stricker, E.M. (1976). The physiological psychology of hunger: a physiological perspective. *Psychol. Rev.,* 83, 409–431.

Frohman, L.A. (1980). Neurotransmitters as regulators of endocrine function. In *Neuroendocrinology* (D.T. Krieger and J.C. Hughes, Eds.), pp. 44–57. Sinauer Associates, Sunderland, Massachusetts.

Frosch, W.A. (1970). Psychoanalytic evaluation of addiction and habituation. *J. Am. Psychoanal. Assoc.,* 18, 209–218.

Fuller, R.G.C. and Forrest, D.W. (1973). Behavioral aspects of cigarette smoking in relation to arousal level. *Psychol. Rep.* 33, 115–121.

Fuller, R.W. and Molloy, B.B. (1974). Recent studies with 4-chloroamphetamine and some analogues. In *Advances in Biochemical Psychopharmacology, Vol. 10* (E. Costa, G.L. Gessa, and M. Sandler, Eds.), pp. 195–206. Raven Press, New York.

Fuller, R.W., Perry, K.W. and Molloy, B.B. (1975a). Reversible and irreversible phases of serotonin depletion by 4-chloroamphetamine. *Eur. J. Pharmacol.,* 33, 119–124.

Fuller, R.W., Perry, K.W. and Molloy, B.B. (1975b). Effect of 3-(p-trifluoromethyl-phenoxy)-N-methyl-3-phenyl-propylamine on the depletion of brain serotonin by

4-chloro-amphetamine. *J. Pharmacol. Exp. Ther.,* 193, 796–803.

Funderburk, W.H., Hazelwood, J.C., Ruckert, R.T. and Ward, J.W. (1971). Is 5-hydroxytryptamine involved in the mechanism of action of fenfluramine? *J. Pharm. Pharmacol.,* 23, 468–470.

Fuxe, K. (1965). Evidence for the existence of monoamine neurons in the central nervous system. IV. Distribution of monoamine nerve terminals in the central nervous system. *Acta Physiol. Scand. (Suppl.* 247), 64, 37–85.

Fuxe, K., Agnati, L.F., Bolme, P., Hökfelt, T., Lidbrink, P., Ljungdahl, A., Perez de la Mora, M. and Örgren, S. (1975). The possible involvement of GABA mechanisms in the action of benzodiazepines on central catecholamine neurons. In *Mechanisms of Action of Benzodiazepines* (E. Costa and P. Greengard, Eds.), pp. 45–51. Raven Press, New York.

Fuxe, K. and Gunne, L.M. (1964). Depletion of amine stores in brain catecholamine terminals on amygdaloid stimulation. *Acta Physiol. Scand.,* 62, 493–494.

Fuxe, K., Hökfelt, T., Agnati, L.F., Johannson, O., Goldstein, M., Perez de la Mora, M., Possani, L., Tapia, R., Teran, L. and Palacios, R. (1978). Mapping out central catecholamine neurons: immunohistochemical studies on catecholamine-synthesizing enzymes. In *Psychopharmacology: A Generation of Progress* (M.A. Lipton, A. DiMascio, K.F. Killam, Eds.), pp. 67–94, Raven Press, New York.

Fuxe, K. and Johnsson, G. (1974). Further mapping of central 5-hydroxytryptamine neurons: studies with the neuroxtoxic dihydroxytryptamines. In *Advances in Biochemical Psychopharmacology. Vol. 10* (E. Costa, G.G. Gessa, and M. Sandler, Eds.), pp. 1–12. Raven Press, New York.

Gaddum, J.H. (1958). 5-Hydroxytryptamine. In *London Symposium, 1957,* (G.P. Lewis, Ed.), p. 195. Pergamon, London.

Gallager, D.W. and Aghajanian, G.K. (1976). Effect of antipsychotic drugs on the firing of dorsal raphe cells, II. Reversal by picrotoxin. *Eur. J. Pharmacol.,* 39, 357–364.

Ganten, D. and Speck, G. (1978). The brain renin-angiotensin system: a model for the synthesis of peptides in the brain. *Biochem. Pharmacol.,* 27, 2379–2389.

Garattini, S., Kato, R., Lamestra, L. and Valzelli, L. (1960). Electroshock, brain serotonin and barbiturate narcosis. *Experientia,* 16, 156–157.

Garattini, S., Mussini, E. and Randall, L.O. (Eds.) (1973). *The Benzodiazepines.* Raven Press, New York.

Garattini, S. and Valzelli, L. (1965). *Serotonin.* Elsevier, New York.

Garver, D.L., Schlemmer, R.F., Maas, J.W. and Davis, J.M. (1975). A schizophreniform behavioral psychosis mediated by dopamine. *Am. J. Psychiat.,* 132, 33–38.

Geller, I. (1962). Use of approach avoidance behavior (conflict) for evaluating depressant drugs. In *Psychosomatic Medicine* (J.H. Nodine and J.H. Moyer, Eds.), pp. 267–274. Lea and Febiger, Philadelphia.

Geller, I., Hartmann, R.J., Croy, D.J. and Haber, B. (1974). Attenuation of conflict behavior with cinanserin, a serotonin antagonist: reversal of the effect with 5-hydroxytryptophan and α-methyl tryptamine. *Res. Commun. Clin. Pathol. Pharmacol.,* 7, 165–174.

Geller, I. and Seifter, J. (1960). The effects of meprobamate, barbiturates, *d*-amphetamine and promazine on experimentally-induced conflict in the rat. *Psychopharmacologia,* 1, 482–492.

German, D.C. and Bowden, D.M. (1974). Catecholamine systems as the neural substrate for intracranial self-stimulation: a hypothesis. *Brain Res.,* 73, 381–419.

Gerner, R.H., Post, R.M., Spiegel, A.M. and Murphy, D.L. (1977). Effects of parathormone and lithium treatment on calcium and mood in depressed patients. *Biol. Psychiatry,* 12, 145–151.

Gessa, G.L. and Tagliamonte, A. (1974). Possible role of brain serotonin and dopamine in controlling male sexual behavior. In *Advances in Biochemical Psychopharmacology, Vol. 11* (E. Costa, G.L. Gessa and M. Sandler, Eds.), pp. 217–228. Raven Press, New York.

Geyer, M.A., Puerto, A., Dawsey, W.J., Knapp, S., Bullard, W.P. and Mandell, A.J. (1976a). Histological and enzymatic studies of the mesolimbic and mesostriatal serotonergic pathways. *Brain Res.,* 106, 241–256.

Geyer, M.A., Puerto, A., Menkes, D.B., Segal, D.S. and Mandell, A.J. (1976b). Behavioral studies following lesions of the mesolimbic and mesostriatal serotonergic pathways. *Brain Res.,* 106, 257–270.

Gilbert, R.F.T., Emson, P.C., Hunt, S.P., Bennett, G.W., Marsden, C.A., Sandberg, B.E.B., Steinbusch, H.W.M. and Verhofstad, A.A.J. (1982). The effects of monoamine neurotoxins on peptides in the rat spinal cord. *Neurosci.* 7, 60–87.

Gillin, J.C., Kaplan, J., Stillman, R. and Wyatt, R.J. (1976). The psychedelic model of schizophrenia: the case of *N,N*–dimethyltryptamine. *Am. J. Psychiatry,* 133, 203–208.

Gillin, J.C., Stoff, D.M. and Wyatt, R.J. (1978). Transmethylation hypothesis: a review. In *Psychopharmacology: A Generation of Progress* (M.A. Lipton, A. DiMascio and K.F. Killam, Eds.), pp. 1097–1112. Raven Press, New York.

Gispen, W.H., Krivoy, W.A., deWied, D. and Zimmerman, E. (1975). Effect of rifampicin on development of tolerance to analgesic actions of morphine. *Life Sci.,* 17, 247–251.

Glick, S.D. (1976). Screening and therapeutics: animal models and human problems. In *Behavioral Pharmacology* (S.D. Glick and J. Goldfarb, Eds.), pp. 339–361. Mosby, St. Louis.

Glowinski, J. and Axelrod, J. (1964). Inhibition of uptake of tritiated noradrenaline in the intact rat brain by imipramine and structurally related compounds. *Nature,* 204, 1318-1319.

Glowinski, J. and Axelrod, J. (1965). Effects of drugs on the uptake, release and metabolism of ³H-norepinephrine in the rat brain. *J. Pharmacol. Exp. Ther.,* 149, 43-49.

Glowinski, J., Hamon, M. and Héry, F. (1973). Regulation of 5-HT synthesis in central serotonergic neurons. In *New Concepts in Neurotransmitter Regulation* (A.J. Mandell, Ed.), pp. 239-257. Plenum Press, New York.

Goddard, J.L. (1973). The medical business. *Sci. Am.* 229, 161-166.

Gluckman, M.I. and Baum, T. (1969). The pharmacology of iprindole, a new antidepressant. *Psychopharmacologia,* 15, 168-185.

Gold, R.M. (1967). Aphagia and adipsia following unilateral and bilateral asymetrical lesions in rats. *Physiol. Beh.,* 2, 211-220.

Goldberg, S.R. (1970). Relapse to opioid dependence: the role of conditioning. In *Drug Dependence* (R.T. Harris, W.M. McIsaac and C.R. Schuster, Eds.), pp. 170-197. Univ. of Texas Press, Austin.

Goldberg, S.R. and Schuster, C.R. (1967). Conditioned suppression by a stimulus associated with nalorphin in morphine-dependent monkeys. *J. Exp. Anal. Beh.,* 10, 235-242.

Goldstein, A. (1976a). Heroin addiction: sequential treatment employing pharmacological supports. *Arch. Gen. Psychiatry,* 33, 353-358.

Goldstein, A. (1976b). Opioid peptides (endorphins) in pituitary and brain. *Science,* 193, 1081-1086.

Goldstein, A., Aronow, L. and Kalman, S.M. (1974). *Principles of Drug Action: The Basis of Pharmacology.* Wiley, New York.

Goldstein, S., Lowney, L.I. and Pal, B.K. (1971). Stereospecific and nonspecific interactions of the morphine congener levorphanol in subcellular fractions of mouse brain. *Proc. Nat. Acad. Sci.,* 68, 1742-1747.

Goldstein, D.B. and Goldstein, A. (1961). Possible role of enzyme induction and regression in drug tolerance and addiction. *Biochem. Pharmacol.,* 8, 48.

Goldstein, M., Lew, J.Y., Matsumoto, Y., Hökfelt, T. and Fuxe, K. (1978). Localization and function of PNMT in the central nervous system. In *Psychopharmacology: A Generation of Progress* (M.A. Lipton, A. DiMascio and K.F. Killam, Eds.), pp. 261-269. Raven Press, New York.

Goodman, L.S. and Gilman, A. (Eds.) (1980). *The Pharmacological Basis of Therapeutics.* MacMillan, New York.

Goodwin, F.K. and Post, R.M. (1974). Brain serotonin, affective illness, and antidepressant drugs: cerebrospinal fluid studies with probenecid. In *Advances in Biochemical Psychopharmacology, Vol. 11* (E. Costa, G.L. Gessa and M. Sandler, Eds.), pp. 341-355. Raven Press, New York.

Goodwin, F.K., Post, R.M., Dunner, D.L. and Gordon, E.K. (1973). Cerebrospinal fluid amine metabolites in affective illness: the probenecid technique. *Am. J. Psychiatry,* 130, 73-79.

Goodwin, F.K. and Potter, W.Z. (1978). The biology of affective illness: amine neurotransmitters and drug response. In *Depression: Biology, Psychodynamics and Treatment* (J.O. Cole, A.F. Schatzberg and S.H. Frazier, Eds.), pp. 41-73. Plenum Press, New York.

Gottesfeld, A., Kelly, J.S. and Renaud, L.P. (1972). The in vivo neuropharmacology of amino-oxyacetic acid in the cerebral cortex of the cat. *Brain Res.,* 42, 319-335.

Graeff, F.G. (1974). Tryptamine antagonists and punished behavior. *J. Pharmacol. Exp. Ther.,* 189, 344-350.

Graeff, F.G. and Schoenfeld, R.I. (1970). Tryptaminergic mechanisms in punished and nonpunished behavior. *J. Pharmacol. Exp. Ther.,* 173, 277-283.

Grandison, L. and Guidotti, A. (1977). Stimulation of food intake by muscimol and beta endorphin. *Neuropharmacol.,* 16, 533-536.

Grant, L.D., Coscina, D.V., Grossman, S.P. and Freedman, D.X. (1972). Muricide after serotonin depleting lesions of midbrain raphe nuclei. *Pharm. Biochem. Behav.,* 1, 77-80.

Gray, E.G. (1959). Axo-somatic and axo-dendritic synapses of the cerebral cortex: an electron microscopic study. *J. Anat.,* 93, 420-423.

Gray, E.G. (1967). The synapse. *Sci. J. (London),* 3, 5, 66-72.

Gray, E.G. (1970). The fine structure of nerve. *Comp. Biochem. Physiol.,* 36, 419-448.

Green, A.R. and Grahame-Smith, D.G. (1975). 5-Hydroxytryptamine and other indoles in the central nervous system. In *Handbook of Psychopharmacology Vol. 3, Biochemistry of Biogenic Amines* (L.L. Iversen, S.D. Iversen, S.H. Snyder, Eds.), pp. 169-245. Plenum Press, New York.

Green, J.P., Johnson, C.L. and Weinstein, H. (1978). Histamine as a neurotransmitter. In *Psychopharmacology: A Generation of Progress* (M.A. Lipton, A. DiMascio and K.F. Killam, Eds.), pp. 319-332. Raven Press, New York.

Green, J.P. and Maayani, S. (1977). Tricyclic antidepressent drugs block histamine H_2 receptors in brain. *Nature,* 269, 163-165.

Greenblatt, D.J. and Shader, R.I. (1974). *Benzodiazepines in Clinical Practice.* Raven Press, New York.

Greenblatt, D.J. and Shader, R.I. (1978). Pharmacotherapy of anxiety with benzodiazepines and β-adrenergic blockers. In *Psychopharmacology: A Generation of Progress* (M.A. Lipton, A. DiMascio and K.F. Killam, Eds.), pp. 1381-1390. Raven Press, New York.

Greengard, P. (1976). Possible role for cyclic nucleotides and phosphorylated membrane proteins in postsynaptic actions of neurotransmitters. *Nature,* 260, 101-108.

Greengard, P. (1979). Some chemical aspects of neurotransmitter action. *Trends Pharmacol. Sci.,* 1, 27-29.

Greengard, P., McAfee, D.A. and Kebabian, J.W. (1972). On the mechanism of action of cyclic AMP and its role in synaptic transmission. In *Advances in Cyclic Nucleotide*

Research, Vol. 1 (P. Greengard and G.A. Robison, Eds.), pp. 337–355. Raven Press, New York.

Gringauz, A. (1978). *Drugs, How They Act and Why*. Mosby, St. Louis.

Grinker, R.R. and Spiegel, J.P. (1945). *Men Under Stress*. Blakiston, Philadelphia.

Gritz, E.R. and Jarvick, M.E. (1978). Nicotine and smoking. In *Handbook of Psychopharmacology, Vol. 11* (L.L. Iversen, S.D. Iversen and S.H. Snyder, Eds.), pp. 425–464. Plenum Press, New York.

Groves, P.M., Wilson, C.J., Young, S.J. and Rebec, G.V. (1975). Selfinhibition by dopaminergic neurons. *Science*, 190, 522–529.

Guidotti, A. (1978). Synaptic mechanisms in the action of benzodiazepines. In *Psychopharmacology: A Generation of Progress* (M.A. Lipton, A. DiMascio and K.F. Killam, Eds.), pp. 1349–1357. Raven Press, New York.

Guidotti, A., Badiani, G. and Pepeu, G. (1972). Taurine distribution in cat brain. *J. Neurochem.*, 19, 431–435.

Guidotti, A., Baraldi, M., Schwartz, J.P. and Costa, E. (1979). Molecular mechanisms regulating the interactions between the benzodiazepines and GABA receptors in the central nervous system. *Pharm. Biochem. Beh.*, 10, 803–807.

Guillemin, R. (1980). Hypothalamic hormones: releasing and inhibiting factors. In *Neuroendocrinology* (D.T. Krieger and J.C. Hughes, Eds.), pp. 23–32. Sinauer Associates, Sunderland, Massachusetts.

Guillemin, R. and Burgus, R. (1972). The hormones of the hypothalamus. *Sci. Am.*, 227, 5, 24–33.

Guillemin, R., Vargo, T., Rossier, J., Minick, S., Ling, W., Rivier, C., Vale, W. and Bloom, F. (1977). β-Endorphin and adrenocorticotropin are secreted concomitantly by the pituitary gland. *Science*, 197, 1367–1369.

Gunne, L.M. (1963). Catecholamines and 5-hydroxytryptamine in morphine tolerance and withdrawal. *Acta Physiol. Scand. (Suppl. 204)*, 58, 204, 1–91.

Gunne, L.M., Lindstrom, L. and Terenius, J. (1977). Naloxone-induced reversal of schizophrenic hallucinations. *J. Neural Transm.*, 40, 13–20.

Guroff, G. (1975). Some aspects of aromatic amino acid metabolism in the brain. In *The Nervous System, Vol. I, The Basic Neurosciences* (Donald B. Tower, Ed.), pp. 553–564. Raven Press, New York.

Haber, E. and Wrenn, S. (1976). Problems in identification of the beta-adrenergic receptor. *Physiol. Rev.*, 56, 2, 317–338.

Hadley, M.E. and Bagnara, J.T. (1975). Regulation of release and mechanism of action of MSH. *Am. Zool.*, 15, Suppl. 1, 81–104.

Hadley, M.E., Davis, M.D. and Morgan, C.M. (1977). Cellular control of melanocyte stimulating hormone secretion. *Front. Horm. Res.*, 4, 94–104.

Haefely, W.E. (1977). Synaptic pharmacology of barbiturates and benzodiazepines, *Agents Actions*, 7/3, 353–359.

Haefely, W.E. (1978). Behavioral and neuropharmacological aspects of drugs in anxiety and related states. In *Psychopharmacology: A Generation of Progress* (M.A. Lipton, A. DiMascio and K.F. Killam, Eds.), pp. 1359–1374. Raven Press, New York.

Haefely, W., Kulcsár, A., Möhler, H., Pieri, L., Polc, P. and Schaffner, R. (1975). Possible involvement of GABA in the central actions of benzodiazepines. In *Advances in Biochemical Psychopharmacology, Vol. 14* (E. Costa and P. Greengard, Eds.), pp. 131–151. Raven Press, New York.

Haggendal, J. and Lindqvist, M. (1964). Disclosure of labile monoamine fractions in brain and their correlation to behavior. *Acta Physiol. Scand.*, 60, 351–362.

Haier, R. (1980). The diagnosis of schizophrenia: a review of recent developments. *Schizophr. Bull.*, 6, 417–428.

Hall, Z.W., Hildebrand, J.G. and Kravitz, E.A. (1974). *Chemistry of Synaptic Transmission*. Chiron Press, Newton, Massachusetts.

Halliwell, G., Quinton, R.M. and Williams, F.E. (1964). A comparison of imipramine, chlorpromazine and related drugs in various tests involving autonomic functions and antagonism of reserpine. *Br. J. Pharmacol.*, 23, 330–350.

Hammer, M., Makiesky-Barrow, S. and Gutwirth, L. (1978). Social networks and schizophrenia. *Schizophr. Bull.*, 4, 522–545.

Hammerschlag, R. and Roberts, E. (1976). Overview of chemical transmission. In *Basic Neurochemistry* (G.J. Siegel, R.W. Albers, R. Katzman and B.W. Agranoff, Eds.), pp. 167–179. Little, Brown, Boston.

Hamon, M., Bourgoin, S., Morot-Gaudry, Y., Héry, F. and Glowinski, J. (1974). Role of active transport of tryptophan in the control of 5-hydroxytryptophan biosynthesis. In *Advances in Biochemical Psychopharmacology, Vol. 11* (E. Costa, G.L. Gessa and M. Sandler, Eds.), pp. 153–162. Raven Press, New York.

Hamori, J. and Szentagothai, J. (1965). The Purkinje cell baskets: ultrastructure of an inhibitory synapse. *Acta Biol. Acad. Sci. Hung.*, 15, 465–479.

Hanbauer, 1., Pradhan, S. and Yang, H.Y.T. (1980). Role of calmodulin in dopaminergic transmission. In *Calmodulin and Cell Function Vol. 356* (D.M. Watterson and F.F. Vincenzi, Eds.), pp. 292–303, N.Y. Acad. Sci. Publ. New York.

Hanson, L. (1967). Evidence that the central action of (+)-amphetamine is mediated via catecholamines. *Psychopharmacologia*, 10, 289–297.

Harper, R.G., Solish, G.I., Purow, H.M., Sang, E. and Panepinto, W.C. (1974). The effect of a methadone treatment program upon pregnant heroin addicts and their newborn infants. *Pediatrics*, 54, 300–305.

Harris, G.W. (1937). The induction of ovulation in the rabbit by electric stimulation of the hypothalamo-hypophyseal stalk. *Proc. Roy. Soc. Br.*, 122, 374–394.

Harris, G.W. (1955). *Neural Control of the Pituitary Gland.* Edward Arnold, London.

Harris, L.S. and Dewey, W.L. (1973). Role of cholinergic systems in the central action of narcotic agonists and antagonists. In *Agonist and Antagonist Actions of Narcotic Analgesic Drugs* (H.W. Kosterlitz, H.O.J. Collier and J.E. Villarreal, Eds.), pp. 198–206. University Park Press, Baltimore.

Harris, R.T. and Balster, R.L. (1970). An analysis of psychological dependence. In *Drug Dependence* (R.T. Harris, W.M. McIsaac and C.R. Shuster, Eds.), pp. 214–226. Univ. of Texas Press, Austin, Texas.

Hartman, E. (1978). Effects of psychotropic drugs on sleep: the catecholamines and sleep. In *Psychopharmacology: A Generation of Progress* (M.A. Lipton, A. DiMascio and K.F. Killam, Eds.), pp. 711–728. Raven Press, New York.

Hartzell, H.C. and Fambrough, D.M. (1982). Acetylcholine receptors: distribution and extrajunctional density in rat diaphragm after denervation correlated with acetylcholine sensitivity. *J. Gen. Physiol.* 60, 248–262.

Harvald, B. and Hauge, M. (1956). Catamnestic investigation of Danish twins. *Dan. Med. Bull.,* 3, 150–158.

Harvey, J.A. and McMaster, S.E. (1977). Fenfluramine: cummulative neurotoxicity after chronic treatment with low dosages in the rat. *Commun. Psychopharmacol.,* 1, 3–17.

Harvey, J.A., Schlosberg, A.J. and Yunger, L.M. (1974). Effect of *p*-chlorophenylalanine and brain lesions on pain sensitivity and morphine analgesia in the rat. In *Advances in Biochemical Psychopharmacology, Vol. 10* (E. Costa, G.L. Gessa and M. Sandler, Eds.), pp. 233–245. Raven Press, New York.

Harvey, S.C. (1975). Hypnotics and sedatives. In *The Pharmacological Basis of Therapeutics* (L.S. Goodman and A. Gilman, Eds.), pp. 102–123. MacMillan, New York.

Havlicek, V. and Friesen, H.G. (1979). Comparison of behavioral effects of somatostatin and β-endorphin in animals. In *Central Nervous System Effects of Hypothalamic Hormones and Other Peptides* (R. Collu, A. Barbeau, J-G. Rochefort and J.R. Ducharme, Eds.), pp. 381–402. Raven Press, New York.

Hayashi, T. (1956). *Chemical Physiology of Excitation in Muscle and Nerve.* Dainihon-Tosho, Tokyo.

Health Consequences of Smoking. A report of the Surgeon General (1980). DHEW Publ. No. (PHS) 79-50066. U.S. Gov't. Printing Office, Washington, D.C.

Hearst, E. (1964). Drug effects on stimulus generalization gradients in the monkey. *Psychopharmacologia,* 6, 57–70.

Held, H. (1897). Beitrage zur struktur der Nervenzellen und ihrer Fortsatze. *Arch. Anat. Physiol. (Leipzig),* 204–294.

Heller, J.M., Pearson, J. and Simon, E.J. (1973). Distribution of stereospecific binding of the potent narcotic analgesic etorphine in the human brain: predominance in the limbic system. *Res. Commun. Chem. Pathol. Pharmacol.,* 6, 1052–1062.

Henderson, G. and Hughes, J. (1976). The effects of morphine on the release of noradrenaline from the mouse vas deferens. *Br. J. Pharmacol.,* 57, 551–557.

Hendley, E.D. and Welch, B.L. (1975). Electroconvulsive shock: sustained decrease in norepinephrine uptake in a reserpine model of depression. *Life Sci.,* 16, 45–54.

Henriksen, S., Dement, W. and Barchas, J. (1974). The role of serotonin in the regulation of a phasic event of rapid eye movement sleep: the pontogeniculo-occipital wave. In *Advances in Biochemical Psychopharmcology, Vol. 11* (E. Costa, G.L. Gessa and M. Sandler, Eds.), pp. 169–179. Raven Press, New York.

Henry, J.L. (1977). Substance P and pain: a possible relation in afferent transmission. In *Substance P* (U.S. von Euler and B. Pernow, Eds.), pp. 231–240. Raven Press, New York.

Heritage, A.S., Stumpf, W.E., Sar, M. and Grant, L.D. (1980). Brainstem catecholamine neurons are target sites for sex steroid hormones. *Science,* 207, 1377–1379.

Herndon, R.M. and Coyle, J.T. (1977). Selective destruction of neurons by a transmitter agonist. *Science,* 198, 71–72.

Herschel, R., Havlicek, V., Rezek, M. and Kroeger, E. (1977). Cerebroventricular administration of somatostatin (SRIF) effect on central levels of cyclic AMP. *Life Sci.,* 20, 821–826.

Héry, F., Pujol, J.F., Lopez, M., Macon, J. and Glowinski, J. (1970). Increased synthesis and utilization of serotonin in the central nervous system of the rat during paradoxical sleep deprivation. *Brain Res.,* 21, 391–403.

Héry, R., Rouer, E., Kan, J.P. and Glowinski, J. (1974). The major role of the tryptophan active transport in the diurnal variations of 5-hydroxytryptamine synthesis in the rat brain. In *Advances in Biochemical Psychopharmacology, Vol. 11* (E. Costa, G.L. Gessa and M. Sandler, Eds.), pp. 163–167. Raven Press, New York.

Herz, A., Albus, K., Metys, J., Schubert, P. and Teschemacher, H. (1970). On the central sites for the antinociceptive action of morphine and fentanyl. *Neuropharmacol.,* 9, 539-551.

Hess, W.R. (1954). Diencephalon, autonomic and extrapyramidal functions. *Monogr. Biol. Med. Vol. 3,* Grune and Stratton, New York.

Heston, L.L. (1970). The genetics of schizophrenia and schizoid disease. *Science,* 167, 249–256.

Heuser, J.E. (1976). Morphology of synaptic vesicle discharge and reformation at the frog neuromuscular junction. In *Motor Innervation of Muscle* (S. Thesleff, Ed.), pp. 51–115. Academic Press, London.

Heuser, J.E. (1977). Synaptic vesicle exocytosis revealed in quick-frozen frog neuromuscular junctions treated with 4-aminopyridine and given a single electric shock. In *Society for Neuroscience Symposia, Vol. II* (W.M. Cowan and J.A. Ferrendelli, Eds.), pp. 215–239. Society for Neuroscience, Bethesda, Maryland.

Heuser, J.E. and Reese, T.S. (1973). Evidence for recycling of synaptic vesicle membrane during transmitter release at the frog neuromuscular junction. *J. Cell Biol.,* 57, 315–344.

Heuser, J.E. and Reese, T.S. (1977). Structure of the synapse. In *Handbook of Physiology, The Nervous System, Vol. 1* (J.M. Brookhart and V.B. Mountcastle, Eds.), pp. 261–294. American Physiological Society, Washington, D.C.

Heuser, J.E., Reese, T.S. and Landis, D.M.D. (1974). Functional changes in frog neuromuscular junction studied with freeze-fracture. *J. Neurocytol.,* 3, 109–131.

Hillarp, N.A., Fuxe, K. and Dahlström, A. (1966). Demonstration and mapping of central neurons containing dopamine, noradrenaline and 5-hydroxytryptamine and their reactions to psychopharmaca. *Pharmacol. Rev.,* 18, 727.

Himmelsbach, C.K. (1943). Can the euphoric analgetic and physical dependence effects of drugs be separated? With reference to physical dependence. *Fed. Proc.,* 2, 201–203.

Ho, A.K.S., Loh, H.H., Craves, F., Hitzemann, R.J. and Gershon, S. (1970). The effect of prolonged lithium treatment on the synthesis rate and turnover of monoamines in brain regions of rats. *Eur. J. Pharmacol.,* 10, 72–78.

Ho, I.K., Loh, H.H. and Way, E.L. (1973). Cyclic adenosine monophosphate antagonism of morphine analgesia. *J. Pharmacol. Exp. Ther.,* 185, 336–346.

Hodgkins, A.L. (1964a). *The Conduction of the Nervous Impulse.* Liverpool Univ. Press, Liverpool.

Hodgkin, A.L. (1964b). The ionic basis of nervous conduction. *Science,* 145, 1148–1153.

Hodgkin, A.L. and Huxley, A.F. (1952). A quantitative description of membrane current and its application to conduction and excitation in nerve. *J. Physiol. (London),* 117, 500–544.

Hofmann, A. (1970). The discovery of LSD and subsequent investigations on natural occurring hallucinogens. In *Discoveries in Biological Psychiatry* (F.J. Ayd and B. Blackwell, Eds.), pp. 93–106. Lippincott, Philadelphia.

Hökfelt, T., Efendik, S., Johansson, O., Luft, R. and Arimura, A. (1974a). Immunohistochemical localization of somatostatin (growth hormone releasing factor) in the guinea pig brain. *Brain Res.,* 80, 165–169.

Hökfelt, T., Elde, R., Johannsson, O., Ljungdahl, Å., Schultzberg, M., Fuxe, K., Goldstein, M., Nilsson, G., Pernow, B., Terenius, L., Ganten, D., Jeffcoate, S.L., Rehfeld, J. and Said, S. (1978). Distribution of peptide-containing neurons. In *Psychopharmacology: A Generation of Progress* (M.A. Lipton, A DiMascio and K.F. Killam, Eds.), pp. 39–66. Raven Press, New York.

Hökfelt, T., Fuxe, K., Goldstein, M. and Johansson, O. (1973). Evidence for adrenaline neurons in the rat brain. *Acta Physiol. Scand.,* 89, 286–288.

Hökfelt, T., Fuxe, K., Johansson, O., Jeffcoate, S. and White, N. (1974b). Distribution of thyrotropin releasing hormone (TRH) in the central nervous system as revealed with immunohistochemistry. *Eur. J. Pharmacol.,* 34, 389–392.

Hökfelt, T., Kellerth, J.O., Nilsson, G. and Pernow, B. (1975a). Experimental immunohistochemical studies on the localization and distribution of substance P in cat primary sensory neurons. *Brain Res.,* 100, 234–252.

Hökfelt, T., Kellerth, J.O., Nilsson, G. and Pernow, B. (1975b). Substance P: localizing in the central nervous system and in some primary sensory neurons. *Science,* 190, 889–890.

Hökfelt, T., Ljungdahl, Å., Fuxe, K. and Johansson, O. (1974c). Dopamine nerve terminals in the rat limbic cortex: aspects of the dopamine hypothesis of schizophrenia. *Science,* 184, 177–179.

Hökfelt, T., Ljungdahl, Å., Terenius, L., Elde, R. and Nilsson, G. (1977). Immunohistochemical analysis of peptide pathways possibly related to pain and anlagesia: enkephalin and substance P. *Proc. Nat. Acad. Sci.,* 74, 3081–3085.

Hollister, A.S., Breese, G.R. and Cooper, B.R. (1974). Comparison of tyrosine hydroxylase and dopamine-β-hydroxylase inhibition with the effects of various 6-OHDA treatments of amphetamine-induced motor activity. *Psychopharmacologia,* 36, 1–16.

Hollister, L.E. (1967). *Chemical Psychosis: LSD and Related Drugs.* Thomas, Springfield, Illinois.

Hollister, L.E. (1973). *Clinical Use of Psychotherapeutic Drugs.* Thomas, Springfield, Illinois.

Hollister, L.E. (1977). Some general thoughts about endogenous psychotogens. In *Neuroregulators and Psychiatric Disorders* (E. Usdin, D.A. Hamburg and J.D. Barchas, Eds.), pp. 550–556. Oxford Univ. Press, New York.

Hollister, L.E. (1978). Psychotomimetic drugs in man. In *Handbook of Psychopharmacology, Vol. 11* (L.L. Iversen, S.D. Iversen and S.H. Snyder, Eds.), pp. 389–424. Plenum Press, New York.

Hollister, L.E. (1980) Dependence on benzodiazepines. In *Benzodiazepines: A Review of Research Results,* (S.I. Szara and J.P. Ludford, Eds.), pp. 70–82. Superintendent of Documents, Washington, D.C.

Hollister, L.E. and Friedhoff, A.J. (1966). Effects of 3,4-dimethoxyphenylethylamine in man. *Nature,* 310, 1377–1378.

Höllt, V., Dum, J., Bläsig, J., Schubert, P. and Herz, A. (1975). Comparison of in vivo and in vitro parameters of opiate receptor binding in naive and tolerant/dependent rodents. *Life Sci.,* 16, 1823–1828.

Holter, H. (1961). How things get into cells. *Sci. Am.,* 205, 3, 167–180.

Holtz, P. (1950). Ueber die sympathicomimetische Wirksamkeit von Gehirnextrackten. *Acta Physiol. Scand.,* 20, 354–362.

Honig, W.K. (Ed.) (1966). *Operant Behavior: Areas of*

Research and Application. Appleton-Century-Crofts, New York.

Horita, A. and Carino, M.A. (1975). Thyrotropin-releasing hormone (TRH)–induced hyperthermia and behavioral excitation in rabbits. *Psychopharmacol. Commun.*, 1, 403–414.

Hornykiewicz, O. (1963). Die topische lokalisation und vehalten von Noradrenalin und Dopamin-(3-Hydroxytyramin) in der Substantia Nigra des Normalin und Parkinsonkranken. *Wien. Klin. Wochenschr.*, 75, 309–312.

Hornykiewicz, O. (1966). Dopamine (3-hydroxytyramine) and brain function. *Pharmacol. Rev.*, 18, 925–964.

Hornykiewicz, O. (1974). The mechanisms of action of L-dopamine in Parkinson's disease. *Life Sci.*, 15, 1249–1259.

Horovitz, Z.P., Piala, J.J., High, J.P., Burke, J.C. and Leaf, R.C. (1966). Effects of drugs on the mouse-killing (muricide) test and its relationship to amygdaloid function. *Int. J. Neuropharmacol.*, 5, 405–411.

Horst, W.D. and Spirt, N. (1974). A possible mechanism for the antidepressant activity of thyrotropin-releasing hormone. *Life Sci.* 15, 1073–1082.

Hosobuchi, Y., Rossier, J., Bloom, F. and Guillemin, R. (1979). Stimulation of human periaqueductal gray for pain relief increases immunoreactive β-endorphin in ventricular fluid. *Science,* 203, 279–281.

Houde, R.W. and Wallenstein, S.L. (1953). A method evaluating analgesia in patients with chronic pain. *Drug Addiction & Narcotics Bull.,* Appendix F., 660–682.

Howell, W.H. (1942). *A Textbook of Physiology, 14th Ed.* Saunders, Philadelphia.

Hsia, Y.E. (1976). Disorders of amino acid metabolism. In *Basic Neurochemistry* (G.J. Siegel, R.W. Albers, R. Katzman and B.W. Agranoff, Eds.), pp. 500–541. Little, Brown, Boston.

Hughes, J. (1975). Search for the endogenous ligand of the opiate receptor. *Neurosci. Res. Prog. Bull.,* 13, 55–58.

Hughes, J., Smith, T.W., Kosterlitz, H.W., Fothergill, L.A., Morgan, B.A. and Morris, H.R. (1975a). Identification of two related pentapeptides from the brain with potent opiate agonist activity. *Nature,* 258, 577–579.

Hughes, J., Smith, T., Morgan, B. and Fothergill, L. (1975b). Purification and properties of enkephalin—the possible endogenous ligand for the morphine receptor. *Life Sci.,* 16, 1753–1758.

Hughes, P.H. and Crawford, G.A. (1972). A contagious disease model for researching and intervening in heroin epidemics. *Arch. Gen. Psychiatry,* 27, 149–155.

Hunt, H.F. and Brady, J.V. (1951). Some effects of electroconvulsive shock on a conditioned emotional response ("anxiety"). *J. Comp. Physiol. Psychol.,* 44, 1, 88–98.

Huntington, G. (1872). On chorea. *Med. Surg. Rep.,* 26, 317.

Huston, J.P. and Staubli, U. (1978). Retrograde amnesia produced by posttrial injection of substance P into substantia nigra. *Brain Res.,* 159, 468–472.

Hutchinson, J.S., Schelling, P. Möhring, J. and Ganten, D. (1976). Effect of intraventricular perfusion of angiotensin II in conscious normal rats and in rats with hereditary hypothalamic diabetes insipidus. *Clin. Sci. Mol. Med.,* 51, 391s–394s.

Huxley, A.F. (1964). Excitation and conduction in nerve: quantitative analysis. *Science,* 145, 1154–1159.

Innes, I.R. and Nickerson, M. (1975). Atropine, scopolamine and related antimuscarinic drugs. In *The Pharmacological Basis of Therapeutics, 5th Edition.* (L.S. Goodman and A. Gilman, Eds.), pp. 514–532. Macmillan, New York.

Isbell, H. (1950). Addiction to barbiturates and barbiturate abstinence syndrome. *Ann. Intern. Med.,* 33, 108–121.

Isbell, H., Altschul, S., Kornetsky, C.H., Eisenman, A.J., Flanary, H.G. and Fraser, H.F. (1950). Chronic barbiturate intoxication. *Arch. Neurol. Psychiatry,* 64, 1–28.

Isbell, H., Miner, E.J. and Logan, C.R. (1959). Cross tolerance between d–2 brom–lysergic acid diethylamide (BOL-148) and d–diethylamide of lysergic acid (LSD-25). *Psychopharmacologia,* 1, 109–116.

Isbell, H., Wolbach, A. and Rosenberg, D. (1962). Observations on direct and cross tolerance with LSD and dextroamphetamine in man. *Fed. Proc.,* 2, 416.

Isbell, H., Wolbach, A.B., Wikler, A. and Miner, E.J. (1961). Cross tolerance between LSD and psilocybin. *Psychopharmacologia,* 2, 147–159.

Iversen, L.L. (1975a). Dopamine receptors in the brain. *Science,* 188, 1084–1089.

Iversen, L.L. (1975b). Uptake processes for biogenic amines. In *Handbook of Psychopharmacology, Vol. 3* (L.L. Iversen, S.D. Iversen and S.H. Snyder, Eds.), pp. 381–442. Plenum Press, New York.

Iversen, L.L. (1978). Biochemical psychopharmacology of GABA. In *Psychopharmacology: A Generation of Progress* (M.A. Lipton, A. Di Mascio and K.F. Killam, Eds.), pp. 25–38. Raven Press, New York.

Iversen, L.L. (1979). The chemistry of the brain. *Sci. Am.,* 241, 3, 134–149.

Iversen, L.L. and Bloom, F.E. (1972). Studies of the uptake of ^{3}H-GABA and ^{3}H-glycine in slices and homogenates of rat brain and spinal cord by electron microscopic autoradiography. *Brain Res.,* 41, 131–143.

Iversen, L.L., Iversen, S.D. and Snyder, S.H. (Eds.) (1978). *Handbook of Psychopharmacology, Vol. 14, Affective Disorders: Drug Actions in Animals and Man.* Plenum Press, New York.

Iversen, L.L., Jessell, T. and Kanazawa, I. (1976). Release and metabolism of substance P in rat hypothalamus. *Nature,* 264, 81–83.

Iversen, S.D. (1974). 6-Hydroxydopamine: a chemical lesion technique for studying the role of amine neurotransmitters in behavior. In *The Neurosciences, Third Study Program* (F.O. Schmitt and F.G. Worden, Eds.), pp. 705–711. MIT Press, Cambridge, Massachusetts.

Iversen, S.D. and Iversen, L.L. (1981). *Behavioral Pharmacology,* Oxford Univ. Press, New York.

Jackman, H.L. and Meltzer, H.Y. (1980). Factors affecting determination of platelet monoamineoxidase activity. *Schizophr. Bull.,* 6, 259–266.

Jackson, I.M.D. and Reichlin, S. (1977). Brain thyrotropin-releasing hormone is independent of the hypothalamus. *Nature,* 267, 853–854.

Jacobowitz, D.M. (1978). Monoaminergic pathways in the central nervous system. In *Psychopharmacology: A Generation of Progress* (M.A. Lipton, A. DiMascio and K.F. Killam, Eds.), pp. 119–129. Raven Press, New York.

Jacobs, B.L. (1973). A multidimensional approach to the study of unit activity in freely moving animals. In *Brain Unit Activity During Behavior* (M.I. Phillips, Ed.), pp. 268–287. Thomas, Springfield, Illinois.

Jacobs, B.L. (1974). Evidence for the functional interaction of two central neurotransmitters. *Psychopharmacologia,* 39, 81–86.

Jacobs, B.L., Wise, W.D. and Taylor, K.M. (1974). Differential behavioral and neurochemical effects following lesions of the dorsal and median raphe nuclei in rats. *Brain Res.,* 79, 353–361.

Jacobson, S. (1972). Neurocytology. In *An Introduction to the Neurosciences* (B.A. Curtis, S. Jacobson and E.M. Marcus), pp. 36–71. Saunders, Philadelphia.

Jacoby, J.H., Shebshelowitz, H., Fernstrom, J.D. and Wurtzman, R.J. (1975). The mechanism by which methiothepin, a putative serotonin receptor antagonist, increased brain 5-hydroxyindole levels. *J. Pharmacol. Exp. Ther.,* 195, 2, 257–264.

Jacquet, Y.F. and Lajtha, A. (1974). Paradoxical effects after microinjection of morphine in the periaqueductal gray matter in the rat. *Science,* 185, 1055–1057.

Jacquet, Y.F. and Marks, N. (1976). The C-fragment of β-lipotropin: an endogenous neuroleptic or antipsychotogen? *Science,* 194, 632–635.

Jacquet, Y.F., Marks, N. and Li, C.H. (1976). Behavioral and biochemical properties of "opioid" peptides. In *Opiates and Endogenous Opiate Peptides* (H. Kosterlitz, Ed.), pp. 411–414. Elsevier/North-Holland, Amsterdam.

Jaffe, J.H. (1970). The implementation and evaluation of new treatments for compulsive drug users. In *Drug Dependence* (R.T. Harris, W.M. McIsaac and C.R. Schuster, Eds.), pp. 229–241. Univ. of Texas Press, Austin.

Jaffe, J.H. (1975). Drug addiction and drug abuse. In *The Pharmacological Basis of Therapeutics, 5th Edition* (L.S. Goodman and A. Gilman, Eds.), pp. 284–324. Macmillan, New York.

Jaffe, J.H. and Jarvik, M.E. (1978). Tobacco use and tobacco use disorder. In *Psychopharmacology: A Generation of Progress* (M.A. Lipton, A. DiMascio and K.F. Killam, Eds.), pp. 1665–1676. Raven Press, New York.

Jaffe, J.H. and Martin, W.R. (1975). Narcotic analgesics and antagonists. In *The Pharmacological Basis of Therapeutics, 5th Edition* (L.S. Goodman and A. Gilman, Eds.), pp. 245–283. Macmillan, New York.

Jaffe, J.H. and Sharpless, S. (1968). Pharmacological denervation supersensitivity in the central nervous system: a theory of physical dependence. *Proc. Assoc. Res. Nerv. Ment. Dis.,* 46, 226–246.

Janowsky, D.S. and Davis, J.M. (1976). Methylphenidate, dextroamphetamine, levoamphetamine effects on schizophrenic symptoms. *Arch. Gen. Psychiatry,* 33, 304–308.

Jarvik, M.E. (1970). Drugs used in the treatment of psychiatric disorders. In *The Pharmacological Basis of Therapeutics* (L.S. Goodman and A. Gilman, Eds.), pp. 151–203. Macmillan, New York.

Jarvik, M.E., Cullen, J.W., Gritz, E.R., Vogt, T.M. and West, L.J. (Eds.) (1977). *Research on Smoking Behavior, NIDA Research Monograph 17.* Supt. of Documents, U.S. Govt, Printing Office, Washington, D.C.

Jequier, E., Lovenberg, W. and Sjoerdsma, A. (1967). Tryptophan hydroxylase inhibition: the mechanism by which *p*-chlorophenylalanine depletes rat brain serotonin. *Mol. Pharmacol.,* 3, 274–278.

Jespersen, S. and Scheel-Krüger, J. (1970). Antagonism by methysergide of the 5-hydroxytryptamine-like action of toxic doses of fenfluramine in dogs. *J. Pharm. and Pharmacol.,* 22, 637–638.

Jespersen, S. and Scheel-Krüger, J. (1973). Evidence for a difference between fenfluramine– and amphetamine–induced anorexia. *J. Pharm. Pharmacol.,* 25, 49–54.

Jessell, T.M. and Iversen, L.L. (1977). Opiate analgesics inhibit substance P release from rat trigeminal nucleus. *Nature,* 268, 549–551.

Jeste, D.V. and Wyatt, R.J. (1979). In search of treatment for tardive dyskinesia: review of the literature. *Schizophr. Bull.,* 5, 251–293.

Johnson, F.N. (1975). *Lithium Research and Therapy.* Academic Press, New York.

Johnson, G.A., Kim, E.G. and Boukma, S.J. (1972). 5-Hydroxyindole levels in rat brain after inhibition of dopamine-β-hydroxylase. *J. Pharmacol. Exp. Ther.,* 180, 539–546.

Johnston, G.A.R. (1975). Biochemistry of glycine, taurine, glutamate, and aspartate. In *Handbook of Psychopharmacology, Vol. 4* (L.L. Iversen, S.D. Iversen and S.H. Snyder, Eds.), pp. 59–81. Plenum Press, New York.

Johnston, J.P. (1968). Some observations upon a new inhibitor of monoamine oxidase in brain tissue. *Biochem. Pharmacol.,* 17, 1285–1297.

Jones, B., Bobillier, P. and Jouvet, M. (1968). Effets de la destruction des neurons contenent des catecholamines du mesencephale sur le cycle veillesommeil de chat. *C.R. Soc. Biol. (Paris),* 163, 176–180.

Jori, A. and Garattini, S. (1965). Interaction between

imipramine-like agents and catecholamine-induced hyperthermia. *J. Pharm. Pharmacol.,* 17, 480–488.

Jouvet, M. (1967). Neurophysiology of the states of sleep. In *The Neurosciences* (G.C. Quarton, T. Melnechuk and F.O. Schmitt, Eds.), pp. 529–544. Rockefeller Univ. Press, New York.

Jouvet, M. (1972). Some monoaminergic mechanisms controlling sleep and waking. In *Brain and Human Behavior* (A.G. Karczmar and J.C. Eccles, Eds.), pp. 131–162, Springer Verlag, Berlin.

Jouvet, M. (1974). Monoaminergic regulation of the sleep-waking cycle in the cat. In *The Neurosciences, 3rd Study Program* (F.O. Schmitt and F.G. Worden, Eds.), pp. 499–508. MIT Press, Cambridge, Mass.

Jouvet, M. and Pujol, J.F. (1974). Effects of central alterations of serotonergic neurons upon the sleep-waking cycle. In *Advances in Biochemical Psychopharmacology, Vol. 11* (E. Costa, G.L. Gessa and M. Sandler, Eds.), pp. 199–209. Raven Press, New York.

Julien, R.M. (1981). A *Primer of Drug Action.* Freeman, San Francisco.

Kales, A. and Scharf, M.B. (1973). Sleep laboratory and clinical studies of the effects of benzodiazepines on sleep: flurazepam, diazepam, or chlordiazepoxide, and Ro 5-4200. In *The Benzodiazepines* (S. Garattini, E. Mussini and L.O. Randall, Eds.), pp. 577–598. Raven Press, New York.

Kales, A., Scharf, M.B. and Kales, J.D. (1978). Rebound insomnia: a new clinical syndrome. *Science,* 201, 1039–1041.

Kanof, P.D. and Greengard, P. (1978). Brain histamine receptors as targets for antidepressant drugs. *Nature,* 272, 329–333.

Kao, I. and Drachman, D.B. (1977). Myasthenic immunoglobulin accelerates acetylcholine receptor degradation. *Science,* 196, 527–529.

Kao, I., Drachman, D.B. and Price, D.L. (1976). Botulinum toxin: mechanism of presynaptic blockade. *Science,* 193, 1256–1258.

Kaplan, J., Mandel, L.R. and Stillman, R. (1974). Blood and urine levels of *N,N*–dimethyl–tryptamine following administration of psychoactive dosages to human subjects. *Psychopharmacologia,* 38, 239–245.

Karczmar, A.G. and Dun, N.J. (1978). Cholinergic synapses: physiological, pharmacological and behavioral considerations. In *Psychopharmacology: A Generation of Progress* (M.A. Lipton, A. DiMascio and K.F. Killam, Eds.), pp. 293–305. Raven Press, New York.

Karli, P., Vergnes, M. and Didiergeorges, F. (1969). Rat-mouse interspecific aggression behaviour and its manipulation by brain ablation and by brain stimulation. In *Aggressive Behaviour* (S. Garattini and E.B. Sigg, Eds.), pp. 47–55. Wiley, New York.

Karobath, M. and Leitich, H. (1974). Antipsychotic drugs and dopamine-stimulated adenylate cyclase prepared from corpus striatum of rat brain. *Proc. Nat. Acad. Sci.,* 71, 2915–2918.

Kastin, A.J., Plotnikoff, N.P., Sandman, C.A. and Spirtes, M.A. (1975). The effects of MSH and MIF on the brain. In *Anatomical Neuroendocrinology* (W.E. Stumpf and L.D. Grant, Eds.), pp. 290–297. Karger, New York.

Kastin, A.J., Sandman, C.A., Stratton, L.O., Schally, A.V. and Miller, L.H. (1975). Behavioral and electrophysiologic changes in rat and man after MSH. *Prog. Brain Res.,* 42, 143–150.

Katz, B. (1966). *Nerve, Muscle and Synapse.* McGraw-Hill, New York.

Katz, B. (1971). Quantal mechanism of neural transmitter release. *Science,* 173, 123–126.

Katz, B. and Miledi, R. (1970). Further study of the role of calcium in synaptic transmission. *J. Physiol.,* 207, 789–801.

Katz, B. and Miledi, R. (1972). The statistical nature of the acetylcholine potential and its molecular components. *J. Physiol.,* 224, 665–699.

Katz, B. and Thesleff, S. (1957). A study of the "densensitization" produced by acetylcholine at the motor end-plate. *J. Physiol. (London),* 138, 63–80.

Katz, R.I., Chase, T.N. and Kopin, I.J. (1968). Evoked release of norepinephrine and serotonin from brain slices: inhibition by lithium. *Science,* 162, 466–467.

Katz, R.I. and Kopin, I.J. (1969). Release of norepinephrine-^{3}H evoked from brain slices by electrical–field stimulation—calcium dependency and the effects of lithium, ouabain, and tetrodotoxin. *Biochem. Pharmacol.,* 18, 1935–1939.

Katzman, R. (1976). Blood–brain–CSF barriers. In *Basic Neurochemistry* (G.J. Siegel, R.W. Albers, R. Katzman and B.W. Agranoff, Eds.), pp. 414–428. Little, Brown, Boston.

Kebabian, J.W. (1978). Dopamine-sensitive adenylate cyclase: a receptor mechanism for dopamine. *Adv. Biochem. Psychopharmacol.,* 19, 131–154.

Kebabian, J.W. and Calne, D.B. (1979). Multiple receptors for dopamine. *Nature,* 277, 93–96.

Kebabian, J.W. and Greengard, P. (1971). Dopamine-sensitive adenyl cyclase: possible role in synaptic transmission. *Science,* 174, 1346–1349.

Kebabian, J.W., Petzold, G.L. and Greengard, P. (1972). Dopamine–sensitive adenylate cyclase in caudate nucleus of rat brain and its similarity to the "dopamine receptor". *Proc. Nat. Acad. Sci.,* 69, 2145–2149.

Kehr, W., Carlsson, A., Lindqvist, M., Magnusson, T. and Atack, C. (1972). Evidence for a receptor-mediated feedback control of striatal tyrosine hydroxylase activity. *J. Pharm. Pharmacol.,* 24, 744–747.

Kelleher, R.T. and Morse, W.H. (1964). Escape behavior and punished behavior. *Fed. Proc.,* 23, 808–817.

Kelly, J.S. and Beart, P.M. (1975). Amino acid receptors in CNS. II. GABA in supraspinal regions. In *Handbook of Psychopharmacology, Vol. 4* (L.L. Iversen, S.D. Iversen and S.H. Snyder, Eds.), pp. 129–209. Plenum Press, New York.

Kemper, T.D. (1978). *A Social Interactional Theory of Emotions.* Wiley-Interscience, New York.

Kessler, S. (1980). The genetics of schizophrenia: a review. *Schizophr. Bull., 6,* 404–416.

Kety, S.S., Rosenthal, D., Wender, P.H., Schulsinger, F. and Jacobsen, B. (1975). Mental illness in the biological and adoptive families of adopted individuals who have become schizophrenic. In *Genetic Research in Psychiatry* (R.R. Fieve, D. Rosenthal and H. Brill, Eds.), pp. 147–165. Johns Hopkins Univ. Press, Baltimore.

Kewitz, H., Wilson, I.B. and Nachmansohn, D. (1956). A specific antidote against lethal alkyl phosphate intoxication. II. Antidotal properties. *Arch. Biochem. Biophys., 64,* 456–465.

Keynes, R.D. (1975). Organization of the ionic channels in nerve membranes. In *The Nervous System, Vol. 1* (D.B. Tower, Ed.), pp. 165–175. Raven Press, New York.

Keynes, R.D. (1979). Ion channels in the nerve cell membrane. *Sci. Am.,* 240, 3, 126–135.

King, C.D. (1974). 5-Hydroxytryptamine and sleep in the cat: a brief overview. In *Advances in Biochemical Psychopharmacology* (E. Costa, G.L. Gessa and M. Sandler, Eds.), pp. 211–216. Raven Press, New York.

Kizer, J.S. and Youngblood, W.W. (1978). Neurotransmitter systems and central neuroendocrine regulation. In *Psychopharmacology: A Generation of Progress* (M.A. Lipton, A. DiMascio and K.F. Killam, Eds.), pp. 465–486. Raven Press, New York.

Klee, W.A. and Streaty, R.A. (1974). Narcotic receptor sites in morphine–dependent rats. *Nature,* 248, 61–63.

Klein, D.F. and Davis, J.M. (1969). *Diagnosis and Drug Treatment of Psychiatric Disorders.* Williams and Wilkins, Baltimore.

Kleitman, N. (1929). Sleep. *Physiol. Rev., 9,* 624–665.

Klerman, G.L. (1977). Better but not well: social and ethical issues in the deinstitutionalization of the mentally ill. *Schizophr. Bull.,* 3, 617–631.

Kobayashi, R.M., Brown, M. and Vale, W. (1977). Regional distribution of neurotensin and somatostatin in rat brain. *Brain Res.,* 126, 584–588.

Koe, B.K. and Weissman, A. (1966). Parachlorophenylalanine: a specific depletor of brain serotonin. *J. Pharmacol. Exp. Ther.,* 154, 499–516.

Koelle, G.B. (1975a). Anticholinesterase agents. In *The Pharmacological Basis of Therapeutics, 5th Edition* (L.S. Goodman and A. Gilman, Eds.), pp. 445–466. Macmillan, New York.

Koelle, G.B. (1975b). Parasympathomimetic agents. In *The Pharmacological Basis of Therapeutics, 5th Edition* (L.S. Goodman and A. Gilman, Eds.), pp. 467–476. Macmillan, New York.

Koelle, G.B. (1975c). Neuromuscular blocking agents. In *The Pharmacological Basis of Therapeutics, 5th Edition* (L.S. Goodman and A. Gilman, Eds.), pp. 575–588. Macmillan, New York.

Kohlschütter, E. (1863). Messungen der Festigkeit des Schlafes. *Zeitschrift f. rationelle Medicin.* Dritte Reihe, Band 17, pp. 209–227.

Koizumi, K. and Brooks, C.M. (1974). The autonomic nervous system and its role in controlling visceral activities. In *Medical Physiology Vol. 1* (V. Mountcastle, Ed.), pp. 783–812. Mosby, St. Louis.

Kolata, G.B. (1981a). Drug found to help heart attack survivors. *Science,* 214, 774–775.

Kolata, G.B. (1981b) Clues to the cause of senile dementia. *Science,* 211, 1032–1033.

Kopin, I.J. (1980). Catecholamine, adrenal hormones and stress. In *Neuroendocrinology* (D.T. Krieger and J.C. Hughes, Eds.), pp. 159–166. Sinauer Associates, Sunderland, Massachusetts.

Koslow, S.H. (1977). Biosignificance of *N*- and *O*-methylated indoles to psychiatric disorders. In *Neuroregulators and Psychiatric Disorders.* (E. Usdin, D.A. Hamburg and J.D. Barchas, Eds.), pp. 210–219. Oxford Univ. Press, New York.

Koster, R., Anderson, M. and DeBeer, E.J. (1959). Acetic acid for analgesic screening. *Fed. Proc.,* 18, 412.

Kosterlitz, H.W. (Ed.) (1976). *Opiates and Endogenous Opiate Peptides.* Elsevier/North-Holland, Amsterdam.

Kosterlitz, H.W., Collier, H.O.J. and Villarreal, J.E. (Eds.) (1973a). *Agonist and Antagonist Actions of Narcotic Analgesic Drugs.* University Park Press, Baltimore.

Kosterlitz, H.W. and Hughes, J. (1975). Some thoughts on the significance of enkephalin, the endogenous ligand. *Life Sci.,* 17, 91–96.

Kosterlitz, H.W., Lord, J.A.H. and Watt, A.J. (1973b). Morphine receptor in the myenteric plexus of the guinea-pig ileum. In *Agonist and Antagonist Actions of Narcotic Analgesic Drugs* (H.W. Kosterlitz, H.O.J. Collier and J.E. Villarreal, Eds.), pp. 45–61. University Park Press, Baltimore.

Kosterlitz, H.W., Lydon, R.J. and Watt, A.J. (1970). The effects of adrenaline, noradrenaline and isoprenaline on inhibitory α- and β-adrenoceptors in the longitudinal muscle of the guinea-pig ileum. *Br. J. Pharmacol.,* 39, 398–413.

Kosterlitz, H.W. and Waterfield, A.A. (1975). In vitro models in the study of structure-activity relationships of narcotic analgesics. *Annu. Rev. Pharmacol.,* 15, 29–47.

Kovacs, G.L., Bohus, B. and Versteeg, D.H.G. (1979). Facilitation of memory consolidation by vasopressin: mediation by terminals of the dorsal noradrenergic bundle? *Brain Res.,* 172, 73–85.

Kraepelin, E. (1913). *Textbook of Psychiatry.* Trans. by R.M. Barclay. Livingston, Edinborough.

Krasnegor, N.A. (Ed.) (1978). *Behavioral Tolerance: Research and Treatment Implications.* NIDA Research Monograph #18. U.S. Gov't Printing Office, Washington, D.C.

Kraulis, I., Foldes, G., Traikov, H., Dubrovsky, B. and Birmingham, M.K. (1975). Distribution, metabolism and biological activity of deoxycorticosterone in the central nervous system. *Brain Res.,* 88, 1–14.

Kravitz, E.A. (1967). Acetylcholine, gamma aminobutyric acid, and glutamic acid: physiological and chemical studies related to their roles as neurotransmitter agents. In *The Neurosciences. A Study Program* (G.C. Quarton, T. Melnecuk, F.O. Schmitt, Eds.), pp. 433–443. Rockefeller Univ. Press, New York.

Kress, J.F. (1905). Veronalismus, *Therapeutische Monatshefte,* 19, 467.

Krieger, D.T. and Hughes J.C. (Eds.) 1980. *Neuroendocrinology.* Sinauer Associates, Sunderland, Mass.

Krnjević, K. (1975). Acetylcholine receptors in vertebrate CNS. In *Handbook of Psychopharmacology, Vol. 6* (L.L. Iversen, S.D. Iversen and S.H. Snyder, Eds.), pp. 97–126. Plenum Press, New York.

Krnjević, K. (1977). Effects of substance P on central neurons in cats. In *Substance P* (U.S. von Euler and B. Pernow, Eds.), pp. 217–230. Raven Press, New York.

Krnjević, K. and Phillis, J.W. (1963). Pharmacologic properties of acetylcholine-sensitive cells in the cerebral cortex. *J. Physiol.,* 166, 328–350.

Krnjević, K., Randie, M. and Straughan, D.W. (1966). Pharmacology of cortical inhibition. *J. Physiol.,* 184, 78–105.

Krnjević, K. and Reinhardt, W. (1979). Choline excites cortical neurons. *Science,* 206, 121–122.

Krogsgaard-Larsen, P., Johnston, G.A.R., Lodge, D. and Curtis, D.R. (1977). A new class of GABA agonists. *Nature,* 268, 53–55.

Kuffler, S.W. and Nicholls, J.G. (1976). *From Neuron to Brain.* Sinauer Associates, Sunderland, Massachusetts.

Kuffler, S.W. and Yoshikami, D. (1975). The number of transmitter molecules in a quantum: an estimate from iontophoretic application of acetylcholine at the neuromuscular synapse. *J. Physiol.,* 251, 465–482.

Kuhar, M.J. (1978). Central cholinergic pathways: physiologic and pharmacologic aspects. In *Psychopharmacology: A Generation of Progress* (M.A. Lipton, A. DiMascio and K.F. Killam, Eds.), pp. 199–203. Raven Press, New York.

Kuhar, M.J., Aghajanian, G.K. and Roth, R.H. (1974). Serotonin neurons: a synaptic mechanism for the reuptake of serotonin. In *Advances in Biochemical Psychopharmacology, Vol. 10* (E. Costa, G.L. Gessa and M. Sandler, Eds.), pp. 287–295. Raven Press, New York.

Kuhar, M.J., Pert, C.B. and Snyder, S.H. (1973a). Regional distribution of opiate receptor binding in monkey and human brain. *Nature,* 245, 447–450.

Kuhar, M.J., Sethy, V.H., Roth, R.H. and Aghajanian, G.K.

(1973b). Choline: selective accumulation by central cholinergic neurons. *J. Neurochem.,* 20, 581–593.

Kuschinsky, K. (1977). Opiate dependence. *Prog. Pharmacol.,* 1, 1–39.

Lader, M. (1978a). Nicotine and smoking behavior. *Br. J. Clin. Pharmacol.,* 5, 289–292.

Lader, M. (1978b). Current psychophysiological theories of anxiety. In *Psychopharmacology: A Generation of Progress* (M.A. Lipton, A. DiMascio and K.F. Killam, Eds.), pp. 1375–1380. Raven Press, New York.

Lakke, J.P.W.F., van Praag, H.M., van Twisk, R., Doorenbos, H. and Witt, F.G.J. (1974). Effects of administration of thyrotropin releasing hormone in Parkinsonism. *Clin. Neurol. Neurosurg.,* 3/4, 1–5.

Lal, H. (1975). Narcotic dependence, narcotic action and dopamine receptors. *Life Sci.,* 17, 483–496.

Lal, H. (Ed.) (1977). *Discriminative Stimulus Properties of Drugs.* Plenum Press, New York.

Lal, H., Gianutsos, G. and Miksic, S. (1977). Discriminable stimuli produced by narcotic analgesics. In *Discriminative Stimulus Properties of Drugs* (H. Lal, Ed.), pp. 23–47. Plenum Press, New York.

Lamotte, C., Perte, C.B. and Snyder, S.H. (1976). Opiate receptor binding in primate spinal cord: distribution and changes after dorsal root section. *Brain Res.,* 112, 407–412.

Lampert, A., Nirenberg, M. and Klee, W.A. (1976). Tolerance and dependence evoked by an endogenous opiate peptide. *Proc. Nat. Acad. Sci.,* 73, 3165–3167.

Lang, D.W., Darrah, H.K., Hedley-Whyte, J. and Laasberg, L.H. (1975). Uptake into brain proteins of ^{35}S-methionine during morphine tolerance. *J. Pharmacol. Exp. Ther.,* 192, 521–530.

Lange, W. and von Krueger, G. (1932). Über Ester der Monofluorophosphosäure. *Ber. Dtsch. Chem. Ges.,* 65, 1598–1601.

Langley, J.N. (1921). *The Autonomic Nervous System.* Cambridge Univ. Press, London.

Langrod, J., Brill, L., Lowinson, J. and Joseph, H. (1972). Methadone maintenance from research to treatment. In *Major Modalities in the Treatment of Drug Abuse* (L. Brill and L. Lieberman, Eds.), pp. 107–141. Behavioral Publications, New York.

Lasagna, L., Mosteller, F., von Felsinger, J.M. and Beecher, H.K. (1954). A study of the placebo response. *Am. J. Med.,* 16, 770–779.

Leaf, R.C., Wnek, D.J., Gay, P.E., Corcia, R.M. and Lamon, S. (1975). Chlordiazepoxide and diazepam induced mouse killing by rats. *Psychopharmacologia,* 44, 23–28.

Lee, T.P., Kuo, J.F. and Greengard, P. (1972). Role of muscarinic cholinergic receptors in regulation of guanosine 3', 5'-cyclic monophosphate content in mammalian brain, heart muscle, and intestinal smooth muscle. *Proc. Nat. Acad. Sci.,* 69, 3287–3291.

Lee, C.Y., Tseng, L.F. and Chiu, T.H. (1967). Influence of denervation on localization of neurotoxins from clopid venoms in rat diaphragm. *Nature*, 215, 1177–1178.

Lees, G.M., Kosterlitz, H.W. and Waterfield, A.A. (1973). Characteristics of morphine-sensitives release of neurotransmitter substances. In *Agonist and Antagonist Actions of Narcotic Analgesic Drugs* (H.W. Kosterlitz, H.O.J. Collier and J.E. Villarreal, Eds.), pp. 142–152. University Park Press, Baltimore.

Lefkowitz, R.J. (1978). Identification and regulation of adrenergic receptors. In *Psychopharmacology: A Generation of Progress* (M.A. Lipton, A. DiMascio and K.F. Killam, Eds.), pp. 389–396. Raven Press, New York.

Lefkowitz, R.J., Mukherjee, C., Coverstone, M. and Caron, M.C. (1974). Stereospecific [³H](-)-alprenolol binding sites, β–adrenergic receptors and adenylate cyclase. *Biochem. Biophys. Res. Commun.*, 60, 703–709.

Legros, J.J., Gilot, P., Seron, X., Claessens, J.J., Adam, A., Moeglen, J.M., Audibert, A. and Berchier, P. (1978). Influence of vasopressin on learning and memory. *Lancet*, 1, 41–42.

Lehninger, A.L. (1975). *Biochemistry - The Molecular Basis of Cell Structure and Function (2nd Edition)*. Worth, New York.

Leibowitz, S.F. (1971). Hypothalamic alpha- and beta-adrenergic systems regulate both thirst and hunger in the rat. *Proc. Nat. Acad. Sci.*, 68, 322–334.

Leibowitz, S.F. (1974a). Adrenergic receptor mechanisms on eating and drinking. In *The Neurosciences, Third Study Program* (F.O. Schmitt and F.G. Worden, Eds.), pp. 713–719. MIT Press, Cambridge.

Leibowitz, S.F. (1974b). Norepinephrine–elicited eating: involvement of neuroendocrine systems of the paraventricular nucleus. In *Society for Neuroscience, Program for 4th Annual Meeting. St. Louis, Mo.*, Abstract, 301. Society for Neuroscience, Bethesda, Maryland.

Lennard, H.L., Epstein, L.J. and Rosenthal, M.S. (1972). The methadone illusion. *Science*, 176, 881–884.

Lerner, P., Nosé, P., Gordon, E.K. and Lovenberg, W. (1977). Haloperidol: effect of long term treatment on rat striatal dopamine synthesis and turnover. *Science*, 197, 181–183.

Levine, R.R. (1973). *Pharmacology of Drug Actions and Reactions*. Little, Brown, Boston.

Lewis, J.W., Sherman, J.E. and Liebeskind, J.C. (1981). Opioid and non-opioid stress analgesia: assessment of tolerance and cross tolerance with morphine. *J. Neurosci.*, 1, 358–363.

Lewis, P.R. and Shute, C.C.D. (1978). Cholinergic pathways in CNS. In *Handbook of Psychopharmacology, Vol. 9* (L.L. Iversen, S.D. Iversen and S.D. Snyder, Eds.), pp. 315–355. Plenum Press, New York.

Lewis, T., Pickering, G.W. and Rothschild, P. (1931). Observations upon muscular pain in intermittent claudication. *Heart*, 15, 359–383.

Li, C.H. and Chung, D. (1976). Isolation and structure of an untriakontapeptide with opiate activity from camel pituitary glands. *Proc. Nat. Acad. Sci.*, 73, 1145–1148.

Libet, B. (1979). Which postsynaptic action is mediated by cAMP? *Life Sci.*, 24, 1043–1058.

Lidbrink, P., Corrodi, H., Fuxe, K. and Olson, L. (1973). The effects of benzodiazepines, meprobamate, and barbiturates on central monoamine neurons. In *The Benzodiazepines* (S. Garattini, E. Mussini, and L.O. Randall, Eds.), pp. 203–223. Raven Press, New York.

Lieberman, L. and Brill, L. (1972). Rational authority. In *Major Modalities in the Treatment of Drug Abuse* (L. Brill and L. Lieberman, Eds.), pp. 67–84. Behavioral Publications, New York.

Liebeskind, J.C., Guilbaud, G., Besson, J.M. and Oliveras, J.L. (1973). Analgesia from electrical stimulation of the periaqueductal gray matter in the cat: behavioral observations and inhibitory effects on spinal cord neurones. *Brain Res.*, 50, 441–446.

Lindsley, D.B. (1958). The reticular system and perceptual discrimination. In *Reticular Formation of The Brain* (H.H. Jasper, L.D. Proctor, R.S. Knighton, W.C. Noshay and R.T. Costello, Eds.), pp. 513–534. Little, Brown, Boston.

Lindvall, O. and Björklund, A. (1974). The organization of the ascending catecholamine neuron systems in the rat brain as revealed by the glyoxylic acid fluorescence method. *Acta Physiol. Scand. Suppl., 412*, 1–48.

Lindvall, O. and Björklund, A. (1978). Organization of catecholamine neurons in the rat central nervous system. In *Handbook of Psychopharmacology, Vol. 9* (L.L. Iversen, S.D. Iversen and S.H. Snyder, Eds.), pp. 139–222. Plenum Press, New York.

Lints, C.E. and Harvey, J.A. (1969). Altered sensitivity to footshock and decreased brain content of serotonin following brain lesions in the rat. *J. Comp. Physiol. Psychol.*, 67, 23–32.

Lipinski, J.F., Schaumberg, H.H. and Baldessarini, R.J. (1973). Regional distribution on histamine in the human brain. *Brain Res.*, 52, 403–408.

Lippa, A.S., Critchett, D., Sano, M.C., Klepner, C.A., Greenblatt, E.N., Coupet, J. and Beer, B. (1979). Benzodiazepine receptors: cellular and behavioral characteristics. *Pharmacol. Biochem. Behav.*, 10, 831–843.

Lipper, S. and Kornetsky, C. (1971). Effect of chlorpromazine on conditional avoidance as a function of CS-US interval length. *Psychopharmacologia*, 22, 144–150.

Litten, W. (1975). The most poisonous mushrooms. *Sci. Am.*, 232, 3, 90–101.

Ljungdahl, Å. and Hökfelt, T. (1973). Autoradiographic uptake patterns of [³H] GABA and [³H] glycine in central nervous tissues with special references to the cat spinal cord. *Brain Res.*, 62, 587–595.

Lloyd, K.G. and Bartholini, G. (1974). The effects of methiothepin on cerebral monoamine neurons. In *Advances in Biochemical Psychopharmacology, Vol. 10* (E.

Costa, G.L. Gessa and M. Sandler, Eds.), pp. 305–309. Raven Press, New York.

Loewi, O. (1921). Ueber humorale Uebertragbarkeit der Herznervenwirkung. *Pflügers Arch.*, 189, 239–242.

Loh, H.H., Tseng, L.F., Wei, E. and Li, C.H. (1976). β-endorphin is a potent analgesic agent. *Proc. Nat. Acad. Sci.*, 73, 2895–2898.

Lovenberg, W., Jequier, E. and Sjoerdsma, A. (1968). Tryptophan hydroxylation in mammalian systems. *Adv. Pharmacol.*, 6A, 21–36.

Lowry, P.J. and Scott, A.P. (1977). Structural relationships and biosynthesis of corticotropin, lipotropin and melanotropin. *Front. Horm. Res.*, 4, 11–17.

Lucchesi, B.R., Schuster, C.R. and Emley, G.S. (1967). The role of nicotine as a determinant of cigarette smoking frequency in man with observations of certain cardiovascular effects associated with the tobacco alkaloids. *Clin. Pharmacol. Ther.*, 8, 789–796.

Ludwig, B.J. and Piech, E.C. (1951). Some anticonvulsant agents derived from 1,3 propanediols. *J. Am. Chem. Soc.*, 73, 5779–5781.

MacDonald, R.L. and Barker, J.L. (1978). Specific antagonism of GABA-mediated post-synaptic inhibition in cultured mammalian spinal cord neurons: a common mode of convulsant action. *Neurology*, 28, 325–330.

MacIntosh, F.C. (1976). Acetylcholine. In *Basic Neurochemistry* (G.J. Siegel, R.W. Albers, R. Katzman and B.W. Agranoff, Eds.), pp. 180–202. Little, Brown, Boston.

MacIntosh, F.C. and Collier, B. (1976). The Neurochemistry of cholinergic terminals. In *Handbook of Experimental Pharmacology: Organization, Function and Pharmacology of the Neuromuscular Junction* (E. Zaimis, and J. MacLagan, Eds.), pp. 99–228. Springer Verlag, Berlin.

Mackerer, C.R., Kochman, R.L., Bierschenk, B.A. and Bremner, S.S. (1978). The binding of ^{3}H–diazepam to rat brain homogenates. *J. Pharmacol. Exp. Ther.*, 206, 405–413.

MacLennan, A.J., Drugan, R.C., Hyson, R.L., Maier, S.F., Madden, J. and Barchas, J.D. (1982). Corticosterone: a critical factor in an opioid form of stress-induced analgesia. *Science*, 215, 1530–1532.

Macon, J.B., Sokoloff, L. and Glowinski, J. (1971). Feedback control of rat brain 5-hydroxytryptamine. *J. Neurochem.*, 18, 323–331.

Magni, F., Moruzzi, G., Rossi, G.F. and Zanchetti, A. (1961). EEG arousal following inactivation of the lower brain stem by selective injection of barbiturate into the vertebral circulation. *Arch. Ital. Biol.*, 99, 33–71.

Mahadik, S.P., Tamir, H. and Rapport, M. (1975). Molecular composition and functional organization of synaptic structures. In *Advances in Neurochemistry, Vol. 3* (B.W. Agranoff and M.H. Aprison, Eds.), pp. 99–163. Plenum Press, New York.

Mahler, H.R. (1977). Proteins of the synaptic membrane. *Neurochem. Res.*, 2, 119–147.

Major, L.F. and Murphy, D.L. (1978). Platelet and plasma amine oxidase activity in alcoholic individuals. *Br. J. Psychiatry*, 132, 548–554.

Majorossy, K., Réthelyi, M. and Szentagothai, J. (1965). The large glomerular synapse of the pulvinar. *J. Hirnforschung*, 7, 415–432.

Maker, H.S., Clarke, D.D. and Lajtha, A.L. (1976). Intermediary metabolism of carbohydrates and amino acids. In *Basic Neurochemistry* (G.J. Siegel, R.W. Katzman and B.W. Agranoff, Eds.), pp. 279–307. Little, Brown, Boston.

Malick, J.B. and Goldstein, J.M. (1977). Analgesic activity of enkephalins following intracerebral administration in the rat. *Life Sci.*, 20, 827–832.

Malthe-Sorenssen, D., Wood, P.L., Cheney, D.L. and Costa, E. (1978). Modulation of the turnover rate of acetylcholine in rat brain by intraventricular injections of thyrotropin releasing hormone, somatostatin, neurotensin and angiotensin II. *J. Neurochem.*, 31, 685–691.

Mandel, A.J. and Morgan, M. (1971). Indole (ethyl) amine N-methyltransferase in human brain. *Nature*, 230, 85–87.

Mao, C.C. and Costa, E. (1978). Biochemical pharmacology of GABA transmission. In *Psychopharmacology: A Generation of Progress* (M.A. Lipton, A. DiMascio and K.F. Killam, Eds.), pp. 307–318. Raven Press, New York.

Mao, C.C., Guidotti, A. and Costa, E. (1975). Evidence for an involvement of GABA in the mediation of the cerebellar cGMP decrease and the anticonvulsant action of diazepam. *Naunyn-Schmiedeberg's Arch. Pharmacol.*, 289, 369–378.

Marangos, P.J., Clark, R., Martino, A.M., Paul, S.M. and Skolnick, P. (1979). Demonstration of two new endogenous "benzodiazepine-like" compounds from the brain. *Psychiatry Res.*, 1, 121–130.

Marchbanks, R.M. (1975). Biochemistry of cholinergic neurons. In *Handbook of Psychopharmacology, Vol. 3* (L.L. Iversen, S.D. Iversen and S.H. Snyder, Eds.), pp. 247–326. Plenum Press, New York.

Marcyznski, T.J. (1976). Serotonin and the central nervous system. In *Chemical Transmission in the Mammalian Central Nervous System* (C.H. Hockman and D. Bieger, Eds.), pp. 349–429. University Park Press, Baltimore.

Marek, K., and Haubrich, D.R. (1977). Thyrotropin-releasing hormone—increased catabolism of catecholamines in brains of thyroidectomized rats. *Biochem. Pharmacol.*, 26, 1817–1818.

Margules, D.L., Moisset, B., Lewis, M.J., Shibuya, H. and Pert, C.B. (1978). β-endorphin is associated with overeating in genetically obese mice (ob/ob) and rats (fa/fa). *Science*, 202, 988–991.

Margules, D.L. and Stein, L. (1967). Neuroleptics vs. tranquilizers: evidence from animal behavior studies of mode and site of action. In *Neuropsychopharmacology* (H. Brill, J.O. Cole, P. Deniker, H. Hippius and P.B. Bradley, Eds.), pp. 108–120. Excerpta Medica Foundation, New York.

Margules, D.L. and Stein, L. (1968). Increase of "antianxiety" activity and tolerance of behavioral depressions during chronic administration of oxazepam. *Psychopharmacologia (Berlin)* 13, 74–80.

Marks, I.M. (1969). *Fears and Phobias.* Academic Press, New York.

Marshall, J.M. (1974). Vertebrate smooth muscle. In *Medical Physiology Vol. 1* (V.B. Mountcastle, Ed.), pp. 121–148. Mosby, St. Louis.

Martin, B.R., Dewey, W.L., Chau-Pham, T. and Prange, A.J., Jr. (1977). Interactions of thyrotropin releasing hormone and morphine sulfate in rodents. *Life Sci., 20,* 715–722.

Martin, J.B., Reichlin, S. and Bick, K.L. (Eds.) (1981). *Neurosecretion and Brain Peptides: Implications for Brain Function and Neurological Disease. Advances in Biochemical Psychopharmacology, Vol. 28.* Raven Press, New York.

Martin, W. (1970). Pharmacological redundancy as an adaptive mechanism in the CNS. *Fed. Proc., 29,* 13–18.

Martin, W.R. (1967). Opioid antagonists. *Pharmacol. Rev., 19,* 463–521.

Martin, W.R., Gorodetzky, C.W. and McClane, T.K. (1966). An experimental study in the treatment of narcotic addicts with cyclazocine. *Clin. Pharmacol. Ther., 7,* 455–465.

Martin, W.R., Sloan, J.W., Christian, S.T. and Clements, H. (1972). Brain levels of tryptamine. *Psychopharmacologia,* 24, 331–346.

Martinez-Hernandez, A., Bell, K.P. and Norenberg, M.D. (1977). Glutamine synthetase: glial localization in brain. *Science,* 195, 1356–1358.

Marx, J.L. (1980). Calmodulin: a protein for all seasons. *Science,* 208, 274–276.

Matthysse, S.W. (1977). The role of dopamine in schizophrenia. In *Neuroregulators and Psychiatric Disorders* (E. Usdin, D.A. Hamburg and J.D. Barchas, Eds.), pp. 3–13. Oxford University Press, New York.

Mattke, D. (1968). A pilot investigation in neuroleptic therapy. *Dis. Nerve. Syst., 29,* 515–524.

Maugh, T.H. (1981). Analgesic from mushrooms begins clinical trials. *Science, 212,* 431.

Maupin, B. (1961). Serotonin determination, metabolism, pharmacology some biological aspects. *Psychopharmacol. Serv. Cent. Bull.,* 15–57.

May, E.L. and Sargent L.J. (1965). Morphine and its modifications. In *Analgetics* (G. de Stevens, Ed.), pp. 123–178. Academic Press, New York.

Mayer, D.J. and Hayes, R.L. (1975). Stimulation-produced analgesia: development of tolerance and cross-tolerance to morphine. *Science,* 188, 941–943.

Mayer, D.J. and Liebeskind, J.C. (1974). Pain reduction by focal electrical stimulation of the brain: an anatomical and behavioral analysis. *Brain Res., 68,* 73–93.

Mayer, N., Lembeck, F., Saria, A. and Gamse, R. (1979). Substance P: characteristics of binding to synaptic vesicles of rat brain. *Naunyn-Schmiedeberg's Arch. Pharmacol., 306,* 45–51.

Maynert, E.W. and Klingman, G.I. (1962). Tolerance to morphine. I. Effects on catecholamines in the brain and adrenal glands. *J. Pharmacol. Exp. Ther., 135,* 285–295.

McAfee, D.A. and Greengard, P. (1972). Adenosine 3', 5'-monophosphate: electrophysiological evidence for a role in synaptic transmission. *Science,* 178, 310–312.

McCauley, R.B. (1981). Monoamine oxidases and the pharmacology of monoamine oxidase inhibitors. In *Neuropharmacology of the CNS and Behavioral Disorders* (G.C. Palmer, Ed.), pp. 93–109. Academic Press, New York.

McElroy, J.F., DuPont, A.F. and Feldman, R.S. (1982). The effects of fenfluramine and fluoxetine on the acquisition of a conditioned avoidance response in rats. *Psychopharmacology,* 77, 356–359.

McElroy, J.F. and Feldman, R.S. (1982). Generalization between benzodiazepine- and triazolopyridazine–elicited discriminative cues. *Pharmacol. Biochem. Behav.,* 17, 709–713.

McGeer, P.L., Eccles, J.C. and McGeer, E.G. (1978). *Molecular Neurobiology of the Mammalian Brain.* Plenum Press, New York.

McGeer, P.L., Hattori, T. and McGeer, E.G. (1975). Chemical and autoradiographic analysis of γ-aminobutyric acid transport in Purkinje cells of the cerebellum. *Exp. Neurol., 47,* 26–41.

McGeer, P.L., McGeer, E.G., Fibiger, H.C. and Wickson, V. (1971). Neostriatal choline acetylase and cholinesterase following selective brain lesions. *Brain Res., 35,* 308–314.

McGivern, R., Berka, C., Berntson, G.G., Walker, J.M. and Sandman, C.A. (1979). Effect of naloxone on analgesia induced by food deprivation. *Life Sci., 25,* 885–888.

McGlothlin, W.H. and Arnold, D.O. (1971). LSD revisited—a ten-year follow-up of medical LSD use. *Arch. Gen. Psychiatry,* 24, 35–49.

McLennan, H. (1970). *Synaptic Transmission, Second Edition.* Saunders, Philadelphia.

McLennan, H. (1975). Excitatory amino acid receptors in the central nervous system. In *Handbook of Psychopharmacology, Vol. 4* (L.L. Iversen, S.D. Iversen and S.H. Snyder, Eds.), pp. 211–228. Plenum Press, New York.

McMillan, D.E. (1975). Determinants of drug effects on punished responding. *Fed. Proc., 34,* 1870–1879.

McMillan, D.E. and Leander, J.D. (1976). Effects of drugs on schedule-controlled behavior. In *Behavioral Pharmacology* (S.D. Glick and J. Goldfarb, Eds.), pp. 85–139. Mosby, St. Louis.

Means, A.R. and Dedman, J.R. (1980). Calmodulin—an intracellular calcium receptor. *Nature,* 285, 73–77.

Medical News. (1975). There's no 'safe trimester' with teratogenic drugs. *J. Am. Med. Assoc.,* 234, 264–265.

Meek, J.L., Fuxe, K. and Carlsson, A. (1971). Blockade of p-chloroamphetamine-induced 5-hydroxytryptamine depletion by chlorimipramine, chlorpheniramine and meperidine. *Biochem. Pharmacol.,* 20, 707–709.

Meek, J.L. and Neff, N.H. (1972). Tryptophan 5-hydroxylase: approximation of half-life and rate and axonal transport. *J. Neurochem.,* 19, 1519–1525.

Meites, J. (1977). The 1977 Nobel prize in physiology or medicine, *Science,* 198, 594–596.

Meltzer, H.Y. (1980). Relevance of dopamine autoreceptors for psychiatry: preclinical and clinical studies. *Schizophr. Bull.,* 6, 456–475.

Meltzer, H.Y., Jackman, H. and Arora, R.C. (1980). Brain and skeletal muscle monoamine oxidase activity in schizophrenia. *Schizophr. Bull.,* 6, 208–212.

Mendelson, W.B., Gillin, J.C. and Wyatt, J.C. (1977). *Human Sleep and its Disorders.* Plenum Press, New York.

Meselson, M. and Robinson, J.P. (1980). Chemical warfare and chemical disarmament. *Sci. Am.,* 242, 4, 38–47.

Meyer, R.E. (1972). *Guide to Drug Rehabilitation.* Beacon Press, Boston.

Meyer, R.E. and Mirin, S.M. (1979). *The Heroin Stimulus.* Plenum Press, New York.

Meyerson, B.J., Carrer, H. and Eliasson, M. (1974). 5-Hydroxytryptamine and sexual behavior in the female rat. In *Advances in Biochemical Psychopharmacology, Vol. 11* (E. Costa, G.L. Gessa and M. Sandler, Eds.), pp. 229–242. Raven Press, New York.

Meyerson, B.J. and Eliasson, M. (1977). Pharmacological and hormonal control of reproductive behavior. In *Handbook of Psychopharmacology, Vol. 8* (L.L. Iversen, S.D. Iversen and S.D. Snyder, Eds.), pp. 159–232. Plenum Press, New York.

Miczek, K.A. (1974). Intraspecies aggression in rats: effects of d-amphetamine and chlordiazepoxide. *Psychopharmacologia,* 39, 275–301.

Miczek, K.A. and Barry, H. (1976). Pharmacology of sex and aggression. In *Behavioral Pharmacology* (S.D. Glick and J. Goldfarb, Eds.), pp. 176–257. Mosby, St. Louis.

Miczek, K.A., Thompson, M.L. and Shuster, L. (1982). Opioid-like analgesia in defeated mice. *Science,* 215, 1520–1522.

Miledi, R. and Potter, L.T. (1971). Acetylcholine receptors in muscle fibers. *Nature,* 233, 599–603.

Miledi, R. and Slater, C.R. (1970). On the degeneration of rat neuromuscular junctions after nerve section. *J. Physiol.,* 207, 507–528.

Miller, R.J. and Iversen, L.L. (1974). Effects of psychoactive drugs on dopamine (3,4-dihydroxyphenylethylamine)-sensitive adenylate cyclase activity in corpus striatum of rat brain. *Biochem. Soc. Trans.,* 2, 256–259.

Minneman, K.P., Pittman, R.N. and Molinoff, P.B. (1981). β-adrenergic receptor subtypes: properties, distribution, and regulation. *Annu. Rev. Neurosci.,* 4, 419–461.

Minz, B. (1955). *The role of Humoral Agents in Nervous Activity.* Thomas, Springfield, Illinois.

Mishler, E.G. and Scotch, N.A. (1963). Sociological factors in the epidemiology of schizophrenia. *Psychiatry,* 26, 315–343.

Miyamoto, M. and Nagawa, Y. (1977). Mesolimbic involvement in the locomotor stimulant action of thyrotropin–releasing hormone (TRH) in rats. *Eur. J. Pharmacol.,* 44, 143–152.

Mohler, H. and Okada, T. (1977a). Benzodiazepine receptor: demonstration in the central nervous system. *Science,* 198, 849–850.

Mohler, H. and Okada, T. (1977b). Properties of [^{3}H] diazepam binding to benzodiazepine receptors in rat cerebral cortex. *Life Sci.,* 20, 2101–2110.

Moja, E., Stoff, D.M., Gillin, J.C. and Wyatt, R.J. (1976). Dose–response effects of β-phenylethylamine on stereotyped behavior in pargyline-treated rats. *Biol. Psychiatry,* 11, 731–742.

Molinoff, P.B. (1974). The use of snake venom toxins to study and isolate cholinergic receptors. In *The Neurosciences, Third Study Program* (F.O. Schmitt and F.G. Worden, Eds.), pp. 759–763. MIT Press, Cambridge, Massachusetts.

Molinoff, P.B. and Potter, L.T. (1972). Isolation of the cholinergic receptor proteins of torpedo electric tissue. In *Advances in Biochemical Psychopharmacology, Vol. 6* (E. Costa, L. Iversen, and R. Paoletti, Eds.), pp. 111–134. Raven Press, New York.

Monachon, M-A., Burkard, W.P., Jalfre, M. and Haefely, W. (1972). Blockade of central 5-hydroxytryptamine receptors by methiothepin. *Naunyn-Schmiedeberg's Arch. Pharmacol.* 274, 192–197.

Moore, J.W., Blaustein, M.P., Anderson, N.C. and Narashashi, T. (1967). Basis of tetrodotoxin's selectivity in blockage of squid axons. *J. Gen. Physiol.,* 50, 1401–1411.

Moore, K.E. (1978). Amphetamines: biochemical and behavioral actions in animals. In *Handbook of Psychopharmacology, Vol. 11* (L.L. Iversen, S.D. Iversen and S.H. Snyder, Eds.), pp. 41–98. Plenum Press, New York.

Moore, K.E. and Kelly, P.H. (1978). Biochemical pharmacology of mesolimbic and mesocortical dopaminergic neurons. In *Psychopharmacology: A Generation of Progress* (M.A. Lipton, A. DiMascio and K.F. Killam, Eds.), pp. 221–234. Raven Press, New York.

Moore, R.Y. (1974). Visual pathways and the central control of diurnal rhythms. In *Neurosciences, Third Study Program* (F.O. Schmitt and F.G. Worden, Eds.), pp. 537–542. MIT Press, Cambridge, Massachusetts.

Moore, R.Y. and Eichler, V.B. (1972). Loss of a circadian adrenal corticosterone rhythm following suprachiasmatic lesions in the rat. *Brain Res.,* 42, 201–206.

Moore, R.Y. and Klein, D.C. (1974). Visual pathways and the central neural control of a circadian rhythm in pineal serotonin N-acetyltransferase activity. *Brain Res.,* 71, 17–33.

Morell, P. (Ed.) (1978). *Myelin.* Plenum Press, New York.

Morell, P. and Norton, W.T. (1980). Myelin. *Sci. Am., 242,* 5, 88–118.

Morse, W.H. (1962). Use of operant conditioning techniques for evaluating the effects of barbiturates on behavior. In *Psychosomatic Medicine* (J.H. Nodine and J.H. Moyer, Eds.), pp. 275–281. Lea and Febiger, Philadelphia.

Moses, A.M. (1980). Diabetes insipidus and ADH regulation. In *Neuroendocrinology* (D.T. Krieger and J.C. Hughes, Eds.), pp. 141–148. Sinauer Associates, Sunderland, Massachusetts.

Mountcastle, V.B. and Baldessarini, R.J. (1974). Synaptic transmission. In *Medical Physiology, Vol. 1* (V.B. Mountcastle, Ed.), pp. 182–223. Mosby, St. Louis.

Moussa, B.H., Youdim, M.H. and Bourgoin, S. (1974). Purification of pig brainstem tryptophan hydroxylase and some of its properties. In *Advances in Biochemical Psychopharmacology, Vol. 11* (E. Costa, G.L. Gessa and M. Sandler, Eds.), pp. 13–17. Raven Press, New York.

Moyer, J.A., Greenberg, L.H., Frazer, A., Brunswick, D.J., Mendels, J. and Weiss, B. (1979). Opposite effects of acute and repeated administration of desmethylimipramine on adrenergic responsiveness in rat pineal gland. *Life Sci., 24,* 2237–2244.

Moyer, K.E. (1968). Kinds of aggression and their physiological basis. *Commun. Beh. Biol.,* A, 2, 65–87.

Mudge, A.W., Leeman, S.E. and Fishbach, G.D. (1979). Enkephalin inhibits release of substance P from sensory neurons in culture and decreases action potential duration. *Proc. Nat. Acad. Sci.,* 76(1), 526–530.

Murphy, D.L., Brodie, H.K.H., Goodwin, F.K. and Bunney, W.E. Jr. (1971). Regular induction of hypomania by L-dopa in "bipolar" manic–depressive patients. *Nature,* 229, 135–136.

Murphy, D.L. and Kalin, N.H. (1980). Biological and behavioral consequences of alterations in monoamine oxidase activity. *Schizophr. Bull.,* 6, 355–367.

Murphy, D.L. and Wyatt, R.J. (1972). Reduced monoamine oxidase in blood platelets from schizophrenic patients. *Nature,* 238, 225–226.

Murphy, D.L. and Wyatt, R.J. (1975). Neurotransmitter-related enzymes in the major psychiatric disorders. In *Biology of the Major Psychoses, Vol. 54* (D.X. Freedman, Ed.), pp. 277–288. Raven Press, New York.

Musacchio, J.M. (1975). Enzymes involved in the biosynthesis and degradation of catecholamines. In *Handbook of Psychopharmacology, Vol. 3* (L.L. Iversen, S.D. Iversen and S.H. Snyder, Eds.), pp. 1–35. Plenum Press, New York.

Musacchio, J.M., Julou, L., Kety, S.S. and Glowinski, J. (1969). Increase in rat tyrosine hydroxylase activity produced by electroconvulsive shock. *Proc. Nat. Acad. Sci.,* 63, 1117–1119.

Myers, R.D. (1974). *Handbook of Drug and Chemical Stimulation of the Brain.* Van Nostrand Reinhold, New York.

Myers, R.D., Metcalf, G. and Rice, J.C. (1977). Identification by microinjection on TRH-sensitive sites in the cat's brain stem that mediate respiratory, temperature, and other autonomic changes. *Brain Res.,* 126, 105–115.

Myrsten, A.L., Post, B., Frankenhaeuser, M. and Elgerot, A. (1975). Immediate effects of cigarette smoking as related to different smoking habits. *Percept. Mot. Skills,* 40, 515–523.

Nagatsu, T., Levitt, M. and Udenfriend, S. (1964). Tyrosine hydroxylase. The initial step in norepinephrine synthesis. *J. Biol. Chem.,* 239, 2910–2917.

Nakata, Y., Kusaka, Y., Segawa, T., Yajima, H. and Kitagawa, K. (1978). Substance P: regional distribution and specific binding to synaptic membranes in rabbit central nervous system. *Life Sci.,* 22, 259–268.

Narasimhachari, N. and Lin, R.L. (1974). A possible mechanism for the antischizophrenic action of chlorpromazine: inhibition of the formation of dimethyltryptamine by chlorpromazine metabolites. *Res. Commun. Chem. Pathol. Pharmacol.,* 8, 341–351.

Nastuk, W.L. (1974). Neuromuscular transmission. In *Medical Physiology, Vol. 1* (V.B. Mountcastle, Ed.), pp. 151–181. Mosby, St. Louis.

Nathanson, J.A. and Greengard, P. (1976). Cyclic nucleotides and synaptic transmission. In *Basic Neurochemistry* (G.J. Siegel, R.W. Albers, R. Katzman and B.W. Agranoff, Eds.), pp. 246–262. Little, Brown, Boston.

Nathanson, J.A. and Greengard, P. (1977). "Second messengers" in the brain. *Sci. Am.,* 237, 2, 108–119.

Nauta, W.J.H., (1975). Anatomical organization of pain pathways in the central nervous system. *Neurosci. Res. Prog. Bull.,* 13, 84–87.

Neff, N.H., Yang, H.-Y.T., Gordis, C. and Bialek, D. (1974). The metabolism of indolealkyamines by type A and B monoamine oxidase of the brain. In *Advances in Biochemical Psychopharmacology, Vol. 11* (E. Costa, G.L. Gessa and M. Sandler, Eds.), pp. 51–58. Raven Press, New York.

Nelsen, J.M. and Goldstein, L. (1972). Improvement of performance on an attention task with chronic nicotine treatment in rats. *Psychopharmacologia,* 26, 347–360.

Nelsen, J.M. and Goldstein, L. (1973). Chronic nicotine treatment in rats: 1. Acquisition and performance of an attention task. *Res. Commun. Chem. Pathol. Pharmacol.,* 5, 681–693.

Nelsen, J.M., Pelley, K. and Goldstein, L. (1973). Chronic nicotine treatment in rats: 2. Electroencephalographic amplitude and variability changes occurring within and between structures. *Res. Commun. Chem. Pathol. Pharmacol.,* 5, 694–704.

Nestoros, J.N. (1980). Ethanol specifically potentiates GABA-mediated neurotransmission in feline cerebral cortex. *Science,* 209, 708–710.

Nichols, J.R. (1963). A procedure which produces sustained

opiate–directed behavior (morphine addiction) in the rat. *Psychol. Rep.,* 13, 895–904.

Nicoll, R.A. (1975). Peptide receptors in the CNS. In *Handbook of Psychopharmacology, Vol. 4* (L.L. Iversen, S.D. Iversen and S.H. Snyder, Eds.), pp. 229–263. Plenum Press, New York.

Nicoll, R.A. (1978a). Physiological studies on amino acids and peptides as prospective transmitters in the CNS. In *Psychopharmacology: A Generation of Progress* (M.A. Lipton, A. DiMascio and K.F. Killam, Eds.), pp. 103–118. Raven Press, New York.

Nicoll, R.A. (1978b). Selective actions of barbiturates on synaptic transmission. In *Psychopharmacology: A Generation of Progress* (M.A. Lipton, A. DiMascio and K.F. Killam, Eds.), pp. 1337–1348. Raven Press, New York.

Nicoll, R.A. (1978c). Pentobarbital: differential postsynaptic action on sympathetic ganglion cells. *Science,* 199, 451–452.

Nicoll, R.A. (1979). Differential postsynaptic effects of barbiturates on chemical transmission. In *The Neurobiology of Chemical Transmission* (M. Otsuka and E.W. Hall, Eds.), pp. 267–278. Wiley, Toronto.

Nicoll, R.A. and Iwamoto, E.T. (1978). Action of pentobarbital on sympathetic ganglion cells. *J. Neurophysiol.,* 41, 4, 977–986.

Nicoll, R.A. and Padjen, A. (1976). Pentylenetetrazol, an antagonist of GABA at primary afferents of the isolated frog spinal cord. *Neuropharmacol.,* 15, 69–71.

Nielsen, M., Braestrup, C. and Squires, R.F. (1978). Evidence for a late evolutionary appearance of brain–specific benzodiazepine receptors: an investigation of 18 vertebrates and 5 invertebrate species. *Brain Res.,* 141, 342–346.

Niemegeers, C.J.E., Verbruggen, F.J. and Janssen, P.A.J. (1969). The influence of various neuroleptic drugs on shock avoidance in rats. *Psychopharmacologia,* 16, 161–182.

Nies, A., Robison, D.S., Harris, L.S. and Lamborn, K.R. (1974). Comparison of monoamine oxidase substrate activities in twins, schizophrenics, depressives and controls. *Adv. Biochem. Psychopharmacol.,* 12, 59–70.

Nies, A., Robinson, D.S., Lamborn, K.R. and Lampert, R.P. (1973). Genetic control of platelet and plasma monoamine oxidase activity. *Arch. Gen. Psychiatry,* 28, 834–838.

Noback, C.R. and Demarest, R.J. (1977). *The Nervous System: Introduction and Review, Second Edition.* McGraw-Hill, New York.

Nobin, A. and Björklund, A. (1973). Topography of the monoamine neuron systems in the human brain as revealed in fetuses. *Acta Physiol. Scand., (Suppl. 388,)* 88, 1–40.

Nordin, G., Ottosson, J.O. and Roos, B.E. (1971). Influence of convulsive therapy on 5-hydroxyindoleacetic acid and homovanillic acid in cerebrospinal fluid in endogenous depression. *Psychopharmacologia,* 29, 315–320.

North, R.A. and Tonini, M. (1976). Hyperpolarization by morphine of myenteric neurons. In *Opiates and En-dogenous Opioid Peptides* (H.W. Kosterlitz, Ed.), pp. 205–212. Elsevier/North Holland, Amsterdam.

North, R.A. and Williams, J.T. (1976). Enkephalin inhibits firing of myenteric neurons. *Nature,* 264, 460–461.

Norton, W.T. (1976). Formation, structure, and biochemistry of myelin. In *Basic Neurochemistry* (G.J. Siegel, R.W. Albers, R. Katzman and B.W. Agranoff, Eds.), pp. 74–99. Little, Brown, Boston.

Nyback, H.V., Walters, J.R., Aghajanian, G.K. and Roth, R.H. (1975). Tricyclic antidepressants: effects on the firing rate of brain noradrenergic neurons. *Eur. J. Pharmacol.,* 32, 302–312.

O'Brien, C.P. (1975). Experimental analysis of conditioning factors in human narcotic addiction. *Pharmacol. Rev.,* 27, 533–543.

O'Brien, C.P., Testa, T., O'Brien, T.J., Brady, J.P. and Wells, B. (1977). Conditioned narcotic withdrawal in humans. *Science,* 195, 1000–1002.

Ochs, S. (1972). Fast transport of materials in mammalian nerve fibers. *Science,* 176, 252–260.

Ochs, S. (1975). Axoplasmic transport. In *The Nervous System, Vol. 1* (D.B. Tower, Ed.), pp. 137–146. Raven Press, New York.

Ochs, S. (1981). Axoplasmic transport. In *Basic Neurochemistry, Third Edition* (C.J. Siegel, R.W. Albers, B.W. Agranoff and R. Katzman, Eds.), pp. 425–442. Little, Brown, Boston.

Okada, Y., Nitsch-Hassler, C., Kim, J.S., Bak, I.J. and Hassler, R. (1971). The role of gamma–aminobutyric acid (GABA) in the extrapyramidal motor system. I. Regional distribution of GABA in rabbit, rat, guinea pig and baboon CNS. *Exp. Brain Res.,* 13, 514–518.

Oldendorf, W.H. (1975). Permeability of the blood-brain barrier. In *The Nervous System, Vol. 1* (D.B. Tower, Ed.), pp. 279–289. Raven Press, New York.

Olds, J. and Milner, P. (1954). Positive reinforcement produced by electrical stimulation of septal area and other regions of rat brain. *J. Comp. Physiol. Psychol.,* 47, 419–427.

Oliver, C., Barnea, A., Warberg, J., Eskay, R. and Porter, J.C. (1977). Distribution, characterization and subcellular localization of MSH in the brain. *Front. Horm. Res.,* 4, 162–166.

Oliverio, A. (1966). Effects of mecamylamine on avoidance conditioning and maze learning of mice. *J. Pharmacol. Exp. Ther.,* 154, 350–356.

Oliveros, J.C., Jandali, M.K., Timsit-Berthier, M., Remy, R., Benghezal, A., Audibert, A. and Moeglen, J.M. (1978). Vasopressin in amnesia. *Lancet,* 1,8054, 42.

Olson, R.W., Greenlee, D., van Ness, P. and Ticku, M.K. (1978). Studies on the gamma–aminobutyric acid receptor/ionophore proteins in mammalian brain. In *Amino Acids as Neurotransmitters* (F. Fonnum, Ed.), pp. 467–486. Plenum Press, New York.

Osborne, H., Przewlocki, R., Höllt, V. and Herz, A. (1979). Release of β-endorphin from rat hypothalamus in vitro. *Eur. J. Pharmacol.*, 55, 425–428.

Osmond, H. and Smythies, J.R. (1952). Schizophrenia: a new approach. *J. Ment. Sci.*, 98, 309–315.

Oswald, I., Lewis, S.A., Tagney, J., Firth, H. and Haider, I. (1973). Benzodiazepines and human sleep. In *The Benzodiazepines* (S. Garattini, E. Mussini and L.O. Randall, Eds.), pp. 613–625. Raven Press, New York.

Otsuka, M. and Konishi, S. (1976). Release of substance P-like immunoreactivity from isolated spinal cord of newborn rat. *Nature,* 264, 83–84.

Overton, D.A. (1971). Discriminative control of behavior by drug states. In *Stimulus Properties of Drugs* (T. Thompson and R. Pickens, Eds.), pp. 87–110. Appleton-Century-Crofts, New York.

Palade, G.E. and Palay, S.L. (1954). Electron microscope obervations of interneuronal and neuromuscular synapses. *Anat. Rec.*, 118, 335.

Palay, S.L. and Palade, G.E. (1955). The fine structure of neurons. *J. Biophys. Biochem. Cytol.*, 1, 69–88.

Palmer, G.C. (Ed.) (1981). *Neuropharmacology of the Central Nervous System.* Academic Press, New York.

Pandey, G., Heinze, W.J., Brown, B.D. and Davis, J.M. (1979a). Electronvulsive shock treatment decreases β-adrenergic receptor sensitivity in rat brain. *Nature,* 280, 234–235.

Pandey, G.N., Dorus, E., Davis, J. and Tosteson, D.C. (1979b). Lithium transport in human red blood cells: Genetic and clinical aspects. *Arch. Gen. Psychiat.*, 36, 902–908.

Pappas, G.D. (1975). Ultrastructural basis of synaptic transmission. In *The Nervous System, Vol. 1* (D.B. Tower, Ed.), pp. 19–30. Raven Press, New York.

Pappas, G.D. and Waxman, S.G. (1972). Synaptic fine structure—morphological correlates of chemical and electrotonic transmission. In *Structure and Function of Synapses* (G.D. Pappas and D.P. Purpura, Eds.), pp. 1–43. Raven Press, New York.

Parsegian, V.A. (1977). Considerations in determining the mode of influence of calcium on vesicle-membrane interaction. In *Society for Neuroscience Symposia, Vol. 11* (W.M. Cowan and J.A. Ferrendelli, Eds.), pp. 161–171. Society for Neuroscience, Bethesda, Maryland.

Pastan, I. (1972). Cyclic AMP. *Sci. Am.*, 227, 2, 97–105.

Pasternak, G.W., Goodman, R. and Snyder, S.H. (1975). An endogenous morphine–like factor in mammalian brain. *Life Sci.*, 16, 1765-1769.

Pasternak, G.W. Simantov, R. and Snyder, S.H. (1976). Characterization of an endogenous morphine–like factor (enkephalin) in mammalian brain. *Mol. Pharmacol.*, 12, 504–513.

Pasternak, G.W., and Snyder, S.H. (1974). Opiate receptor

binding. Effects of enzymatic treatments. *Mol. Pharmacol.*, 10, 183–193.

Paton, W. (1969). A pharmacologic approach to drug dependence and drug tolerance. In *Scientific Basis of Drug Dependence* (H. Steinberg, Ed.), pp. 31–47. J.A. Churchill, London.

Paul, M.I., Ditzion, B.R., Pauk, G.L. and Janowski, D.S. (1970). Urinary adenosine 3'5'-monophosphate excretion in affective disorders. *Am. J. Psychiatry,* 126, 1493–1497.

Paul, S.M. (1977). Movement and madness. Towards a biological model of schizophrenia. In *Psychopathology: Experimental Models* (J.D. Maser and M.E.P. Seligman, Eds.), pp. 358–386. Freeman, San Francisco.

Pavlov, I. (1972). *Conditioned reflexes.* Translated by G.V. Anrep. Oxford Univ. Press, New York.

Peach, M.J. (1975). Cations: calcium, magnesium, barium, lithium, and ammonium. In *The Pharmacological Basis of Therapeutics, Fifth Edition* (L.S. Goodman and A. Gilman, Eds.), pp. 782–797. Macmillan, New York.

Penfield, W.G. (1932). Neuroglia, normal and pathological. In *Cytology and Cellular Pathology of the Nervous System. Vol. 11* (W.G. Penfield, Ed.), pp. 423–479. Hoeber, New York.

Penfield, W.G. and Jasper, H.H. (1954). *Epilepsy and the Functional Anatomy of the Human Brain.* Little, Brown, Boston.

Peroutka, S.J. and Snyder, S.H. (1980). Long–term antidepressant treatment decreases spiroperidol-labeled serotonin receptor binding. *Science,* 210, 88–90.

Pert, C.B., Kuhar, M.J. and Snyder, S.H. (1975). Autoradiographic localization of the opiate receptor in rat brain. *Life Sci.*, 16, 1849–1854.

Pert, C.B., Snowman, A.M. and Snyder, S.H. (1974). Localization of opiate binding in synaptic membranes of rat brain. *Brain Res.*, 70, 184–188.

Pert, C.B. and Snyder, S.H. (1973). Properties of opiate-receptor binding in rat brain. *Proc. Nat. Acad. Sci.*, 70, 2243-2247.

Pert, C.B. and Snyder, S.H. (1974). Opiate receptor binding of agonists and antagonists affected differentially by sodium. *Mol. Pharmacol.*, 10, 868–879.

Petrusz, O., Sar, M., Crossman, G.H. and Kizer, J.S. (1977). Synaptic terminals with somatostatin–like immunoreactivity in the rat brain. *Brain Res.*, 137, 181–187.

Phillips, A.G., Carter, D.A. and Fibiger, H.C. (1976). Dopaminergic substrates of intracranial self-stimulation in the caudate-putamen. *Brain Res.*, 104, 221–232.

Phillips, M.I. (1978). Angiotensin in the brain. *Neuroendocrinol.*, 25, 354–377.

Phillips, M.I. and Hoffman, W.E. (1977). Sensitive sites in the brain for the blood pressure and drinking responses to angiotensin II. In *Central Actions of Angiotensin and Related Hormones* (J.P. Buckley and C.M. Ferrario, Eds.), pp. 325–356. Pergamon Press, Elmsford, New York.

Phillis, J.W. (1976a). Acetylcholine and synaptic transmission in the central nervous system. In *Chemical Transmission in the Mammalian Nervous System* (C.H. Hockman and D. Bieger, Eds.), pp. 159–213. University Park Press, Baltimore.

Phillis, J.W. (1976b). Is β–(4-chlorophenyl)–GABA a specific antagonist of substance P on cerebral cortical neurons? *Experientia, 32,* 593–594.

Phillis, J.W. (1977). Substance P and related peptides. In *Society for Neuroscience Symposia, Vol. II.* (W.M. Cowan and J.A. Ferendelli, Eds.), pp. 241–264. Society for Neuroscience, Bethesda, Maryland.

Pickel, V.M., Reis, D.J. and Leeman, S.E. (1977). Ultrastructural localization of substance P in neurons in rat spinal cord. *Brain Res., 122,* 534–540.

Pierce, E.T., Foote, W.E. and Hobson, J.A. (1976). The efferent connection of the nucleus raphe dorsalis. *Brain Res., 107,* 137–144.

Pijnenburg, A.J.J., Honig, W.M.M. and van Rossum, J.M. (1975). Antagonism of apomorphine- and d-amphetamine-induced stereotyped behaviour by injection of low doses of haloperidol into the caudate nucleus and the nucleus accumbens. *Psychopharmacologia, 45,* 65–71.

Pletscher, A. (1968). Monoamine oxidase inhibiters: effects related to psychostimulation. In *Psychopharmacology: A Review of Progress 1957–1967* (D.H. Efron, Ed.), Pub 1836, pp. 649–654. U.S. Gov't. Printing Office, Washington D.C.

Plotnikoff, N.P., Prange, A.J., Breese, G.R. and Wilson, I.C. (1974). Thyrotropin releasing hormone: enhancement of dopa activity in thyroidectomized rats. *Life Sci., 14,* 1271–1278.

Polc, P., Mohler, H. and Haefely, W. (1974). The effect of diazepam on spinal cord activities: possible sites and mechanisms of action. *Naunyn-Schmiedeberg's Arch. Pharmacol., 284,* 319–337.

Pollin, W., Cardon, P. and Kety, S. (1961). Effects of amino acid feedings in schizophrenic patients treated with iproniazid. *Science, 133,* 104–105.

Poritsky, R. (1969). Two and three dimensional ultrastructure of boutons and glial cells on the motoneuronal surface in the cat spinal cord. *J. Comp. Neurol., 135,* 423–452.

Post, R.M., Fink, E., Carpenter, W.T. and Goodman, F.K. (1975). Cerebrospinal fluid amine metabolites in acute schizophrenia. *Arch. Gen. Psychiatry, 32,* 1063–1069.

Post, R.M., Kotin, J. and Goodwin, F.K. (1974). The effects of cocaine on depressed patients. *Am. J. Psychiatry, 131,* 511–517.

Potter, L.T. (1973). Acetylcholine receptors in vertebrate skeletal muscles and electric tissues. In *Drug Receptors* (H.P. Rang, Ed.), pp. 295–310. University Park Press, Baltimore.

Powley, T.L. and Keesey, R.E. (1970). Relationship of body body weight to the lateral hypothalamic feeding syndrome. *J. Comp. Physiol. Psychol., 70,* 25–36.

Pradhan, S.N. and Dutta, S.N. (1970). Behavioral effects of arecoline in rats. *Psychopharmacologia, 17,* 49–58.

Prange, A.J., Jr., Breese, G.R., Cott, J.M., Martin, B.R., Cooper, B.R., Wilson, I.C. and Plotnikoff, N.P. (1974). Thyrotropin releasing hormone: antagonism of pentobarbital in rodents. *Life Sci., 14,* 447–455.

Prange, A.J., Jr., Nemeroff, C.B. and Lipton, M.A. (1978a). Behavioral effects of peptides: basic and clinical studies. In *Psychopharmacology: A Generation of Progress* (M.A. Lipton, A. DiMascio, and D.F. Killam, Eds.), pp. 441–458. Raven Press, New York.

Prange, A.J., Jr., Nemeroff, C.B., Lipton, M.A., Breese, G.R. and Wilson, I.C. (1978b). Peptides and the central nervous system. In *Handbook of Psychopharmacology, Vol. 13* (L.L. Iversen, S.D. Iversen and S.H. Snyder, Eds.), pp. 1–107. Plenum Press, New York.

Prange, A.J., Jr., Nemeroff, C.B., Loosen, P.T., Bissett, G., Osbahr, A.J., Wilson, I.C. and Lipton, M.A. (1979). Behavioral effects of thyrotropin-releasing hormone in animals and man: a review. In *Central Nervous System Effects of Hypothalamic Hormones and Other Peptides* (R. Collu, A. Barbeau, J.R. Ducharme and J.G. Rochefort, Eds.), pp. 75–96. Raven Press, New York.

Prange, A.J., Jr. and Wilson, I.C. (1972). Thyrotropin-releasing hormone (TRH) for the immediate relief of depression: a preliminary report. *Psychopharmacologia, 26,* 82.

Prange, A.J., Jr., Wilson, I.C., Knox, A., McClane, T.K. and Lipton, M.A. (1970). Enhancement of imipramine by thyroid stimulating hormone: clinical and theoretical implications. *Am. J. Psychiatry, 127,* 191–199.

Prasad, C., Matsui, T., Williams, J. and Peterkofsky, A. (1978). Thermoregulation in rats: opposing effects of thyrotropin releasing hormone and its metabolite histidyl–proline diketopiperazine. *Biochem. Biophys. Res. Commun., 85,* 1582–1587.

Price, H.L. (1975). General anesthetics: intravenous anesthetics. In *The Pharmacological Basis of Therapeutics, Fifth Edition* (L.S. Goodman and A. Gilman, Eds.), pp. 97–101. Macmillan, New York.

Puig, M.M., Gascon, P., Craviso, G.L. and Musacchio, J.M. (1977). Endogenous opiate receptor ligand: electrically induced release in the guinea pig ileum. *Science, 195,* 419–420.

Purpura, D.P. (1974). Dendritic spine "dysgenesis" and mental retardation. *Science, 186,* 1126–1128.

Quarles, R.H. (1975). Glycoproteins in the nervous system. In *The Nervous System, Vol. 1* (D.B. Tower, Ed.), pp. 493–501. Raven Press, New York.

Quenzer, L.F. and Feldman, R.S. (1975). The mechanism of anti-muricidal effects of chlordiazepoxide. *Pharmacol. Biochem. Behav., 3,* 567–571.

Quenzer, L.F. and Feldman, R.S. (1976). Chlordiazepoxide

effects on brain amines and cAMP in suppression of aggression. In *Neuropsychopharmacology, Proc. IX Congress* (J.R. Bossier, H. Hippius and R. Pichet, Eds.), pp. 698–714. Excerpta Medica, Amsterdam.

Quenzer, L.F., Feldman, R.S. and Moore, J.W. (1974). Toward a mechanism of the anti-aggression effects of chlordiazepoxide in rats. *Psychopharmacologia,* 34, 81–94.

Quenzer, L., Yahn, D., Alkadhi, K. and Volle, R.L. (1979). Transmission blockade and stimulation of ganglionic adenylate cyclase by catecholamines. *J. Pharmacol. Exp. Ther.,* 208, 31–36.

Rahe, R.H. (1975). The pathway between subjects' recent life changes and their near-future illness reports: representative results and methodological issues. In *Stressful Life Events: Their Nature and Effects* (B.S. Dohrenwend and B.P. Dohrenwend, Eds.), pp. 73–86. Wiley, New York.

Rahe, R.H. (1979). Life change events and mental illness: an overview. *J. of Hum. Stress,* 5, 2–10.

Rahe, R.H. and Arthur, R.J. (1978). Life changes and illness studies: past history and future directions. *J. of Hum. Stress,* 4, 3–15.

Ramsey, T.A. (1981). Manic-depressive illness and the pharmacology of lithium. In *Neuropharmacology of the CNS and Behavioral Disorders* (G.C. Palmer, Ed.), pp. 111–121. Academic Press, New York.

Randall, L.O., Heise, G.A., Schallek, W., Bagdon, R.E., Banziger, R., Boris, A., Moe, R.A. and Abrams, W.B. (1961). Pharmacological and clinical studies on valium, a new psychotherapeutic agent of the benzodiazepine class. *Curr. Ther. Res. Clin. Exp.,* 3, No. 9, 405–425.

Randall, L.O. and Kapell, B. (1973). Pharmacological activity of some benzodiazepines and their metabolites. In *The Benzodiazepines* (S. Garattini, E. Mussini and L.O. Randall, Eds.), pp. 27–51. Raven Press, New York.

Randall, L.O., Schallek, W., Heise, G.A., Keith, E.F. and Bagdon, R.E. (1960). The psychosedative properties of methaminodiazepoxide. *J. Pharmacol. Exp. Ther.,* 129, 163–171.

Randall, L.O., Schallek, W., Sternbach, L.H. and Ning, R.Y. (1974). Chemistry and pharmacology of the 1,4–benzodiazepines. In *Psychopharmacological Agents, Vol. 3* (M. Gordon, Ed.), pp. 175–281. Academic Press, New York.

Randic, M. and Miletic, V. (1977). Effect of substance P in cat dorsal horn neurons activated by noxious stimuli. *Brain Res.,* 128, 164–169.

Randrup, A. and Munkvad, I. (1967). Stereotyped activities produced by amphetamine in several animal species and man. *Psychopharmacologia,* 11, 300–310.

Randrup, A., Munkvad, I., Fog, R. and Ayhan, I.H. (1975). Catecholamines in activation, stereotypy, and level of mood. In *Catecholamines and Behavior, Vol. 1* (A.J. Friedhoff, Ed.), pp. 89–107. Plenum Press, New York.

Rapport, M.M., Green, A.A. and Page, I.H. (1948). Crystal-line serotonin. *Science,* 108, 329–330.

Rastogi, R.B. (1979). Thyrotropin-releasing hormone influences on behavior: possible involvement of brain monoaminergic systems. In *Central Nervous System Effects of Hypothalamic Hormones and Other Peptides* (R. Collu, A Barbeau, J.G. Rochefort and J.R. Ducharme, Eds.), pp. 123–140. Raven Press, New York.

Rech, R.H. (1968). Effects of cholinergic drugs on poor performance of rats in a shuttle-box. *Psychopharmacologia,* 12, 371–383.

Rehfeld, J.F. (1980). Cholecystokinin. *Trends Neurosci.,* March, 65–67.

Reich, T., Clayton, P.J. and Winokur, G. (1969). Family history studies V: the genetics of mania. *Am. J. Psychiatry,* 125, 1358–1369.

Reis, D.J., Rifkin, M. and Corvelli, A. (1971). Effect of morphine on cat brain norepinephrine in regions with daily monoamine rhythms. *Eur. J. Pharmacol.,* 8, 149–152.

Reiter, R.J. (1976). Pineal and associated neuroendocrine rhythms. *Psychoneuroendocrinol.,* 1, 255–263.

Remmer, H. (1962). Drugs as activators of drug enzymes. In *Metabolic Factors Controlling Duration of Drug Action, Vol. 6* (B.B.Brodie and E.G. Erdos, Eds.), p. 235f. Macmillan, New York.

Renaud, L.P. (1978). Peptides as neurotransmitters or neuromodulators. In *Psychopharmacology: A Generation of Progress* (M.A. Lipton, A. DiMascio and K.F. Killam, Eds.), pp. 423–430. Raven Press, New York.

Renaud, L.P. and Martin, J.B. (1975). Thyrotropin releasing hormone (TRH): depressant action on central neuronal activity. *Brain Res.,* 86, 150–154.

Renaud, L.P., Martin, J.B., and Brazeau, P. (1975a). Depressant action of TRH, LH-RH, and somatostatin on activity of central neurons. *Nature,* 255, 233–235.

Rexed, B. (1954). A cytoarchitectonic atlas of the spinal cord in the cat. *J. Comp. Neurol.,* 100, 297–379.

Reynolds, A.K. and Randall, L.O. (1957). *Morphine and Allied Drugs.* Univ. of Toronto Press, Toronto.

Reynolds, G.S. (1975). *A Primer of Operant Conditioning.* Scott Foresman, Glenview, Illinois.

Rickels, K. (1980). Benzodiazepines: clinical use patterns. In *Benzodiazepines: Review of Research Results 1980* (S.I. Szara and S. Ludford, Eds.), pp. 43–60. NIDA Research Monograph Series, No. 33. Supt. of Documents, Washington D.C.

Ritchie, J.M. (1975a). The aliphatic alcohols. In *The Pharmacological Basis of Therapeutics* (L.S. Goodman and A. Gilman, Eds.), pp. 137–151. Macmillan, New York.

Ritchie, J.M. (1975b). Central nervous system stimulants. The xanthines. In *The Phamacological Basis of Therapeutics* (L.S. Goodman and A. Gilman, Eds.), pp. 367–378. Macmillan, New York.

Ritchie, J.M. and Cohen, P.J. (1975). Cocaine, procaine and other synthetic local anesthetics. In *The Pharmacological*

Basis of Therapeutics (L.S. Goodman and A. Gilman, Eds.), pp. 379–403. Macmillan, New York.

Roberts, E. (1956). Formation and liberation of γ-aminobutyric acid in brain. In *Progress in Neurobiology. I. Neurochemistry* (S.R. Korey and J.I. Nurnberger, Eds.), pp. 11–25. Hoeber-Harper, New York.

Roberts, E. (1972). An hypothesis suggesting that there is a defect in the GABA system in schizophrenia. *Neurosci. Res. Prog. Bull.*, 10, 468–482.

Roberts, E. (1974). γ-Aminobutyric acid and nervous system function—a perspective. *Biochem. Pharmacol.*, 23, 2637–2649.

Roberts, E. (1975). GABA in nervous system function—an overview. In *The Nervous System Vol. 1* (D.B. Tower, Ed.), pp. 541–552. Raven Press, New York.

Roberts, E. (1978). Immunocytochemical visualization of GABA neurons. In *Psychopharmacology, A Generation of Progress* (M.A. Lipton, A. DiMascio and K.F. Killam, Eds.), pp. 95–102. Raven Press, New York.

Roberts, E., Chase, T. and Tower, D.B. (Eds.) (1975). *GABA and Nervous System Function*. Raven Press, New York.

Roberts, E. and Frankel, S. (1950). γ-Aminobutyric acid in brain: its formation from glutamic acid. *J. Biol. Chem.*, 187, 55–63.

Roberts, E. and Hammerschlag, R. (1976). Amino acid transmitters. In *Basic Neurochemistry* (C.J. Siegel, R.W. Albers, R. Katzman and B.W. Agranoff, Eds.), pp. 218–245. Little, Brown, Boston.

Roberts, P.J., Woodruff, G.N. and Iversen, L.L. (Eds.) (1978). *Advances in Biochemical Psychopharmacology, Vol. 9, Dopamine*. Raven Press, New York.

Robertson, J.D. (1975). Membrane models: theoretical and real. In *The Nervous System Vol. 1* (D.B. Towers, Ed.), pp. 43–58. Raven Press, New York.

Robichaud, R.C. and Sledge, K.L. (1969). The effects of *p*-chlorophenylalanine on experimentally induced conflict in the rat. *Life Sci.*, 8, 965–696.

Robinson, D.S. and Nies, A. (1980). Demographic, biologic, and other variables affecting monoamine oxidase activity. *Schizophr. Bull.*, 6, 298–307.

Robison, G.A., Butcher, R.W. and Sutherland, E.W. (1971). *Cyclic AMP*. Academic Press, New York.

Robison, G.A., Coppen, A.J., Whybrow, P.C. and Prange, A.J. (1970). Cyclic AMP in affective disorders. *Lancet*, 2, 1028–1029.

Roffman, M., Reddy, C. and Lal, H. (1972). Alleviation of morphine-withdrawal symptoms by conditional stimuli: possible explanation for "drug hunger" and "relapse." In *Drug Addiction: Experimental Pharmacology* (J.M. Singh, L. Miller and H. Lal, Eds.), pp. 223–226. Futura, Mt. Kisco, New York.

Roll, S.K. (1970). Intracranial self-stimulation and wakefulness: effect of manipulating ambient brain catecholamines. *Science*, 168, 1370–1372.

Rolls, E.T., Kelly, P.H. and Shaw, S.G. (1974). Noradrenaline, dopamine and brain stimulation reward. *Pharmacol. Biochem. Behav.*, 2, 735–740.

Rondeau, D.B., Jolicoeur, F.B., Belanger, F. and Barbeau, A. (1978). Motor activity induced by substance P in rats. *Pharmacol. Biochem. Behav.*, 9, 769–775.

Rosecrans, J.A. and Glennon, R.A. (1979). Drug-induced cues in studying mechanisms of drug action. *Neuropharmacol.*, 18, 981–989.

Roseman, S. (1974). Complex carbohydrates and intercellular adhesion. In *The Cell Surface in Development* (A. Moscona, Ed.), pp. 255–271. Wiley, New York.

Rosenthal, D., Wender, P.H., Kety, S.S. and Welner, J. (1971). The adopted-away offspring of schizophrenics. *Am. J. Psychiatry*, 128, 307–311.

Rosenzweig, M.R., Bennett, E.L. and Diamond, M.C. (1972). Brain changes in response to experience. *Sci. Am.*, 226, 2, 22–29.

Rosloff, N. and Davis, J.M. (1974). Effect of iprindole on norepinephrine turnover and transport. *Psychopharmacologia*, 40, 53–64.

Rossier, J., Rogers, J., Shibaski, T., Guillemin, R. and Bloom, F.E. (1979). Opioid peptides and α-melanocyte-stimulating hormone in genetically obese (ob/ob) mice during development. *Proc. Nat. Acad. Sci.*, 76, 2077–2080.

Rossier, J., Vargo, T.M., Minick, S., Ling, N., Bloom, F.E. and Guillemin, R. (1977). Regional dissociation of β-endorphin and enkephalin contents in rat brain and pituitary. *Proc. Nat. Acad. Sci.*, 74, 5162–5165.

Roszak, T. (1969). *The Making of a Counter Culture*. Doubleday, Garden City, New York.

Roth, R.H., Morgenroth, V.H. and Salzman, P.M. (1975). Tyrosine hydroxylase: allosteric activation induced by stimulation of central noradrenergic neurons. *Naunyn-Schmiedeberg's Arch. Pharmacol.*, 289, 327–343.

Roth, R.H., Salzman, P.M. and Nowycky, M.C. (1978). Impulse flow and short-term regulation of transmitter biosynthesis in central catecholamine neurons. In *Psychopharmacology: A Generation of Progress* (M.A. Lipton, A. DiMascio and K.F. Killam, Eds.), pp. 185–198. Raven Press, New York.

Rothman, J.E. (1981). The Golgi apparatus: two organelles in tandem. *Science*, 213, 1212–1219.

Roy, A.C. and Collier, H.O.J. (1975). Prostaglandins, cyclic AMP and the mechanisms of opiate dependence. *Life Sci.*, 17, 85–90.

Rubovits, R. and Klawans, H.L. (1972). Implications of amphetamine stereotyped behavior as a model for tardive dyskinesia. *Arch. Gen. Psychiatry*, 27, 502–507.

Ruda, M.A. (1982). Opiate and pain pathways: demonstration of enkephalin synapses on dorsal horn projection neurons. *Science*, 215, 1523–1524.

Ryall, R.W. (1975). Amino acid receptors in CNS. I. GABA and glycine in spinal cord. In *Handbook of Psychophar-*

macology, Vol. 4 (L.L. Iversen, S.D. Iversen and S.H. Snyder, Eds.), pp. 83–128. Plenum Press, New York.

Saavedra, J.M. (1977). Tryptamine and dimethyltryptamine: are they related to psychiatric disorders? In *Neuroregulators and Psychiatric Disorders* (E. Usdin, D.A. Hamburg, and J.D. Barchas, Eds.), pp. 201–209. Oxford Univ. Press, New York.

Saavedra, J.M. and Axelrod, J. (1973). Effect of drugs on the tryptamine content of rat tissues. *J. Pharmacol. Exp. Ther.,* 185, 523–529.

Saavedra, J.M. and Axelrod, J. (1976). Octopamine as a putative neurotransmitter. In *Advances in Biochemical Psychopharmacology, Vol. 15* (E. Costa, E. Giacobini and R. Paoletti, Eds.), pp. 95–110. Raven Press, New York.

Saavedra, J.M., Palkovits, M., Brownstein, M.J. and Axelrod, J. (1974). Serotonin distribution in the nuclei of the rat hypothalamus and preoptic region. *Brain Res.,* 77, 157–165.

Saito, K., Konishi, S. and Otsuka, M. (1975). Antagonism between lioresal and substance P in rat spinal cord. *Brain Res.,* 97, 177–180.

Salmoiraghi, G.C. and Bloom, F.E. (1964). Pharmacology of individual neurons. *Science,* 144, 493–499.

Samanin, R., Gumulka, W. and Valzelli, L. (1970). Reduced effect of morphine in midbrain raphe lesioned rats. *Eur. J. Pharmacol.,* 10, 339–343.

Sanders-Bush, E., Gallager, D.A. and Sulser, F. (1974). On the mechanism of brain 5–hydroxytryptamine depletion by *p*-chloroamphetamine and related drugs and the specificity of their action. In *Advances in Biochemical Psychopharmacology, Volume 10* (E. Costa, G.L. Gessa and M. Sandler, Eds.), pp. 185–194. Raven Press, New York.

Sargant, W. and Slater, E. (1972). *An Introduction to Physical Methods of Treatment in Psychiatry*. Science House, New York.

Satyamurti, S., Drachman, D.B. and Sloane, F. (1975). Blockade of acetycholine receptors: a model of myasthenia gravis. *Science,* 187, 955–977.

Schallek, W., Horst, W.D. and Schlosser, W. (1979). Mechanisms of action of benzodiazepines. In *Advances in Pharmacology and Chemotherapy, Vol. 16* (S. Garattini, A. Goldin, F. Hawking and I.J. Kopin, Eds.), pp. 45–87. Academic Press, New York.

Schally, A.V. (1978). Aspects of hypothalamic regulation of the pituitary gland. *Science,* 202, 18–28.

Schally, A.V., Arimura, A. and Kastin, A.J. (1973). Hypothalamic regulatory hormones. *Science,* 179, 341–350.

Schanberg, S.M., Schildkraut, J.J. and Kopin, I.J. (1967). The effects of psychoactive drugs on norepinephrine-³H metabolism in brain. *Biochem. Pharmacol.,* 16, 393–399.

Schecter, M.D. and Rosecrans, J.A. (1971). CNS effect of nicotine as the discriminative stimulus for the rat in a T-maze. *Life Sci.,* 10, 821–832.

Scheibel, M.E. and Scheibel, A.B. (1967). Anatomical basis of attention mechanisms in vertebrate brains. In *The Neurosciences, A Study Program* (G.C. Quarton, T. Melnechuk and F.O. Schmitt, Eds.), pp. 577–602. Rockefeller Univ. Press, New York.

Schelling, P., Hutchinson, J.J., Ganten, U., Sponer, G. and Ganten, D. (1976). Impermeability of the blood—cerebrospinal fluid barrier for angiotensin II in rats. *Clin. Sci. Mol. Med.,* 51, 355–377.

Schildkraut, J.J. (1965). The catecholamine hypothesis of affective disorders: a review of supporting evidence. *Am. J. Psychiatry,* 122, 509–522.

Schildkraut, J.J. (1973). Pharmacology—the effects of lithium on biogenic amines. In *Lithium, Its Role in Psychiatric Research and Treatment* (S. Gershon and B. Shopsin, Eds.), pp. 51–74. Plenum Press, New York.

Schildkraut, J.J., Herzog, J.M., Orsulak, P.J., Edelman, S.E., Shein, H.M. and Frazier, S.H. (1976). Reduced platelet monoamine oxidase activity in a subgroup of schizophrenic patients. *Am. J. Psychiatry,* 133, 438–440.

Schildkraut, J.J. and Keeler, B.A. (1973). MHPG excretion in depressive disorders: relation to clinical subtypes and desynchronized sleep. *Science,* 181, 762–764.

Schildkraut, J.J. and Kety, S.S. (1967). Biogenic amines and emotion. *Science,* 156, 21–30.

Schildkraut, J.J., Orsulak, P.J., Schatzberg, A.F. and Herzog, J.M. (1980). Platelet monoamine oxidase activity in subgroups of schizophrenic disorders. *Schizophr. Bull.,* 6, 220–225.

Schildkraut, J.J., Schanberg, S.M., Breese, G.R. and Kopin, I.J. (1967). Norepinephrine metabolism and drugs used in the affective disorders: a possible mechanism of action. *Am. J. Psychiatry,* 124, 600–608.

Schildkraut, J.J., Schanberg, S.M. and Kopin, I.J. (1966). The effects of lithium ion on [³H]norepinephrine metabolism in brain. *Life Sci.,* 5, 1479–1483.

Schildkraut, J.J., Winokur, A., Draskoczy, P.R. and Hensle, J.H. (1972). Changes in norepinephrine turnover in rat brain during chronic administration of imipramine and protriptyline: a possible explanation for the delay in onset of clinical antidepressant effect. *Am. J. Psychiatry,* 127, 1032–1039.

Schmitt, F.O., Dev, P. and Smith, B.H. (1976). Electrotonic processing of information by brain cells. *Science,* 193, 114–120.

Schubert, P., Höllt, V. and Herz, A. (1975). Autoradiographic evaluation of the intracerebral distribution of [³H]etorphine in the mouse brain. *Life Sci.,* 16, 1855–1856.

Schultes, R.E. (1970). Botanical and chemical distribution of hallucinogens. *Am. Rev. Plant Physiol.,* 21, 571–598.

Schultes, R.E. (1978). Plant and plant constituents as mind-altering agents throughout history. In *Handbook of Psychopharmacology, Vol. 11* (L.L. Iversen, S.D. Iversen and S.H. Snyder, Eds.), pp. 219–242. Plenum Press, New York.

Schultz, J. (1976). Psychoactive drug effects on a system which generates cyclic AMP in brain. *Nature,* 261, 417–418.

Schulz, S.C., van Kammen, D.P., Balow, J.E., Flye, M.W. and Bunney, W.E., Jr. (1981). Dialysis in schizophrenia: a double-blind evaluation. *Science,* 211, 1066–1068.

Schuster, C.R. and Thompson, T. (1969). Self administration of and behavioral dependence on drugs. *Annu. Rev. Pharmacol.,* 9, 483–502.

Schwab, R.S., England, A.C., Jr., Poskanzer, D.C. and Young, R.Y. (1969). Amantadine in the treatment of Parkinson's disease. *J. Am. Med. Assoc.,* 208, 1168–1170.

Schwartz, J.H. (1980). The transport of substances in nerve cells. *Sci. Am.,* 242, 4, 152–171.

Scientific American (1979). *The Brain.* Freeman, San Francisco.

Sedvall, G. (1975). Receptor feedback and dopamine turnover in CNS. In *Handbook of Psychopharmacology, Vol. 6* (L.L. Iversen, S.D. Iversen and S.H. Snyder, Eds.), pp. 127–177. Plenum Press, New York.

Seeman, P. and Lee, T. (1975). Antipsychotic drugs: direct correlation between clinical potency and presynaptic action on dopamine neurons. *Science,* 188, 1217–1219.

Seiden, L.S. and Dykstra, L.A. (1977). *Psychopharmacology, A Biochemical and Behavioral Approach.* Van Nostrand Reinhold, New York.

Selikoff, I.J., Robitzek, E.H. and Ornstein, G.G. (1952). Toxicity of hydrazine derivatives of isonicotinic acid in the chemotherapy of human tuberculosis. *Quart. Bull. Seaview Hosp.,* 13, 17–26.

Sepinwall, J. and Cook, L. (1978). Behavioral pharmacology of antianxiety drugs. In *Handbook of Psychopharmacology, Vol. 13* (L.L. Iversen, S.D. Iversen and S.H. Snyder, Eds.), pp. 345–393. Plenum Press, New York.

Serra, G., Argiolas, A., Klimek, V., Fadda, F. and Gessa, G.L. (1979). Chronic treatment with antidepressants prevents the inhibitory effect of small doses of apomorphine on dopamine synthesis and motor activity. *Life Sci.,* 25, 415–424.

Sessions, G.R., Kant, G.J. and Koob, G.F. (1976). Locus ceruleus lesions and learning in the rat. *Physiol. Behav.,* 17, 5, 853–860.

Sethy, V.H. and Van Woert, M.H. (1974). Modification of striatal acetylcholine concentration by dopamine receptor agonists. *Res. Commun. Chem. Pathol. Pharmacol.,* 8, 13–28.

Severs, W.B. and Daniels-Severs, A.E. (1973). Effects of angiotensin on the central nervous system. *Pharmacol. Rev.,* 25, 415–449.

Severs, W.B., Summy-Long, J., Taylor, J.S. and Connor, J.D. (1970). A central effect of angiotensin: release of pituitary pressor material. *J. Pharmacol. Exp. Ther.,* 174, 27–34.

Shader, R.I. and Greenblatt, D.J. (1977). Clinical implications of benzodiazepines pharmacokinetics. *Am. J. Psychiatry,* 134, 652–656.

Sharma, S.K., Klee, W.A. and Nirenberg, M. (1975a). Dual regulation of adenylate cyclase accounts for narcotic dependence and tolerance. *Proc. Nat. Acad. Sci.,* 72, 3092–3096.

Sharma, S.K., Nirenberg, M. and Klee, W.A. (1975b). Morphine receptors as regulators of adenylate cyclase activity. *Proc. Nat. Acad. Sci.,* 72, 590–594.

Sharpe, L.G., Garnett, J.E. and Cicero, T.J. (1974). Analgesia and hyperactivity produced by intracranial microinjections of morphine into the periaqueductal gray matter of the rat. *Behav. Biol.,* 11, 303–313.

Sharpless, S.K. (1970). Hypnotics and sedatives: 1. The barbiturates. In *The Pharmacological Basis of Therapeutics* (L.S. Goodman and A. Gilman, Eds.), pp. 98–120. Macmillan, New York.

Shaw, D.M. (1975). Lithium and amine metabolites. In *Lithium Research and Therapy* (F.N. Johnson, Ed.), pp. 411–423. Academic Press, New York.

Shaw, D.M., Camps, F. and Eccleston, E.G. (1967). 5-Hydroxytryptamine in the hindbrains of depressive suicides. *Br. J. Psychiatry,* 113, 1407–1411.

Sheard, M.H. (1969). The effect of *p*–chlorophenylalanine on behavior in rats: relation to brain serotonin and 5–hydroxyindoleacetic acid. *Brain Res.* 15, 524–528.

Sheard, M.H. (1974). The effect of *p*–chloroamphetamine on single raphe neurons. In *Advances in Biochemical Psychopharmacology, Volume 10* (E. Costa, G.L. Gessa and M. Sandler, Eds.), pp. 179–184. Raven Press, New York.

Shepard, J.F. (1914). *The Circulation and Sleep.* Univ. of Michigan Studies, Scientific Series, Ann Arbor, Michigan.

Sherrington, C.S. (1897). The central nervous system. In *A Textbook of Physiology, Vol. 3* (M. Foster, Ed.), Macmillan, London.

Shih, J.C., Eiduson, S., Geller, E. and Costa, E. (1974). Serotonin–binding proteins isolated by affinity chromatography. In *Advances in Biochemical Psychopharmacology, Volume 10* (E. Costa, G.L. Gessa and M. Sandler, Eds.), pp. 101–104. Raven Press, New York.

Shopsin, B., Friedman, E. and Gershon, J. (1976). Parachlorophenylalanine reversal of tranylcypromine effects in depressed patients. *Arch. Gen. Psychiatry,* 33, 811–822.

Shulgin, A.T. (1978). Psychotomimetic drugs: structure-activity relationships. In *Handbook of Psychopharmacology, Vol. 11* (L.L. Iversen, S.D. Iversen and S.H. Snyder, Eds.), pp. 243–333. Plenum Press, New York.

Sidman, M. (1953). Avoidance conditioning with brief shock and no exteroceptive warning stimulus. *Science,* 118, 157–158.

Siegel, G.J., Albers, R.W., Agranoff, B.W. and Katzman, R. (Eds.) (1981). *Basic Neurochemistry,* Little, Brown, Boston.

Siegel, S. (1975). Evidence from rats that morphine tolerance is a learned response. *J. Comp. Physiol. Psychol.,* 89, 498-506.

Siegel, S. (1976). Morphine analgesic tolerance: its situation specificity supports a Pavlovian conditioning model. *Science,* 193, 323-325.

Siegel, S., Hinson, R.E. and Krank, M.D. (1981). Morphine-induced attenuation of morphine tolerance. *Science,* 212, 1533-1534.

Siegmund, E., Cadmus, R. and Lu, G. (1957). A method for evaluating both non-narcotic and narcotic analgesics. *Proc. Soc. Exp. Biol. Med.,* 95, 729-731.

Siggins, G.R., Hoffer, B.J. and Ungerstedt, U. (1974). Electrophysiological evidence for involvement of cyclic adenosine monophosphate in dopamine responses of caudate neurons. *Life Sci.,* 15, 779-792.

Simantov, R., Kuhar, M.J., Pasternak, G.W. and Snyder, S.H. (1976). The regional distribution of a morphine-like factor enkephalin in monkey brain. *Brain Res.,* 106, 189-197.

Simon, E.J. (1975). Opiate receptor binding with [³H] etorphine. *Neurosci. Res. Prog. Bull.,* 13, 43-50.

Simon, E.J. (1976). The opiate receptors. *Neurochem. Res.,* 1, 3-28.

Simon, E.J., Heller, J.M. and Edelman, I. (1973). Stereospecific binding of the potent narcotic analgesic [³H]etorphine to rat brain homogenate. *Proc. Nat. Acad. Sci.,* 70, 1947-1949.

Simon, J.R., Contrera, J.F. and Kuhar, M.J. (1976). Binding of [³H]kainic acid, an analogue of *L*-glutamate, to brain membranes. *J. Neurochem.,* 26, 141-147.

Sims, K.L. (1974). Biochemical characteristics of mammalian brain 5-hydroxytryptophan decarboxylase activity. In *Advances in Biochemical Psychopharmacology, Vol. 11* (E. Costa, G.L. Gessa and M. Sandler, Eds.), pp. 43-50. Raven Press, New York.

Sims, K.L. and Bloom, F.E. (1973). Rat brain *L*-3,4-dihydroxyphenylalanine and *L*-5-hydroxytryptophan decarboxylase activities. Differential effect of 6-hydroxydopamine. *Brain Res.,* 49, 165-175.

Singer, S.J. and Nicolson, G.L. (1972). The fluid mosaic model of the structure of cell membranes. *Science,* 175, 720-731.

Sirette, N.E., McLean, A.S., Bray, J.J. and Hubbard, J.I. (1977). Distribution of angiotensin II receptors in rat brain. *Brain Res.,* 122, 299-312.

Skirboll, L.R., Grace, A.A. and Bunney, B.S. (1979). Dopamine auto- and postsynaptic receptors: electrophysiological evidence for differential sensitivity to dopamine agonists. *Science,* 206, 80-82.

Skolnick, P., Marangos, P.J., Syapin, P., Goodwin, F.K. and Paul, S.M. (1979). CNS benzodiazepine receptors: physiological studies and putative endogenous ligands. *Pharmacol. Biochem. Behav.,* 10, 815-823.

Smith, C.B., Sheldon, M.I., Bednarczyk, J.H. and Villarreal, J.E. (1972). Morphine-induced increases in the incorporation of ¹⁴C-tyrosine into ¹⁴C-dopamine and ¹⁴C-norepinephrine in the mouse brain: antagonism by naloxone and tolerance. *J. Pharmacol. Exp. Ther.,* 180, 547-577.

Smith, C.M. (1972). The release of acetylcholine from rat hippocampus. *Br. J. Pharmacol.,* 45, 172P.

Smith, R.J. (1979). Study finds sleeping pills overprescribed. *Science,* 204, 287-288.

Smoking and Health, a Report from the Surgeon General (1980). DHEW Publ. No. (PHS) 79-50066. U.S. Gov't Printing Office, Washington, D.C.

Snyder, S.H. (1972). Catecholamines and serotonin. In *Basic Neurochemistry* (R.W. Albers, G.J. Siegel, R. Katzman and B.W. Agranoff, Eds.), pp. 89-104. Little, Brown, Boston.

Snyder, S.H. (1974). Catecholamines as mediators of drug effects in schizophrenia. In *The Neurosciences, Third Study Program* (F.O. Schmitt and F.G. Worden, Eds.), pp. 721-232. MIT Press, Cambridge, Massachusetts.

Snyder, S.H. (1975a). Amino acid neurotransmitters: biochemical pharmacology. In *The Nervous System, Vol. 1* (D.B. Tower, Ed.), pp. 355-361. Raven Press, New York.

Snyder, S.H. (1975b). Neurotransmitter and drug receptors in the brain. *Biochem. Pharmacol.,* 24, 1371-1374.

Snyder, S.H. (1977). Opiate receptors and internal opiates. *Sci. Am.,* 236, 3, 44-56.

Snyder, S.H. (1980a). *Biological Aspects of Mental Disorders,* Oxford Univ. Press, New York.

Snyder, S.H. (1980b). Brain peptides as neurotransmitters. *Science,* 209, 976-983.

Snyder, S.H., Banerjee, S.P., Yamamura, H.I. and Greenberg, D. (1974). Drugs, neurotransmitters, and schizophrenia. *Science,* 184, 1243-1253.

Snyder, S.H., Creese, I. and Burt, D.R. (1977). Dopamine receptor binding in the mammalian brain: revelance to psychiatry. In *Neuroregulators and Psychiatric Disorders* (E. Usdin, D.A. Hamburg and J. Barchas, Eds.), pp. 526-537. Oxford Univ. Press, New York.

Snyder, S.H. and Enna, S.J. (1975). The role of central glycine receptors in the pharmacologic actions of benzodiazepines. In *Mechanisms of Action of Benzodiazepines* (E. Costa and P. Greengard, Eds.), pp. 81-91. Raven Press, New York.

Snyder, S.H. and Goodman, R.R. (1980). Multiple transmitter receptors. *J. Neurochem.,* 35, 5-15.

Snyder, S.H., Pasternak, G.W. and Pert, C.B. (1975). Opiate receptor mechanisms. In *Handbook of Psychopharmacology, Vol. 5* (L.L. Iversen, S.D. Iversen and S.H. Snyder, Eds.), pp. 329-360. Plenum Press, New York.

Snyder, S.H. and Pert, C.B. (1975). Regional distribution of the opiate receptor. *Neurosci. Res. Prog. Bull.,* 13, 35-38.

Snyder, S.H. and Yamamura, H.I. (1977). Antidepressants and the muscarinic acetylcholine receptor. *Arch. Gen. Psychiatry,* 34, 236-239.

Snyder, S.H., Young, A.B., Bennet, J.P. and Mulder, A.H. (1973). Synaptic biochemistry of amino acids. *Fed. Proc.,* 32, 2039-2047.

Soubrie, P., Thiebot, M.-H. and Simon, P. (1979). Enhanced suppressive effects of aversive events induced in rats by picrotoxin: possibility of a GABA control on behavior inhibition. *Pharmacol. Biochem. Behav.,* 10, 463-469.

Southgate, P.J., Mayer, S.R., Boxall, E. and Wilson, A.B. (1971). Some 5-hydroxytryptamine-like actions of fenfluramine: a comparison with (+)-amphetamine and diethylproprion. *J. Pharm. Pharmacol.,* 23, 600-605.

Spanos, N.P. and Gottlieb, J. (1976). Ergotism and the Salem village witch trials. *Science,* 194, 1390-1394.

Spatz, H. (1951). Neues über Verknüpfung von Hypophyse und Hypothalamus. *Acta Neuroveg.,* 3, 5-49.

Spector, S., Shore, P.A. and Brodie, B.B. (1960). Biochemical and pharmacological effects of the monoamine oxidase inhibitors, iproniazid, 1-phenyl-2-hydrazinopropane (JB516), and 1-phenyl-3-hydrazinobutane (JB835). *J. Pharmacol. Exp. Ther.,* 128, 15-21.

Spector, S., Sjoerdsma, A. and Udenfriend, S. (1965). Blockade of endogenous norepinephrine synthesis by 1-methyltyrosine, an inhibitor of tyrosine hydroxylase. *J. Pharmacol. Exp. Ther.,* 147, 86-95.

Spirtes, M.A., Christensen, C.W., Harston, C.T. and Kastin, A.J. (1978). *L*-MSH and MIF-1 effects on cGMP levels in various rat brain regions. *Brain Res.,* 144, 189-193.

Squires, R.F., Benson, D.I., Braestrup, C., Coupet, J., Klepner, C.A., Myers, V. and Beer, B. (1979). Some properties of brain specific benzodiazepine receptors: new evidence for multiple receptors. *Pharmacol. Biochem. Behav.,* 10, 825-830.

Squires, R.F. and Braestrup, C. (1977). Bezodiazepine receptors in rat brain. *Nature,* 266, 732-734.

Starr, M.S., James, T.A. and Gayetten, D. (1978). Behavioral depressant and antinociceptive properties of substance P in the mouse: possible implication of brain monoamines. *Eur. J. Pharmacol.,* 48, 203-212.

Stavinoha, W.B. and Weintraub, S.J. (1974). Choline content of rat brain. *Science,* 183, 964-965.

Stein, L. (1968). Chemistry of reward and punishment. In *Psychopharmacology, A Review of Progress; 1957-1967* (D.H. Efron, Eds.), pp. 105-123. U.S. Government Printing Office, Washington, D.C.

Stein, L. (1978). Reward transmitters: catecholamines and opioid peptides In *Psychopharmacology: A Generation Of Progress* (M.A. Lipton, A. DiMascio and K.F. Killam, Eds.), pp. 569-581. Raven Press, New York.

Stein, L., Belluzzi, J.D., Ritter, S. and Wise, C.D. (1974). Self-stimulation reward pathways: norepinephrine vs. dopamine. *J. Psychiat. Res.,* 11, 115-124.

Stein, L., Belluzzi, J.D. and Wise, C.D. (1977a). Benzodiazepines: behavioral and neurochemical mechanisms. *Am. J. Psychiatry,* 134, 665-669.

Stein, L. and Seifter, J. (1961). Possible mode of antidepressive action of imipramine. *Science,* 134, 286-287.

Stein, L. and Wise, C.D. (1970). Mechanism of the facilitating effects of amphetamine on behavior. In *Psychotomimetic Drugs* (D.H. Efron, Ed.), pp. 123-149. Raven Press, New York.

Stein, L. and Wise, C.D. (1974). Serotonin and behavioral inhibition. In *Advances in Biochemical Pharmacology, Vol. 11* (E. Costa, G.L. Gessa and M. Sandler, Eds.), pp. 281-291. Raven Press, New York.

Stein, L., Wise, C.D. and Belluzzi, J.D. (1975). Effects of benzodiazepines on central serotonergic mechanisms. In *Mechanisms of Action of Benzodiazepines* (E. Costa and P. Greengard, Eds.), pp. 29-44. Raven Press, New York.

Stein, L., Wise, C.D. and Belluzzi, J.D. (1977b). Neuropharmacology of reward and punishment. In *Handbook of Psychopharmacology, Vol. 8* (L.L. Iversen, S.D. Iversen and S.H. Snyder, Eds.), pp. 25-53. Plenum Press, New York.

Stein, L., Wise, C.D. and Berger, B.D. (1973). Antianxiety actions of benzodiazepines: decrease in activity of serotonin neurons in the punishment system. In *The Benzodiazepines* (S. Garattini, E. Mussini and L.O. Randall, Eds.), pp. 299-326. Raven Press, New York.

Sternbach, L.H. (1973). Chemistry of 1,4-benzodiazepines and some aspects of the structure-activity relationship. In *The Benzodiazepines* (S. Garattini, E. Mussini and L.O. Randall, Eds.), pp. 1-26. Raven Press, New York.

Sternbach, L.H., Randall, L.O. and Gustafson, S.R. (1964). 1,4-Benzodiazepines (chlordiazepoxide and related compounds). In *Psychopharmacological Agents* (M. Gordon, Ed.), pp. 137-224. Academic Press, New York.

Stewart, J.M., Getto, C.J., Neldner, K., Reeve, E.B., Krivoy, W.A. and Zimmermann, E. (1976). Substance P and analgesia. *Nature,* 262, 784-785.

Stillman, R.C., Wyatt, R.J., Murphy, D.L. and Rauscher, F.P. (1978). Low platelet monoamine oxidase activity and chronic marijuana use. *Life Sci.,* 23, 1577-1582.

Stinus, L., Kelly, A.E. and Iversen, S.D. (1978). Increased spontaneous activity following substance P infusion into A10 dopaminergic area. *Nature,* 276, 616-618.

Stoll, W.A. (1974). Lysergsaure-diethyl-amid, ein phantasticum aus der Mutterkorngruppe. *Schweiz. Arch. Neurol. Psychiatr.,* 60, 279-323.

Stone, T.W., Taylor, D.A. and Bloom, F.E. (1975). Cyclic AMP and cyclic GMP may mediate opposite neuronal responses in the rat cerebral cortex. *Science,* 187, 845-847.

Strauss, J.S. and Carpenter, W.T. (1981). *Schizophrenia.* Plenum Press, New York.

Stricker, E.M., Friedman, M.I. and Zigmond, M.J. (1975). Glucoregulatory feeding by rats after intraventricular 6-hydroxydopamine on lateral hypothalamic lesions. *Science,* 189, 895-897.

Stricker, E.M. and Zigmond, M.J. (1974). Effects on homeostasis of intraventricular injections of 6-hydroxydopamine in rats. *J. Comp. Physiol. Psychol.,* 86, 973–994.

Strömbom, U. (1977) Antagonism by haloperidol of locomotor depression induced by small doses of apomorphine. *J. Neural Transm.,* 40, 191–194.

Sugrue, M.F. (1973). Effects of morphine and pentazocine on the turnover of noradrenaline and dopamine in various regions of the rat brain. *Br. J. Pharmacol.,* 47, 644P.

Sullivan, J.L., Coffey, C.E., Sullivan, P.D., Taska, R., Mahorny, S. and Cavenar, J.C. (1980). Metabolic factors affecting monoamine oxidase activity. *Schizophr. Bull.,* 6, 308–313.

Sulser, F., Bickel, M.H. and Brodie, B.B. (1964). The action of desmethylimipramine in counteracting sedation and cholinergic effects of reserpine-like drugs. *J. Pharmacol. Exp. Ther.,* 144, 321–330.

Sulser, F., Vetulani, J. and Mobley, P.L. (1978). Mode of action of antidepressant drugs. *Biochem. Pharmacol.,* 27, 257–261.

Sutherland, E.W. (1972). Studies on the mechanism of hormone action. *Science,* 177, 401–408.

Suzuki, K. (1975). Sphingolipids of the nervous system. In *The Nervous System, Vol. 1* (D.B. Tower, Ed.), pp. 483–491. Raven Press, New York.

Swanson, L.W., Kucharczyk, J. and Mogenson, G.J. (1978). Autoradiographic evidence for pathways from the medial preoptic area to the midbrain involved in the drinking response to angiotensin II. *J. Comp. Neurol.,* 178, 645–659.

Szara, S. (1956). Dimethyltryptamine: its metabolism in man: the relation of its psychotic effect to serotonin metabolism. *Experientia,* 12, 441–442.

Tagliamonte, A., Tagliamonte, P., Gessa, G.L. and Brodie, B.B. (1969). Compulsive sexual activity induced by *p*-chlorophenylalanine in normal and pinealectomized male rats. *Science,* 166, 1433–1435.

Tagliamonte, D., Perez-Cruet, J. and Tagliamonte, A. (1970). Differential effect of *p*-chorophenylalanine (PCPA) on the sexual behavior and the electrocorticogram of male rabbits. *Pharmacologist,* 12, 205.

Takemori, A.E. (1975). Neurochemical bases for narcotic tolerance and dependence. *Biochem. Pharmacol.,* 24, 2121–2126.

Takeuchi, A. and Takeuchi, N. (1966). On the permeability of the presynaptic terminal of the crayfish neuromuscular junction during synaptic inhibition and the action of gamma-aminobutyric acid. *J. Physiol., (London),* 183, 433–449.

Tallman, J.F., Paul, S.M., Skolnick, P. and Gallager, D.W. (1980). Receptors for the age of anxiety: pharmacology of the benzodiazepines. *Science,* 207, 274–281.

Tamminga, C.A., Schaffer, M.H., Smith, R.C. and Davis, J.M. (1978). Schizophrenia symptoms improve with apomorphine. *Science,* 200, 567–568.

Tapia, R. (1975). Biochemical pharmacology of GABA in CNS. In *Handbook of Psychopharmacology, Vol. 4* (L.L. Iversen, S.D. Iversen and S.H. Snyder, Eds.), pp. 1–58. Plenum Press, New York.

Taube, H.D., Borowski, E., Endo, T. and Starke, K. (1976). Enkephalin: a potential modulator of noradrenaline release in rat brain. *Eur. J. Pharmacol.,* 38, 377–380.

Taylor, K.M., Gfeller, E. and Snyder, S.H. (1972). Regional localization of histamine and histidine in the brain of the rhesus monkey. *Brain Res.,* 41, 171–179.

Taylor, K.M. and Laverty, R. (1973). The interaction of chlordiazepoxide, diazepam, and nitrazepam with catecholamines and histamine in regions of the rat brain. In *The Benzodiazepines* (S. Garattini, E. Mussini and L.O. Randall, Eds.), pp. 191–202. Raven Press, New York.

Tebecis, A.K. (1972). Antagonism of 5-hydroxytryptamine by methiothepin shown in microiontophoretic studies of neurons in the lateral geniculate nucleus. *Nature,* 238, 63–64.

Telegdy, G. and Kovacs, G.L. (1979). Role of monoamines in mediating the action of ACTH, vasopressin, and oxytocin. In *Central Nervous System Effects of Hypothalamic Hormones and Other Peptides* (R. Collu, A. Barbeau, J.-G. Rochefort and J.R. Ducharme, Eds.), pp. 189–205. Raven Press, New York.

Tenen, S.S. (1967). The effects of *p*-chlorophenylalanine, a serotonin depletor, on avoidance acquisition, pain sensitivity and related behavior in the rat. *Psychopharmacologia,* 10, 204–219.

Tenen, S.S. (1968). Antagonism of the analgesic effect of morphine and other drugs by *p*-chlorophenylalanine, a serotonin depletor. *Psychopharmacologia,* 12, 278–285.

Terenius, L. (1973). Stereospecific interaction between narcotic analgesics and a synaptic plasma membrane fraction of rat cerebral cortex. *Acta Pharmacol. Toxicol.,* 32, 317–320.

Terenius, L. and Wahlstrom, A. (1974). Inhibitor(s) of narcotic receptor binding in brain extracts and cerebrospinal fluid. *Acta Pharmacol. Toxicol., 35 (Suppl. 1),* 87 (Abst.).

Terenius, L. and Wahlstrom, A. (1975). Morphine-like ligand for opiate receptors in human CSF. *Life Sci.,* 16, 1759–1764.

Teschemacher, H., Opheim, K.E., Cox, B.M. and Goldstein, A. (1975). A peptide-like substance from pituitary that acts like morphine. 1. Isolation. *Life Sci.,* 16, 1771–1776.

Tester-Dalderup, C.B.M. (1980). Hypotensive drugs. In *Side Effects of Drugs, Annual 4* (M.N.G. Dukes, Ed.), pp. 144–157. Excerpta Medica, Princeton, New Jersey.

Thierry, A.M., Feketee, M. and Glowinski, J. (1968). Effects of stress on the metabolism of noradrenaline, dopamine and serotonin (5-HT) in the central nervous system of the rat. II. Modifications of serotonin metabolism. *Eur. J. Pharmacol.,* 4, 384–389.

Thierry, A.M., Stinus, L., Blanc, G. and Glowinski, J. (1973). Some evidence for the existence of dopaminergic neurons in the rat cortex. *Brain Res.,* 50, 230–234.

Thompson, T. and Pickens, R. (1970). Stimulant self-administration by animals: some comparisons with opiate self-administration. *Fed. Proc.,* 29, 6–12.

Thompson, T., Pickens, R. and Meisch, R.A. (Eds.) (1970). *Readings in Behavioral Pharmacology.* Appleton-Century-Crofts, New York.

Thompson, T. and Schuster, C.R. (1964). Morphine self-administration, food reinforced and avoidance behaviors in rhesus monkeys. *Psychopharmacologia,* 5, 87–94.

Thompson, T. and Schuster, C.R. (1968). *Behavioral Pharmacology.* Prentice-Hall, Englewood Cliffs, New Jersey.

Thorner, M.W. (1935). The psycho-pharmacology of sodium-amytal. *J. Nerv. Ment. Dis.,* 81, 161–167.

Tinklenberg, J.R. (1977). Antianxiety medications and the treatment of anxiety. In *Psychopharmacology—From Theory to Practice* (J.D. Barchas, P.A. Berger, R.D. Ciaranello and G.R. Elliott, Eds.), pp. 226–241. Oxford Univ. Press, New York.

Tower, D.B. (Ed.) (1975). *The Nervous System, Vol. 1, The Basic Neurosciences.* Raven Press, New York.

Traber, J., Fisher, K., Latzin, S. and Hamprecht, B. (1974). Morphine antagonizes the action of prostaglandin in neuroblastoma cells but not of prostaglandin and noradrenalin in glioma and glioma x fibroblast hybrid cells. *FEBS Lett.,* 49, 260–263.

Traber, J., Fisher, K., Latzin, S. and Hamprecht, B. (1975). Morphine antagonizes action of prostaglandin in neuroblastoma and neuroblastoma X glioma hybrid cells. *Nature,* 253, 120–122.

Trulson, M.E. and Jacobs, B.L. (1979). Dissociation between the effects of LSD on behavior in raphe unit activity in freely moving cats. *Science,* 205, 3, 515–518.

Tuček, S. (Ed.) (1979). *The Cholinergic Synapse. Progress in Brain Research, Vol. 49.* Elsevier, New York.

Twarog, B.M. and Page, I.H. (1953). Serotonin content of some mammalian tissues and a method for its determination. *Am. J. Physiol.,* 157–161.

Uchizono, K. (1965). Characteristics of excitatory and inhibitory synapses in the central nervous system of the cat. *Nature,* 207, 642–643.

Uchizono, K. (1967). Synaptic organization of the Purkinje cells in the cerebellum of the cat. *Exp. Brain Res.,* 4, 97–113.

Ulrich, R. (1967). Pain, aggression and aversive control. In *Neuropsychopharmacology* (H. Brill, J.O. Cole, P. Deniker, H. Hippius and P.B. Bradley, Eds.), pp. 766–773. Excerpta Medica Foundation, New York.

Ulrich, R. and Azrin, N. (1962). Reflexive fighting in response to aversive stimulation. *J. Exp. Anal. Behav.,* 5, 511–520.

Ungerstedt, U. (1971a). Stereotaxic mapping of the mono-amine pathway in the rat brain. *Acta Physiol. Scand.,* 82, Suppl. 367, 1–48.

Ungerstedt, U. (1971b). Postsynaptic supersensitivity after 6-hydroxydopamine induced degeneration in the nigro-striatal dopamine system in the rat brain. *Acta Physiol. Scand.,* 82, Suppl. 367, 69–93.

Ugerstedt, U. (1971c). Striatal dopamine release after amphetamine or nerve degeneration revealed by rotational behavior. *Acta Physiol. Scand.,* 82, Suppl. 367, 49–68.

Ungerstedt, U. (1974a). Functional dynamics of central monoamine pathways. In *The Neurosciences, Third Study Program* (F.O. Schmitt and F.G. Worden, Eds.), pp. 979–988. MIT Press, Cambridge, Massachusetts.

Ungerstedt, U. (1974b). Brain dopamine neurons and behavior. In *The Neurosciences, Third Study Program* (F.O. Schmitt and F.G. Worden, Eds.), pp. 695–703. MIT Press, Cambridge, Massachusetts.

U'Prichard, D.C., Greenberg, D.A., Sheehan, P.P. and Snyder, S.H. (1978). Tricyclic antidepressents: therapeutic properties and affinity for α-noradrenergic receptor binding sites in the brain. *Science,* 199, 197–198.

Urban, I., Lopes da Silva, F.H., van Leeuwen, S. and de Wied, D. (1974). A frequency shift in the hippocampal theta activity. *Brain Res.,* 69, 361–365.

Usdin, E. and Bunney, W.E., Jr., (Eds.) (1975). *Pre- and Postsynaptic Receptors.* Marcell Dekker, New York.

Usdin, E., Hamburg, D.A. and Barchas, J.D. (Eds.) (1977). *Neuroregulators and Psychiatric Disorders.* Oxford Univ. Press, New York.

Vaillant, G.E. (1964). Antagonism between physostigmine and atropine on the behavior of the pigeon. *Naunyn-Schmiedeberg's Arch. Pharmacol.,* 248, 406–416.

Vaillant, G.E. (1967). A comparison of antagonists of physostigmine-induced suppression of behavior. *J. Pharmacol. Exp. Ther.,* 157, 636–648.

Vakil, R.T. (1949). Clinical trials of rauwolfia serpentina in essential hypertension. *Br. Heart J.,* 11, 350–355.

Valzelli, L. (1974). 5-Hydroxytryptamine in aggressiveness. In *Advances in Biochemical Psychopharmacology, Vol. 11* (E. Costa, G.L. Gessa and M. Sandler, Eds.), pp. 255–263. Raven Press, New York.

Valzelli, L. (Ed.) (1978). *Psychopharmacology of Aggression.* Karger, New York.

Van Wimersma Greidanus, T.B. (1977). Effects of MSH and related peptides on avoidance behavior in rats. *Front. Horm. Res.,* 4, 129–139.

Van Wimersma Greidanus, T.B. (1979). Neuropeptides and avoidance behavior with special reference to the effects of vasopressin, ACTH, and MSH on memory processes. In *Central Nervous System Effects of Hypothalmic Hormones and Other Peptides* (R. Collu, A. Barbeau, J.-G. Rochefort and J.R. Ducharme, Eds.), pp. 177–187. Raven Press, New York.

Van Wimersma Greidanus, T.B., Bohus, B. and de Wied, D. (1975a). CNS sites of action of ACTH, MSH and vasopressin in relation to avoidance behavior. In

Anatomical Neuroendocrinology (W.E. Stumpf and L.O. Grant, Eds.), pp. 284–289. Karger, New York.

Van Wimersma Greidanus, T.B. and de Wied, D. (1976). Modulation of passive avoidance behavior of rats by intracerebroventricular administration of anti-vasopressin serum. *Behav. Biol.,* 18, 325–333.

Van Wimersma Greidanus, T.B., Dogteram, J. and de Wied, D. (1975b). IVT administration of anti-vasopressin serum inhibits memory consolidation in rats. *Life Sci.,* 16, 637–644.

Vetulani, J., Stawarz, R.J., Dingell, J.V. and Sulser, F. (1976a). A possible common mechanism of action of antidepressant treatments. *Naunyn-Schmiedeberg's Arch. Pharmacol.,* 293, 109–114.

Vetulani, J., Stawarz, R.J. and Sulser, F. (1976b). Adaptive mechanisms of the noradrenergic cAMP generating system in limbic forebrain of the rat: adaptation to persistant changes in the availability of norepinephrine. *J. Neurochem.,* 27, 661–666.

Vetulani, J. and Sulser, F. (1975). Action of various antidepressant treatment reduces reactivity of noradrenergic cyclic AMP-generating system in limbic forebrain. *Nature,* 257, 495–496.

Vogel, R.A., Cooper, B.R., Barlow, T.S., Prange, A.J., Mueller, R.A. and Breese, G.R. (1979). Effects of thyrotropin-releasing hormone on locomotor activity, operant performance and ingestive behavior. *J. Pharmacol. Exp. Ther.,* 208, 161–168.

Vogt, M. (1954). The concentration of sympathin in different parts of the central nervous system under normal conditions and after the administration of drugs. *J. Physiol.,* 123, 451–481.

Vogt, M. (1974). The effect of lowering the 5-hydroxytryptamine content of the rat spinal cord on analgesia produced by morphine. *J. Physiol.,* 236, 483–498.

Volkmann, R. and Cressey, D.R. (1963). Differential association and the rehabilitation of drug addicts. *Am. J. Sociol.,* 69, 129–142.

Volle, R.L. and Koelle, G.B. (1975). Ganglionic stimulating and blocking agents. In *The Pharmacological Basis of Therapeutics* (L.S. Goodman and A. Gilman, Eds.), pp. 565–575. Macmillan, New York.

von Euler, U.S. (1935). Über die spezifische blutdrucksenkende Substanz des menschlichen Prostata- und Samenblasensekretes. *Klin. Wschr.* 14, 1182–1183.

von Euler, U.S. (1946a). The presence of a substance with sympathin properties in spleen extracts. *Acta Physiol. Scand.,* 11, 168–186.

von Euler, U.S. (1946b). A specific sympathomimetic ergone in adrenergic nerve fibers (sympathin) and its relations to adrenaline and noradrenaline. *Acta Physiol. Scand.,* 12, 73–97.

von Euler, U.S. (1948). Noradrenaline and histamine in autonomic nerves. *Acta Physiol. Scand.,* Suppl. 53, 20–21.

von Euler, U.S. (1971). Adrenergic neurotransmitter function. *Science,* 173, 202–206.

von Euler, U.S. and Gaddum, J.H. (1931). An unidentified depressor substance in certain tissue extracts. *J. Physiol.,* 72, 74–87.

Von Voigtlander, P.F. and Moore, K.E. (1971). Dopamine: release from the brain in vivo by amantadine. *Science,* 174, 408–409.

Wade, N. (1978a). Guillemin and Schally: the years in the wilderness. *Science,* 200, 279–282.

Wade, N. (1978b). Guillemin and Schally: the three-lap race to Stockholm. *Science,* 200, 411–415.

Wade, N. (1978c). Guillemin and Schally: a race spurred by rivalry. *Science,* 200, 510–513.

Wagemaker, H. and Cade, R. (1977). The use of hemodialysis in chronic schizophrenia. *Am. J. Psychiatry,* 134, 684–685.

Walker, J.B. (1974). The effect of lithium on hormone–sensitive adenylate cyclase from various areas of rat brain. *Biol. Psychiatry,* 8, 245–251.

Ward, I.L., Crowley, W.R., Zemlan, F.P. and Margules, D.L. (1975). Monoaminergic mediation of female sexual behavior. *J. Comp. Physiol. Psychol.,* 88, 53–61.

Wasacz, J. (1981). Natural and synthetic narcotic drugs. *Am. Sci.,* 69, 318–324.

Wasman, M. and Flynn, J.P. (1962). Directed attack elicited from hypothalamus. *Arch. Neurol.,* 6, 220–227.

Watkins, L.R. and Mayer, D.J. (1982). Organization of endogenous opiate and nonopiate pain control systems. *Science,* 216, 1185–1192.

Watson, S.J. (1977). Hallucinogens and other psychotomimetics: biological mechanisms. In *Psychopharmacology* (J.D. Barchas, P.A. Berger, R.D. Ciaranello and G.R. Elliott, Eds.), pp. 341–354. Oxford Univ. Press, New York.

Watson, S.J., Barchas, J.D. and Li, C.H. (1977). β-Lipotropin: localization of cells and axons in rat brain by immunocytochemistry. *Proc. Nat. Acad. Sci.,* 74, 5155–5158.

Watterson, D.M. and Vincenzi, F.F. (Eds.) (1980). *Calmodulin and Cell Function. Ann. N.Y. Acad. Sci.,* Vol. 356. New York Academy of Science, New York.

Watzman, N. and Barry, H., III. (1968). Drug effects on motor coordination. *Psychopharmacologia,* 12, 414–423.

Wauquier, A. and Niemegeers, C.J.E. (1972). Intracranial self-stimulation in rats as a function of various stimulus parameters. II. Influence of haloperidol, pimozide, and pipamperone on medial forebrain bundle stimulation with monopolar electrodes. *Psychopharmacologia,* 27, 191–202.

Weeks, J.R. (1964). Experimental narcotic addiction. *Sci. Am.,* 210, 46–52.

Weeks, J.R. and Collins, R.J. (1964). Factors affecting voluntary morphine intake in self-maintained addicted rats. *Psychopharmacologia,* 6, 267–279.

Wei, E, and Loh, H. (1976a). Physical dependence on opiatelike peptides. *Science,* 193, 1262–1263.

Wei, E. and Loh, H. (1976b). Chronic intracerebral infusion of morphine and peptides with osmotic minipumps, and the development of physical dependence. In *Opiates and Endogenous Opioid Peptides* (H.W. Kosterlitz, Ed.), pp. 303–310. Elsevier/North-Holland, Amsterdam.

Wei, E., Loh, H.H. and Way, E.L. (1972). Neuroanatomical correlates of morphine dependence. *Science, 177,* 616–617.

Wei, E., Sigel, S., Loh, H. and Way, E.L. (1975). Thyrotropin–releasing hormone and shaking behavior in rat. *Nature, 253,* 739–740.

Weiner, H. (1975). Schizophrenia: etiology. In *Comprehensive Textbook of Psychiatry, Vol. 11* (A.M. Freedman, H.I. Kaplan and B.J. Sadock, Eds.), pp. 866–899. Williams and Wilkins, Baltimore.

Weinswig, M.H. (1973). *Use and Misuse of Drugs Subject to Abuse.* Pegasus, New York.

Weiss, B. and Kidman, A.D. (1969). Neurobiological significance of cyclic 3',5'-adenosine monophosphate. In *Advances in Biochemical Psychopharmacology, Vol. 1* (E. Costa and P. Greengard, Eds.), pp. 131–164. Raven Press, New York.

Weiss, B. and Laties, V.G. (1961). Changes in brain tolerance and other behavior produced by salicylates. *J. Pharmacol. Exp. Ther., 113,* 120–129.

Weiss, B. and Laties, V.G. (1964). Drug effects on the temporal patterning of behavior. *Fed. Proc., 23,* 801–807.

Weissman, A., Koe, B.K. and Tenen, S.S. (1966). Antiamphetamine effects following inhibition of tyrosine hydroxylase. *J. Pharmacol. Exp. Ther., 151,* 329–352.

Welch, A.S. and Welch, B.L. (1968). Effect of stress and parachlorophenylalanine upon brain serotonin, 5-hydroxyindoleacetic acid and catecholamines in grouped and isolated mice. *Biochem. Pharmacol., 17,* 699–708.

Welch, B.L. and Welch, A.S. (1969). Aggression and the biogenic amine neurohumors. In *Aggressive Behavior* (S. Garattini and E.B. Sigg, Eds.), pp. 188–202. Excerpta Medica Foundation, Amsterdam.

Wells, B. (1973). *Psychedelic Drugs.* Penguin Books, Baltimore.

Welsh, J.H. (1954). Marine invertebrate preparations useful in the bioassay of acetylcholine and 5-hydroxytryptamine. *Nature, 173,* 955–956.

Wender, P.H., Rosenthal, D., Kety, S.S., Schulsinger, F. and Welner, J. (1974). Cross–fostering: a research strategy for clarifying the role of genetic and experimental factors in the etiology of schizophrenia. *Arch. Gen. Psychiatry, 30,* 121–128.

Whittaker, V.P. and Gray, E.G. (1962). The synapse: biology and morphology, *Br. Med. Bull., 18,* 223–228.

Wikler, A. (1965). Conditioning factors in opiate addiction and relapse. In *Narcotics* (D.M. Wilner and G.G. Kasselbaum, Eds.), pp. 85–100. McGraw Hill, New York.

Wikler, A. (1968). Diagnosis and treatment of drug dependence of the barbiturate type. *Am. J. Psychiatry, 125,* 758–765.

Wikler, A. (1973). Dynamics of drug dependence. Implications of a conditioning theory for research and treatment. *Arch. Gen. Psychiatry, 28,* 611–616.

Williams, B.J. and Pirch, J.H. (1974). Correlation between brain adenyl cyclase activity and spontaneous motor activity in rats after chronic reserpine treatment. *Brain Res., 68,* 227–234.

Williamson, M.J., Paul, S.M. and Skolnick, P. (1978). Demonstration of [^{3}H]diazepam binding to benzodiazepine receptors in vivo. *Life Sci., 23,* 1935–1940.

Wilson, I.C., Prange, A.J., Jr., McClane, T.K., Rabon, A.M. and Lipton, M.A. (1970). Thyroid hormone enhancement of imipramine in nonretarded depressions. *N. Engl. J. Med., 282,* 1063–1067.

Winokur, A. and Beckman, A.L. (1978). Effects of thyrotropin releasing hormone, norepinephrine and acetylcholine on the activity of neurons in the hypothalamus, septum and cerebral cortex of the rat. *Brain Res., 150,* 205–209.

Winokur, A., Davis, R. and Utiger, R.D. (1977). Subcellular distribution of thyrotropin releasing hormone (TRH) in rat brain and hypothalamus. *Brain Res., 120,* 423–434.

Winokur, A. and Utiger, R.D. (1974). Thyroptropin–releasing hormone: regional distribution in rat brain. *Science, 185,* 265–269.

Winter, C.A. (1965). The physiology and pharmacology of pain and its relief. In *Analgetics* (G. de Stevens, Ed.), pp. 10–74. Academic Press, New York.

Wise, C.D., Baden, M.M. and Stein, L. (1974). Post-mortem measurement of enzymes in human brain: evidence of a central noradrenergic deficit in schizophrenia. *J. Psychiatr. Res., 11,* 185–198.

Wise, C.D., Berger, B.D. and Stein, L. (1972). Benzodiazepines: anxiety-reducing activity by reduction of serotonin turnover in the brain. *Science, 177,* 180–183.

Wise, C.D., Berger, B.D. and Stein, L. (1973). Evidence of α–noradrenergic reward receptors and serotonergic punishment receptors in the rat brain. *Biol. Psychiatry, 6,* 3–21.

Wise, C.D., Potkin, S.G., Bridge, T.P., Phelps, B.H., Cannon-Spoor, H.E. and Wyatt, R.J. (1980). Sources of error in the determination of platelet monoamine oxidase: a review of methods. *Schizophr. Bull., 6,* 245–253.

Wise, C.D. and Stein, L. (1969). Facilitation of brain self–stimulation by central administration of norepinephrine. *Science, 163,* 299–301.

Wise, R.A. (1978). Neuroleptic attenuation of intracranial self-stimulation: reward or performance deficits? *Life Sci., 22,* 535–542.

Wolfe, B.B., Harden, T.K., Sporn, J.R. and Molinoff, P.B. (1978). Presynaptic modulation of beta adrenergic receptors in rat cerebral cortex after treatment with antidepressants. *J. Pharmacol. Exp. Ther., 207,* 446–457.

Wong, D.T., Horng, J.S., Bymaster, F.P., Hauser, K.L. and Molloy, B.B. (1974). A selective inhibitor of serotonin uptake: Lilly 110140, 3-(p-fluoromethylphenoxy)-N-methyl-3-phenylpropylamine. *Life Sci., 15,* 471–479.

Woodbury, J.W. (1966). The cell membrane: ionic and potential gradients and active transport. In *Physiology and Biophysics* (T.C. Ruch, and H.D. Patton, Eds.), pp. 1–25. Saunders, Philadelphia.

Woods, J.H. and Schuster, C.R. (1968). Reinforcement properties of morphine, cocaine, and SPA as a function of unit dose. *Int. J. Addict.,* 3, 231–237.

Woods, J.H. and Schuster, C.R. (1970). Regulation of drug self-administration. In *Drug Dependence* (R.T. Harris, W.M. McIsaac and C.R. Shuster, Eds.), pp. 158–169. Univ. of Texas Press, Austin, Texas.

Woolfe, G. and MacDonald, A.D. (1944). The evaluation of the analgesic action of pethidine hydrochloride (Demerol). *J. Pharmacol. Exp. Ther.,* 80, 300–307.

Wurtman, R.J. (1980). The pineal as a neuroendocrine transducer. In *Neuroendocrinology* (D.T. Krieger and J.C. Hughes, Eds.), pp. 102–108. Sinauer Associates, Sunderland, Massachusetts.

Wurtman, R.J. and Axelrod, J. (1966). Control of enzymatic synthesis of adrenaline in the adrenal medulla by adrenal cortical steroids. *J. Biol. Chem.,* 241, 2301–2305.

Wurtman, R.J., Larin, F., Mostafapour, S. and Fernstrom, J.D. (1974). Brain catechol synthesis: control by brain tyrosine concentration. *Science,* 185, 183–184.

Wyatt, R.J. (1976). Biochemistry and schizophrenia IV. The neuroleptics—their mechanism of action. A review of the biochemical literature. *Psychopharmacol. Bull.,* 12, 5–50.

Wyatt, R.J., Gillin, J.C., Stoff, D.M., Moja, E.A. and Tinklenberg, J.R. (1977). β-Phenylethylamine and the neuropsychiatric disturbances. In *Neuroregulators and Psychiatric Disorders* (E. Usdin, D. Hamburg and J. Barchas, Eds.), Oxford Univ. Press, New York.

Wyatt, R.J. and Murphy, D.L. (1975). Neurotransmitter-related enzymes in the major psychiatric disorders: II. MAO and DBH in schizophrenia. In *Biology of the Major Psychoses* (D.X. Freedman, Ed.), pp. 289–297. Raven Press, New York.

Wyatt, R.J., Murphy, D.L., Belmaker, R., Cohen, S., Donnelly, C.H. and Pollin, W. (1973a). Reduced monoamine oxidase activity in platelets: a possible genetic marker for vulnerability to schizophrenia. *Science,* 179, 916–918.

Wyatt, R.J., Potkin, S.G., Bridge, T.P., Phelps, B.H. and Wise, C.D. (1980). Monoamine oxidase in schizophrenia: an overview. *Schizophr. Bull.,* 6, 199–207.

Wyatt, R.J., Potkin, S.G. and Murphy, D.L. (1979). Platelet monoamine oxidase activity in schizophrenia: a review of the data. *Am. J. Psychiatry,* 136, 377–385.

Wyatt, R.J., Saavedra, J.M. and Axelrod, J. (1973b). A dimethyltryptamine (DMT) forming enzyme in human blood. *Am. J. Psychiatry,* 130, 754–760.

Wyatt, R.J., Schwartz, M.A., Erdelyi, E. and Barchas, J.B. (1975). Dopamine-β-hydroxylase activity in brains of chronic schizophrenic patients. *Science,* 187, 368–370.

Yaksh, T.L., Farb, D.H., Leeman, S.E. and Jessell, T.M. (1979). Intrathecal capsaicin depletes substance P in the rat spinal cord and produces prolonged thermal analgesia. *Science,* 206, 481–483.

Yalow, R.S. (1978). Radioimmunoassay: a probe for the fine structure of biologic systems. *Science,* 200, 1236–1245.

Yang, H.-Y.T. and Neff, N.H. (1974). The monoamine oxidases of brain: selective inhibition with drugs and the consequences for the metabolism of biogenic amines. *J. Pharmacol. Exp. Ther.,* 189, 733–740.

Yarbrough, G.G. (1976). TRH potentiates excitatory actions of acetylcholine on cerebral cortical neurons. *Nature,* 263, 523–524.

Yen, C.I., Stranger, R.L. and Millman, N. (1959). Ataractic suppression of isolation-induced aggressive behavior. *Arch. Int. Pharm. Ther.,* 123, 179–185.

Young, A.B., Oster-Granite, M.L., Herndon, R.M. and Snyder, S.H. (1974). Glutamic acid: selective depletion by viral-induced granule cell loss in hamster cerebellum. *Brain Res.,* 73, 1–13.

Young, A.B. and Snyder, S.H. (1974). The glycine synaptic receptor: evidence that strychnine binding is associated with the ionic conductance mechanism. *Proc. Nat. Acad. Sci.,* 71, 4002–4005.

Young, A.B., Zukin, S.R. and Snyder, S.H. (1974). Interactions of benzodiazepines with central nervous system receptors: possible mechanism of action. *Proc. Nat. Acad. Sci.,* 71, 2246–2250.

Zbinden, G. and Randall, L.O. (1967). Pharmacology of benzodiazepines: laboratory and clinical correlations. In *Advances in Pharmacology, Vol. 5* (S. Garattini and P.A. Shore, Eds.), pp. 213–291. Academic Press, New York.

Zeller, E.A., Barsky, J., Fouts, J.R., Kirschheimer, W.F. and Van Orden, L.S. (1952). Influence of isonicotinic acid hydrazide (INH) and 1-isonicotinyl-2-isopropyl hydrazine (IIH) on bacterial and mammalian enzymes. *Experientia,* 8, 349–350.

Zemlan, F.P. (1978). Influence of *p*-chloroamphetamine and *p*-chlorophenylalanine on female mating behavior. *Ann. N.Y. Acad. Sci.,* 305, 621–626.

Zigmond, M.J. and Stricker, E.M. (1974). Ingestive behavior following damage to central dopamine neurons: implications for homeostasis and recovery of function. In *Neuropsychopharmacology of Monoamines and Their Regulatory Enzymes* (E. Usdin, Ed.), pp. 385–402. Raven Press, New York.

Zimmerman, H. (1979). On the vesicle hypothesis. *Trends Neurosci.,* November, 282–284.

Zornetzer, S.F. (1978). Neurotransmitter modulation and memory: a new neuropharmacological phrenology? In *Psychopharmacology: A Generation of Progress* (M.A. Lipton, A. DiMascio and K.F. Killam, Eds.), pp. 637–649. Raven Press, New York.

Index

This book was set in Compugraphic English Times at A&B Typesetters. Format and production by Joseph Vesely, illustrations by Fredric J. Schoenborn. The book was manufactured by R. R. Donnelley & Sons.